Veterinary Toxicology and Immunology

Veterinary Toxicology and Immunology

Edited by **Shawn Kiser**

⬜ SYRAWOOD
PUBLISHING HOUSE

New York

Published by Syrawood Publishing House,
750 Third Avenue, 9th Floor,
New York, NY 10017, USA
www.syrawoodpublishinghouse.com

Veterinary Toxicology and Immunology
Edited by Shawn Kiser

© 2016 Syrawood Publishing House

International Standard Book Number: 978-1-68286-137-0 (Hardback)

Printed in the United States of America.

Contents

Preface

The purpose of the book is to provide a glimpse into the dynamics and to present opinions and studies of some of the scientists engaged in the development of new ideas in the field from very different standpoints. This book will prove useful to students and researchers owing to its high content quality.

Toxicology and immunology explore the infections, diseases, agents as well as antidotes affecting living organisms and form a crucial part of veterinary sciences. Over the past few decades, remarkable progress has been made in these disciplines. This book lucidly discusses topics like evaluation of new vaccines, systemic immunology, infections, host-pathogen interactions, etc. The students of veterinary sciences and veterinary pathology will find in this book an ideal guide. It will enable them to arrive at a comprehensive diagnosis. This book strives to provide a fair idea about this discipline and helps develop a better understanding of the latest advances within this field.

At the end, I would like to appreciate all the efforts made by the authors in completing their chapters professionally. I express my deepest gratitude to all of them for contributing to this book by sharing their valuable works. A special thanks to my family and friends for their constant support in this journey.

Editor

Cytokine profiles in pregnant gilts experimentally infected with porcine reproductive and respiratory syndrome virus and relationships with viral load and fetal outcome

Andrea Ladinig[1*], Joan K Lunney[2], Carlos JH Souza[2,3], Carolyn Ashley[1], Graham Plastow[4] and John CS Harding[1]

Abstract

In spite of extensive research, immunologic control mechanisms against Porcine Reproductive and Respiratory Syndrome virus (PRRSv) remain poorly understood. Cytokine responses have been exhaustively studied in nursery pigs and show contradictory results. Since no detailed reports on cytokine responses to PRRSv in pregnant females exist, the objectives of this study were to compare host cytokine responses between PRRSv-infected and non-infected pregnant gilts, and to investigate relationships between cytokine levels in infected gilts and viral load or fetal mortality rate. Serum samples and supernatants of peripheral blood mononuclear cells (PBMC) either stimulated with PRRSv or phorbol myristate acetate/Ionomycin (PMA/Iono) were analyzed for cytokines/chemokines: interleukins (IL) 1-beta (IL1β), IL4, IL8, IL10, IL12, chemokine ligand 2 (CCL2), interferon alpha (IFNα) and interferon gamma (IFNγ). Three cytokines (IFNα, CCL2, IFNγ) in gilt serum differed significantly in inoculated versus control gilts over time. In supernatants of PRRSv stimulated PBMC from PRRSv-infected gilts, levels of IFNα were significantly decreased, while IL8 secretion was significantly increased. PRRSv infection altered the secretion of all measured cytokines, with the exception of IFNα, from PBMC after mitogen stimulation, indicating a possible immunomodulatory effect of PRRSv. IFNα, CCL2, and IFNγ in serum, and IFNγ in supernatants of PMA/Iono stimulated PBMC were significantly associated with viral load in tissues, serum or both. However, only IFNα in supernatants of PRRSv stimulated PBMC was significantly associated with fetal mortality rate. We conclude that of the eight cytokines tested in this study IFNα was the best indicator of viral load and severity of reproductive PRRSv infection.

Introduction

Cytokines and chemokines play a key role in the regulation of the innate, humoral (T-helper 2 [Th2]) and cellular (T-helper 1 [Th1]) immune responses [1]. *Early cytokines* including the type I interferons and pro-inflammatory cytokines (interleukins 1 (IL1), IL6 and tumor necrosis factor-alpha (TNFα)), and *late cytokines* such as interferon-gamma (IFNγ), are important regulators of adaptive immune responses [2]. Two important chemokines are interleukin 8 (IL8 or CXCL8), a potent recruiter of neutrophils to sites of infection, and chemokine ligand 2 (CCL2), which induces the migration of monocytes from blood to become tissue macrophages [3]. Antiviral or type I interferons are produced by a variety of cells, with plasmacytoid dendritic cells (pDC) or interferon producing cells (IPCs) being specialists in this task [3]. Type II interferon, IFNγ, and IL12 are key inducers of Th1 immune responses [2,3]. The functions of IL10 are diverse, but principally aimed at immune regulation [3,4]. Unlike in human or mouse, in which IL4 is the major Th2 cytokine [5-7], the role of IL4 in pigs is not completely clear and its expression in vivo following viral infection is usually low or undetectable [8-10].

Recently, bead-based multiplex assays, also known as Fluorescent Microsphere Immunoassays (FMIA), became available for measurement of cytokines in porcine specimens. FMIA allows high throughput, simultaneous detection and quantification of multiple analytes and

---

* Correspondence: andrea.ladinig@usask.ca
[1]Department of Large Animal Clinical Sciences, Western College of Veterinary Medicine, University of Saskatchewan, Saskatoon, SK, Canada
Full list of author information is available at the end of the article

significantly reduced time and sample volume requirements [11,12]. For detection of cytokines, FMIA technology relies on the availability of capture and detection antibodies (Abs) enabling specific and sensitive measurement of the respective analytes. Because a limited number of swine antibodies are available and not all work well in multiplex FMIA the use of FMIA to detect swine cytokines is presently limited [13].

Cytokine responses to Porcine Reproductive and Respiratory Syndrome virus (PRRSv) infection have been exhaustively studied using both in vivo and in vitro models. A thorough review is beyond the scope of the present paper. However, reports on cytokine responses to PRRSv infection in vivo contain contradictory results and were mainly performed in nursery pigs using respiratory models. Rowland et al. [14] used a reproductive model to investigate cytokine responses in PRRSv-infected fetuses but not in dams. To our knowledge, no detailed reports of cytokine responses to PRRSv infection in pregnant sows or gilts exist. Therefore, the objectives of the present study were: 1) to compare host cytokine responses between PRRSv-infected and non-infected gilts following experimental infection in the third trimester of gestation; 2) to investigate relationships between cytokine levels and viral load in gilt serum and gilt tissues; and 3) to investigate relationships between cytokine levels and fetal mortality rate defined at the level of the gilt as percent dead fetuses per litter. Three specific host responses were evaluated over 19 days post inoculation (dpi): 1) cytokine production in gilt serum, 2) cytokine production in supernatants of PRRSv-stimulated peripheral blood mononuclear cells (PBMC), and 3) cytokine production in supernatants of phorbol myristate acetate/Ionomycin (PMA/Iono) stimulated PBMC.

Materials and methods
Animal experiment and sample collection
The experimental infection protocol is described in detail in Ladinig et al. [15]. Briefly, on experimental day 0 (D0), 114 pregnant Landrace gilts (gestation day 85 ± 1 over 12 biweekly replicates) were inoculated with PRRSv isolate NVSL 97–7895 (1×10^5 $TCID_{50}$; 2 mL intramuscular and 1 mL into each nostril) (INOC), while 19 control gilts were similarly sham inoculated (CTRL). PRRSv negativity of gilts was confirmed before delivery to the University of Saskatchewan by ELISA (IDEXX PRRS X3 Ab test, IDEXX laboratories, Inc., Maine, USA) and PCR (Tetracore PRRS real-time PCR kit, Tetracore, Inc., Rockville, USA). Furthermore, all gilts were negative for PRRSv RNA by a strain-specific in-house quantitative reverse transcription polymerase chain reaction (qRT-PCR) in serum on D0 [15]. Serum and whole blood samples were collected on D0, D2, D6, D19 and D21. On D21 (gestation day 106 ± 1), gilts were humanely euthanized and

necropsy examinations were performed on gilts and their fetuses. Fetal preservation status was recorded and the percent dead fetuses were calculated for each litter. PRRSv RNA concentrations were measured in gilt serum and gilt tissue samples (lung, tonsil, reproductive and tracheobronchial lymph node) collected at termination using qRT-PCR [15]. The experiment was approved by the University of Saskatchewan's Animal Research Ethics Board, and adhered to the Canadian Council on Animal Care guidelines for humane animal use (permit #20110102).

PBMC stimulation
PBMC were isolated from whole blood collected on D0, D2, D6 and D19 by gradient centrifugation using lymphocyte separation medium (Ficoll-Paque™ PLUS, GE Healthcare). Cells were re-suspended in RPMI medium 1640 (RPMI) (Life Technologies, Burlington, ON, Canada) supplemented with antibiotics (1% Pen/Strep) and 10% fetal bovine serum (FBS) (Life Technologies, Burlington, ON, Canada). On the day of isolation, freshly isolated PBMC were seeded in 48-well tissues culture plates (1×10^6 cells/ well, total volume 500 µL). Duplicate wells for each stimulation time point were stimulated with either 10 ng/mL PMA (Sigma-Aldrich, Oakville, ON, Canada) and 250 ng/mL ionomycin (Sigma-Aldrich, Oakville, ON, Canada) (PMA/Iono) or with PRRSv isolate NVSL 97–7895 (multiplicity of infection =1). Unstimulated cells were seeded in duplicate wells containing cell culture medium only. Plates were incubated at 37 °C in 5% CO_2 for either 36 h (PMA/Iono stimulation) or 60 h (PRRSv stimulation). Cells and supernatants from duplicate wells were pooled and centrifuged ($400\,g$, 10 min). Supernatant aliquots were stored frozen at −80 °C until further testing.

Cytokine testing
Serum samples (D0, D2, D6, D21) and PBMC supernatants (D0, D2, D6, D19) were analysed for the following innate, regulatory, Th1 and Th2 cytokines/chemokines by FMIA: IL1β, IL8, CCL2, IFNα, IL10, IL12, and IL4. Due to the lack of availability of antibodies suitable for FMIA, an enzyme-linked immunosorbent assay (ELISA) was used to measure IFNγ.

Multiplex fluorescent microsphere immunoassay (FMIA)
For serum samples, a 7-plex in-house FMIA assay was developed as previously described with several modifications [12]. Beads, standards and Ab pairs used for the different cytokines are listed in Table 1. Briefly, capture antibodies were covalently coupled to magnetic beads (Biorad, Mississauga, ON, Canada). Coupling efficiency was tested by staining newly coupled beads with goat anti-mouse IgG-Phycoerythrin labeled Ab (Life Technologies, Burlington, ON, Canada) and comparing fluorescence

Table 1 Standards, capture and detection antibodies used by FMIA and ELISA

Cytokine (bead region)	Standard (source)	Capture Ab (source)	Detection Ab (source)
IL1β (26)	DY681, part 841042 (RD)	DY681, part 841040 (RD)	BAF 681 (RD)
IL8 (27)	SD061 (L)	MCA1660 (C)	MAB5351 (RD)
CCL2 (53)	RP0017S-025 (C)	Anti-poCCL2 clone 5–2 (Lu)	Anti-poCCL2 clone 18–1 (Lu)
IFNα (45)	17105-1 (C)	GTX11408 (GT)	27105-1 (C)
IL10 (28)	CSC0103, part SD064 (L)	ASC0104 (L)	ASC9109 (L)
IL12 (36)	DY912, part 841099 (RD)	MA0413S-500 (C)	BAM9122 (RD)
IL4 (34)	CSC1283, part 5S.128.10 (L)	CSC1283, part 5S.128.09 (L)	ASC0849 (L)
IFNγ (ELISA)	CSC4033, part SD066 (L)	CSC4033, part ASC4934D (L)	CSC4033, part ASC4839D (L)

(RD) R&D Systems, Minneapolis, MN, USA; (L) Life technologies, Burlington, ON, Canada; (C) Cedarlane, Burlington, ON, Canada; (GT) GeneTex, Irvine, CA, USA; (Lu) Lunney lab, Beltsville, MD, USA (Lunney et al., manuscript in preparation).

intensity of the newly coupled beads with existing batches (generously provided by Dr C. Souza, USDA, Beltsville, MD, USA). Serum from a healthy, non-infected gilt with no measurable levels of relevant cytokines by FMIA was used to prepare serial dilutions of cytokine standards (Figure 1A). The same serum was used as negative control on each FMIA plate. All serum samples were tested at a 1:3 dilution in phosphate buffered saline (PBS, pH 7.4) supplemented with 1% bovine serum albumin (BSA) and 0.05% sodium azide (PBS-BN). Samples and standards were incubated with magnetic beads in duplicate wells of a 96-well plate for 2 h. All incubations were performed in the dark (aluminum foil cover) at room temperature on a rotating plate shaker (500 rpm). A 96-well plate washer (Bio-Plex Pro™ II Wash Station, Biorad, Mississauga, ON, Canada) was used to perform 3 washes with PBS +0.05% Tween 20 (PBST) after each incubation step. Fifty µL of anti-cytokine, biotinylated, secondary antibody (Ab) diluted in PBS-BN were added to each well and plates were incubated for 90 min. The optimal concentration of each biotinylated detection Ab was determined by titration. Finally, beads in each well were incubated in 50 µL of a solution containing 10 ug/mL of Strepavidin-R-Phycoerythrin (SAPE, PJRS20 Prozyme, Hayward, CA, USA) for 30 min, washed, and re-suspended in 100 µL PBST. Coupled microspheres were analyzed on a Bio-Plex® 200 system (Biorad, Mississauga, ON, Canada) and analyzed with the Bio-Plex Manager software version 6.1 (Biorad, Mississauga, ON, Canada). All mean fluorescence intensity (MFI) measurements were background corrected by subtracting the MFI of the negative control (control serum diluted 1:3 in PBS-BN) from the MFI for the relevant analyte in each sample.

PBMC supernatants were tested in a similar manner. However, due to high cytokine concentrations present after either PRRSv or PMA/Iono stimulation, a higher sample dilution was required for certain analytes and use of a 7-plex assay was therefore not feasible. For supernatants of PRRSv stimulated PBMC, CCL2 was analyzed as a single-plex assay at a 1:100 dilution, while the remaining

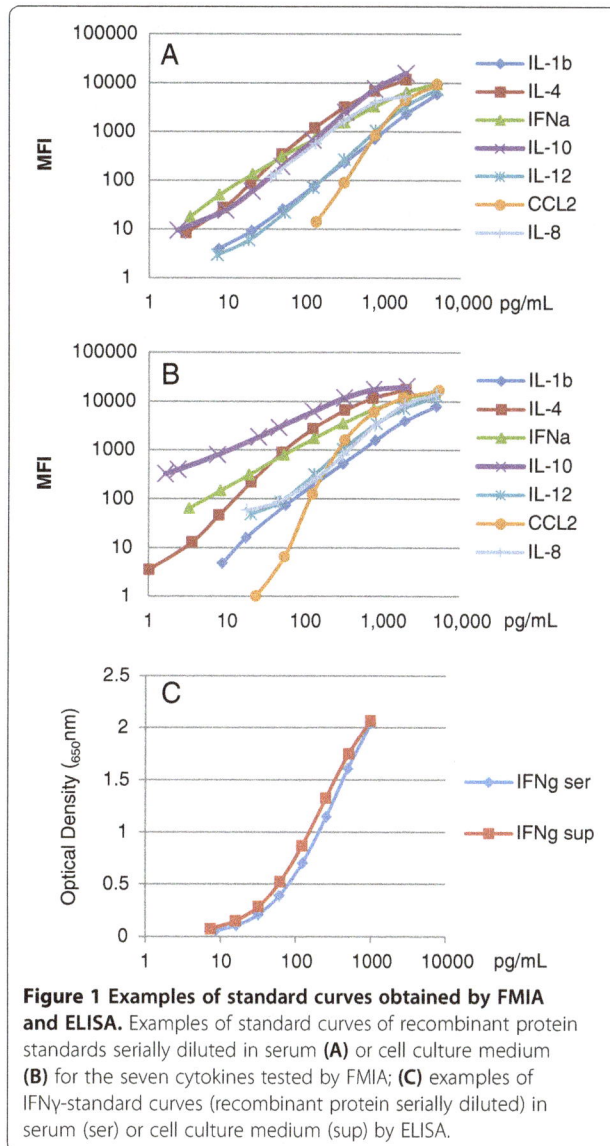

Figure 1 Examples of standard curves obtained by FMIA and ELISA. Examples of standard curves of recombinant protein standards serially diluted in serum **(A)** or cell culture medium **(B)** for the seven cytokines tested by FMIA; **(C)** examples of IFNγ-standard curves (recombinant protein serially diluted) in serum (ser) or cell culture medium (sup) by ELISA.

analytes were tested in a 6-plex assay at a 1:5 dilution. For supernatants of PMA/Iono stimulated PBMC, IL-8 was analyzed at a 1:20 dilution, while the remaining analytes were tested in a 6-plex assay at a 1:5 dilution. Cell culture medium (RPMI +10% FBS +1% Pen/Strep) at the relevant dilution in PBS-BN was used as negative control and to prepare standard curves (Figure 1B). Biotinylated detection Abs were titrated in order to determine the optimal concentration to use in testing PBMC supernatants. Results from supernatants of PRRSv or PMA/Iono stimulated PBMC were adjusted by subtracting the cytokine levels in supernatants of unstimulated cells cultured for the same time point (36 or 60 h). These are reported as "adjusted" cytokine values herein.

IFN-γ ELISA

The assay was carried out using the Novex Swine IFNγ antibody duoset kit (Life Technologies Inc., Burlington, ON, Canada) according to the manufacturer's instructions. Low coefficient of variation (CV) Immulon 4 HBX 96 well plates (VWR International, Mississauga, ON, Canada) were coated with capture Ab diluted in Coating Buffer B (Life Technologies Inc., Burlington, ON, Canada). 5X Assay Buffer (Novex Antibody Pair Buffer Set, Life Technologies Inc., Burlington, ON, Canada) diluted in ddH$_2$O was used as a blocking solution and for dilution of detection and Streptavidin-HRP Abs and samples as appropriate. Plates were washed with PBST using a Bio-Plex Pro II Wash Station. Peroxidase-labeled conjugates were detected by the addition of SureBlue Reserve TMB Microwell Substrate (Mandel Scientific Company Inc, Guelph, ON, Canada). Color was developed in the dark until the optical density of the highest standard reached approximately 2.0 at a wavelength of 650 nm without addition of Stop Solution. Plates were read in a Vmax Microplate Reader (Molecular Devices Corporation, Downingtown, PA, USA) using SoftMaxPro software Version 1.1 (Sunnyvale, CA, USA). The standard curve (1000 pg/mL to 8 pg/mL) was constructed using doubling dilutions (Figure 1C). Concentrations of IFNγ in samples were estimated by comparison with a 4-parameter standard curve generated by the software. Serum samples were diluted 1:3 in assay buffer whereas the standard diluent was a 1:3 solution of control gilt serum in assay buffer. Supernatants of PRRSv and PMA/Iono stimulated PBMC were tested at 1:3 and 1:100 dilutions, respectively, in assay buffer. The standard diluent was a corresponding dilution of cell culture medium in assay buffer. As above, IFNγ levels in PBMC supernatants were adjusted by subtracting the IFNγ levels in supernatants of unstimulated cells; adjusted IFNγ values are compared and reported herein.

Cytokine quality control (QC)

Protein standards (Table 1) were used to prepare high and low concentration quality controls in either control serum or cell culture media at the relevant dilution in PBS-BN. Both high and low quality controls were run in duplicate on each FMIA and ELISA plate. Process behavior control charts were used to monitor the inter-plate variation of each cytokine concentration in the QC samples, as well as the MFI of the highest and lowest standard on each FMIA plate. Plates were repeated if values fluctuated above or below the 3-sigma natural process limits on the appropriate control charts. Individual samples were repeated if the replicate CV was >20% as calculated by the instrument's software.

Statistical analysis

Separate statistical analyses were conducted using Stata 13 (STATA Corp, College Station, Texas, USA) to address each of three objectives. To meet the key model assumptions, data were transformed (logarithm base$_{10}$ or zero-skewness (lnskew0 function in STATA)) as appropriate. First, to determine if cytokine levels differed between INOC and CTRL gilts, multilevel mixed-effects linear regression models were developed. These models used gilt as a random effect and accounted for repeated measures by day. All remaining analyses used data from INOC gilts only and specifically focused on the cytokines that differed statistically between INOC and CTRL gilts. Our second objective was to determine potential relationships between cytokine levels (serum and supernatants) and PRRS viral load in serum and tissues. For these analyses, multilevel mixed-effects linear regression models controlling for experimental replicate were used. The area under the curve (AUC) for PRRSv RNA (target copies/μL, D0-D21) and cytokine protein (pg/mL) in serum (D0-D21) and supernatants (D0-D19) over time was calculated using the formula $AUC = (t_1\text{-}t_0)(a_1 + a_0)/2 + (t_2\text{-}t_1)(a_1 + a_2)/2 + \ldots + (t_n\text{-}t_{n-1})(a_{n-1} + a_n)/2$. Our third objective was to determine potential associations between cytokine levels in serum (AUC) and fetal survival rate (percentage of dead fetuses per litter). For all analyses, cytokine levels in sera or adjusted cytokine levels in supernatants (as described above) were used.

To account for multiple comparisons, all associations were considered statistically significant if $P < 0.01$. All final models were evaluated to ensure normality and homoscedasticity of residuals.

Results

Cytokine differences between inoculated and control gilts

Examples of standard curves of recombinant protein standards serially diluted in either serum or cell culture medium for the seven cytokines tested by FMIA are presented in Figures 1A and 1B. Examples of standard curves for the IFNγ ELISA are presented in Figure 1C.

Cytokine levels showed a high degree of variation between individual gilts in all sample types (Additional file 1, Additional file 2 and Additional file 3). Serum levels of CCL2, IFNα and IFNγ differed significantly between INOC and CTRL gilts over time ($P < 0.001$ for all). INOC gilts showed a significant increase in CCL2 and IFNα in sera collected on D2 and D6, whereas IFNγ was increased significantly on D2 only (Figure 2). IFNγ levels measured in serum of INOC gilts on D21 were lower than CTRL gilts; however, differences were not statistically significant. High serum levels of IL1β and IL8 at all 4 time points were measured in individual INOC and CTRL gilts, but PRRSv inoculation had no effect on these analytes over time (Additional file 1). Levels of IL12, IL10 and IL4 were very low in serum of both INOC and CTRL gilts and did not significantly differ over time (Additional file 1).

In supernatants of PRRSv stimulated PBMC, levels of IFNα and IL8 differed significantly between INOC and CTRL gilts over time ($P \leq 0.001$). PRRSv stimulation induced high levels of IFNα in PBMC from CTRL gilts and from INOC gilts before inoculation. Levels of IFNα were highly variable, ranging from 62 to 17025 pg/mL. A significant reduction in IFNα was detected in stimulated PBMC from INOC gilts compared to CTRL on D2, D6, and D19 (Figure 3A). Decreased levels were detected in all INOC gilts but to varying degrees. IL8 levels in supernatants of PRRSv stimulated PBMC were significantly increased on D2, D6, and D19 in INOC versus CTRL gilts (Figure 3B). Levels of IL1β, CCL2, IFNγ, IL4, IL10 and IL12 in supernatants of PRRSv stimulated PBMC were either not detectable or low, and did not significantly differ between INOC and CTRL gilts over time (Additional file 2).

IFNα was not induced by PMA/Iono stimulation. All other cytokines from PMA/Iono stimulated PBMC differed between INOC and CTRL gilts over time ($P < 0.001$ for all except IFNγ where only a trend was reported ($P = 0.039$)) (Additional file 3). Among the 7 cytokines measured, four discrete patterns were observed reflecting the potential effects of gilt PRRSv infection on PBMC PMA/Iono

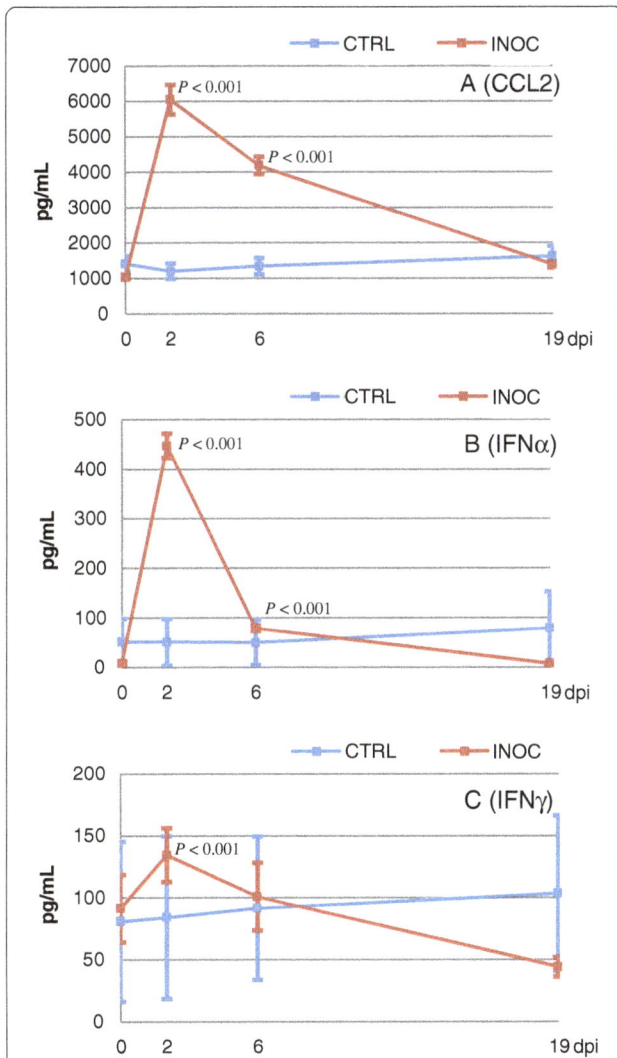

Figure 2 CCL2, IFNα and IFNγ levels in gilt serum over time. Mean (± SEM) CCL2 **(A)**, IFNα **(B)** and IFNγ **(C)** levels in serum from 111 INOC and 19 CTRL gilts across respective study days; P-values indicate significant differences between INOC and CTRL gilts on individual days.

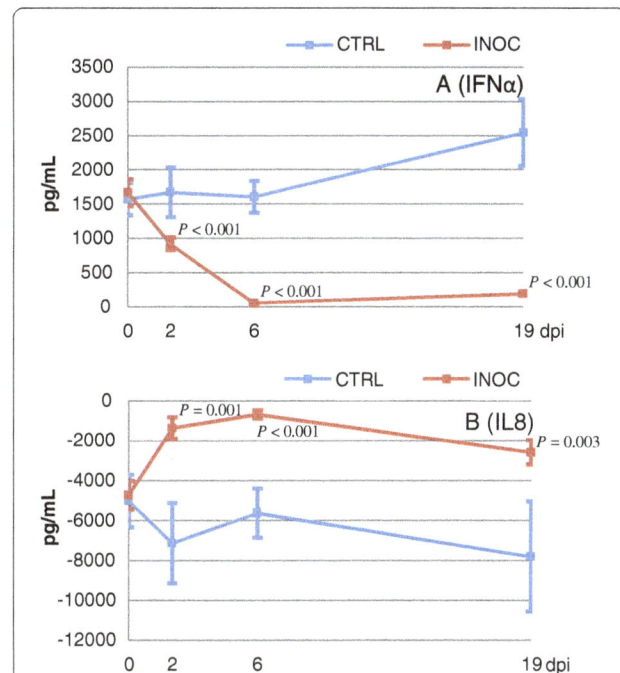

Figure 3 Adjusted IFNα and IL8 levels in supernatants of PRRSv stimulated PBMC over time. Mean (± SEM) adjusted IFNα **(A)** and IL8 **(B)** levels in supernatants of PRRSv stimulated PBMC from 111 INOC and 19 CTRL gilts across respective study days. P-values indicate significant differences between INOC and CTRL gilts on individual days. Adjusted cytokine levels were calculated by subtracting values in supernatants of unstimulated cells from PRRSv stimulated cells.

responsiveness. First, PRRSv infection resulted in a significantly increased CCL2 response to PMA/Iono stimulation
on D2 and D6 but not on D19 (early induction; Figure 4A).
These statistical differences however, are the result of a
single outlier CTRL gilt with massive spontaneous production of CCL2 from unstimulated PBMC on day 2.
With this outlier removed, CCL2 production significantly
differed between INOC and CTRL over time ($P = 0.01$)
with levels in INOC increased on D2 and D6 compared
to CTRL. After adjusting for multiple comparison this
was considered a trend (D2 $P = 0.027$, D6 $P = 0.019$). By
contrast, levels of IL8, IL10, and IL12 were significantly
decreased on D2 in INOC compared to CTRL gilts (early
suppression; Figures 4B-D). Following PMA/Iono stimulation, levels of IL1β decreased similarly on D2, but were

significantly increased in PBMC from INOC versus CTRL
gilts on D6 (early suppression with rebound; Figure 4E).
Finally, IL4 demonstrated late suppression with levels
from PMA/Iono stimulated PBMC significantly decreased
in INOC versus CTRL on D19. Prior to D19, IL4 levels
numerically increased in INOC gilts (Figure 4F). Similarly,
IFNγ levels decreased in INOC gilts on D19; however, differences were not significant but rather a trend ($P = 0.023$;
Additional file 3).

Relationships between cytokines levels and PRRS viral load
Detailed results on viral loads in gilt serum and tissues
can be found in Ladinig et al. [15]. Briefly, all INOC gilts
were viremic on D2 and D6, and 94/111 (84.7%) remained
viremic until termination. The percentage of tissues that

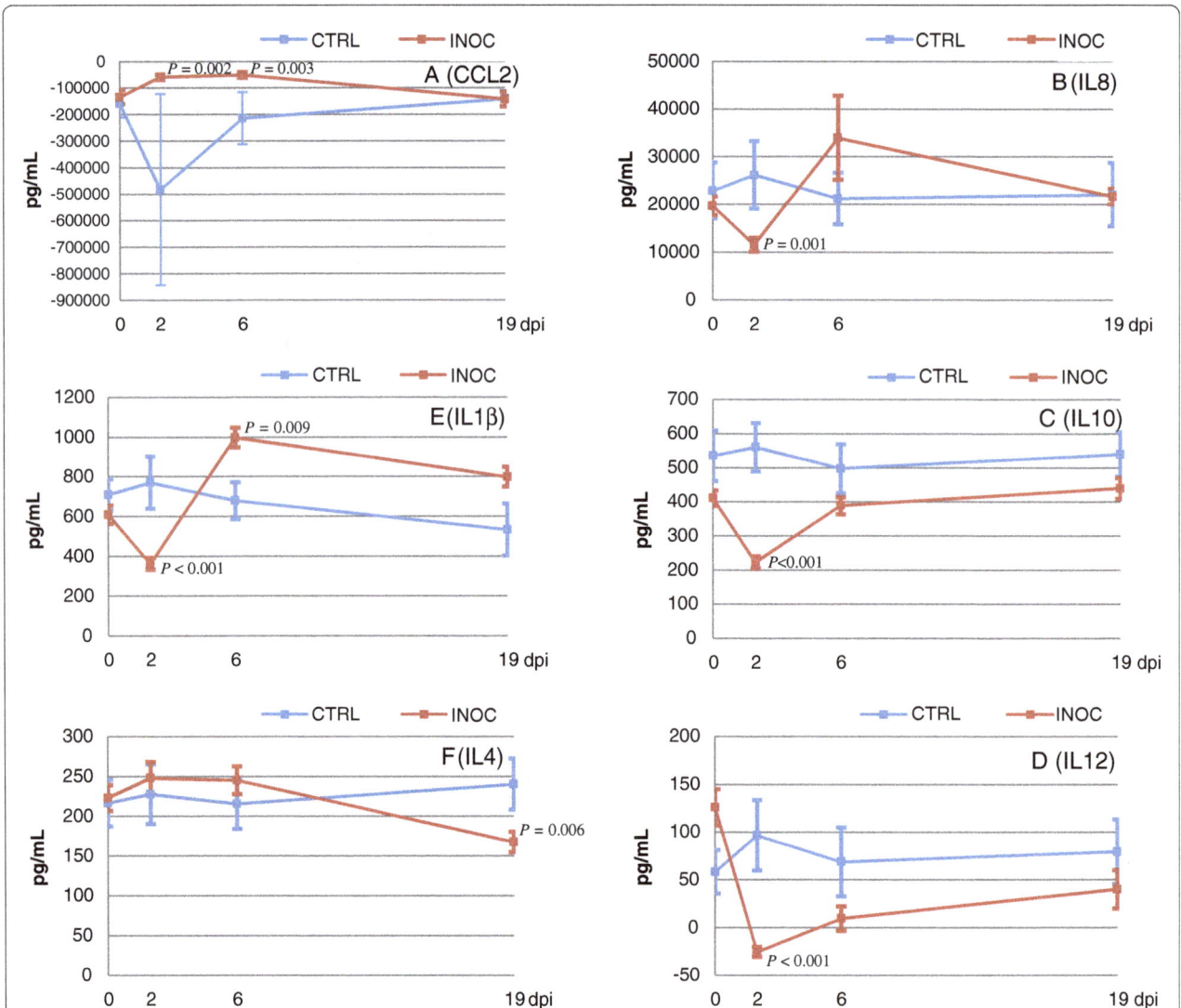

Figure 4 Adjusted CCL2, IL8, IL10, IL12, IL1β, and IL4 levels in supernatants of PMA/Iono stimulated PBMC over time. Mean (± SEM) adjusted CCL2 **(A)**, IL8 **(B)**, IL10 **(C)**, IL12 **(D)**, IL1β **(E)**, and IL4 **(F)** levels in supernatants of PMA/Iono stimulated PBMC from 111 INOC and 19 CTRL gilts across respective study days. P-values indicate significant differences between INOC and CTRL gilts on individual days. Adjusted cytokine levels were calculated by subtracting values in supernatants of unstimulated cells from PMA/Iono stimulated cells.

tested positive by PRRSv qRT-PCR at termination (D21) from INOC gilts were 90.1 (lung), 99.1 (tonsil), 100 (reproductive lymph node), and 99.1 (tracheobronchial lymph node), respectively. The mean viral loads of positive samples were 3.5 ($\pm$1.2) $\log_{10}$ RNA copies/mg in lung, 5.6 ($\pm$0.8) $\log_{10}$ RNA copies/mg in tonsil, 5.8 ($\pm$0.8) $\log_{10}$ RNA copies/mg in reproductive lymph node, and 4.8 ($\pm$0.9) $\log_{10}$ RNA copies/mg in tracheobronchial lymph node. AUC of IFNα and CCL2 in serum were positively associated with the AUC for viral load in serum (Table 2, Figures 5A and B). As shown in Figure 5, this association was mainly driven by gilts with high cytokine levels and high viral load over time, represented in the upper right quadrant. Importantly, no gilts had high cytokine levels but low viral loads over time (lower right quadrant). A positive association was detected between the AUC for CCL2 in serum and the viral load in lung. IFNα levels in serum trended to be positively associated with viral load in tonsil, while IFNγ levels showed a significant, but negative association (Table 2). No associations could be found for cytokine levels in serum with viral load in tracheobronchial lymph node. Although none of the cytokines measured in supernatants of PRRSv stimulated PBMC were associated with viral load in serum or tissues, levels of IFNγ in supernatants of PMA/Iono stimulated PBMC showed a negative association with viral load in reproductive lymph node (Table 2).

Relationships between cytokines and fetal mortality rate

In INOC gilts, the percentage of dead fetuses 21 days post inoculation varied from 0% to 94.4% (mean 41.0 $\pm$ 22.8%). AUC of IFNα in supernatants of PRRSv stimulated PBMC was significantly associated with percent dead (β = 0.001, P = 0.006) (Figure 5C), similarly AUC of IFNα in serum trended to be positively associated with fetal death (β = 0.0035, P = 0.060). For cytokine levels in

supernatants, a negative trend was detected between the AUC of IL10 in PMA/Iono stimulated PBMC and percent dead fetuses (β = −0.001, P = 0.045). For the remaining analytes, levels in serum or in supernatants were not associated with fetal death.

Discussion

The results presented herein are part of an extensive and complex dataset obtained in a large scale, multi-institutional project aimed at finding phenotypic and genotypic predictors of PRRSv resistance in pregnant gilts. The objectives of this present study were to investigate cytokine responses in serum and supernatants of PBMC, either stimulated with PRRSv or a nonspecific mitogen (PMA/Iono), and to determine possible associations with the outcome of infection in a reproductive model. In order to investigate genotypic variation in the severity of reproductive PRRS, a large number of gilts were experimentally inoculated in the third trimester of gestation, while the number of CTRL gilts was reduced to the minimum needed to provide baseline data.

PMA, a diester of phorbol and potent tumor promoter which activates the signal transduction enzyme protein kinase C, is often used in conjunction with ionomycin, an ionophore inducing calcium transport into the cell, in order to stimulate immune responses in vitro [3,16]. In the present experiment, PMA/Iono stimulation of PBMC induced the secretion of all cytokines tested with the exception of IFNα. Four distinct patterns were observed in the way PRRSv infection altered PBMC cytokine secretions after PMA/Iono stimulation. The altered secretion of cytokines by PMA/Iono stimulated PBMC from INOC gilts after infection indicates a PRRSv immunomodulatory effect. However, the biological meaning of these findings is difficult to interpret. When testing the associations between cytokine levels in supernatants of PMA/Iono

Table 2 Associations between cytokine levels and viral load in serum and tissues following PRRSv infection in pregnant gilts

PRRSv RNA concentration ($\log_{10}$/µL or mg)	Serum cytokine levels (AUC)			PMA/Iono supernatant (AUC)
	IFNα	CCL2	IFNγ	IFNγ
Serum (AUC)	P = 0.003	P < 0.001	ns	ns
	β = 0.002134	β = 0.000104		
Lung	ns	P = 0.010	ns	ns
		β = 0.000010		
Tonsil	P = 0.016	ns	P < 0.001	ns
	β = 0.000185		β = −0.000115	
Repro LN	ns	ns	ns	P = 0.002
				β = −0.0000004

The associations between cytokine levels over time (represented as area under curve (AUC)) and viral load in gilt serum and tissues are presented. P-values (regression coefficients, β) were obtained by univariate, multilevel mixed-effects regression models. Only analytes that were found to be significantly associated with viral load in either serum or any of the tested tissues are included. No association was found among cytokines in supernatants of PRRSv stimulated PBMC and viral load. Repro LN = reproductive lymph node. PMA/Iono supernatant AUC = AUC of IFNγ levels secreted from PMA/Iono stimulated PBMC from PRRSv infected gilts. ns = not significant (P > 0.01).

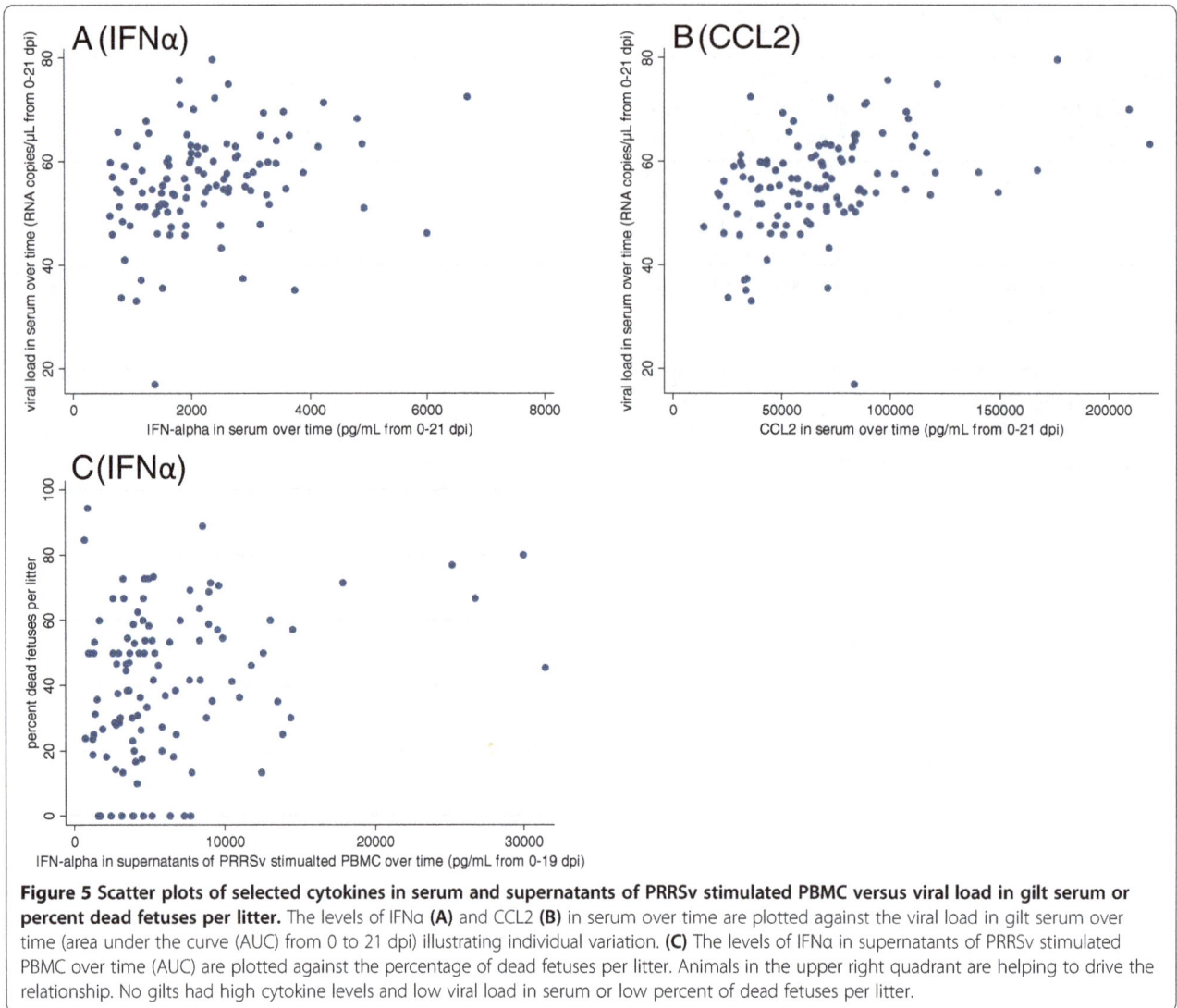

Figure 5 Scatter plots of selected cytokines in serum and supernatants of PRRSv stimulated PBMC versus viral load in gilt serum or percent dead fetuses per litter. The levels of IFNα **(A)** and CCL2 **(B)** in serum over time are plotted against the viral load in gilt serum over time (area under the curve (AUC) from 0 to 21 dpi) illustrating individual variation. **(C)** The levels of IFNα in supernatants of PRRSv stimulated PBMC over time (AUC) are plotted against the percentage of dead fetuses per litter. Animals in the upper right quadrant are helping to drive the relationship. No gilts had high cytokine levels and low viral load in serum or low percent of dead fetuses per litter.

stimulated PBMC and viral load or fetal mortality rate, the only significant association was between IFNγ and viral load in reproductive lymph node, where higher levels of IFNγ were associated with a lower viral burden.

Serum IFNγ levels were significantly increased in INOC gilts early in infection. This finding agrees with several reports of either numeric or significant increases in the number of IFNγ secreting cells by enzyme-linked immunospot (ELISPOT) assay, or in the protein levels measured in serum of pigs after PRRSv inoculation [12,17-24]. IFNγ levels in supernatants of PRRSv stimulated PBMC also showed a slight increase on D2, which was not statistically significant. Unlike IFNα and CCL2, no association was found between IFNγ levels in serum and viral load in gilt serum over time. On the other hand, viral loads in tonsil were negatively associated with IFNγ levels in serum

indicating a possible protective effect of IFNγ. However, IFNγ levels over time were not associated with fetal death. In contrast, Lowe et al. [25] showed that a strong cell mediated immune response determined by use of an IFNγ ELISPOT was correlated with protection against reproductive PRRS in 3 of 4 investigated farms.

The present study found IFNα to be one of the most relevant cytokines in PRRSv infection. High levels of IFNα were produced by PRRSv stimulated PBMC from CTRL gilts and INOC gilts before inoculation, which is in contrast to previous reports [26,27]. IFNα production, however, was significantly decreased in PBMC collected at all time points following PRRSv inoculation. The levels of IFNα in supernatants of PRRSv stimulated PBMC were positively associated with fetal mortality. Interestingly, it was previously demonstrated that North American type

PRRS viruses are potent inhibitors of type 1 interferon production in pDC [28], which are a major source of IFNα and play a key role in the early control of virus replication and the development of adaptive antiviral immune responses [29]. By contrast, a recent study showed that various type 1 and type 2 PRRSv strains induced IFNα secretion by pDC and showed either no or only weak suppression of IFNα secretion [27]. These recent data corroborate our findings of increased levels of IFNα in serum from INOC gilts. However, results of IFNα measurements in serum from PRRSv infected pigs are quite inconsistent. While some studies could not detect significant IFNα increases in serum of PRRSv inoculated pigs within one week of infection [12,18], others did [19,30]. Increased levels of IFNα might have negative effects in regards to PRRSv infection, since it was previously shown that IFNα up-regulated the expression of sialoadhesin and therefore enhanced PRRSv infection of monocytes [31].

In agreement with our results, Souza et al. [32] found significant increases in serum IFNα and CCL2 levels of nursery piglets within the first 2 weeks after inoculation with PRRSv 97–7895, the same virus strain as used for this study. IFNα and CCL2 levels in serum were also associated with PRRSv RNA concentration and growth performance where piglets with low concentration in serum showed a faster return to basal levels of IFNα and CCL2 in serum compared to highly viremic animals. Although we demonstrate the biological importance of INFα in the reproductive PRRSv model herein, the relevance of CCL2 responses in reproductive PRRS is questionable. Although serum CCL2 levels were positively associated with viral burden in serum and lung tissue in the present study, no association was detected between CCL2 levels and fetal death. We propose the role of CCL2 in PRRSv infection primarily involves monocyte recruitment in lung, and is unrelated to mechanisms of fetal death or survival.

Although IL8 levels significantly increased in supernatants of PRRSv stimulated PBMC from INOC gilts after infection, this finding did not have any biological relevance as IL8 levels were not associated with any measured outcome, including PRRSv viral levels or fetal mortality rate. In agreement with previous reports [12,19], no significant increase in serum IL8 levels was detected in INOC compared to CTRL gilts.

In conclusion, PRRSv infection increased IFNα, CCL2, and IFNγ levels in serum but only before 7 dpi. Viral load in gilt serum was positively associated with serum IFNα and CCL2 levels. Although CCL2 and IFNγ were not associated with fetal outcome, IFNα levels in serum trended to be positively associated with fetal mortality rate. The importance of IFNα in regards to PRRSv infection was demonstrated by the significant inhibition of IFNα secretion by PRRSv stimulated PBMC from INOC

gilts after infection, and a significant positive association between fetal mortality rate and levels of IFNα in supernatants from PRRSv stimulated PBMC. Therefore, IFNα secretion could be used as a possible indicator of viral load and severity of reproductive PRRS. By contrast, IL8 was not associated with viral load or fetal death even though IL8 secretion by PRRSv stimulated PBMC from INOC gilts was significantly increased at all investigated time points after infection. Finally, levels of IFNγ in supernatants of PMA/Iono stimulated PBMC were suppressed by 21 days post-inoculation, and were negatively associated with viral load in reproductive lymph node. Together with the fact that IFNγ levels in serum were negatively associated with viral load in tonsil, this suggests a protective effect of IFNγ in PRRSv pathogenesis.

Additional files

Additional file 1: Mean cytokine levels (SD) in serum. Mean cytokine (SD) levels in serum are presented for the 8 analysed cytokines from 111 INOC and 19 CTRL gilts on respective study days post inoculation. If the repeated measures, multilevel mixed-effects regression model demonstrated values in INOC significantly differed from CTRL gilts over all experimental days (DAY*INOC), group differences on individual days were compared (INOC_CTRL). Due to multiple comparisons, $P < 0.01$ was considered statistically significant. ns = not significant.

Additional file 2: Mean cytokine levels (SD) in supernatants of unstimulated and PRRSv stimulated PBMC. Mean (SD) cytokine levels in supernatants of unstimulated and PRRSv stimulated PBMC are presented for the 8 analysed cytokines from 111 INOC and 19 CTRL gilts on the respective study days post inoculation. Adjusted values were calculated by subtracting values in supernatants of unstimulated cells from PRRS stimulated cells and used in statistical analyses. Statistics determined whether values in INOC significantly differed from CTRL gilts over all experimental days (DAY*INOC), or on individual days (INOC_CTRL). Due to multiple comparisons, $P < 0.01$ was considered statistically significant; ns = not significant.

Additional file 3: Mean cytokine levels (SD) in supernatants of unstimulated and PMA/Iono stimulated PBMC. Mean (SD) cytokine levels in supernatants of unstimulated and phorbol myristate acetate/ Ionomycin (PMA/Iono) stimulated PBMC are presented for the 8 analysed cytokines from 111 INOC and 19 CTRL gilts on the respective study days post inoculation. Adjusted values were calculated by subtracting values in supernatants of unstimulated cells from PMA/Iono stimulated cells and used in statistical analyses. Statistics determined whether values in INOC significantly differed from CTRL gilts over all experimental days (DAY*INOC) or on individual days (INOC_CTRL). Due to multiple comparisons, $P < 0.01$ was considered statistically significant. ns = not significant.

Abbreviations
(Ab): Antibody; (APC): Antigen-presenting cells; (AUC): Area under the curve; (BSA): Bovine serum albumin; (CCL2): Chemokine ligand 2; (CV): Coefficient of variation; (DC): Dendritic cells; (ELISA): Enzyme-linked immunosorbent assay; (ELISPOT): Enzyme-linked immunospot assay; (FBS): Fetal bovine serum; (FMIA): Fluorescent Microsphere Immunoassays; (INOC): Gilts inoculated with PRRSv; (CTRL): Gilts that were sham inoculated; (IFNα): Interferon alpha; (IFNγ): Interferon gamma; (IPCs): Interferon producing cells; (IL): Interleukins; (MHC): Major histocompatibility complex; (MFI): Mean fluorescence intensity; (NK cells): Natural killer cells; (PBMC): Peripheral blood mononuclear cells; (PMA/Iono): Phorbol myristate acetate/Ionomycin; (PBS): Phosphate buffered saline; (PBS-BN): PBS with 0.05% sodium azide; (PBST): PBS +0.05% Tween 20; (pDC): Plasmacytoid dendritic cells; (PRRSv): Porcine Reproductive and Respiratory Syndrome virus; (QC): Quality control; (qRT-PCR): Quantitative reverse transcription polymerase chain reaction; (Th1): T-helper 1; (Th2): T-helper 2; (SAPE): Strepavidin-R-Phycoerythrin; (TNFα): Tumor necrosis factor-alpha.

Competing interests
The authors declare that they have no competing interests.

Authors' contributions
AL and JH conducted the research, led the interpretation of results and drafted the manuscript. GP and JKL assisted in the experimental design and interpretation. JH, AL and CA led the animal infection trials including animal care, collection of samples and PCR assays. JKL and CS helped develop the cytokine assays. JH and AL coordinated and oversaw statistical analysis of the data. All co-authors reviewed and contributed to writing of the manuscript. All authors read and approved the final manuscript.

Acknowledgements
The authors wish to acknowledge the numerous technicians and students from the Western College of Veterinary Medicine, Vaccine and Infectious Disease Organization, Prairie Diagnostic Services, Inc. and the University of Alberta who assisted with this project. We offer special thanks to Samuel Abrams for the help in the development of the FMIA assay, and to Ian Dohoo for his guidance with statistical analyses. Pregnant gilts were provided and bred by Fast Genetics Inc, Spiritwood, Canada, with management support of Dawn Friesen, Connie Heisler, Donell Wingerter and Benny Mote. Funding for the project was generously provided by grants from Genome Canada and Genome Prairie (grant number 2209-F), with administrative support from Genome Alberta.

Author details
[1]Department of Large Animal Clinical Sciences, Western College of Veterinary Medicine, University of Saskatchewan, Saskatoon, SK, Canada. [2]U.S. Department of Agriculture, Animal Parasitic Diseases Laboratory, Beltsville Agricultural Research Center, Agricultural Research Service, Beltsville, MD, USA. [3]EMBRAPA Pesca e Aquicultura, Palmas, TO, Brazil. [4]Department of Agricultural, Food, and Nutritional Science, Faculty of Agricultural, Life and Environmental Sciences, University of Alberta, Edmonton, AB, Canada.

References
1. Dinarello CA (2000) Proinflammatory cytokines. Chest 118:503–508
2. van Reeth K, Nauwynck H (2000) Proinflammatory cytokines and viral respiratory disease in pigs. Vet Res 31:187–213
3. Murphy KP (2012) *Janeway's Immunobiology*. Garland Science, Taylor & Francis Group, LLC, New York, USA
4. Moore KW, de Waal MR, Coffman RL, O'Garra A (2001) Interleukin-10 and the interleukin-10 receptor. Annu Rev Immunol 19:683–765
5. Howard M, Farrar J, Hilfiker M, Johnson B, Takatsu K, Hamaoka T, Paul WE (1982) Identification of a T cell-derived B cell growth factor distinct from interleukin 2. J Exp Med 155:914–923
6. Zhou Y, Lin G, Baarsch MJ, Scamurra RW, Murtaugh MP (1994) Interleukin-4 suppresses inflammatory cytokine gene transcription in porcine macrophages. J Leukocyte Biol 56:507–513
7. Zhou Y, Lin G, Murtaugh MP (1995) Interleukin-4 suppresses the expression of macrophage NADPH oxidase heavy chain subunit (gp91-phox). Biochim Biophys Acta 1265:40–48
8. Diaz I, Mateu E (2005) Use of ELISPOT and ELISA to evaluate IFN-gamma, IL-10 and IL-4 responses in conventional pigs. Vet Immunol Immunopathol 106:107–112
9. Murtaugh MP, Baarsch MJ, Zhou Y, Scamurra RW, Lin G (1996) Inflammatory cytokines in animal health and disease. Vet Immunol Immunopathol 54:45–55
10. Murtaugh MP, Johnson CR, Xiao Z, Scamurra RW, Zhou Y (2009) Species specialization in cytokine biology: is interleukin-4 central to the T(H)1-T(H)2 paradigm in swine? Dev Comp Immunol 33:344–352
11. Christopher-Hennings J, Araujo KP, Souza CJ, Fang Y, Lawson S, Nelson EA, Clement T, Dunn M, Lunney JK (2013) Opportunities for bead-based multiplex assays in veterinary diagnostic laboratories. J Vet Diagn Invest 25:671–691
12. Lawson S, Lunney J, Zuckermann F, Osorio F, Nelson E, Welbon C, Clement T, Fang Y, Wong S, Kulas K, Christopher-Hennings J (2010) Development of an 8-plex Luminex assay to detect swine cytokines for vaccine development: assessment of immunity after porcine reproductive and respiratory syndrome virus (PRRSV) vaccination. Vaccine 28:5356–5364
13. U.S. Veterinary Immune Reagent Network. [www.vetimm.org]
14. Rowland RR (2010) The interaction between PRRSV and the late gestation pig fetus. Virus Res 154:114–122
15. Ladinig A, Wilkinson J, Ashley C, Detmer SE, Lunney JK, Plastow G, Harding JC (2014) Variation in fetal outcome, viral load and ORF5 sequence mutations in a large scale study of phenotypic responses to late gestation exposure to type 2 porcine reproductive and respiratory syndrome virus. PLoS One 9:e96104
16. Gao Y, Flori L, Lecardonnel J, Esquerre D, Hu ZL, Teillaud A, Lemonnier G, Lefevre F, Oswald IP, Rogel-Gaillard C (2010) Transcriptome analysis of porcine PBMCs after in vitro stimulation by LPS or PMA/ionomycin using an expression array targeting the pig immune response. BMC Genomics 11:292
17. Diaz I, Darwich L, Pappaterra G, Pujols J, Mateu E (2005) Immune responses of pigs after experimental infection with a European strain of porcine reproductive and respiratory syndrome virus. J Gen Virol 86:1943–1951
18. Gomez-Laguna J, Salguero FJ, De Marco MF, Pallares FJ, Bernabe A, Carrasco L (2009) Changes in lymphocyte subsets and cytokines during European porcine reproductive and respiratory syndrome: increased expression of IL-12 and IL-10 and proliferation of CD4(−)CD8(high). Viral Immunol 22:261–271
19. Guo B, Lager KM, Henningson JN, Miller LC, Schlink SN, Kappes MA, Kehrli ME, Jr, Brockmeier SL, Nicholson TL, Yang HC, Faaberg KS (2013) Experimental infection of United States swine with a Chinese highly pathogenic strain of porcine reproductive and respiratory syndrome virus. Virology 435:372–384
20. Meier WA, Galeota J, Osorio FA, Husmann RJ, Schnitzlein WM, Zuckermann FA (2003) Gradual development of the interferon-gamma response of swine to porcine reproductive and respiratory syndrome virus infection or vaccination. Virology 309:18–31
21. Miguel JC, Chen J, Van Alstine WG, Johnson RW (2010) Expression of inflammatory cytokines and Toll-like receptors in the brain and respiratory tract of pigs infected with porcine reproductive and respiratory syndrome virus. Vet Immunol Immunopathol 135:314–319
22. Petry DB, Lunney J, Boyd P, Kuhar D, Blankenship E, Johnson RK (2007) Differential immunity in pigs with high and low responses to porcine reproductive and respiratory syndrome virus infection. J Anim Sci 85:2075–2092
23. Wang G, Song T, Yu Y, Liu Y, Shi W, Wang S, Rong F, Dong J, Liu H, Cai X, Zhou EM (2011) Immune responses in piglets infected with highly pathogenic porcine reproductive and respiratory syndrome virus. Vet Immunol Immunopathol 142:170–178
24. Wesley RD, Lager KM, Kehrli ME, Jr (2006) Infection with porcine reproductive and respiratory syndrome virus stimulates an early gamma interferon response in the serum of pigs. Can J Vet Res 70:176–182
25. Lowe JE, Husmann R, Firkins LD, Zuckermann FA, Goldberg TL (2005) Correlation of cell-mediated immunity against porcine reproductive and respiratory syndrome virus with protection against reproductive failure in sows during outbreaks of porcine reproductive and respiratory syndrome in commercial herds. J Am Vet Med Assoc 226:1707–1711
26. Albina E, Carrat C, Charley B (1998) Interferon-alpha response to swine arterivirus (PoAV), the porcine reproductive and respiratory syndrome virus. J Interferon Cytokine Res 18:485–490
27. Baumann A, Mateu E, Murtaugh MP, Summerfield A (2013) Impact of genotype 1 and 2 of porcine reproductive and respiratory syndrome viruses on interferon-a responses by plasmacytoid dendritic cells. Vet Res 44:33
28. Calzada-Nova G, Schnitzlein WM, Husmann RJ, Zuckermann FA (2011) North American porcine reproductive and respiratory syndrome viruses inhibit type I interferon production by plasmacytoid dendritic cells. J Virol 85:2703–2713
29. Colonna M, Trinchieri G, Liu YJ (2004) Plasmacytoid dendritic cells in immunity. Nat Immunol 5:1219–1226
30. Dwivedi V, Manickam C, Binjawadagi B, Linhares D, Murtaugh MP, Renukaradhya GJ (2012) Evaluation of immune responses to porcine reproductive and respiratory syndrome virus in pigs during early stage of infection under farm conditions. Virol J 9:45
31. Delputte PL, Van Breedam W, Barbe F, Van Reeth K, Nauwynck HJ (2007) IFN-alpha treatment enhances porcine Arterivirus infection of monocytes via upregulation of the porcine Arterivirus receptor sialoadhesin. J Interferon Cytokine Res 27:757–766
32. Souza CJH, Choi I, Araujo KPC, Abrams SM, Kerrigan M, Rowland RR, Lunney JK (2013) Comparative serum immune responses of pigs after a challenge with porcine reproductive and respiratory syndrome virus (PRRSV). In: Proceedings of the 10th IVIS International Veterinary Immunology Symposium. Milan, Italy, p 47

2

Highly pathogenic avian influenza virus infection in chickens but not ducks is associated with elevated host immune and pro-inflammatory responses

Suresh V Kuchipudi[1*], Meenu Tellabati[1], Sujith Sebastian[1], Brandon Z Londt[2], Christine Jansen[3], Lonneke Vervelde[3,4], Sharon M Brookes[2], Ian H Brown[2], Stephen P Dunham[1] and Kin-Chow Chang[1]

Abstract

Highly pathogenic avian influenza (HPAI) H5N1 viruses cause severe infection in chickens at near complete mortality, but corresponding infection in ducks is typically mild or asymptomatic. To understand the underlying molecular differences in host response, primary chicken and duck lung cells, infected with two HPAI H5N1 viruses and a low pathogenicity avian influenza (LPAI) H2N3 virus, were subjected to RNA expression profiling. Chicken cells but not duck cells showed highly elevated immune and pro-inflammatory responses following HPAI virus infection. HPAI H5N1 virus challenge studies in chickens and ducks corroborated the in vitro findings. To try to determine the underlying mechanisms, we investigated the role of signal transducer and activator of transcription-3 (STAT-3) in mediating pro-inflammatory response to HPAIV infection in chicken and duck cells. We found that *STAT-3* expression was down-regulated in chickens but was up-regulated or unaffected in ducks in vitro and in vivo following H5N1 virus infection. Low basal STAT-3 expression in chicken cells was completely inhibited by H5N1 virus infection. By contrast, constitutively active STAT-3 detected in duck cells was unaffected by H5N1 virus infection. Transient constitutively-active STAT-3 transfection in chicken cells significantly reduced pro-inflammatory response to H5N1 virus infection; on the other hand, chemical inhibition of STAT-3 activation in duck cells increased pro-inflammatory gene expression following H5N1 virus infection. Collectively, we propose that elevated pro-inflammatory response in chickens is a major pathogenicity factor of HPAI H5N1 virus infection, mediated in part by the inhibition of STAT-3.

Introduction

Avian influenza A viruses continue to spread globally causing millions of poultry deaths and are significant zoonotic pathogens [1]. In particular, Eurasian lineage highly pathogenic avian influenza (HPAI) H5N1 virus infection causes severe disease in humans with a fatality rate of about 60% [2]. Most human influenza pandemics of the 20th century had been caused by influenza A viruses (IAVs) that originated, either wholly or in part, from avian influenza A viruses [3]. Ducks and waterfowl are reservoirs for most IAVs, including the hemagglutinin (HA) and neuraminidase (NA) subtypes that have caused previous human pandemics [4]. Despite being susceptible to infection with a wide range of IAVs, such birds often show little or no clinical signs [5,6].

In contrast, most HPAI H5N1 virus strains produce very severe disease in chickens, turkeys and quails often causing up to 100% mortality within 2–3 days [7,8]. With their natural resistance, ducks support genetic reassortment of influenza viruses providing a mechanism of evolution of genetically diverse IAVs including HPAI H5N1 viruses [9-11]. The rapid onset of fatal disease in chickens and no evidence of clinical disease in ducks suggests that there are potential differences in the innate immune mechanisms between these two important avian hosts. Recent evidence shows that the resistance of ducks to HPAI virus infection is not absolute. Contemporary

* Correspondence: suresh.kuchipudi@nottingham.ac.uk
[1]School of Veterinary Medicine and Science, University of Nottingham, Sutton Bonington Campus, College Road, Loughborough, Nottingham, Leicestershire LE12 5RD, UK
Full list of author information is available at the end of the article

Eurasian lineage HPAI H5N1 viruses have caused large numbers of deaths in both poultry and water fowl including ducks. Experimental infection of Pekin ducks (*Anas platyrhynchos*) with a HPAI H5N1 clade 2.2.1 virus (A/turkey/Turkey/1/2005) causes fatal infection [12], suggesting that certain clades of contemporary Eurasian lineage HPAI H5N1 viruses are able to overcome the natural innate resistance of ducks.

The unusual severity of HPAI H5N1 virus infection in humans, in contrast to seasonal H3N2 or H1N1 influenza viruses, has been regarded to be due to hyper-acute induction of pro-inflammatory cytokines often referred as hypercytokinemia or cytokine storm [13-15]. Pigs show mild or no clinical signs following HPAI H5N1 virus infection [16]. We recently showed that the innate resistance of pigs to HPAI H5N1 virus is mediated through reduced pro-inflammation and infectious virus release [17]. These findings indicate that dysregulation of host pro-inflammatory response to infection is a key contributing factor to the morbidity and mortality of virulent influenza virus infections. Similarly a recent study found that excessive delayed inflammatory cytokine responses may contribute to the severe pathogenicity of HPAI H7N1 in chickens [18]. However, the pathophysiology of H5N1 virus infection in chickens and ducks remains unclear. To further our molecular understanding of the pathogenesis of HPAI H5N1 virus infection in chickens and ducks, we examined differences in host gene response to IAV infection between chickens and ducks in vitro (in lung cells) and in vivo.

Materials and methods
Viruses
A low pathogenicity avian influenza virus (A/mallard duck/England/7277/06, referred to as LPAI-H2N3), a classical HPAI H5N1 virus strain (A/turkey/England/50-92/91, referred to as H5N1-tyEng91) and a contemporary Eurasian lineage clade 2.2.1 HPAI H5N1 virus (A/turkey/Turkey/1/05, referred to as H5N1-tyTR05) were used in this study. While the "classical" H5N1 virus typically causes non-lethal infection in ducks [19], the contemporary Eurasian lineage (clade 2.2.1) H5N1 virus may cause severe disease with mortality in ducks [12]. All viruses were grown in 10-day-old embryonated chicken eggs by allantoic inoculation.

Primary cells and virus infection
Primary cell cultures were isolated from lungs of 4-week-old broiler chickens and 4-week-old Pekin ducks as previously described [20]. Cells were grown in collagen coated cell culture flasks (Costar, Corning, UK) in Dulbecco's Modified Eagle's Medium (DMEM) and Ham's F12 (1:1) supplemented with 2% chicken embryo extract (Biosera, Uckfield, UK), 5% fetal bovine serum, 1% insulin-transferrin

selenium (Life Technologies, Paisley, UK) and antibiotics. Monolayers of primary cells in 6 well cell culture plates (Costar) were infected with LPAI or HPAI viruses at multiplicity of infection (MOI) of 1.0. Three wells of avian cells were used for each virus infection. Mock infections were performed without virus in triplicate wells for each cell type. Cells were rinsed with phosphate buffered saline (PBS) and infected with appropriate amount of the virus in serum free infection medium comprising 2% Ultroser G (Pal Biosepra, Cedex, France), 500 ng/mL TPCK trypsin (Sigma-Aldrich, Dorset, UK) and antibiotics in Ham's F12 medium. After 2 h incubation with the virus, the cells were washed three times with PBS and fresh medium was added.

Immuno-staining for virus nucleoprotein (NP)
To determine the pattern of virus infection, virus and mock infected cells were fixed in acetone:methanol at 6 hours post-infection (hpi) and were subjected to viral nucleoprotein detection by a primary mouse monoclonal antibody (Abcam, Cambridge, UK) followed by visualization with Envision + system-HRP (DAB; Dako, Ely, UK). Cell culture supernatants form infected cells were titrated in MDCK cells to determine focus forming units (ffu) using an immuno-cytochemical focus assay as previously described [20].

Microarray gene expression profiling
At 24 hpi, total RNA from each well was extracted using RNeasy Plus Mini - QIAshredder Kit (Qiagen, Manchester, UK) and the quality of the total RNA samples was determined using a RNA 6000 nano kit (Agilent 2100 Bioanalyzer, Agilent Technologies, Stockport, UK) following the manufacturer's instructions. Microarray expression analysis was carried out using GeneChip chicken genome arrays (Affymetrix, High Wycombe, UK). Duplicate RNA samples from each of virus or mock infected chicken and duck cells were used for microarray analysis and a total of 16 array chips (3 viruses × 2 avian species × duplicate, plus 2 chicken and 2 duck mock infected) were used in the study.

Microarray expression data were analyzed using GeneSpring GX11 expression analysis software (Agilent Technologies) [21,22]. Functional clustering of data was carried out using DAVID bioinformatics resources version 6.7 [23,24].

To take into account the specificity of heterologous hybridization (between labelled duck targets on chicken probes), a well-established analytical tool was used which involved the hybridization of duck genomic DNA to the chicken chip to establish specific probe binding for duck transcriptome analysis using chicken GeneChip arrays.

Cross species array analysis was performed by generating a probe masking file to select probe-sets on the chicken chip for subsequent duck transcriptome analyses if the probe-set was represented by perfect match (PM) probes with duck gDNA hybridization intensities above an experimentally set threshold [25-27]. An additional file shows the detailed protocols of microarray expression study including the cross species hybridization data analysis (see Additional file 1).

Quantitative reverse transcription PCR (qRT-PCR) for viral and host genes

Viral RNA was extracted from culture media using QIAamp Viral RNA Mini Kit (Qiagen). One-step qRT-PCR to quantify influenza viral matrix gene was performed as previously described [20]. Based on the comparison of global gene expression profiles of chicken and duck cells, key pro-inflammatory and antiviral genes were selected and validated by qRT-PCR using the same total RNA samples as that used for the microarray experiment.

Oligonucleotide primers and hydrolysis probes for TaqMan assays were designed from published sequences using Primer Express software version 3.0.1 (Applied Biosystems, Life Technologies). All primers were provided by Eurofins Genomics (Edersberg, Germany) and all probes were supplied by Sigma Aldrich. Primer and probe sequences are shown in Table 1. qRT-PCR assays for lipopolysaccharide induced TNF alpha factor (*LITAF*) and *STAT-3* genes were performed using SYBR green method using same set of primers for both chicken and duck. Melting curve analysis was performed to ensure the specificity of the SYBR green PCR. qRT-PCR of cDNA samples converted from total RNA (Superscript III First-strand cDNA synthesis system, Life Technologies) was performed on a the *LightCycler* 480 (Roche, Burges Hill, UK), and using a relative standard curve method normalized *to 18S* ribosomal RNA (18SrRNA) expression.

HPAI H5N1 virus challenge in chickens and ducks

Three-week-old Lohmann Brown chickens kept in containment level 3 facilities (AHVLA, Weybridge) were infected with HPAI H5N1-tyTR05 virus. Chickens were inoculated intranasally and intraocularly with 0.1 mL of 1×10^6 EID$_{50}$ virus diluted in PBS. Birds were killed at 24 h after infection (three birds each from virus and control groups), lung and spleen tissues were collected and stored at −80 °C prior to RNA extraction. Three-weeks- old Pekin ducks were inoculated with 0.1 mL of 1×10^6 EID$_{50}$ of H5N1-tyTR05 virus intranasally and intraocularly. Birds were killed humanely at 24 hpi (three birds each from virus and control groups), lung and spleen tissues were collected and stored at −80 °C prior to RNA extraction. Tissues were homogenized using GentleMacs Dissociator (Miltenyi Biotec, Bisley, UK) and total RNA was extracted from the homogenized tissues using RNeasy Mini-Kit (Qiagen) following the

Table 1 Primer and probe sequences for quantitative reverse transcription PCR assays

Gene	GenBank acc. No	Primer sequence	Probe sequence
Chicken			
18S rRNA	AF173612.1	Fwd :TGTGCCGCTAGAGGTGAAATT	5' (6FAM) TTGGACCGGCGCAAGACGAAC 3' (TAMRA)
		Rev: TGGCAAATGCTTTCGCTTT	
IL-6	EU170468	Fwd :CACGATCCGGCAGATGGT	5' (6FAM)ATAAATCCCGATGAAGTGGTCATCC 3' (TAMRA)
		Rev: TGGGCGGCCGAGTCT	
IL-8 /CXCLi1(K60)	NM_205018.1	Fwd :CCCTCGCCACAGAACCAA	5' (6FAM)CCCAGGTGACACCCGGAAGAAACA 3' (TAMRA)
		Rev: CAGCCTTGCCCATCATCTTT	
IFN-α	EU367971	Fwd :CTTCCTCCAAGACAACGATTACAG	5' (6FAM)CCTGCGCCTGGGAACACGTCC 3' (TAMRA)
		Rev: AGGAACCAGGCACGAGCTT	
LITAF	AY765397	Fwd :CCCTTCTGAGGCATTTGGAA	
		Rev: CAGCCTGCAAATTTTGTCTTCTT	
STAT-3	NM_001030931.1	Fwd: TGGGTGGAGAAGGACATCA	
		Rev: CATGGGCAGGTCAATGGTAT	
Duck			
Duck IL-6	AB191038	Fwd :CCAAGGTGACGGAGGAAGAC	5' (6FAM)TGTCTCCTGGCTGGCTTCGACGA 3' (TAMRA)
		Rev: TGGAGAGTTTCTTCAAGCATTTCTC	
Duck IL-8	AB236334.1	Fwd :AGCCTGGTAAGGATGGGAAAC	5' (6FAM)AGCTCCGGTGCCAGTGCATAAGCA 3' (TAMRA)
		Rev: GGGTGGGATGAACTTCGAGTGA	
Duck IFN-α	DQ861429	Fwd :AACCAGCTTCAGCACCACATC	5' (6FAM)TGCTTCCCAGCCGACGCC 3' (TAMRA)
		Rev: TGTGGTTCTGGAGGAAGTGTTG	

manufacturer's instructions. HPAI H5N1 virus challenge studies were performed with AHVLA committee ethical approval and in accordance with the UK 1986 Animal Scientific Procedure Act and AHVLA code of practice for performance of scientific studies using animals [License number 70/7062].

STAT-3 over-expression and chemical inhibition

Based on the high sequence identity of STAT-3 protein (97%) between chicken and mouse, we used a mouse STAT-3 expression plasmid for this study. Primary chicken embryo cells in 6-well culture plates (Costar) were transiently transfected with constitutively active mouse STAT-3 expression plasmid [Stat3-C Flag pRc/CM V, plasmid 8722, Addgene, USA] or empty pRc/CMV vector (Invitrogen) using TransIT-LT1 reagent (Mirus Bio, Cambridge, UK). At 80% cell confluence, transfection mixture containing 250 µL Optimem, 2.5 µg plasmid DNA and 7.5 µL of TransIT reagent were added. Three days post-transfection, cells were infected with H5N1-tyEng91 virus at MOI of 1.0.

Primary duck embryo cells were treated with STAT-3 inhibitor S3I-201 (Calbiochem, Merck, Nottingham, UK), a cell-permeable amidosalicylic acid compound that binds STAT3-SH2 domain and prevents STAT3 phosphorylation/activation, dimerization and DNA-binding, at a final concentration of 100 µM [28] or vehicle (DMSO) control, one day before infection. Duck cells were pre-incubated with H5N1- tyEng91 virus at MOI of 1.0 for 2 h without S3I-201, after two hours the medium was removed, cells were rinsed with PBS and fresh medium with S3I-201 was replaced. At 24 hpi, cell lysates were harvested for protein and total RNA extractions. Western blotting was performed to detect phospho-STAT-3 (#9131, Cell Signaling Technology, Hitchin, UK) and influenza nucleoprotein (NP) (AA5H, #ab 20343, Abcam).

Statistical analysis

qRT-PCR data was subjected to statistical analysis by a randomization test with a pair-wise reallocation using relative expression analysis software tool (REST©) [29].

Results
Comparable susceptibility to influenza virus infection and viral RNA accumulation in chicken and duck cells

Infection of primary chicken and duck lung cells with LPAI-H2N3, H5N1-tyEng91 or H5N1-tyTR05 at 1.0 multiplicity of infection (MOI) based on MDCK cell titration resulted in comparable levels of virus infection as determined by virus NP detection by immunocytochemistry at 6 hpi (Figure 1A to H). Influenza virus matrix gene expression at 24 hpi with LPAI-H2N3, H5N1-tyEng91 and H5N1-tyTR05 viruses was comparable in chicken and duck cells (Figure 1).

More immune-related genes in chicken cells than duck cells were induced by influenza virus infection

A DNA microarray based global gene expression approach with a chicken GeneChip array (Affymetrix) was used to identify differences in gene expression between chicken and duck primary lung cells in response to 24 h of infection with LPAI H2N3, H5N1-tyEng91 or H5N1-tyTR05 viruses. Microarray datasets are available on the gene expression omnibus (GEO) site under accession number GSE33389 [30]. "Probe mask file" generated with a duck genomic DNA hybridization intensity threshold of 200 provided the highest sensitivity for duck expression analysis on the chicken GeneChip platform (Figure 2). Probe masking resulted in a loss of 5639 transcripts out of the total 38 535 transcripts represented in the original chicken GeneChip technology.

With one-way ANOVA and filtering at a $p < 0.05$ from hybridization results of all 3 virus subtypes, 18 783 out of 38 535 transcripts (48.74%) in chicken cells and, but only 7686 out of 32 896 transcripts (23.36%) in duck cells, were differentially regulated relative to corresponding controls.

The overlap among filtered genes based on fold change difference of virus infected (all three viruses) against mock infected samples provided a quantitative view of genes that were differentially expressed in chicken (Figure 3A) and duck (Figure 3B) cells following infection. Of the total number of differentially expressed genes, 12 891 genes (33.45%) in chicken cells and 3132 genes (9.52%) in duck cells were common to all three viruses. Further comparative analysis showed that 546, 754 and 1361 genes were unique to LPAI H2N3, H5N1-tyEng91 and H5N1-tyTR05 infected chicken cells respectively (Figure 3C). In duck cells, 645, 534 and 625 genes were unique to LPAI H2N3, H5N1-tyEng91 and H5N1-tyTR05 infection respectively (Figure 3D). Gene expression profiles were further analysed using the functional annotation tool in DAVID bioinformatics resources 6.7. Genes representing cytokines, chemokines, members of immunoglobulin super family, major histocompatibility complex (MHC), genes involved in T and B lymphocyte function and components of immune signalling pathways such as toll like receptor (TLR) pathway, and janus kinase (JAK) - signal transducer and activator of transcription (STAT) (JAK-STAT) pathway were classified as "immune" genes.

Several genes involved in key biological functions such as enzymes and transcription factors were down-regulated in HPAI H5N1virus infected chicken cells while most of these genes were either up-regulated or not affected in HPAI H5N1 virus infected duck cells (Table 2).

Many more immune-related genes were differentially regulated in chicken cells than in ducks cells in response to infection with the two HPAI H5N1 viruses. Of the 75 immune-related genes that were significantly up-regulated

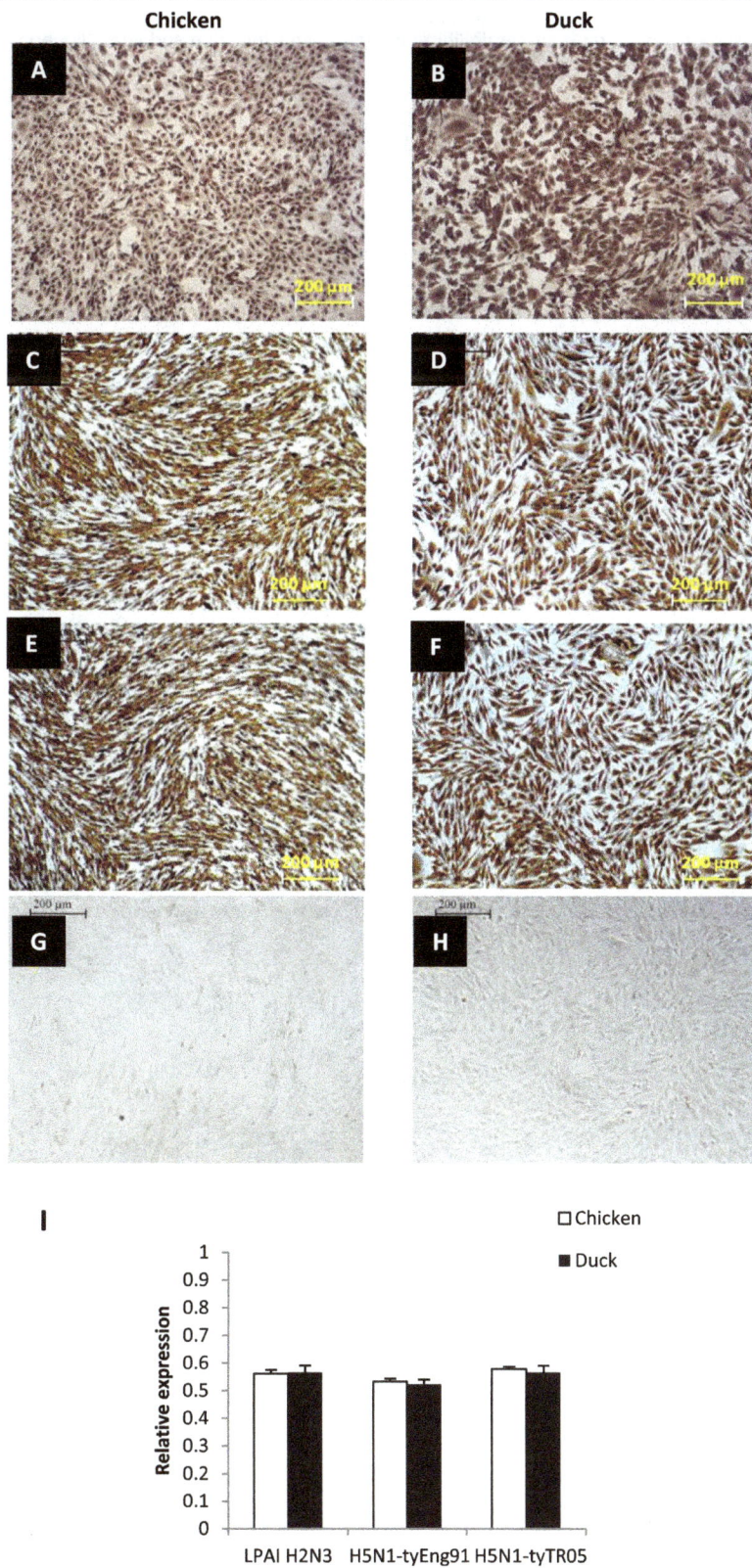

Figure 1 (See legend on next page.)

(See figure on previous page.)
Figure 1 Chicken and duck cells showed comparable susceptibility to influenza virus infection and viral RNA accumulation. At 6 hpi
with LPAI H2N3, H5N1 tyEng91 or H5N1 tyTR05 virus infection at MOI 1.0, similar accumulation of influenza nucleoprotein (NP) was evident in
chicken **(A,C,E)** and duck **(B,D,F)** cells as detected by immunocytochemistry. Mock-infected chicken **(G)** and duck **(H)** cells show no staining.
Comparable accumulation of viral matrix gene RNA between chicken and duck cells at 24 hpi at 1.0 MOI with LPAI H2N3, H5N1-tyEng91 or
H5N1 tyTR05 viruses **(I)**. Data were derived from biological replicates of 3 total RNA samples and the data points are mean relative expression
values normalized to 18SrRNA expression.

in HPAI H5N1-tyEng91 virus infected chicken cells (fold change ≥ 1.3 and $p < 0.05$), expression of 63 genes (84%) was not significantly affected ($p > 0.05$) and 12 genes (16%) were significantly down-regulated ($p < 0.05$) in corresponding duck cells. Full list of immune related genes that were differentially regulated between H5N1 virus infected chicken and duck cells is provided as an additional file (see Additional file 2). A similar difference in immune related gene expression was also observed between chicken and duck cells at 24 h H5N1-tyTR05 virus infection (see Additional file 2). However, some of these immune genes were down-regulated in chicken cells infected with LPAI H2N3 and the genes that were up-regulated showed a lower fold increase than those in the HPAI infected chicken cells (see Additional file 2).

Pro-inflammatory genes were up-regulated in infected chickens (lung cells and in vivo) but not in ducks

Pro-inflammatory cytokine genes, *interleukin* (*IL*)- *6*, *IL-8* (CXCLi1) and *IL-10*, were highly up-regulated in both HPAI H5N1 virus infected chicken cells; in contrast, *IL-8* expression was unchanged, and *IL-6* and *IL-10* were down

regulated in infected duck cells with the same viruses (Table 3). Expression of *IL-18* was up-regulated in duck cells but was down-regulated in chicken cells following infection with H5N1-tyEng91 or H5N1-tyTR05 viruses (Table 3).

Messenger RNA expression levels of *LITAF*, *IL-6* and *IL-8* were significantly up-regulated ($p < 0.05$) in chicken cells infected with LPAI-H2N3 (Figure 4A), H5N1-tyEng91 (Figure 4C) or H5N1-tyTR05 viruses (Figure 4E). However, higher fold increase in the expression was observed in HPAI viral infections (Figures 4C and E) compared with LPAI virus infection (Figure 4A) in chicken cells. In contrast, the three pro-inflammatory genes were either significantly down-regulated ($p < 0.05$) or not significantly altered ($p > 0.05$) in duck cells infected with LPAI H2N3 (Figure 4B), H5N1-tyEng91 (Figure 4D) or H5N1-tyTR05 viruses (Figure 4 F).

Significant up-regulation ($p < 0.05$) of *LITAF* (Figure 5A), *IL-6* (Figure 5B) and *IL-8* (Figure 5C) was also detected in lung and spleen tissues from three-week-old chickens at 24 h of infection with H5N1-tyTR05 or H5N1-tyEng91 HPAI viruses (data not shown), along with abundance of

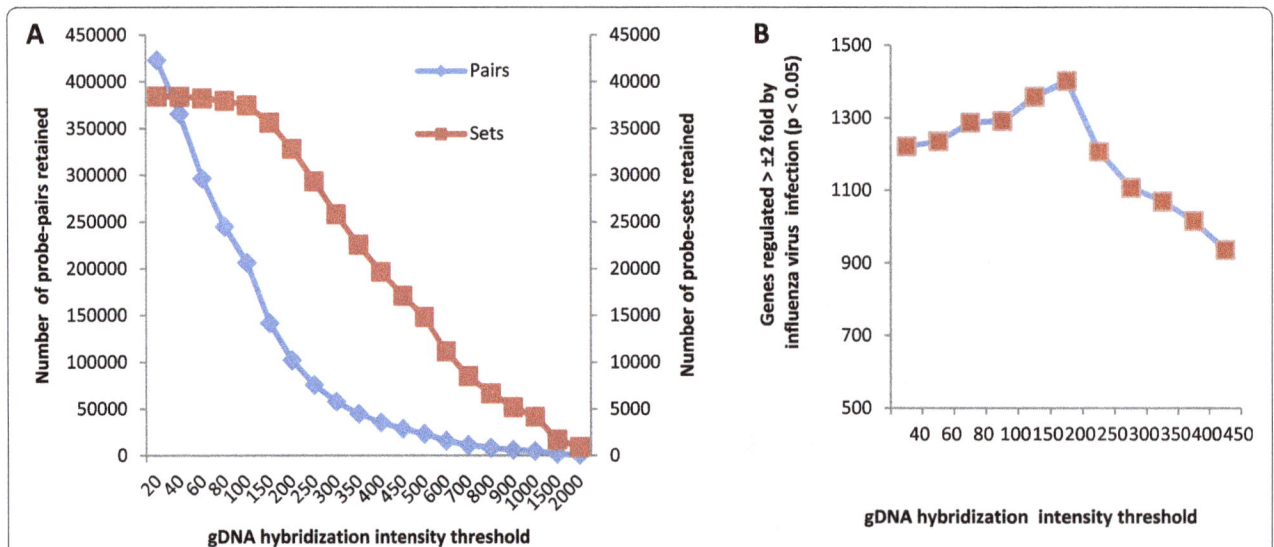

Figure 2 Genomic DNA (gDNA) hybridization intensity threshold of 200 provided the highest sensitivity for duck transcriptomic analysis on the chicken GeneChip. (A) The retention of whole probe-sets from duck gDNA hybridization on the chicken GeneChip array, representing transcripts, was less sensitive to the increase in gDNA hybridization intensities as only a minimum of one probe pair is required to retain a probe-set. **(B)** gDNA hybridization intensity threshold of 200 gave the highest number of significantly differentially regulated genes at ±2 fold ($p ≤ 0.05$) at 24 h following influenza virus infection compared with mock-infected controls. Data derived from hybridizing infected and mock-infected control duck RNA samples on chicken array.

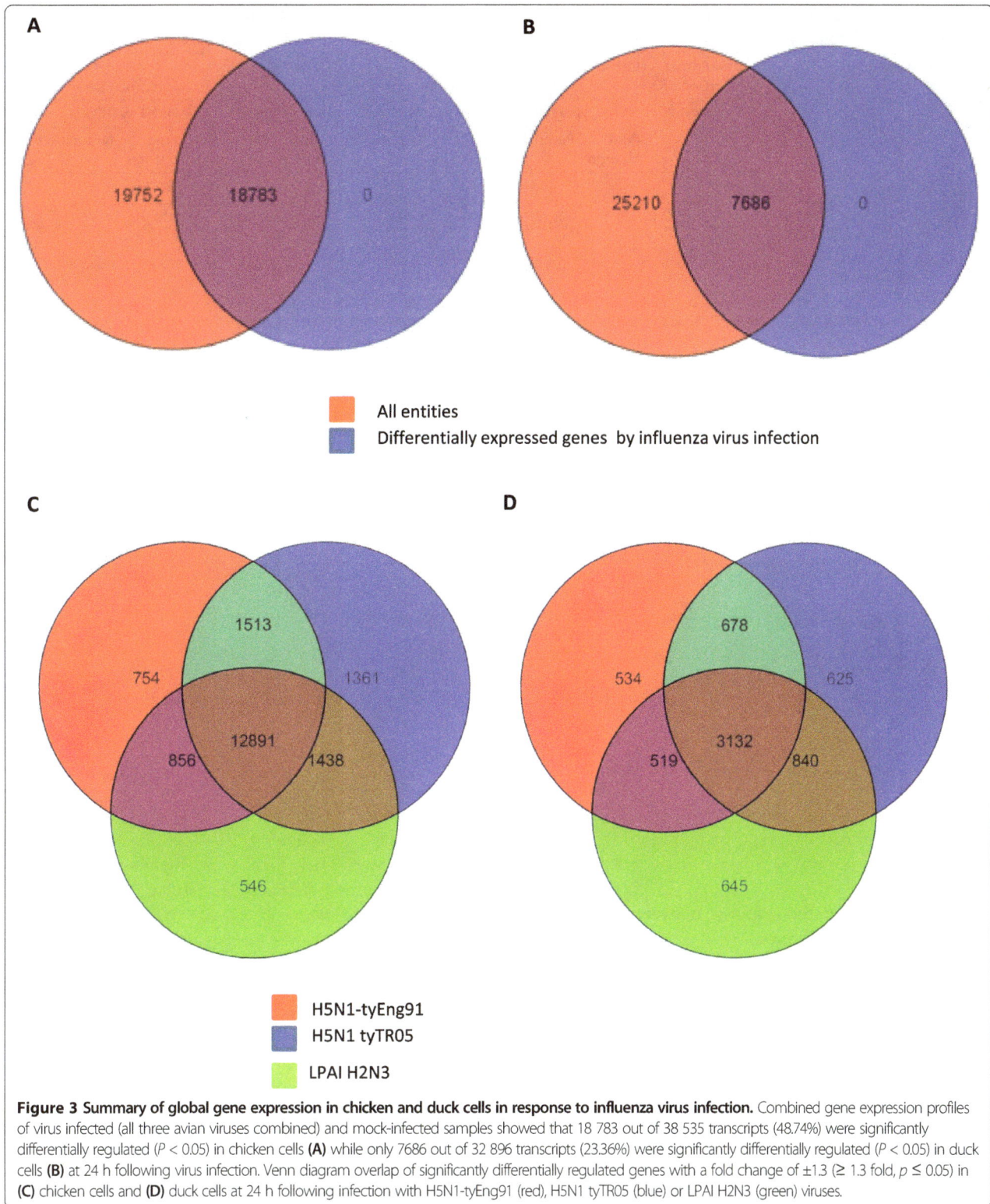

Figure 3 Summary of global gene expression in chicken and duck cells in response to influenza virus infection. Combined gene expression profiles of virus infected (all three avian viruses combined) and mock-infected samples showed that 18 783 out of 38 535 transcripts (48.74%) were significantly differentially regulated ($P < 0.05$) in chicken cells **(A)** while only 7686 out of 32 896 transcripts (23.36%) were significantly differentially regulated ($P < 0.05$) in duck cells **(B)** at 24 h following virus infection. Venn diagram overlap of significantly differentially regulated genes with a fold change of ±1.3 (≥ 1.3 fold, $p \leq 0.05$) in **(C)** chicken cells and **(D)** duck cells at 24 h following infection with H5N1-tyEng91 (red), H5N1 tyTR05 (blue) or LPAI H2N3 (green) viruses.

virus matrix gene expression (Figure 5D). In lung and spleen tissues of 3-week-old Pekin ducks taken at 24 h of infection with H5N1-tyTR05 virus, despite the detection of virus matrix gene expression (Figure 5H), *LITAF*

(Figure 5E) expression was significantly down-regulated ($p < 0.05$); *IL-6* (Figure 5F) and *IL-8* (Figure 5G) expression was not significantly affected ($p > 0.05$). In summary, similar elevated pro-inflammatory response in chickens but

Table 2 Differential expression of genes involved in key biological functions between HPAIV infected chicken and duck cells (detected by microarray)

Gene symbol	Gene name	Entrez Gene ID	Chicken cells				Duck cells			
			H5N1-tyEng91		H5N1-tyTR05		H5N1-tyEng91		H5N1-tyTR05	
			Fold change	Regulation	Fold change	Regulation	Fold change	Regulation	Fold change	Regulation
Signal transduction										
PRKAR2A	Protein kinase, cAMP-dependent, regulatory, type II, alpha	416062	2.27	up	4.59	down	3.96	down	5.86	down
IPO7	Importin 7	423046	-	unchanged	2.21	down	4.83	up	2.99	down
GTPase inhibitor activity										
GPS1	G protein pathway suppressor 1	417382	2.86	down	3.01	down	2.21	up	3.2	up
Lipid metabolism, production of ROS										
ACOX1	Acyl-Coenzyme A oxidase 1, palmitoyl	417366	4.33	down	2.88	down	-	unchanged	3.24	up
Enzymes										
B4GALNT3	Beta-1,4-N-acetyl-galactosaminyl transferase 3	418150	2.07	down	1.33	up	2.58	up	2.08	up
DNPEP	Aspartyl aminopeptidase	424200	2.38	up	1.3	up	-	unchanged	1.44	down
Catalytic activity (vit B6 metabolism)										
PSAT1	Phosphoserine aminotransferase 1	427263	4.38	down	3.9	down	11.44	up	11.69	up
Transcription factor										
RREB1	Ras responsive element binding protein 1	395920	3.41	down	2.26	down	2.73	up	7.31	up
Isoleucyl-tRNA aminoacylation										
IARS2	Isoleucyl-tRNA synthetase 2, mitochondrial	421346	17.58	down	22.92	down	14.52	up	38.82	up
Peptidolysis, IL-4 biosynthesis										
MMP28	Matrix metallopeptidase 28	417523	2.66	down	1.93	down	3.31	up	10.38	up

subdued pro-inflammatory response in ducks was observed in vitro and in vivo.

Comparable type I Interferon response between influenza virus infected chickens and ducks

Interferon alpha (*IFN-α*) expression was up-regulated in chicken (Figure 6A) and duck (Figure 6B) cells at 24 h of infection with LPAI-H2N3, H5N1-tyEng91 or H5N1-tyTR05 virus. Similar significant up-regulation of *IFN-α* expression was observed in the lung and spleen tissues of chickens at 24 h post-challenge with H5N1-tyTR05 (Figure 7B) or H5N1-tyEng91 HPAI viruses (data not shown). Up-regulation of *IFN-α* was also found in the lung and spleen tissues of ducks 24 h post-challenge with H5N1-tyTR05 HPAI virus (Figure 7D).

Differential regulation of key components of JAK-STAT pathway between influenza virus infected chicken and duck cells

Contrasting transcriptional regulation of JAK-STAT pathway between infected chicken and duck cells was observed by microarray (Table 3). Following 24 h of infection with H5N1-tyEng91 or H5N1-tyTR05 virus, members of JAK-STAT signalling pathway (*JAK1, IFN-α receptor 1* [*IFNAR1*], *STAT-3* and *protein inhibitor of activated STAT 2* [*PIAS2*]) were down-regulated in chicken cells. In duck cells, expression of *IFNAR1*, *PIAS2* and *STAT-3* was up-regulated by LPAI H2N3 or H5N1-tyEng91 virus infection. Duck *JAK1* gene was removed during the probe masking procedure and hence its expression was not determined. Notably, in duck cells infected with H5N1-tyTR05 virus, *PIAS2* expression was down-regulated, *STAT3* was unchanged and *IFNAR1* was up-regulated.

STAT-3 mRNA expression was validated in chicken and duck cells by qRT-PCR using the same total RNA samples that were used for microarray analysis. While *STAT-3* expression was not significantly affected (*P* > 0.05) by LPAI H2N3 virus infection, its expression was significantly reduced to half as much (*P* < 0.05) by H5N1-tyEng91 or H5N1-tyTR05 virus in infected chicken cells (Figure 6C). In duck cells, by contrast, *STAT-3* expression was significantly up-regulated (*P* < 0.05) by LPAI H2N3

Table 3 Differential expression of key immune related genes between HPAIV infected chicken and duck cells (detected by microarray)

Gene symbol	Gene name	Entrez Gene ID	Chicken cells				Duck cells			
			H5N1-tyEng91		H5N1-tyTR05		H5N1-tyEng91		H5N1-tyTR05	
			Fold change	Regulation	Fold change	Regulation	Fold change	Regulation	Fold change	Regulation
JAK-STAT Pathway										
STAT3	signal transducer and activator of transcription 3	420027	2.33	down	2.72	down	1.39	up	-	unchanged
JAK1	Janus kinase 1 (a protein tyrosine kinase)	554219	2.79	down	3.21	down	-	Removed*	-	Removed*
IFNAR1	Interferon (alpha, beta and omega) receptor 1	395665	8.02	down	16.65	down	13.91	up	1.37	up
PIAS2	Protein inhibitor of activated STAT, 2	416383	5.05	down	3.86	down	1.62	up	3.7	down
Cytokines and Chemokines										
IL8/ CXCLi1 (K60)	interleukin 8	395872	232.8	up	2.96	up	-	unchanged	-	unchanged
IL6	interleukin 6 (interferon, beta 2)	395337	131.08	up	10.66	up	2.92	down	-	unchanged
IL10	interleukin 10	428264	1.39	up	1.6	up	1.39	down	-	unchanged
IL18	interleukin 18 (interferon-gamma-inducing factor)	395312	4.7	down	4.14	down	3.02	up	2.4	up

*Transcript removed during probe masking.

and H5N1-tyEng91 virus infection; *STAT-3* expression was not significantly affected ($P > 0.05$) by H5N1-tyTR05 virus infection (Figure 6D). Similarly, *STAT-3* mRNA expression was down-regulated in the lung and spleen tissues of chickens challenged with H5N1-tyTR05 virus (Figure 7A) or H5N1-tyEng91 virus (data not shown). STAT-3 mRNA expression in the lung and spleen tissues was not significantly different ($p > 0.05$) in ducks challenged with H5N1-tyTR05 HPAI virus compared with controls (Figure 7C). In summary HPAI H5N1 virus infection resulted in down-regulation of key members of the JAK-STAT signalling pathway in chicken cells but not duck cells.

STAT-3 appears to negatively regulate virus-induced pro-inflammatory response and promote virus replication in chicken and duck cells

We examined the phospho-STAT-3 protein expression in chicken and duck cells using a monoclonal antibody that is specific to pSTAT-3 at tyrosine-705. Phospho-STAT-3 protein in primary duck cells was expressed constitutively and remained strongly expressed at 24 h of infection with H5N1-tyEng91 or H5N1-tyTR05 virus (Figure 6E). In primary chicken cells, by contrast, phospho-STAT-3 was weakly expressed before infection and undetectable at 24 hpi with H5N1-tyEng91 or H5N1-tyTR05 virus (Figure 6E).

To demonstrate a possible functional role of phospho-STAT-3 in mediating host pro-inflammatory response

during influenza virus infection, primary chicken cells were transiently transfected with a phospho-STAT-3 expression plasmid, and duck cells were treated with STAT3 Inhibitor VI (S3I-201) prior to challenge with the H5N1-tyEng91 virus. High expression of p-STAT-3 protein in chicken cells over-expressing pSTAT-3 and reduced p-STAT-3 expression in duck cells treated with S3I-201 at 24 h following virus infection was detected by western blotting (Figure 8A).

Chicken cells transiently transfected with phospho-STAT-3 showed a significant ($p < 0.05$) reduction in *LITAF, IL-6* and *IL-8* mRNA expression following 24 h of H5N1-tyEng91 virus infection (Figure 8B). In duck cells treated with S3I-201, a significant ($p < 0.05$) increase of *LITAF, IL-6* and *IL-8* mRNA expression was observed at 24 h post H5N1-tyEng91 virus infection (Figure 8C). STAT-3 over expression in chicken cells or inhibition in duck cells had no significant ($p > 0.05$) effect on the expression of *IFN-α* expression following H5N1-tyEng91 virus infection. Chicken cells over- expressing phospho STAT-3 showed marginal increase in viral nucleo-protein (NP) expression (Figure 8A), significantly increased ($p < 0.05$) matrix gene mRNA expression (Figure 8D) and infectious virus release in culture supernatant (Figure 8E) at 24 h post H5N1-tyEng91 virus infection. STAT-3 inhibition had no effect on virus NP (Figure 8A), matrix gene expression ($p > 0.05$) (Figure 8D) or infectious virus production at 24 h post H5N1-tyEng91 virus infection in duck cells. In summary STAT-3 over-expression in chicken cells

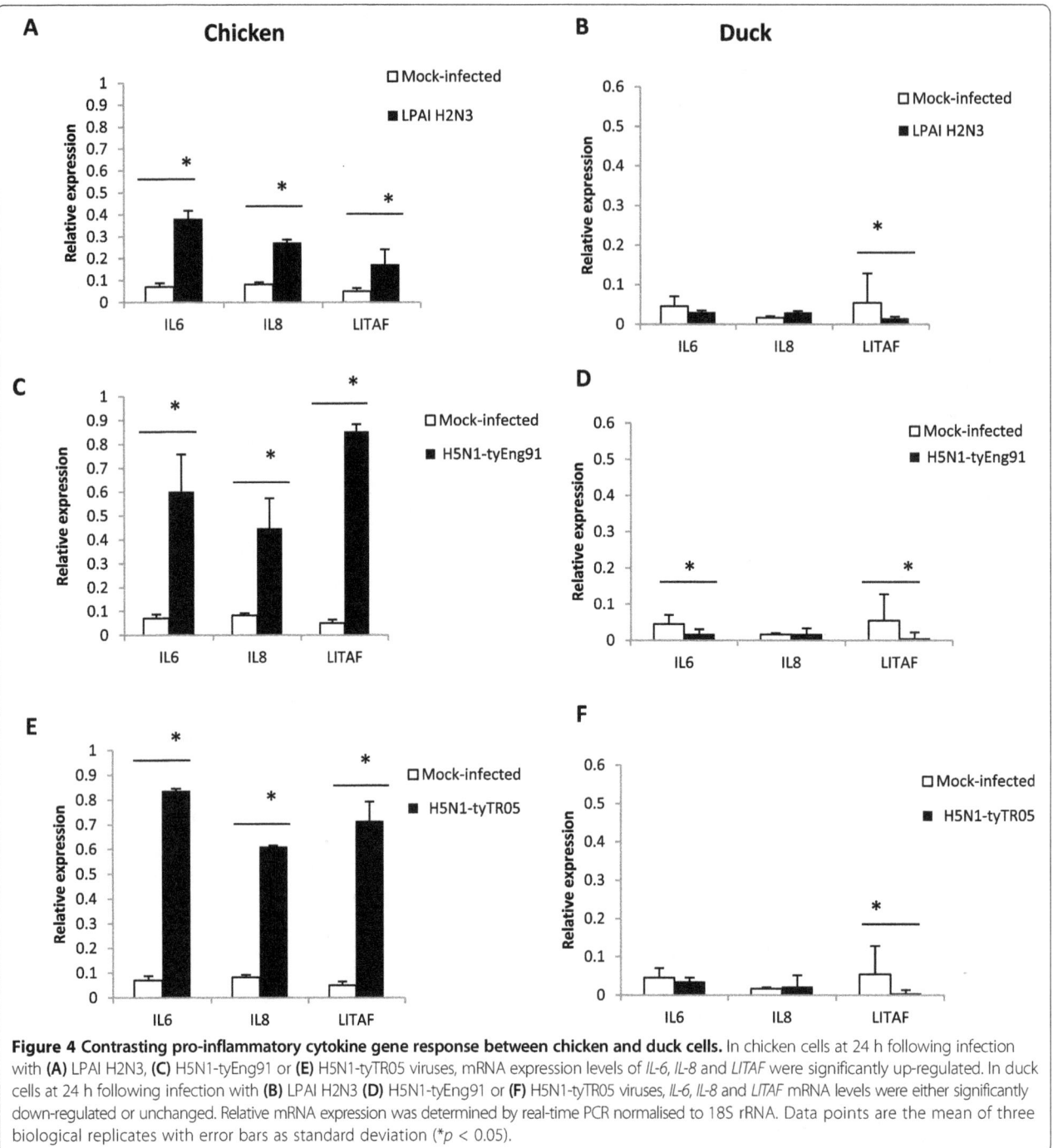

Figure 4 Contrasting pro-inflammatory cytokine gene response between chicken and duck cells. In chicken cells at 24 h following infection with **(A)** LPAI H2N3, **(C)** H5N1-tyEng91 or **(E)** H5N1-tyTR05 viruses, mRNA expression levels of *IL-6*, *IL-8* and *LITAF* were significantly up-regulated. In duck cells at 24 h following infection with **(B)** LPAI H2N3 **(D)** H5N1-tyEng91 or **(F)** H5N1-tyTR05 viruses, *IL-6*, *IL-8* and *LITAF* mRNA levels were either significantly down-regulated or unchanged. Relative mRNA expression was determined by real-time PCR normalised to 18S rRNA. Data points are the mean of three biological replicates with error bars as standard deviation (*$p < 0.05$).

resulted in significant reduction whereas chemical inhibition of STAT-3 in duck cells resulted in significant increase in the proinflammatory gene response to H5N1 virus infection.

Discussion

Microarray global gene expression analysis is a useful tool to gain important insights into the effects of influenza virus infection on host gene expression that could

contribute to influenza pathogenesis [31]. As commercial high density microarray platforms are not yet available for many avian species, cross species hybridization using chicken oligonucleotide microarray is a useful tool to investigate gene expression in a range of avian species [32]. In this study, we successfully demonstrated that the Chicken GeneChip array could be used for the analysis of duck transcriptome as in the previous studies with woodchuck RNA on human microarrays [33] and pig

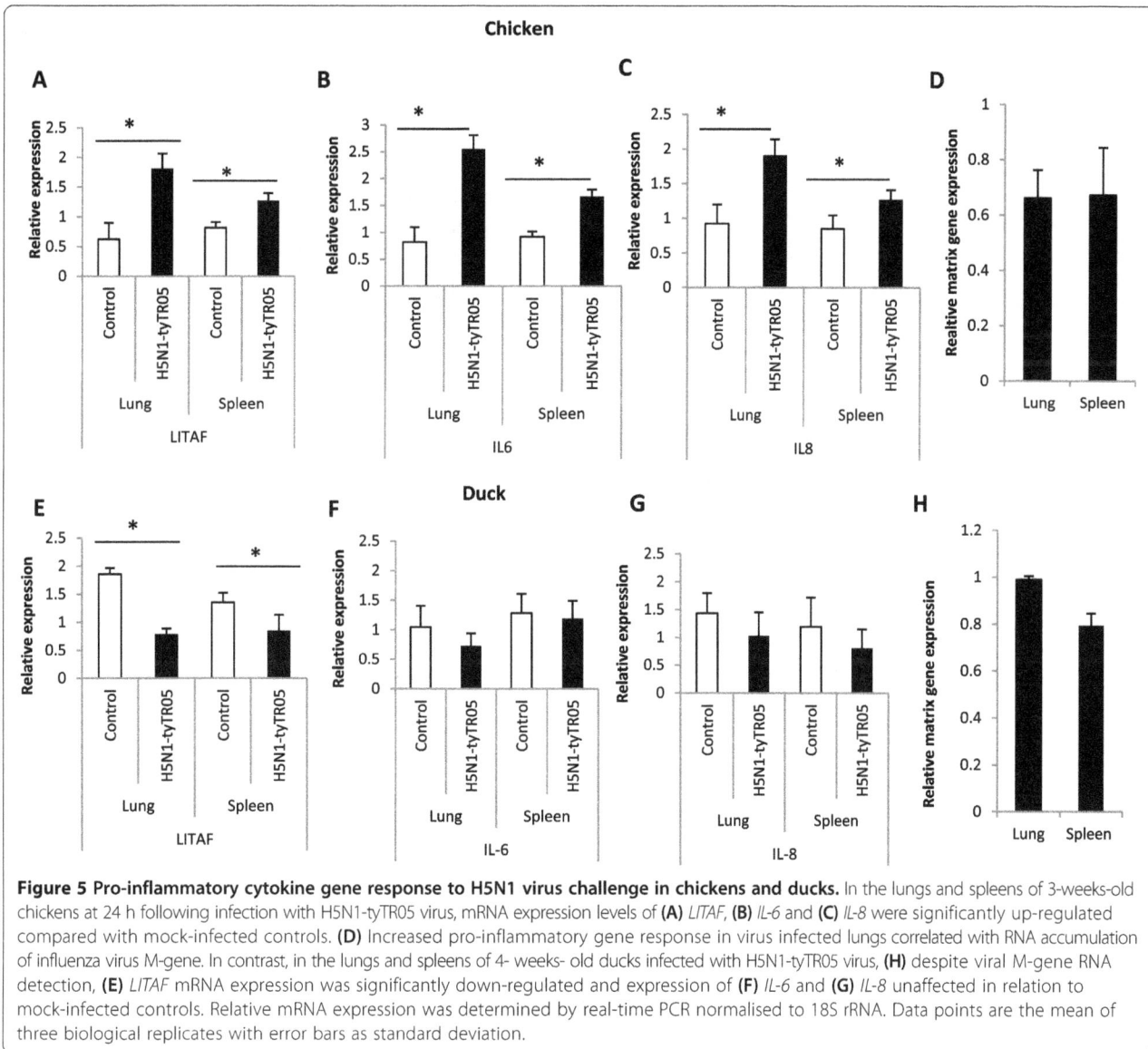

Figure 5 Pro-inflammatory cytokine gene response to H5N1 virus challenge in chickens and ducks. In the lungs and spleens of 3-weeks-old chickens at 24 h following infection with H5N1-tyTR05 virus, mRNA expression levels of **(A)** *LITAF*, **(B)** *IL-6* and **(C)** *IL-8* were significantly up-regulated compared with mock-infected controls. **(D)** Increased pro-inflammatory gene response in virus infected lungs correlated with RNA accumulation of influenza virus M-gene. In contrast, in the lungs and spleens of 4- weeks- old ducks infected with H5N1-tyTR05 virus, **(H)** despite viral M-gene RNA detection, **(E)** *LITAF* mRNA expression was significantly down-regulated and expression of **(F)** *IL-6* and **(G)** *IL-8* unaffected in relation to mock-infected controls. Relative mRNA expression was determined by real-time PCR normalised to 18S rRNA. Data points are the mean of three biological replicates with error bars as standard deviation.

RNA on human nylon microarrays [31]. However, direct high-throughput sequencing approach (RNA-Seq) is increasingly becoming popular. RNA-seq approach provides considerable advantages for examining transcriptome fine structure such as detection of allele-specific expression and splice junctions [34]. However, microarrays remain useful and accurate tools for measuring gene expression levels especially for cross-species studies where the full genome sequence and/or annotation are not available.

We found that influenza virus infection caused differential regulation of a greater number of genes involved in key biological functions in chicken cells compared with that in duck cells. Such changes in vivo could well account for the alterations in the function of infected cells and the pathogenesis of influenza virus in chicken. The relatively fewer changes in differential gene

expression in infected duck cells suggest that cellular function was affected to a lesser degree than in chickens. HPAI viruses like H5N1 cause severe clinical disease in chickens and cause differential regulation of many genes involved in protein metabolism, translation, transcription, host defence/immune response, ubiquitination and the cell cycle [35].

Lethal influenza virus infections have been previously shown to cause an aberrant host innate immune response [18,36]. In this study we showed that HPAI virus infection caused an elevated immune gene response in chicken cells but not in duck cells. We previously showed that a moderated pro-inflammatory response plays an important role in mediating innate host resistance of pigs to H5N1 virus infection [17]. The present study found an elevated pro-inflammatory gene

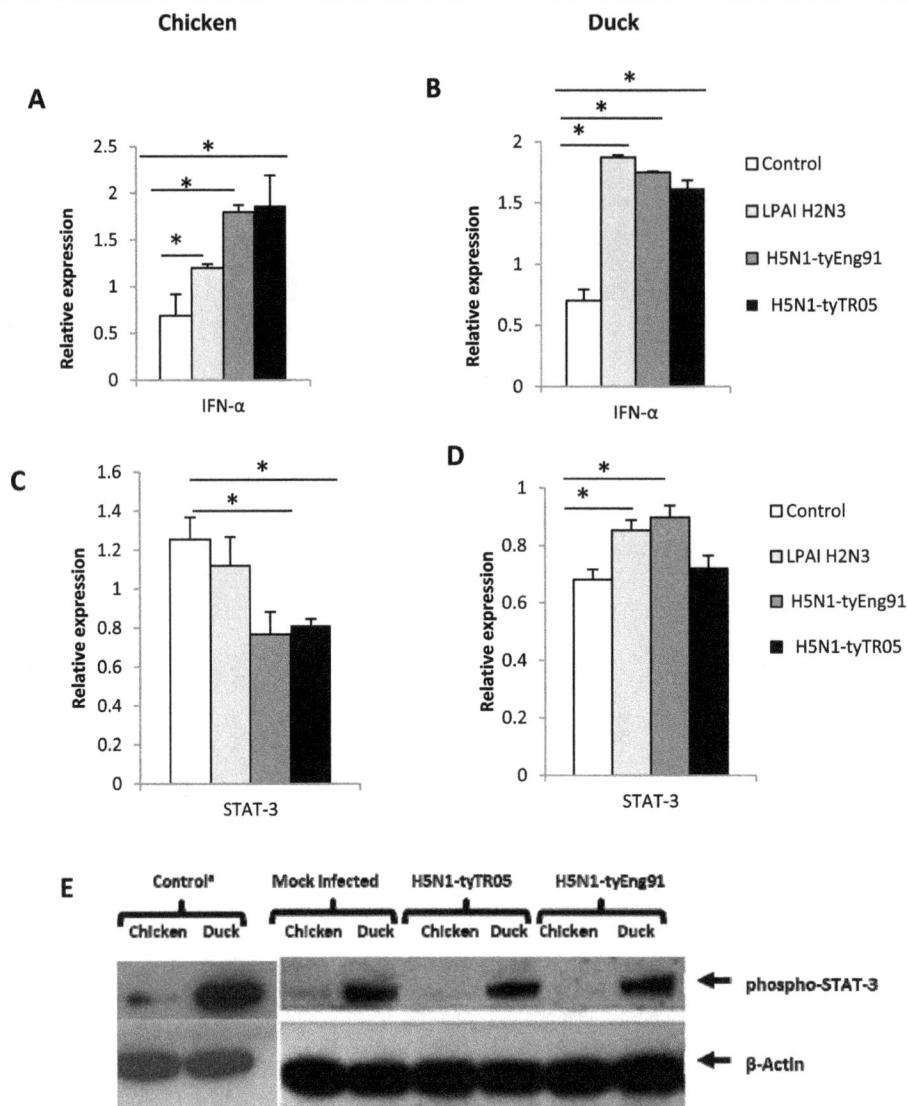

Figure 6 Infected chicken and duck cells showed differential regulation of STAT-3. *IFN-α expression was significantly up-regulated in chicken* **(A)** *and duck* **(B)** *cells at 24 h following infection with LPAI-H2N3, H5N1-tyEng91 or H5N1-tyTR05 viruses.* **(C)** *While STAT-3 expression in chicken cells was not significantly affected by LPAI-H2N3 virus infection it was significantly down-regulated in H5N1-tyEng91 and H5N1-tyTR05 virus infections.* **(D)** *In contrast STAT-3 expression in duck cells was significantly up-regulated by LPAI-H2N3 or H5N1-tyEng91 viruses but was not affected by H5N1-tyTR05 virus infection. Relative mRNA expression was determined by real-time PCR normalised to 18S rRNA. Data points are the mean of three biological replicates with error bars as standard deviation (*p < 0.05).* **(E)** *Strong constitutive phospho-STAT-3 protein expression was detected in duck cells which was unaffected at 24 h following infection with H5N1-tyEng91 and H5N1-tyTR05 viruses. In chicken mock-infected cells, phospho-STAT3 protein expression was scarcely detectable and remained absent at 24 h following virus infection. ªLonger (5 min) exposure showing pSTAT-3 in chicken cells.*

response in infected chickens and an attenuated inflammatory response in ducks following 24 h of infection with HPAI virus. The unusual severity of clinical human cases of H5N1 HPAI virus infection has been suggested to be linked to the hyperacute dysregulation of pro-inflammatory cytokines often referred as cytokine storm [14,15,37]. Tumour Necrosis Factor alpha (*TNF-α*) plays a major role in the development of clinical signs like fever and contributes to the lung lesions in humans [38] and pigs [39] during influenza virus

infections. Due to absence of a "conventional" *TNF-α* gene in birds, expression of a lipopolysaccharide induced TNF alpha factor (*LITAF*) was analyzed in this study. LITAF gene has been previously shown to be very highly up regulated along with other pro-inflammatory cytokines following experimental inoculation of *E.coli* and *Salmonella* endotoxins [40] and LPAIV [41,42]. It is likely that the downstream pathways activated by *LITAF* might have a similar function as *TNF-α* in other species. We found an increased expression of *LITAF* in chickens and a down-regulated *LITAF* expression in ducks infected with H5N1-tyEng91 or H5N1-tyTR05 viruses. Similar increased expression of other pro-inflammatory cytokines *IL-6* and *IL-8* was observed in chickens, but not in ducks, infected with HPAIV [43].

However, pro-inflammatory response in ducks to different H5N1 virus strains could be inherently different. For example, a number of innate immune genes are up-regulated in the lungs of duck infected with a HPAI H5N1 virus (A/duck/Hubei/49/05), a LPAI H5N1 virus (A/goose/Hubei/65/05) [44] and a HPAI H5N1 virus (A/Vietnam/1203/04) [45]. In theory, the lack of such robust innate immune activation in ducks in vitro and in vivo following H5N1-tyTR05 virus could be due to inability of virus replication, or inherent differences in ducks response to different viral strains. However, H5N1-tyTR05 virus replicates to high titres in ducks with detectable viral shedding in oropharyngeal and cloacal swabs [12] and in vitro as shown by NP staining and M gene quantification. Hence, it is likely that there are inherent differences in the response of ducks to different subtypes of HPAI H5N1 viruses.

A previous study suggested that relative susceptibility of chickens to influenza virus, compared with ducks, could be due to the absence of RIG-I in chickens, a cytoplasmic RNA sensor that plays a key role in IFN mediated anti-viral responses [46]. However, a reduced IFN-β response in chicken cells in comparison with duck cells does not always seem to be a consistent observation in all influenza virus infections. Chicken peripheral blood mononuclear cells (PBMC) showed up-regulation of IFN-β while the levels of IFN-β are unaffected in duck PBMCs infected with a low pathogenic LPAI H11N9 influenza virus [47]. Type I interferon (IFN) response to AIV infection in chicken cells is mediated through melanoma differentiation-associated protein 5 (MDA-5) which chicken use to sense IAV infection [48]. Role of host IFN-α/β response in regulating virus replication is complex. In mice IFN-α/β causes either suppression or enhancement of hepatitis B virus (HBV) replication depending on the viral load [49]. Furthermore, a high host interferon IFN response to H5N1 HPAI virus may not, by itself, be sufficient to prevent a severe disease outcome. Conversely, host immune responses to HPAI H5N1 virus infection may contribute to disease pathogenesis. In human cases of HPAI H5N1 virus infection, higher levels of cytokines and chemokines were found in the blood of patients who died than those who survived [50-52].

The present study did not find any difference in IFN-α expression in chickens and ducks following H5N1 HPAI virus infection both in vitro and in vivo, raising a possibility that an IFN-α response by itself may not be sufficient to protect the host against virulent influenza virus infection. A study found strong up-regulation of IFN-γ mRNA in the lung and bursa of ducks but not chicken

following infection with a LPAI H7N1 virus [53]. It is possible that IFN-γ rather than IFN-α or β could be important in protection against virulent influenza infection in avian hosts which warrants further studies.

In summary, we showed that host pro-inflammatory responses could be a key contributing factor to the pathogenesis of H5N1 influenza viruses and that the fatal outcome of H5N1 HPAI virus infection in chickens could be mediated by hyper-acute dysregulation of pro-inflammatory cytokines or the cytokine storm similar to human H5N1 HPAI virus infections. Furthermore, ducks showed attenuated pro-inflammation following infection with both the H5N1 viruses used in this study. However, to evaluate virus subtype specific differences, further comparative studies are required to assess the differences in cytokine response between ducks infected with different H5N1 virus isolates.

We found that *IL-18* was up-regulated in duck cells, but was down regulated in chicken cells infected with HPAIV. *IL-18* is involved in the control of influenza virus replication in the lungs of infected mice, especially at an early stage of infection, through activation of the innate immune mechanisms such as IFN and natural killer (NK) cells [54] and improves the early defence system by augmenting NK cell-mediated cytotoxicity. *IL-18* plays a critical role in the development of protective immunity against various intracellular pathogens including *Mycobacterium tuberculosis*, *Yersinia enterocolitica*, *Cryptococcus neoformans* and herpes simplex virus [55-58]. Recent studies demonstrated that recombinant vaccines simultaneously expressing influenza antigens along with IL-18 significantly enhance the protective efficacy of influenza vaccines in chicken [9]. A study also found that LPAI but not HPAI infection is associated with enhanced NK cell response in lungs of chicken [59], suggesting a crucial role of NK cell response in influenza virus pathogenesis. This evidence warrants further functional studies to investigate the mechanisms underlying the protective role of IL-18 and NK cell response during influenza virus infections in chicken.

The JAK-STAT signalling pathway is activated by the type I (IFN-α and IFN-β) and type II (IFN-γ) interferons [60] and is critical for a successful IFN-α antiviral response against virus infections [61]. This study found that key genes in JAK-STAT signalling pathway were down-regulated in chicken cells but were either up-regulated or unchanged in duck cells at 24 h following HPAIV infection. STAT-3, a key constituent of this pathway plays a critical role in the IFN signalling pathways and is required for a robust IFN-induced antiviral response [62].

STAT family proteins are activated by phosphorylation by JAKs on a single tyrosine in the C-terminus at position 705 that enables their homo- or hetero-dimerization. Dimerized STAT proteins subsequently migrate to the nucleus and stimulate transcription [63]. Hence

Chicken

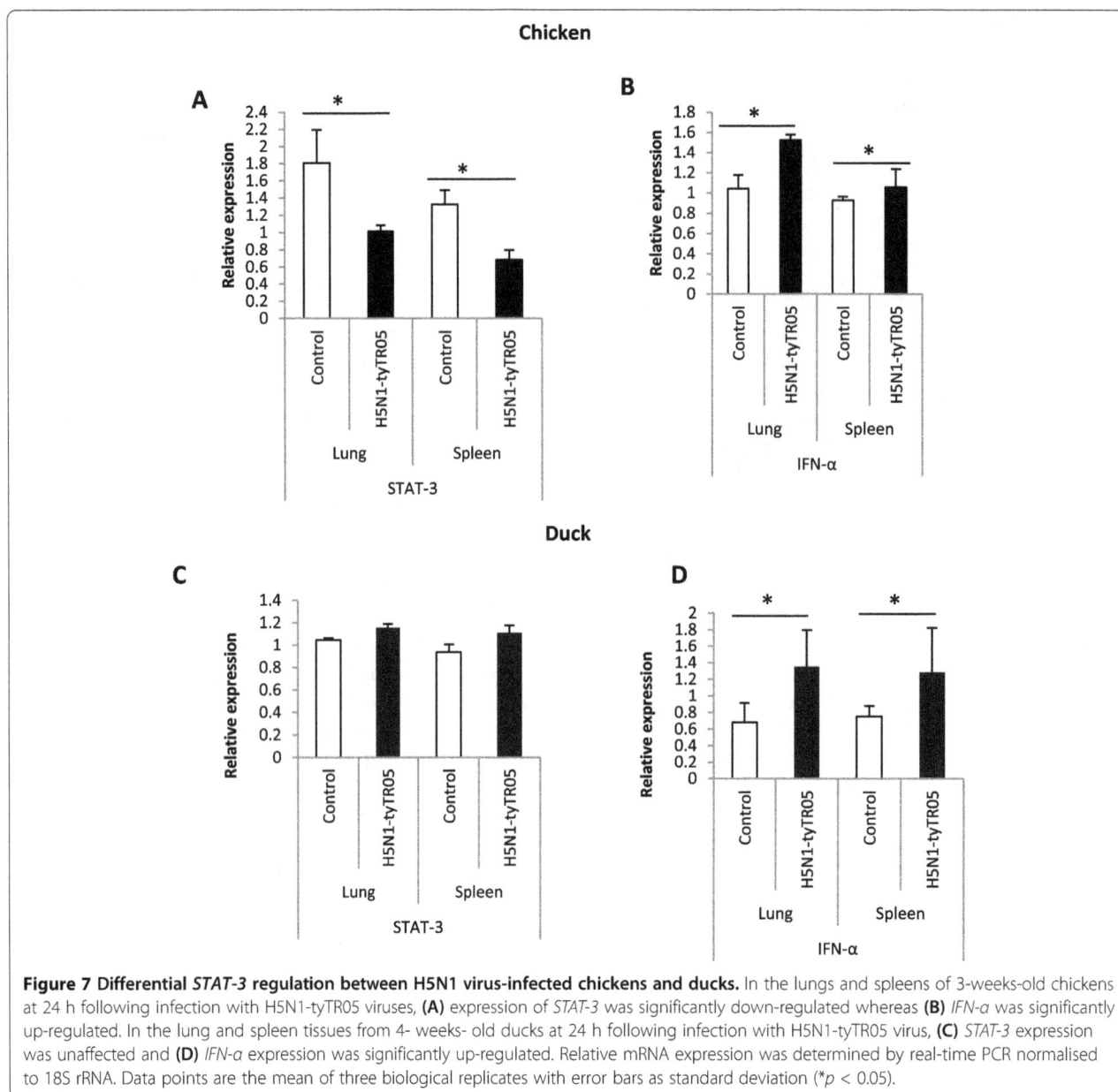

Figure 7 Differential *STAT-3* regulation between H5N1 virus-infected chickens and ducks. In the lungs and spleens of 3-weeks-old chickens at 24 h following infection with H5N1-tyTR05 viruses, **(A)** expression of *STAT-3* was significantly down-regulated whereas **(B)** *IFN-α* was significantly up-regulated. In the lung and spleen tissues from 4- weeks- old ducks at 24 h following infection with H5N1-tyTR05 virus, **(C)** *STAT-3* expression was unaffected and **(D)** *IFN-α* expression was significantly up-regulated. Relative mRNA expression was determined by real-time PCR normalised to 18S rRNA. Data points are the mean of three biological replicates with error bars as standard deviation (*$p < 0.05$).

phosphorylation of STAT-3 at tyrosine- 705 is a key indicator of its DNA binding ability and activity as a transcription factor. We found that duck cells had a high basal expression of pSTAT-3 (Tyr705) compared with chicken cells. pSTAT-3 (Tyr705) protein expression was undetectable in chicken cells 24 h after infection with HPAI H5N1 virus while it was unaffected during infection of duck cells. We could not verify STAT-3 protein expression in-vivo due to unavailability of protein samples from HPAI infected chickens and ducks. The transcriptional down-regulation of *STAT-3* with corresponding lack of pSTAT-3 protein expression in chicken cells suggests that H5N1 HPAI virus infection inhibits STAT-3 mediated gene

transcription and/or activation. An important function of STAT-3 is its antagonistic effect on the inflammatory response. Activation of the STAT-3 signaling pathway promotes a strong anti-inflammatory response thereby blocking the inflammatory cytokine response [64]. Hence, it is likely that the excessive pro-inflammatory response in H5N1 HPAI virus infected chickens could be mediated through the inhibition of STAT-3 and a functional STAT-3 corresponds to an attenuated pro-inflammation in H5N1 virus infected ducks. In addition, *IL-18* stimulation results in enhanced tyrosine phosphorylation of STAT-3 [65]. In the present study *IL-18* activation correlated with increased STAT-3 phophorylation in duck cells while

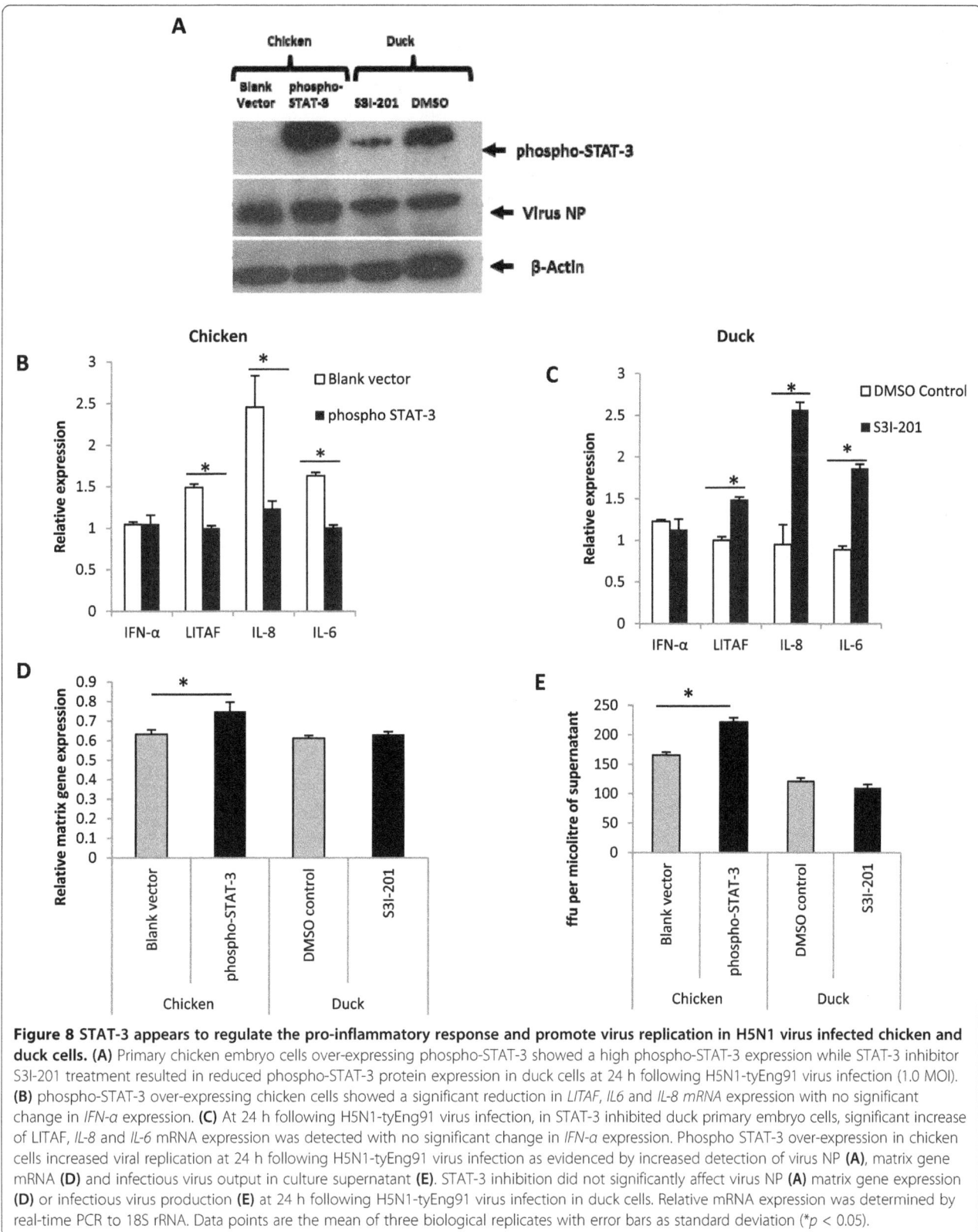

Figure 8 STAT-3 appears to regulate the pro-inflammatory response and promote virus replication in H5N1 virus infected chicken and duck cells. (A) Primary chicken embryo cells over-expressing phospho-STAT-3 showed a high phospho-STAT-3 expression while STAT-3 inhibitor S3I-201 treatment resulted in reduced phospho-STAT-3 protein expression in duck cells at 24 h following H5N1-tyEng91 virus infection (1.0 MOI). **(B)** phospho-STAT-3 over-expressing chicken cells showed a significant reduction in *LITAF*, *IL6* and *IL-8 mRNA* expression with no significant change in *IFN-α* expression. **(C)** At 24 h following H5N1-tyEng91 virus infection, in STAT-3 inhibited duck primary embryo cells, significant increase of LITAF, *IL-8* and *IL-6* mRNA expression was detected with no significant change in *IFN-α* expression. Phospho STAT-3 over-expression in chicken cells increased viral replication at 24 h following H5N1-tyEng91 virus infection as evidenced by increased detection of virus NP **(A)**, matrix gene mRNA **(D)** and infectious virus output in culture supernatant **(E)**. STAT-3 inhibition did not significantly affect virus NP **(A)** matrix gene expression **(D)** or infectious virus production **(E)** at 24 h following H5N1-tyEng91 virus infection in duck cells. Relative mRNA expression was determined by real-time PCR to 18S rRNA. Data points are the mean of three biological replicates with error bars as standard deviation (*$p < 0.05$).

down-regulation of *IL-18* in H5N1virus infected chicken cells correlated with reduced pSTAT-3 detection.

Chicken cells over-expressing constitutively active STAT-3 showed significantly lower *LITAF, IL-6* and *IL-8* mRNA levels compared with the blank plasmid transfected cells at 24 h post H5N1-tyEng91 virus infection. Duck cells treated with S3I-201 that inhibits the transcriptional activity of STAT-3, resulted in increased expression of *LITAF, IL-6* and *IL-8* compared with control cells at 24 h post H5N1-tyEng91 virus infection. Previous studies showed that constitutively active STAT3 can suppress both *IL-6* and *TNF-α* production in lipopolysaccharide-stimulated macrophages [66]. The sum of this evidence raise a strong possibility that STAT-3 mediated gene transcription could play a central role in suppressing pro-inflammatory responses during H5N1 virus infection in ducks. Furthermore the ability of HPAI viruses to inhibit STAT-3 in chickens correlates with excessive pro-inflammatory response and the development of fatal disease. Further studies would help to identify candidate genes that suppress pro-inflammation during HPAI H5N1 virus infection and are transcriptionally regulated by STAT-3.

Surprisingly, we found that STAT-3 over-expression significantly increased H5N1 HPAI virus replication in chicken cells while STAT-3 inhibition had no significant effect on virus replication in duck cells. The increase in influenza virus replication in chicken cells over-expressing STAT-3 could be due to inhibition of type I IFN-mediated antiviral response. However, STAT-3 over-expression or inhibition did not significantly affect *IFN-α* mRNA expression in chicken and duck cells respectively. Conversely, STAT3 has been suggested as an important upstream element in type I IFN signal transduction and in the induction of antiviral activities [62]. The role of STAT-3 in virus replication appears to be complex. For example STAT-3 induction promotes varicella-zoster virus replication [67], activates anti-hepatitis C virus (HCV) activity in liver cells [68] and promotes HCV RNA replication [69]. Findings of the present study suggest that STAT-3 could promote influenza virus replication in chicken cells but not in duck cells. We showed previously that duck cells produce significantly less infectious influenza virus compared with chicken cells which correlated with rapid cell death [20]. It is likely that other mechanisms independent of STAT-3 could contribute to the antiviral effects observed in duck cells. As STAT-3 is a transcription factor and known to mediate the expression of a variety of genes, it is likely that STAT-3 over-expression or inhibition may affect a number of cellular signalling pathways. Hence, further studies are needed to identify candidate genes that play an important role in mediating pro-inflammation and influenza virus replication in chickens and ducks.

Additional files

Additional file 1: Preparation of RNA target and hybridization on to GeneChip expression arrays. Protocol describing sample preparation and hybridization on to Genechip and probe masking for cross species hybridization of duck RNA onto chicken Genechip.

Additional file 2: List of key immune related genes that were differentially regulated between chicken and duck cells following influenza virus infection. List of key immune related genes that were differentially regulated in chicken and duck cells following infection with LPAI H2N3, H5N1-tyEng91 and H5N1-tyTR05 viruses.

Competing interests
The authors declare that they have no competing interests.

Authors' contributions
Conceived and designed the experiments: SVK, SPD and KCC. Performed the experiments and microarray data analysis: SVK. In vivo challenge studies: BZ and SB (duck challenge experiments); CJ and LV (chicken challenge experiments). Planning and organization of HPAI infection experiments: SVK, SB and IB. Analysed qPCR data: SVK, MT and SS. Contributed to the writing of the manuscript: SVK, KCC, SPD, SB, IB and LV. All authors read and approved the final manuscript.

Acknowledgements
We are grateful to colleagues at AHVLA for their valuable support, Fanny Garcon and Vivian Coward (technical assistance); Bethany Nash, Jonathan Ridgeon and Michael Kelly (laboratory support). This work was part funded by the BBSRC grant BB/E010849/1, the University of Nottingham (pump prime grant to SVK) and DEFRA grant SE0782 (BZL, SMB and IHB). In vivo chicken experiment: This study was financially supported by the Netherlands Organization for Scientific Research (NWO) Veni grant 016.096.049, the EU sixth framework program Flupath (grant 04220) and by the "Impulse Veterinary Avian Influenza Research in The Netherlands, Dutch Ministry of Agriculture, Nature and Food Quality (CAJ and LV).

Author details
[1]School of Veterinary Medicine and Science, University of Nottingham, Sutton Bonington Campus, College Road, Loughborough, Nottingham, Leicestershire LE12 5RD, UK. [2]Virology Department, Animal and Plant Health Agency, Weybridge, Addlestone, Surrey KT15 3NB, UK. [3]Department of Infectious Diseases and Immunology, Faculty of Veterinary Medicine, University of Utrecht, Utrecht, The Netherlands. [4]Current address: The Roslin Institute and R(D)SVS, University of Edinburgh, Easter Bush, Midlothian, Edinburgh EH25 9RG, UK.

References
1. Gibbs AJ, Armstrong JS, Downie JC: **From where did the 2009 'swine-origin' influenza A virus (H1N1) emerge?** *Virol J* 2009, **6:**207.
2. Thitithanyanont A, Engering A, Uiprasertkul M, Ekchariyawat P, Wiboon-Ut S, Kraivong R, Limsalakpetch A, Kum-Arb U, Yongvanitchit K, Sa-Ard-Iam N, Rukyen P, Mahanonda R, Kawkitinarong K, Auewarakul P, Utaisincharoen P, Sirisinha S, Mason CJ, Fukuda MM, Pichyangkul S: **Antiviral immune responses in H5N1-infected human lung tissue and possible mechanisms underlying the hyperproduction of interferon-inducible protein IP-10.** *Biochem Biophys Res Commun* 2010, **398:**752–758.
3. Katz JM, Veguilla V, Belser JA, Maines TR, Van Hoeven N, Pappas C, Hancock K, Tumpey TM: **The public health impact of avian influenza viruses.** *Poult Sci* 2009, **88:**872–879.
4. Sharp GB, Kawaoka Y, Jones DJ, Bean WJ, Pryor SP, Hinshaw V, Webster RG: **Coinfection of wild ducks by influenza A viruses: distribution patterns and biological significance.** *J Virol* 1997, **71:**6128–6135.
5. Isoda N, Sakoda Y, Kishida N, Bai GR, Matsuda K, Umemura T, Kida H: **Pathogenicity of a highly pathogenic avian influenza virus, A/chicken/Yamaguchi/7/04 (H5N1) in different species of birds and mammals.** *Arch Virol* 2006, **151:**1267–1279.

6. Perkins LEL, Swayne DE: Pathogenicity of a Hong Kong-origin H5N1 highly pathogenic avian influenza virus for emus, geese, ducks, and pigeons. *Avian Dis* 2002, **46**:53–63.

7. Jeong OM, Kim MC, Kim MJ, Kang HM, Kim HR, Kim YJ, Joh SJ, Kwon JH, Lee YJ: Experimental infection of chickens, ducks and quails with the highly pathogenic H5N1 avian influenza virus. *J Vet Sci* 2009, **10**:53–60.

8. Saito T, Watanabe C, Takemae N, Chaisingh A, Uchida Y, Buranathai C, Suzuki H, Okamatsu M, Imada T, Parchariyanon S, Traiwanatam N, Yamaguchi S: Pathogenicity of highly pathogenic avian influenza viruses of H5N1 subtype isolated in Thailand for different poultry species. *Vet Microbiol* 2009, **133**:65–74.

9. Chen HY, Shang YH, Yao HX, Cui BA, Zhang HY, Wang ZX, Wang YD, Chao AJ, Duan TY: Immune responses of chickens inoculated with a recombinant fowlpox vaccine coexpressing HA of H9N2 avain influenza virus and chicken IL-18. *Antiviral Res* 2011, **91**:50–56.

10. Guan Y, Peiris M, Kong KF, Dyrting KC, Ellis TM, Sit T, Zhang LJ, Shortridge KF: H5N1 influenza viruses isolated from geese in Southeastern China: evidence for genetic reassortment and interspecies transmission to ducks. *Virology* 2002, **292**:16–23.

11. Wibawa H, Henning J, Wong F, Selleck P, Junaidi A, Bingham J, Daniels P, Meers J: A molecular and antigenic survey of H5N1 highly pathogenic avian influenza virus isolates from smallholder duck farms in Central Java, Indonesia during 2007–2008. *Virol J* 2011, **8**:425.

12. Londt BZ, Nunez A, Banks J, Nili H, Johnson LK, Alexander DJ: Pathogenesis of highly pathogenic avian influenza A/turkey/Turkey/1/2005 H5N1 in Pekin ducks (Anas platyrhynchos) infected experimentally. *Avian Pathol* 2008, **37**:619–627.

13. Ramos I, Fernandez-Sesma A: Innate immunity to H5N1 influenza viruses in humans. *Viruses* 2012, **4**(12):3363–3388.

14. Cheung CY, Poon LL, Lau AS, Luk W, Lau YL, Shortridge KF, Gordon S, Guan Y, Peiris JS: Induction of proinflammatory cytokines in human macrophages by influenza A (H5N1) viruses: a mechanism for the unusual severity of human disease? *Lancet* 2002, **360**:1831–1837.

15. Lipatov AS, Andreansky S, Webby RJ, Hulse DJ, Rehg JE, Krauss S, Perez DR, Doherty PC, Webster RG, Sangster MY: Pathogenesis of Hong Kong H5N1 influenza virus NS gene reassortants in mice: the role of cytokines and B- and T-cell responses. *J Gen Virol* 2005, **86**:1121–1130.

16. Lipatov AS, Kwon YK, Sarmento LV, Lager KM, Spackman E, Suarez DL, Swayne DE: Domestic pigs have low susceptibility to H5N1 highly pathogenic avian influenza viruses. *PLoS Pathog* 2008, **4**:e1000102.

17. Nelli RK, Dunham SP, Kuchipudi SV, White GA, Baquero-Perez B, Chang P, Ghaemmaghami A, Brookes SM, Brown IH, Chang KC: Mammalian innate resistance to highly pathogenic avian influenza H5N1 virus infection is mediated through reduced proinflammation and infectious virus release. *J Virol* 2012, **86**:9201–9210.

18. Cornelissen JB, Vervelde L, Post J, Rebel JM: Differences in highly pathogenic avian influenza viral pathogenesis and associated early inflammatory response in chickens and ducks. *Avian Pathol* 2013, **42**:347–364.

19. Wood GW, Parsons G, Alexander DJ: Replication of influenza A viruses of high and low pathogenicity for chickens at different sites in chickens and ducks following intranasal inoculation. *Avian Pathol* 1995, **24**:545–551.

20. Kuchipudi SV, Dunham SP, Nelli R, White GA, Coward VJ, Slomka MJ, Brown IH, Chang KC: Rapid death of duck cells infected with influenza: a potential mechanism for host resistance to H5N1. *Immunol Cell Biol* 2012, **90**:116–123.

21. Irizarry RA, Hobbs B, Collin F, Beazer-Barclay YD, Antonellis KJ, Scherf U, Speed TP: Exploration, normalization, and summaries of high density oligonucleotide array probe level data. *Biostatistics* 2003, **4**:249–264.

22. Irizarry RA, Bolstad BM, Collin F, Cope LM, Hobbs B, Speed TP: Summaries of Affymetrix GeneChip probe level data. *Nucleic Acids Res* 2003, **31**:e15.

23. da Huang W, Sherman BT, Lempicki RA: Systematic and integrative analysis of large gene lists using DAVID bioinformatics resources. *Nat Protoc* 2009, **4**:44–57.

24. da Huang W, Sherman BT, Lempicki RA: Bioinformatics enrichment tools: paths toward the comprehensive functional analysis of large gene lists. *Nucleic Acids Res* 2009, **37**:1–13.

25. Hammond JP, Broadley MR, Craigon DJ, Higgins J, Emmerson ZF, Townsend HJ, White PJ, May ST: Using genomic DNA-based probe-selection to improve the sensitivity of high-density oligonucleotide arrays when applied to heterologous species. *Plant Methods* 2005, **1**:10.

26. X-species Version 2.1 [http://affymetrix.arabidopsis.info/xspecies/]

27. CDF_masking.Zip [http://affymetrix.arabidopsis.info/xspecies/CDF_masking.zip]

28. Siddiquee K, Zhang S, Guida WC, Blaskovich MA, Greedy B, Lawrence HR, Yip ML, Jove R, McLaughlin MM, Lawrence NJ, Sebti SM, Turkson J: Selective chemical probe inhibitor of Stat3, identified through structure-based virtual screening, induces antitumor activity. *Proc Natl Acad Sci U S A* 2007, **104**:7391–7396.

29. Pfaffl MW, Horgan GW, Dempfle L: Relative expression software tool (REST) for group-wise comparison and statistical analysis of relative expression results in real-time PCR. *Nucleic Acids Res* 2002, **30**:e36.

30. Expression data from low- and high-pathogenicity avian influenza-infected chicken and duck cells. [http://www.ncbi.nlm.nih.gov/geo/query/acc.cgi?acc=GSE33389]

31. Moody DE, Zou Z, McIntyre L: Cross-species hybridisation of pig RNA to human nylon microarrays. *BMC Genomics* 2002, **3**:27.

32. Crowley TM, Haring VR, Burggraaf S, Moore RJ: Application of chicken microarrays for gene expression analysis in other avian species. *BMC Genomics* 2009, **10**(Suppl 2):S3.

33. Anderson PW, Tennant BC, Lee Z: Cross-species hybridization of woodchuck hepatitis virus-induced hepatocellular carcinoma using human oligonucleotide microarrays. *World J Gastroenterol* 2006, **12**:4646–4651.

34. Malone JH, Oliver B: Microarrays, deep sequencing and the true measure of the transcriptome. *BMC Biol* 2011, **9**:34.

35. Sarmento L, Afonso CL, Estevez C, Wasilenko J, Pantin-Jackwood M: Differential host gene expression in cells infected with highly pathogenic H5N1 avian influenza viruses. *Vet Immunol Immunopathol* 2008, **125**:291–302.

36. Kobasa D, Jones SM, Shinya K, Kash JC, Copps J, Ebihara H, Hatta Y, Kim JH, Halfmann P, Hatta M, Feldmann F, Alimonti JB, Fernando L, Li Y, Katze MG, Feldmann H, Kawaoka Y: Aberrant innate immune response in lethal infection of macaques with the 1918 influenza virus. *Nature* 2007, **445**:319–323.

37. Chan MC, Cheung CY, Chui WH, Tsao SW, Nicholls JM, Chan YO, Chan RW, Long HT, Poon LL, Guan Y, Peiris JS: Proinflammatory cytokine responses induced by influenza A (H5N1) viruses in primary human alveolar and bronchial epithelial cells. *Respir Res* 2005, **6**:135.

38. Kaiser L, Fritz RS, Straus SE, Gubareva L, Hayden FG: Symptom pathogenesis during acute influenza: interleukin-6 and other cytokine responses. *J Med Virol* 2001, **64**:262–268.

39. Kim B, Ahn KK, Ha Y, Lee YH, Kim D, Lim JH, Kim SH, Kim MY, Cho KD, Lee BH, Chae C: Association of tumor necrosis factor-alpha with fever and pulmonary lesion score in pigs experimentally infected with swine influenza virus subtype H1N2. *J Vet Med Sci* 2009, **71**:611–616.

40. Hong YH, Lillehoj HS, Lee SH, Park D, Lillehoj EP: Molecular cloning and characterization of chicken lipopolysaccharide-induced TNF-alpha factor (LITAF). *Dev Comp Immunol* 2006, **30**:919–929.

41. Reemers SS, Groot Koerkamp MJ, Holstege FC, van Eden W, Vervelde L: Cellular host transcriptional responses to influenza A virus in chicken tracheal organ cultures differ from responses in in vivo infected trachea. *Vet Immunol Immunopathol* 2009, **132**:91–100.

42. Reemers SS, van Haarlem DA, Groot Koerkamp MJ, Vervelde L: Differential gene-expression and host-response profiles against avian influenza virus within the chicken lung due to anatomy and airflow. *J Gen Virol* 2009, **90**:2134–2146.

43. Karpala AJ, Bingham J, Schat KA, Chen LM, Donis RO, Lowenthal JW, Bean AG: Highly pathogenic (H5N1) avian influenza induces an inflammatory T helper type 1 cytokine response in the chicken. *J Interferon Cytokine Res* 2011, **31**:393–400.

44. Huang Y, Li Y, Burt DW, Chen H, Zhang Y, Qian W, Kim H, Gan S, Zhao Y, Li J, Yi K, Feng H, Zhu P, Li B, Liu Q, Fairley S, Magor KE, Du Z, Hu X, Goodman L, Tafer H, Vignal A, Lee T, Kim KW, Sheng Z, An Y, Searle S, Herrero J, Groenen MA, Crooijmans RP, *et al*: The duck genome and transcriptome provide insight into an avian influenza virus reservoir species. *Nat Genet* 2013, **45**:776–783.

45. Vanderven HA, Petkau K, Ryan-Jean KE, Aldridge JR Jr, Webster RG, Magor KE: Avian influenza rapidly induces antiviral genes in duck lung and intestine. *Mol Immunol* 2012, **51**:316–324.

46. Barber MR, Aldridge JR Jr, Webster RG, Magor KE: Association of RIG-I with innate immunity of ducks to influenza. *Proc Natl Acad Sci U S A* 2010, **107**:5913–5918.

47. Adams SC, Xing Z, Li J, Cardona CJ: Immune-related gene expression in response to H11N9 low pathogenic avian influenza virus infection in chicken and Pekin duck peripheral blood mononuclear cells. *Mol Immunol* 2009, **46**:1744–1749.

48. Liniger M, Summerfield A, Zimmer G, McCullough KC, Ruggli N: **Chicken cells sense influenza A virus infection through MDA5 and CARDIF signaling involving LGP2.** *J Virol* 2012, **86:**705–717.

49. Tian Y, Chen WL, Ou JH: **Effects of interferon-alpha/beta on HBV replication determined by viral load.** *PLoS Pathog* 2011, **7:**e1002159.

50. de Jong MD, Simmons CP, Thanh TT, Hien VM, Smith GJ, Chau TN, Hoang DM, Chau NV, Khanh TH, Dong VC, Qui PT, Cam BV, Ha do Q, Guan Y, Peiris JS, Chinh NT, Hien TT, Farrar J: **Fatal outcome of human influenza A (H5N1) is associated with high viral load and hypercytokinemia.** *Nat Med* 2006, **12:**1203–1207.

51. Peiris JS, Yu WC, Leung CW, Cheung CY, Ng WF, Nicholls JM, Ng TK, Chan KH, Lai ST, Lim WL, Yuen KY, Guan Y: **Re-emergence of fatal human influenza A subtype H5N1 disease.** *Lancet* 2004, **363:**617–619.

52. To KF, Chan PK, Chan KF, Lee WK, Lam WY, Wong KF, Tang NL, Tsang DN, Sung RY, Buckley TA, Tam JS, Cheng AF: **Pathology of fatal human infection associated with avian influenza A H5N1 virus.** *J Med Virol* 2001, **63:**242–246.

53. Cornelissen JB, Post J, Peeters B, Vervelde L, Rebel JM: **Differential innate responses of chickens and ducks to low-pathogenic avian influenza.** *Avian Pathol* 2012, **41:**519–529.

54. Liu B, Mori I, Hossain MJ, Dong L, Takeda K, Kimura Y: **Interleukin-18 improves the early defence system against influenza virus infection by augmenting natural killer cell-mediated cytotoxicity.** *J Gen Virol* 2004, **85:**423–428.

55. Bohn E, Sing A, Zumbihl R, Bielfeldt C, Okamura H, Kurimoto M, Heesemann J, Autenrieth IB: **IL-18 (IFN-gamma-inducing factor) regulates early cytokine production in, and promotes resolution of, bacterial infection in mice.** *J Immunol* 1998, **160:**299–307.

56. Fujioka N, Akazawa R, Ohashi K, Fujii M, Ikeda M, Kurimoto M: **Interleukin-18 protects mice against acute herpes simplex virus type 1 infection.** *J Virol* 1999, **73:**2401–2409.

57. Kawakami K, Qureshi MH, Zhang T, Okamura H, Kurimoto M, Saito A: **IL-18 protects mice against pulmonary and disseminated infection with Cryptococcus neoformans by inducing IFN-gamma production.** *J Immunol* 1997, **159:**5528–5534.

58. Sugawara I, Yamada H, Kaneko H, Mizuno S, Takeda K, Akira S: **Role of interleukin-18 (IL-18) in mycobacterial infection in IL-18-gene-disrupted mice.** *Infect Immun* 1999, **67:**2585–2589.

59. Jansen CA, de Geus ED, van Haarlem DA, van de Haar PM, Londt BZ, Graham SP, Gobel TW, van Eden W, Brookes SM, Vervelde L: **Differential lung NK cell responses in avian influenza virus infected chickens correlate with pathogenicity.** *Sci Rep* 2013, **3:**2478.

60. Ho HH, Ivashkiv LB: **Role of STAT3 in type I interferon responses. Negative regulation of STAT1-dependent inflammatory gene activation.** *J Biol Chem* 2006, **281:**14111–14118.

61. Hazari S, Chandra PK, Poat B, Datta S, Garry RF, Foster TP, Kousoulas G, Wakita T, Dash S: **Impaired antiviral activity of interferon alpha against hepatitis C virus 2a in Huh-7 cells with a defective Jak-Stat pathway.** *Virol J* 2010, **7:**36.

62. Yang CH, Murti A, Pfeffer LM: **STAT3 complements defects in an interferon-resistant cell line: evidence for an essential role for STAT3 in interferon signaling and biological activities.** *Proc Natl Acad Sci U S A* 1998, **95:**5568–5572.

63. Paulson M, Pisharody S, Pan L, Guadagno S, Mui AL, Levy DE: **Stat protein transactivation domains recruit p300/CBP through widely divergent sequences.** *J Biol Chem* 1999, **274:**25343–25349.

64. El Kasmi KC, Holst J, Coffre M, Mielke L, de Pauw A, Lhocine N, Smith AM, Rutschman R, Kaushal D, Shen Y, Suda T, Donnelly RP, Myers MG Jr, Alexander W, Vignali DA, Watowich SS, Ernst M, Hilton DJ, Murray PJ: **General nature of the STAT3-activated anti-inflammatory response.** *J Immunol* 2006, **177:**7880–7888.

65. Kalina U, Kauschat D, Koyama N, Nuernberger H, Ballas K, Koschmieder S, Bug G, Hofmann WK, Hoelzer D, Ottmann OG: **IL-18 activates STAT3 in the natural killer cell line 92, augments cytotoxic activity, and mediates IFN-gamma production by the stress kinase p38 and by the extracellular regulated kinases p44erk-1 and p42erk-21.** *J Immunol* 2000, **165:**1307–1313.

66. Williams LM, Sarma U, Willets K, Smallie T, Brennan F, Foxwell BM: **Expression of constitutively active STAT3 can replicate the cytokine-suppressive activity of interleukin-10 in human primary macrophages.** *J Biol Chem* 2007, **282:**6965–6975.

67. Sen N, Che X, Rajamani J, Zerboni L, Sung P, Ptacek J, Arvin AM: **Signal transducer and activator of transcription 3 (STAT3) and survivin induction by varicella-zoster virus promote replication and skin pathogenesis.** *Proc Natl Acad Sci U S A* 2012, **109:**600–605.

68. Zhu H, Shang X, Terada N, Liu C: **STAT3 induces anti-hepatitis C viral activity in liver cells.** *Biochem Biophys Res Commun* 2004, **324:**518–528.

69. Waris G, Turkson J, Hassanein T, Siddiqui A: **Hepatitis C virus (HCV) constitutively activates STAT-3 via oxidative stress: role of STAT-3 in HCV replication.** *J Virol* 2005, **79:**1569–1580.

3

Spatiotemporal interactions between wild boar and cattle: implications for cross-species disease transmission

Jose A Barasona[1*], M Cecilia Latham[2], Pelayo Acevedo[1], Jose A Armenteros[1], A David M Latham[2], Christian Gortazar[1], Francisco Carro[3], Ramon C Soriguer[3] and Joaquin Vicente[1]

Abstract

Controlling infectious diseases at the wildlife/livestock interface is often difficult because the ecological processes driving transmission between wildlife reservoirs and sympatric livestock populations are poorly understood. Thus, assessing how animals use their environment and how this affects interspecific interactions is an important factor in determining the local risk for disease transmission and maintenance. We used data from concurrently monitored GPS-collared domestic cattle and wild boar (*Sus scrofa*) to assess spatiotemporal interactions and associated implications for bovine tuberculosis (TB) transmission in a complex ecological and epidemiological system, Doñana National Park (DNP, South Spain). We found that fine-scale spatial overlap of cattle and wild boar was seasonally high in some habitats. In general, spatial interactions between the two species were highest in the marsh-shrub ecotone and at permanent water sources, whereas shrub-woodlands and seasonal grass-marshlands were areas with lower predicted relative interactions. Wild boar and cattle generally used different resources during winter and spring in DNP. Conversely, limited differences in resource selection during summer and autumn, when food and water availability were limiting, resulted in negligible spatial segregation and thus probably high encounter rates. The spatial gradient in potential overlap between the two species across DNP corresponded well with the spatial variation in the observed incidence of TB in cattle and prevalence of TB in wild boar. We suggest that the marsh-shrub ecotone and permanent water sources act as important points of TB transmission in our system, particularly during summer and autumn. Targeted management actions are suggested to reduce potential interactions between cattle and wild boar in order to prevent disease transmission and design effective control strategies.

Introduction

Most pathogens of concern to livestock are able to cross-infect multiple host species, including wildlife, and therefore in areas where wildlife and livestock co-occur (i.e. interface areas), pathogens can emerge and establish in these sympatric host populations [1]. For example, foot and mouth disease, rabies, anthrax, brucellosis and bovine tuberculosis (TB) have all been shown to be reciprocally transmissible between livestock and wildlife [2-6]. In this context, the demography and behaviour of the hosts' populations can play an important role in intra- and interspecific pathogen transmission by determining contact rates

and environmental exposure [7]. If resources that are commonly used by both domestic and wild species are aggregated, this can result in high spatial and/or temporal overlap between two or more species [6-9], further increasing the probability of disease transmission. How habitat use by hosts affects direct and indirect interactions among hosts is fundamental in understanding multi-host disease transmission [5], and is critical for designing scientifically-based disease control strategies [10]. Nonetheless, the role that spatial and temporal interactions between livestock and wildlife play in exposure to pathogens and disease transmission remains mostly unknown [11,12].

Tuberculosis caused by the *Mycobacterium tuberculosis* complex is an important re-emerging zoonotic disease shared between domestic cattle and wildlife, and the control of this disease is largely limited by the existence of

* Correspondence: joseangel.barasona@uclm.es
[1]SaBio (Health and Biotechnology), IREC, National Wildlife Research Institute (CSIC-UCLM-JCCM), Ciudad Real, Spain
Full list of author information is available at the end of the article

wildlife reservoirs [13-15]. In the United Kingdom, for instance, cattle may become infected with TB by using farm buildings (feed stores and cattle sheds) and grazing on grass that has been contaminated with urine, faeces, sputum or wound exudates of badgers (*Meles meles*) [16,17]. In the United States, white-tailed deer (*Odocoileus virginianus*) and cattle often share rangeland resources, including water sources and feeders, although temporal segregation between these species is often observed [9]. In the Iberian Peninsula, wild boar (*Sus scrofa*) are the main wild maintenance host of TB [18]. Recent studies from Spain suggest that TB infection can spread not only by direct contact among individuals but also by indirect transmission [19], with water sources being high risk areas where pathogen transmission can occur between wildlife and cattle through consumption of short-term infected water [20]. However, epidemiological studies at the interface between livestock and important disease-carrying wildlife, such as wild boar, remain scarce.

Despite compulsory testing and culling of infected cattle, TB infection rates in cattle populations are persistently high in Doñana National Park (DNP), southern Spain [21]. The TB-host community of DNP includes wild boar, red deer (*Cervus elaphus*) and fallow deer (*Dama dama*), all of which occur sympatrically in areas used for traditional cattle husbandry. Interestingly, the populations of these three wildlife hosts exhibit common spatial patterns of TB infection across DNP, which may be explained by resource use and behaviour of these species [21,22]. Recent advances in global positioning system (GPS) technology for monitoring wildlife has proven useful for assessing fine-scale spatiotemporal interactions among species [23], and thus may provide a fundamental understanding of the risk of TB transmission at the wildlife/livestock interface. We deployed GPS technology on cattle and wild boar in DNP to test the hypothesis that patterns of resource selection and spatiotemporal overlap between these two species increase the local risk of interspecific disease transmission. Specifically, we aimed to determine where and when the activity patterns of cattle and wild boar overlapped and whether areas with the greatest potential overlap corresponded with areas with high incidence of TB in cattle.

Material and methods

Study area

We conducted the study in DNP (37°0′ N, 6°30′ W), a protected nature reserve located on the Atlantic coast of southern Spain (Figure 1). The region has a Mediterranean climate, classified as dry sub-humid with marked seasons. In the wet season (December–May), marshlands are flooded and ungulates graze in elevated shrublands. Ungulates in DNP are mostly food limited during summer (June–September), when wetlands and natural water bodies dry up causing senescence of herbaceous vegetation. However, a north–south humid ecotone habitat exists year-round between the elevated shrublands and the low dry marshlands; vegetation within this ecotone is dominated by *Scirpus maritimus* and *Galiopalustris sp.* with *Juncus maritimus* associations (see Additional file 1 for further details on habitat types).

The study area has moderate to high densities of red deer, fallow deer and wild boar throughout DNP. A traditional breed of cattle (locally called "marismeña") is farmed within five cattle management areas in DNP (Figure 1). Coto del Rey (CR) is the northern border of DNP and contains no cattle husbandry. The central area includes three cattle enclosures: SO ($n = 350$ cattle; density = 5.7 cattle/km^2), BR ($n = 168$ cattle; density = 2.6 cattle/km^2), and PU ($n = 152$ cattle; density =4.0 cattle/km^2). Marismillas (MA) is the southern-most area ($n = 318$ cattle; density = 3.1 cattle/km^2). Each cattle management area is surrounded by a cattle-proof fence, which limits the movements of each herd to within their designated management area. However, social groups (overwhelmingly females) showing individual ranging behaviour may be differentiated within each cattle management area [24]. The incidence of TB in cattle is high within DNP (9.23% per year on average), and TB prevalence in wild boar (45–52%), red deer, and fallow deer (14–19%) populations is also high [21,22]. DNP has been proposed as a natural scenario for describing the epidemiology of shared diseases in wild and domestic ungulates [21,22,25].

Animal capture and monitoring

We used data from 18 wild boar and 12 head of cattle from the marismeña breed that were equipped with GPS radio-collars between July 2011 and October 2013. Animal capture followed a protocol approved by the Animal Experiment Committee of Castilla-La Mancha University and by the Spanish Ethics Committee, and designed and developed by scientists (B and C animal experimentation categories) in accordance with EC Directive 86/609/EEC for animal handling and experiments. We captured wild boar using six padded foothold cage traps monitored using camera traps (see [26] for further details). Captured wild boar were anaesthetized, weighed, ear tagged, radio-collared and assessed for condition, age and sex. The anaesthetic protocol (3 mg/kg of tiletamine-zolazepam and 0.05 mg/kg of medetomidine) followed Barasona et al. [26]. Of the collared wild boar, 11 were males (3 sub-adults, < 24 months; 8 adults) and seven were females (2 subadults; 5 adults). All collared cattle were adult females. We captured wild boar in different trapping areas across DNP in order to collar a sample of animals from multiple social groups. Cattle from different social groups were radio-collared during routine veterinary inspections of cattle restrained in the farm's cattle yards. Although

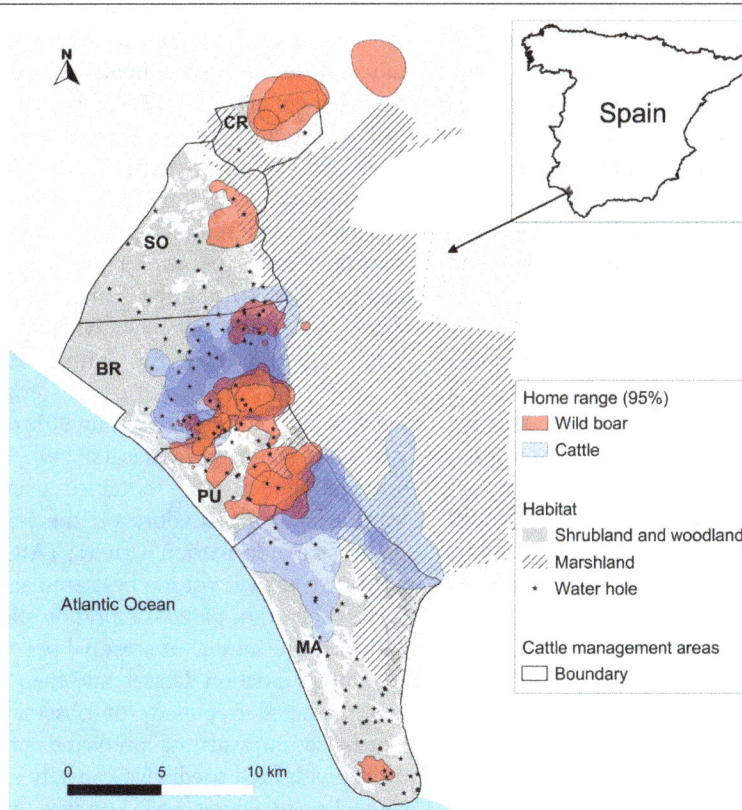

Figure 1 Study area. Location of the study area, Doñana National Park (DNP), Huelva province, southern Spain. Home ranges (defined as the 95% isopleth of kernel density estimators) of 18 wild boar and 12 domestic cattle GPS-collared between July 2011 and October 2013 within five cattle management areas are shown.

cattle were collared in several cattle management areas, the intense trapping efforts were carried out in BR cattle management area, where both species were concurrently monitored (Figure 1).

Radiocollars were programmed to acquire one GPS location per hour and to transmit accumulated packets of 20 locations using GSM (Microsensory System, Spain) [27]. Data collected included date, time, geographic coordinates, and location acquisition time (LAT, which is a measure of the precision of a fix and ranges between 0–160 s). First, we screened GPS locations with LAT ≥ 154 s to detect anomalous fixes (manufacturer's technical data; Microsensory System, Spain). Using this criterion, 189 and 66 GPS fixes were considered anomalous and thus removed from wild boar and cattle databases, respectively. We also discarded GPS locations obtained during the day of collar deployment and of collar retrieval to avoid possible anomalous behaviour associated with handling procedures, even though differences in behaviour post-handling were not detected elsewhere [26]. Positional error associated with GPS locations averaged 26.6 m (SD = 23.5 m), based on stationary tests from 19 collars (1637 locations in total) carried out in the centre of our study area (i.e., open sky). Fix-rate success averaged

81.2% and 94.0% for wild boar and cattle, respectively. We explored whether the lower fix-rate success obtained for wild boar introduced habitat-induced biases [28] or dial-induced biases (e.g., due to wild boar using dense vegetation as rest sites during the day [29,30]. However, no significant differences were found in mean LAT values among habitats (Kruskal-Wallis test, $z = 48.00$, $p > 0.05$) or between day and night ($z = -1.88$, $p > 0.05$). Consequently, we did not correct for habitat-induced fix-rate bias.

Coarse-scale spatial overlap between wild boar and cattle
We estimated annual and seasonal (winter, spring, summer and autumn) home-ranges (HR; 95% Utilization Distribution, UD; [31]) and core-areas (CA; 50% UD) used by each collared animal using the fixed-kernel function from the ADEHABITAT package [32] in R version 2.15.2 [33]. Kernels were estimated using the reference bandwidth method [34] because the least-squares cross-validation method failed to converge for six animals with large sample sizes [35]. Fixed-kernel density estimators allow identification of disjunct areas of activity [34], which can be particularly important for assessing interspecific patterns of space use in heterogeneous environments like DNP.

Home ranges and CA for each individual animal were used to estimate annual and seasonal spatial overlap [36] between wild boar and cattle within the BR cattle management area (Figure 1), where both species were concurrently monitored. Spatial overlap was calculated as the area of overlap in HR or CA between wild boar and cattle divided by (1) the total area of HR or CA for wild boar (i.e., overlap for wild boar relative to cattle), or (2) the total area of HR or CA for cattle (i.e., overlap for cattle relative to wild boar).

Fine-scale spatial interaction between wild boar and cattle

The extent of overlap in HR and CA provides only a coarse indicator of the potential interactions between two species because HR and CA estimators represent only the outline of a distribution of locations [36]. To assess annual and seasonal fine-scale interactions and differences in the use of available resources between cattle and wild boar, we estimated latent selection difference functions (LSDs) [37,38]. The GPS locations were transformed into 26 m radius circular buffers (to account for GPS positional error) [39], and within each buffer we calculated: straight-line distance (km) to nearest artificial water hole (DW); straight-line distance (km) to nearest marsh–shrub ecotone (DE); proportional cover of dense scrub (LT1); proportional cover of low-clear shrubland (LT2); proportional cover of herbaceous grassland (LT3); proportional cover of woodland (LT4); proportional cover of bare land (LT5); and proportional cover of watercourse vegetation (LT6; see Additional file 1). These predictor variables were selected because of their biological relevance for explaining ungulate distribution in DNP (see [40]). Landcover data was obtained from Andalusia Environmental Information [41]. Collinearity among predictor variables was screened using a Spearman's pairwise correlation coefficient value of $|r| > 0.5$ [42].

We estimated LSDs using logistic regression [43] and the "RMS" package [44] in R. For this analysis, we coded locations from cattle as 1 and those from wild boar as 0, i.e. we assessed cattle resource selection or avoidance relative to wild boar. In this analysis, landcover variables with significant positive coefficients indicate those most preferred by cattle relative to wild boar, whereas those with significant negative coefficients indicate those most avoided by cattle relative to wild boar. Distance to-variables, however, should be interpreted the opposite way. Variables with non-significant coefficients represent those habitats with the highest potential for interspecific interactions, because there is no difference in the use or selection of these resources between the two species. The results from LSD analyses can then be used to make inferences about the differences or similarities in fine-scale habitat use and spatial overlap between the two species. The main assumption of LSDs is that all resources should be equally available to both species within the study area. To fulfill this assumption, we only used locations from collared animals located in the central cattle management area (BR; 13 wild boar and 10 cattle; Figure 1) that occurred within annual and seasonal inter-species CA (50% UD) overlap contours, i.e. the area where the greatest inter-species interactions could occur. To account for an unbalanced sampling design and non-independence of observations from the same individual, we estimated robust standard errors using the Huber–White sandwich estimator [45], grouping data by individual.

We randomly split the annual and seasonal datasets, using 70% of locations to parameterize the models (training datasets) and the remaining 30% of locations for model validation (validation datasets) [46]. The best annual and seasonal models were obtained using a forwards–backwards stepwise procedure on the training datasets based on Akaike Information Criteria (AIC) [47]. We assessed predictive capacity of the best annual and seasonal models using calibration plots. Calibration plots were constructed by testing the annual or seasonal best models on the corresponding validation dataset, and then plotting the observed and predicted frequency of observations in each of 10 equal-size intervals of predicted probabilities (0–1). A model with high predictive capacity should show perfectly aligned points along a 45° line (see [48]). We also assessed the predictive capacity of each model with the area under the receiver operating characteristic curve (AUC), to rate the ability of the models to correctly discriminate between cattle and wild boar locations. The AUC ranges from 0.5 for models with no discrimination ability to 1 for models with perfect discrimination ability [48].

Annual and seasonal best LSD models were used to spatially map the relative probability of use (P) by cattle relative to wild boar. Areas with values of P of approx. 0.5 were considered as those where the highest relative probability of spatial interaction between both species could occur [38]. Accordingly, we constructed a spatial interspecific interaction (SII) index for the whole of BR using the rule: SII = $(1 − P)$ if $P \geq 0.5$, and SII = P if $P < 0.5$. Further, because models estimating resource use by a species can be used to predict the species' distribution in other geographical areas (e.g. [49]), we used models trained with data from BR to extrapolate P and derived SII index within 1 ha cells across the whole of DNP. Predicted SII values across DNP were correlated with TB epidemiological data (see below).

Sampling and TB diagnosis

Between 2006 and 2013, 570 wild boar were opportunistically shot by park rangers in DNP, and necropsied as part of the DNP health-monitoring programme (see [21] for details). We recorded the location where animals were shot, the year in which they were sampled, and their TB lesion score, gender and age. Necropsies were performed by qualified wildlife veterinarians that had extensive experience in the diagnosis of macroscopic TB-compatible lesions. Veterinarians performed detailed inspections of the entire animal, including lymph nodes and abdominal and thoracic organs [50]. Cultures using pyruvate-enriched Löwenstein-Jensen medium were performed to confirm TB infection. During the same time period and as part of the TB control programme in DNP, cattle populations within the SO, BR, PU and MA management areas were tested for TB by veterinary authorities using skin tests, and slaughtered if found positive. Prevalence and incidence (as used for cattle because the entire population was tested during annual sanitary campaigns) of TB were estimated for each cattle management area for wild boar and cattle populations, respectively. Finally, we assessed whether there were significant differences in the SII index (annually as well as seasonally) among cattle management areas with high and low TB-incidence in cattle using Mann–Whitney U-tests. All statistical analyses were performed in R version 2.15.2 [33].

Results

Interspecific interactions

We collected 44 699 locations from wild boar and 47 213 locations from cattle during the study period. Collared wild boar were distributed across all five cattle management areas, whereas collared cattle were only present in BR and MA (Figure 1). The GPS locations were homogeneously collected throughout the study period for all seasons and for both species (see Additional file 2).

There was a stark contrast between estimated annual HR and CA sizes for cattle and wild boar (Figure 2), with cattle using significantly larger areas (average ± SE,

HR = 1787.78 ± 826 ha; CA = 346.24 ± 174 ha) than wild boar (HR = 551.33 ± 260 ha; CA = 86 ± 77 ha), (ANOVA, $F_{1, 28}$ = 16.57 for HR; $F_{1, 28}$ = 15.21 for CA; both $p < 0.001$). There were significant seasonal differences in HR sizes for cattle ($F_{3, 8}$ = 3.69, $p = 0.023$), but not for wild boar ($F_{3, 14}$ = 2.47, $p > 0.05$) (Figure 3). The percent overlap in HR and CA between cattle and wild boar varied among seasons, with percent overlap being highest in autumn and lowest in winter (Table 1). Overall, > 60% of wild boar HR overlapped areas used by cattle, whereas ≤ 40% of the HR of cattle overlapped areas used by wild boar. Wild boar CA showed high overlap with areas used by cattle in spring, summer and autumn (66–78% overlap) but not in winter (only 23%).

Fine-scale assessment of spatial interactions between wild boar and cattle revealed that the environmental variables explaining relative habitat selection by cattle and wild boar differed among seasons (Table 2). During winter and spring, cattle used areas significantly further from water sources (DW) than wild boar; however, use of water sources did not differ significantly between the two species during summer and autumn. Cattle and wild boar selection for the marsh–shrub ecotone (DE) did not differ in any of the seasons analyzed. Conversely, cattle showed consistent avoidance of areas with a higher proportion of dense scrub (LT1) relative to wild boar across all seasons. Relative to wild boar, cattle showed avoidance of areas with higher proportions of low-clear shrubland (LT2), herbaceous grassland (LT3) and watercourse vegetation (LT6) during winter and spring. However, during summer and autumn, cattle and wild boar did not differ in their use of these three habitats. Annually, cattle and wild boar did not differ in their selection for areas close to water sources (DW) or for the marsh–shrub ecotone

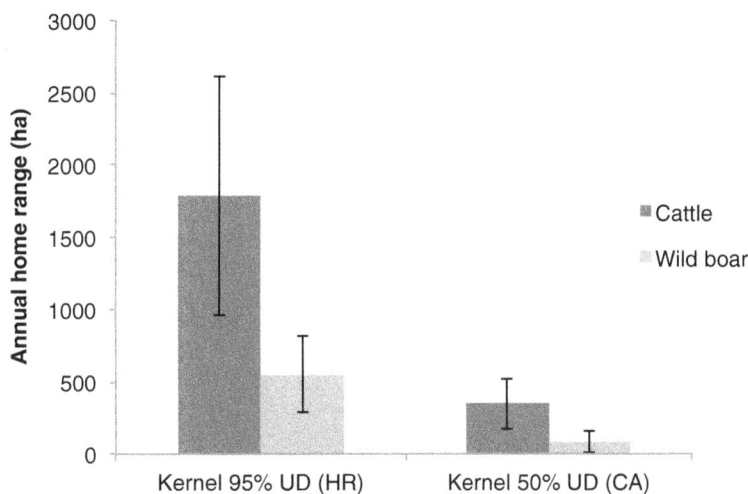

Figure 2 Comparison of mean annual domestic cattle and wild boar home ranges. Home range sizes (ha) derived using fixed-kernel density estimators for 95% utilization distribution (UD) and 50% UD. Kernels were estimated using data from 12 cattle and 18 wild boar GPS-collared between July 2011 and October 2013 in Doñana National Park, Spain. Error bars indicate SE.

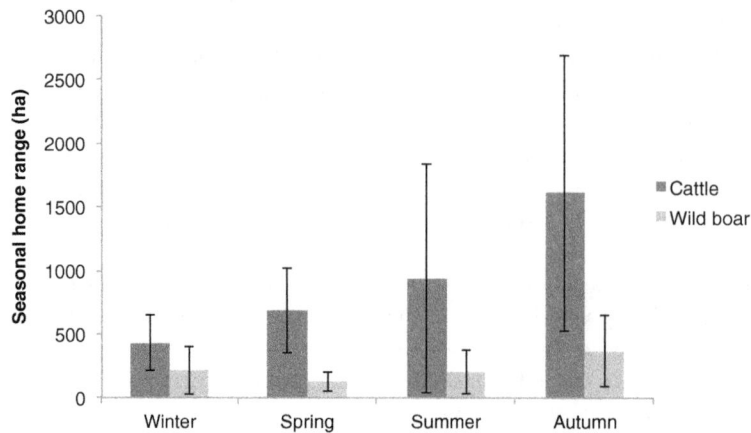

Figure 3 Comparison of mean seasonal domestic cattle and wild boar home ranges. Home range sizes (ha) derived using fixed-kernel density estimators for 95% utilization distribution. Kernels were estimated using data from 12 cattle and 18 wild boar GPS-collared between July 2011 and October 2013 in Doñana National Park, Spain. Error bars indicate SE.

(DE). Validation of LSD models showed that all had good discriminatory power (all AUC > 0.7) and predictive reliability (Additional file 3), supporting their use in extrapolating spatial patterns of SII across the whole of DNP (Figure 4; see also Additional file 4 for annual SII). In general, areas with a high probability of use by both species (high potential interaction) were mostly associated with the marsh-shrub ecotone and permanent water sources (Table 2 and Additional file 4), especially during summer and autumn (dark areas in Figure 4), whereas shrub-woodlands and temporal grass-marshlands had a low probability of interaction.

TB and spatial overlap
Based on culture confirmed lesions, infection was detected in 55.7% (SE = 4.1%; n = 570) of wild boar tested. The prevalence of TB in wild boar was 45.9% (SE = 3.8%; n = 174) in MA, 64.7% (SE = 5.8%; n = 68) in PU, 46.6% (SE = 3.7%; n = 174) in BR, 73.9% (SE = 4.6%; n = 92) in SO, and 72.6% (SE = 5.7%; n = 62) in CR. Official skin testing of 1,139 cattle in DNP from 2006 to 2013 revealed a mean incidence of 9.0% TB reactors (SE = 4.9%). Mean prevalence of TB in wild boar differed significantly among cattle management areas when these areas were grouped into low (MA = 4.1% and BR = 5.6% TB-incidence in cattle; average$_{wild boar TB-prevalence}$ = 46.3%)

or high (PU = 18.1% and SO = 11.8% TB-incidence in cattle; average$_{wild boar TB-prevalence}$ = 69.3%) TB-incidence in cattle ($F_{1, 2}$ = 24.96; $p < 0.05$). Interestingly, the mean predicted value of annual SII (fine-scale spatial interspecific interaction) was also significantly higher in high TB-incidence areas than in low TB-incidence areas (Z = 88; $p < 0.05$; Figure 5). These differences were significant in spring, summer and autumn but not in winter (Figure 5).

Discussion
We assessed fine-scale spatiotemporal interactions between wild and domestic hosts of TB in order to better understand what role resource selection may play in cross-species disease transmission. To our knowledge, this is the first study that has conducted a fine-scale spatial analysis aimed at explaining the patterns of disease transmission at the wild boar/cattle interface. We found that similar use of water resources by cattle and wild boar resulted in high potential interspecific interaction around these landscape features, especially during the dry season. This high spatial overlap at such small spatial extents (e.g. waterholes are only 15 m in diameter) could influence interspecific transmission rates of TB in this Mediterranean system. Our research contributes to an applied understanding of multi-host disease ecology and will help to better target actions

Table 1 Seasonal and annual coarse-scale overlap

	Between-species overlap (%)				
	Season				Annual
	Winter	Spring	Summer	Autumn	
Wild boar relative to cattle (HR; **CA**)	62.9; **23.0**	85.8; **66.4**	76.4; **70.0**	96.2; **77.7**	96.6; **63.4**
Cattle relative to wild boar (HR; **CA**)	35.7; **9.0**	21.8; **14.6**	21.9; **17.2**	40.1; **24.7**	35.5; **21.2**

Spatial overlap between wild boar and domestic cattle within the BR cattle management area (see Figure 1). Percent overlap was estimated using fixed-kernel density estimators for 95% (HR) and 50% (CA; in bold) utilization distribution. Kernels were estimated using data from 12 cattle and 18 wild boar GPS-collared between July 2011 and October 2013 in Doñana National Park, Spain.

Table 2 Result of the models

	LSD seasonal models								LSD annual model	
	Winter (AUC = 0.83)		Spring (AUC = 0.86)		Summer (AUC = 0.76)		Autumn (AUC = 0.71)		AUC = 0.75	
	β	SE	β	SE	β	SE	β	SE	β	SE
Intercept	2.72***	1.608	1.16*	0.481	1.75	1.06	1.11	1.291	2.31*	1.095
DW	2.46*	0.001	2.11*	0.001	1.26 ns	0.001	1.09 ns	0.001	1.46 ns	0.001
DE	−1.46 ns	0.003	−1.26 ns	0.001	−0.79 ns	0.001	0.80 ns	0.001	−1.59 ns	0.001
LT1	−2.90**	0.018	−2.36*	0.009	−3.12**	0.010	−2.19*	0.011	−3.75***	0.009
LT2	−3.37***	0.016	−2.69**	0.007	−0.87 ns	0.012	−1.22 ns	0.012	−3.22**	0.009
LT3	−3.13**	0.017	−3.17**	0.008	−1.18 ns	0.010	−0.88 ns	0.010	−2.25*	0.010
LT4	−1.36 ns	0.015	−4.19***	0.007	−1.46 ns	0.011	−2.12*	0.012	−2.55*	0.009
LT6	−2.95**	0.022	−3.57***	0.008	−1.41 ns	0.012	−1.34 ns	0.011	−3.34***	0.010

Model coefficients (β), standard errors (SE) and area under receiver operating characteristic curve (AUC) from latent selection difference (LSD) functions used for determining relevant factors explaining differences in habitat use by wild boar (coded as 0) and cattle (coded as 1) in Doñana National Park, Spain, July 2011–October 2013. Variable names are described in Additional file 1 and in the methods section. Habitat selection by cattle relative to wild boar was assessed seasonally and annually.
P-values are shown as: ns = $p > 0.05$, * = $p < 0.05$, ** = $p < 0.01$, *** = $p < 0.001$.

and implement control strategies for TB at the wildlife/livestock interface.

We found that cattle had larger HR and CA than wild boar, indicating that these two species have different space use requirements as well as ranging behaviours. Large-scale ranging behaviour in "marismeña" cattle within DNP is mostly determined by human decisions rather than by species-specific traits [24]. Each cattle management area contains a free-ranging cattle herd which is controlled and

regulated according to the Cattle Use Plan [51]. The mean HR and CA for wild boar recorded in our study area are somewhat lower than those reported in previous studies in other Mediterranean areas [52,53]. Differences may be related to food availability, population density, activity behaviour and/or composition of social groups [29,53]. Additional research would be required to elucidate which factors regulate ungulate spatial behaviour in DNP. The spatial distribution of cattle (using 95% or 50% UD)

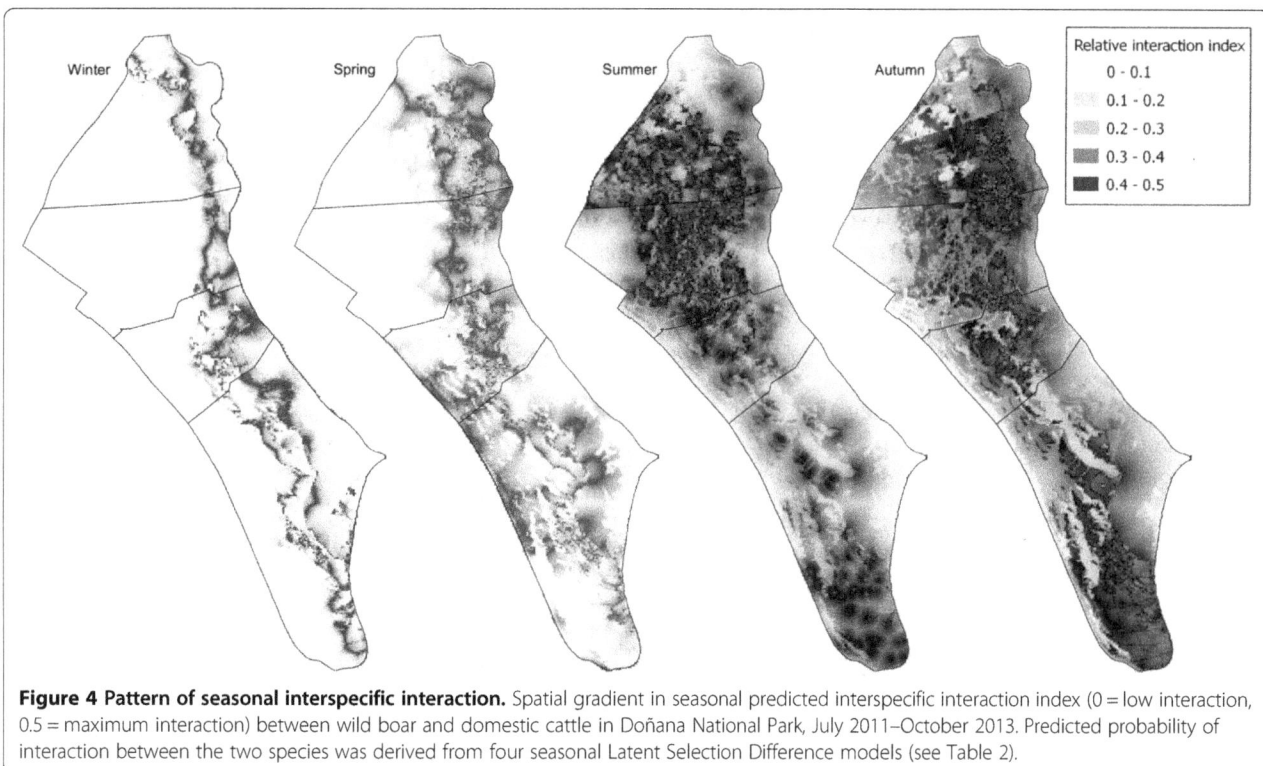

Figure 4 Pattern of seasonal interspecific interaction. Spatial gradient in seasonal predicted interspecific interaction index (0 = low interaction, 0.5 = maximum interaction) between wild boar and domestic cattle in Doñana National Park, July 2011–October 2013. Predicted probability of interaction between the two species was derived from four seasonal Latent Selection Difference models (see Table 2).

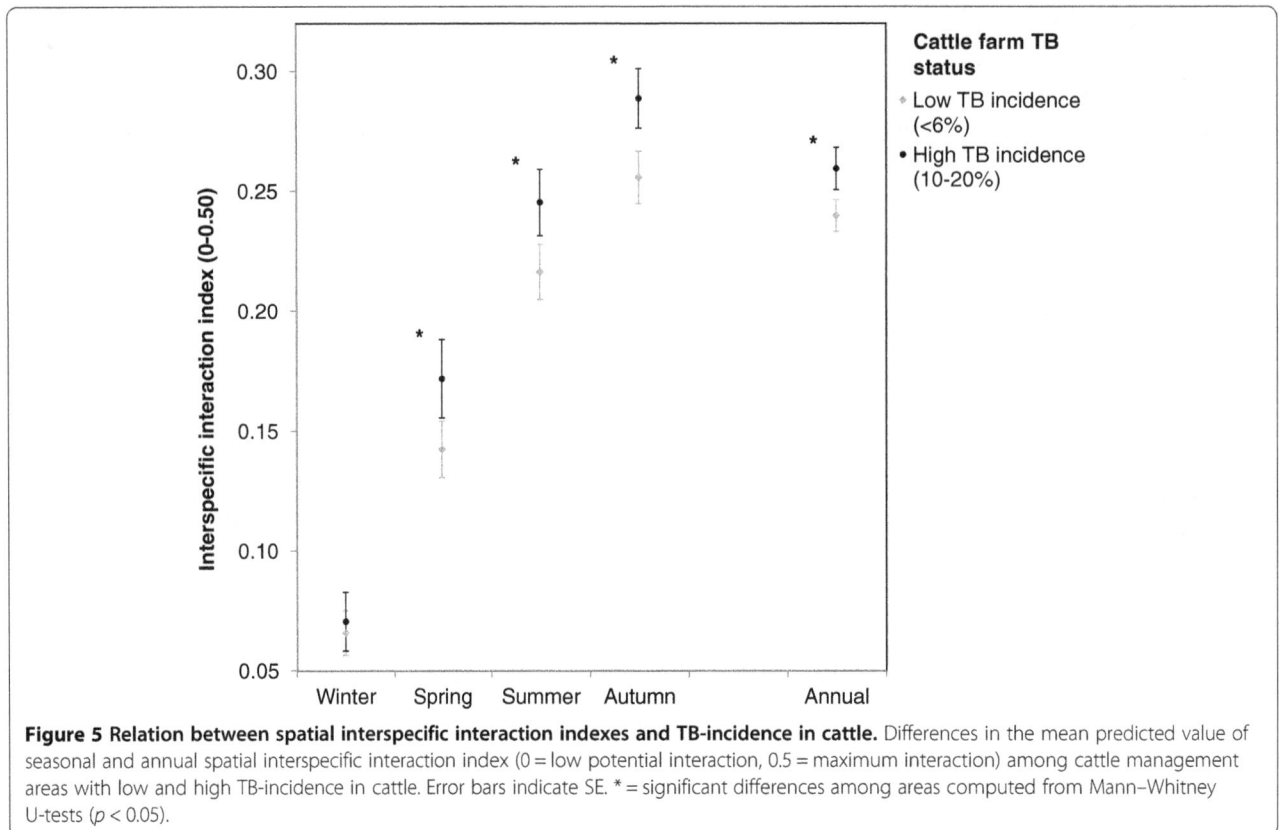

Figure 5 Relation between spatial interspecific interaction indexes and TB-incidence in cattle. Differences in the mean predicted value of seasonal and annual spatial interspecific interaction index (0 = low potential interaction, 0.5 = maximum interaction) among cattle management areas with low and high TB-incidence in cattle. Error bars indicate SE. * = significant differences among areas computed from Mann–Whitney U-tests ($p < 0.05$).

overlapped a large proportion of wild boar HR (97%) and CA (63%), and cattle frequently traversed areas used intensively by wild boar. Given that wild boar HR and CA were comparatively smaller than those of cattle, the concentration of important resources and cattle activity within areas commonly used by wild boar created situations that facilitated interaction (or at least spatial overlap) between the two species. Additionally, fine-scale spatial analyses suggest that within areas intensively used by wild boar there was limited spatial interspecific avoidance (also see [19,20]).

Although there were some similarities in the patterns of resource use in all seasons, wild boar and cattle generally used different resources during winter and spring in DNP. Conversely, limited differences in resource selection during summer and autumn resulted in negligible spatial segregation, and thus probably high encounter rates, between the two species during these seasons. This suggests that interspecific contact and subsequent disease transmission between cattle and wild boar is likely to be highest in drier seasons. Interestingly, the spatial distribution of the interspecific interaction index was consistently high at the marsh–shrub ecotone during all seasons. This is probably because this heterogenous habitat offers important resources for ungulates throughout the year, such food and

shelter (also see [40]). Furthermore, the predicted increase in spatial overlap and fine-scale interactions between wild boar and cattle during summer and autumn is likely related to the increased use of areas where forage and water are still available, when seasonal drought severely reduces the availability of resources in Mediterranean areas [54].

Characterizing and quantifying the potential interactions and the likelihood of disease transmission between domestic and wild hosts is crucial to understanding the complex dynamics of multi-host systems [11,12]. The results from our assessment of the spatial ecology and interactions of wild boar and cattle suggest that environmental and/or interspecific behavioural factors could favour disease transmission at the livestock/wildlife interface. We found that spatial variation in the incidence of TB in cattle in DNP was positively associated with the prevalence of TB in necropsied wild boar, which is consistent with the hypothesis that TB transmission occurs among ungulates, as has previously been argued from both field and molecular epidemiology [21,22]. In the case of wild boar, the high disease prevalence based on culture (up to 50%) observed in DNP is remarkable and indicative of a high risk of disease transmission [22,55], with about one third of pigs in a random sample expected to be actively excreting mycobacteria by several routes (mainly oro-nasally) [56].

The epidemiological interaction between the two host species described above was further supported by the fact that areas with high TB-incidence in cattle were also the areas with higher predicted spatial interaction between cattle and wild boar. This suggests that the dynamics of disease transmission in DNP are partly driven by the presence of environmental features that facilitate spatiotemporal overlap between hosts, as indicated by LSD models. The humid marsh–shrub ecotone and the surrounding water holes were the habitats with the highest potential interaction between wild boar and cattle. These landscape features may act as potential sources of *M. tuberculosis* complex for the host community [19,20,57]. For instance, Kukielka et al. [19] showed that shared water resources in South Central Spain were risky points where TB transmission could occur by indirect contact. Interestingly, we found that the predicted spatial interspecific interaction was highest in areas with high TB-incidence in cattle (and high TB-prevalence in wild boar) during summer and autumn, i.e. the time of year when species are most water-limited. These complex epidemiological scenarios have also been described in dry areas from Africa where cattle share water holes and diseases with wildlife [58]. In South Spain, a recent study reviewed the environmental persistence of *M. tuberculosis* complex and found that wildlife/livestock interactions occur much more often at water sources than would be expected by chance alone [19]. Aggregation of ungulates is promoted around water points, and this subsequently enhances the opportunities for transmission of diseases [59,60]. This may arise because ungulates come into contact with either a higher proportion of individuals from the same or different species, or with a more heavily contaminated environment (i.e. direct and/or indirect mycobacteria transmission). Spread of TB may occur indirectly from contaminated vegetation, water, mud or fomites [61]. Wild boar activity around these water sources (such as wallowing, brushing, drinking, defecating, urinating, and mating) is likely to result in environmental contamination and TB transmission to other hosts.

We used GPS telemetry data from concurrently monitored domestic cattle and wild boar to describe spatiotemporal interactions by means of new analytical procedures [37,38] and from these inferred associated implications for TB transmission. Within this framework, we considered fine-scale spatial overlap in habitats selected by cattle and wild boar as a proxy of interspecific contact. Although we did not measure contact directly, the difficulty of estimating realistic frequency of contact between species, most of which are predicted to be indirect, has been highlighted previously (e.g. [6,62]). However, recent studies have attempted to measure interspecific contact rates in relation to the dynamics of disease transmission. For example, contact rates have been estimated by direct observation of domestic and wild animals in open habitats

where they are easily observed, such as alpine meadows (e.g. [63]). However, this approach was not feasible in our study area because visibility is impeded by closed scrub. Other recent studies using telemetry data have defined critical time and space windows between pairs of GPS locations, and thus only assumed that interspecific contact had occurred within this critical window [62]. Approaches based on proximity loggers potentially have the ability to estimate contact rates between individuals often to within a few meters; however, the performance of these devices is often poor, providing data that is only indicative of contact rates rather than actual contact rates where interactions occur [64]. Further, within an epidemiological context, their utility is constrained to direct rather than indirect disease transmission. The LSD modelling procedure [37] we used proved a reliable tool to estimate annual and seasonal similarities in the use of shared resources, which is valuable for the study of diseases for which direct as well as indirect interactions among sympatric species are of importance in transmission dynamics, as our case [19]. However, the approach was limited in that we could not demonstrate that the spatial overlap between cattle and wild boar occurred within a sufficiently fine-scale temporal window to be directly related to the transmission of TB. Despite this limitation, the LSD approach can provide spatial predictions which can be extrapolated to a larger area where hypotheses related to the spatial risk of interspecific disease transmission can be tested. Additionally, future research could use a combination of proximity loggers and GPS technology to validate rates of interspecific contact, quantify the potential for indirect disease transmission, and identify habitats where both these events occur most frequently.

Epidemiologists and policy makers need to understand the complex interspecific interactions among potential hosts to identify risk factors for disease transmission and prescribe targeted management actions [65]. Our results highlight aspects of the hosts' ecology and behaviour that are likely to affect the probability of interspecific disease transmission. Further, our results identify factors that need to be considered in order to prevent interactions between wild and domestic ungulates at key disease reservoir sources, such as permanent water sources in ecosystems with marked dry seasons. Although welfare of wild animals must be considered, it may be possible to segregate livestock and wild ungulates in areas surrounding permanent water sources. For example, farm biosecurity measures, like small-scale fencing, exclusion gates or deterrents [66], could be implemented at points such as water sources to prevent wild ungulate access to these areas. Recent innovations in South Spain showed that effective segregation strategies of wild ungulates at water points have the potential to reduce interspecific contact and TB transmission at the wildlife/cattle interface [20].

Furthermore, research is being conducted currently into field vaccination of wild boar against *M. bovis* using oral baits [67]. Ideally, tools from several fields of study should be combined into integrated control plans to minimize pathogen transmission [17] and to improve the cost-effectiveness of strategies such as host population control through random or selective culling or through habitat management [68].

Additional files

Additional file 1: Covariates used in the spatial analysis.
Environmental predictors, descriptions, mean values (M) and standard deviations (SD) of GPS locations buffers versus total study area grids used in the analysis of resource separation patterns between cattle and wild boar at Doñana National Park.

Additional file 2: GPS data collection throughout the study period.
Duration of the GPS data collection for each collared wild boar and cattle throughout the study period in Doñana National Park, Spain.

Additional file 3: Calibration plots of the predictive performance of the models. Assessment of the predictive performance of the best seasonal and annual models (see Table 2). Each plot shows the relationship between the predicted probability to be used by cattle in relation to wild boar and the observed proportion of cattle locations on the validation dataset.

Additional file 4: Pattern of annual interspecific interaction. Spatial gradient in predicted annual interspecific interaction index (0 = low interaction, 0.5 = maximum interaction) between domestic cattle and wild boar in Doñana National Park, Spain, July 2011–October 2013. Predicted probability of interaction between the two species was derived from an annual Latent Selection Difference model (see Table 2).

Competing interests
The authors declare that they have no competing interests.

Authors' contributions
JAB, JV contributed to the conception, design, data collection, laboratory work, data analysis, drafting and writing of the manuscript. MCL, PA, ADML contributed to design, data analysis and drafting of the manuscript. JAA, CG, FC, RCS participated in the data collection and drafting of the manuscript. All authors have read and approved the final manuscript.

Acknowledgements
Authors would like to acknowledge many students and collaborators who contributed to field work over the study period, also wish to express their gratitude to the Doñana National Park, the monitoring team of EBD-CSIC for their help with the fieldwork and ICTS of Doñana Biological Station. The present work has benefited from the financial aid of research grants JCCM (PEII10-0262-7673), EU (FP7 grant 613779 WildTBVac) and MINECO (AGL2013-48523-C3-1-R). JAB holds an FPU pre-doctoral scholarship. PA is supported by MINECO-UCLM through "Ramón y Cajal" contract (RYC-2012-11970) and partly by EMIDA-ERA-NET grant APHAEA (219235-FP7-ERA-NET-EMIDA). We also thank Graham Nugent (Landcare Research, Lincoln, New Zealand) for his valuable comments on the study.

Author details
[1]SaBio (Health and Biotechnology), IREC, National Wildlife Research Institute (CSIC-UCLM-JCCM), Ciudad Real, Spain. [2]Landcare Research, PO Box 69040, Lincoln, Canterbury 7640, New Zealand. [3]Estación Biológica de Doñana, Consejo Superior de Investigaciones Científicas (CSIC), Sevilla, Spain.

References
1. Gortázar C, Ferroglio E, Höfle U, Frölich K, Vicente J: Diseases shared between wildlife and livestock: a European perspective. *Eur J Wildl Res* 2007, 53:241–256.
2. Frölich K, Thiede S, Kozikowski T, Jakob W: A review of mutual transmission of important infectious diseases between livestock and wildlife in Europe. *Ann N Y Acad Sci* 2002, 969:4–13.
3. Artois M: Wildlife infectious disease control in Europe. *J Mt Ecol* 2003, 7:89–97.
4. Ward AI, Tolhurst BA, Delahay RJ: Farm husbandry and the risks of disease transmission between wild and domestic mammals: a brief review focusing on bovine tuberculosis in badgers and cattle. *Anim Sci* 2006, 82:767–773.
5. Cooper SM, Scott HM, de la Garza GR, Deck AL, Cathey JC: Distribution and interspecies contact of feral swine and cattle on rangeland in south Texas: implications for disease transmission. *J Wildl Dis* 2010, 46:152–164.
6. Proffitt KM, Gude JA, Hamlin KL, Garrott RA, Cunningham JA, Grigg JL: Elk distribution and spatial overlap with livestock during the brucellosis transmission risk period. *J Appl Ecol* 2011, 48:471–478.
7. Dobson A: Population dynamics of pathogens with multiple host species. *Am Nat* 2004, 164:64–78.
8. Nunn CL, Thrall PH, Kappeler PM: Shared resources and disease dynamics in spatially structured populations. *Ecol Model* 2014, 272:198–207.
9. Cooper SM, Perotto-Baldivieso HL, Owens MK, Meek MG, Figueroa-Pagan M: Distribution and interaction of white-tailed deer and cattle in a semi-arid grazing system. *Agricult Ecosys Environ* 2008, 127:85–92.
10. Hudson PJ, Rizzoli AP, Grenfell BT, Heesterbeek JAP, Dobson AP: *Ecology of Wildlife Diseases.* Oxford: Oxford University Press; 2002:1–5.
11. Böhm M, Hutchings M, White P: Contact networks in a wildlife-livestock host community: identifying high-risk individuals in the transmission of bovine TB among badgers and cattle. *PLoS One* 2009, 4:e5016.
12. Martin C, Pastoret PP, Brochier B, Humblet MF, Saegerman C: A survey of the transmission of infectious diseases/infections between wild and domestic ungulates in Europe. *Vet Res* 2011, 42:70.
13. Phillips C, Foster C, Morris P, Teverson R, Foster C, Morris P, Teverson R: The transmission of Mycobacterium bovis infection to cattle. *Res Vet Sci* 2003, 74:1–15.
14. Gortazar C, Delahay RJ, Mcdonald RA, Boadella M, Wilson GJ, Gavier-Widen D, Acevedo P: The status of tuberculosis in European wild mammals. *Mammal Rev* 2012, 42:193–206.
15. Martínez-López B, Barasona JA, Gortázar C, Rodríguez-Prieto V, Sánchez-Vizcaíno JM, Vicente J: Farm-level risk factors for the occurrence, new infection or persistence of tuberculosis in cattle herds from South-Central Spain. *Prev Vet Med* 2014,116:268–278.
16. Garnett BT, Delahay RJ, Roper TJ: Use of cattle farm resources by badgers (*Meles meles*) and risk of bovine tuberculosis (*Mycobacterium bovis*) transmission to cattle. *Proc Biol Sci* 2002, 269:1487–1491.
17. Delahay RJ, Smith GC, Ward AI, Cheeseman CL: Options for the management of bovine tuberculosis transmission from badgers (*Meles meles*) to cattle: evidence from a long-term study. *Mamm Study* 2005, 30(Suppl 1):S73–S81.
18. Naranjo V, Gortazar C, Vicente J, de la Fuente J: Evidence of the role of European wild boar as a reservoir of *Mycobacterium tuberculosis* complex. *Vet Microbiol* 2008, 127:1–9.
19. Kukielka E, Barasona JA, Cowie CE, Drewe JA, Gortazar C, Cotarelo I, Vicente J: Spatial and temporal interactions between livestock and wildlife in South Central Spain assessed by camera traps. *Prev Vet Med* 2013, 112:213–221.
20. Barasona JA, VerCauteren KC, Saklou N, Gortazar C, Vicente J: Effectiveness of cattle operated bump gates and exclusion fences in preventing ungulate multi-host sanitary interaction. *Prev Vet Med* 2013, 111:42–50.
21. Gortazar C, Torres MJ, Acevedo P, Aznar J, Negro JJ, de la Fuente J, Vicente J: Fine-tuning the space, time, and host distribution of mycobacteria in wildlife. *BMC Microbiol* 2011, 11:27.
22. Gortázar C, Torres MJ, Vicente J, Acevedo P, Reglero M, de la Fuente J, Negro JJ, Aznar-Martín J: Bovine tuberculosis in Doñana biosphere reserve: the role of wild ungulates as disease reservoirs in the last Iberian lynx strongholds. *PLoS One* 2008, 3:e2776.
23. Latham ADM, Latham MC, Anderson DP, Cruz J, Herries D, Hebblewhite M: The GPS craze: six questions to address before deciding to deploy GPS technology on wildlife. *New Zeal J Ecol*, in press.

24. Lazo A: **Ranging behaviour of feral cattle (*Bos taurus*) in Donana National Park, SW Spain.** *J Zool* 1995, **236**:359–369.

25. Romero B, Aranaz A, Sandoval Á, Álvarez J, de Juan L, Bezos J, Sánchez C, Galka M, Fernández P, Mateos A, Domínguez L: **Persistence and molecular evolution of *Mycobacterium bovis* population from cattle and wildlife in Doñana National Park revealed by genotype variation.** *Vet Microbiol* 2008, **132**:87–95.

26. Barasona JA, López-Olvera JR, Beltrán-Beck B, Gortázar C, Vicente J: **Trap-effectiveness and response to tiletamine-zolazepam and medetomidine anaesthesia in Eurasian wild boar captured with cage and corral traps.** *BMC Vet Res* 2013, **9**:107.

27. Cano-Manuel J, Granados JE, Castillo A, Serrano E, Pérez JM, Soriguer RC, Fandos P, Travesí R: **Nuevas tecnologías aplicadas al seguimiento de ungulados silvestres en Sierra Nevada: Collares GPS-GSM.** In *Biodiversidad y Conservación de Fauna y Flora en Ambientes Mediterráneos.* Edited by Barea JM, Ballesteros E, Luzón JM, Moleón M, Tierno JM. Granada, Spain: Sociedad Granatense de Historia Natural Sierra Nevada; 2007:691–705.

28. Frair JL, Nielsen SE, Merrill EH, Lele SR, Boyce MS, Munro RH, Stenhouse GB, Beyer HL: **Removing GPS collar bias in habitat selection studies.** *J Appl Ecol* 2004, **41**:201–212.

29. Lemel J, Truvé J, Söderberg B: **Variation in ranging and activity behaviour of European wild boar *Sus scrofa* in Sweden.** *Wildl Biol* 2003, **9**(Suppl 1):29–36.

30. DeCesare NJ, Squires JR, Kolbe JA: **Effect of forest canopy on GPS-based movement data.** *Wildl Soc Bull* 2005, **33**:935–941.

31. Sodeikat G, Pohlmeyer K: **Escape movements of family groups of wild boar *Sus scrofa* influenced by drive hunts in Lower Saxony.** *Germany Wildl Biol* 2003, **9**(Suppl 1):43–49.

32. Calenge C: **The package adehabitat for the R software: a tool for the analysis of space and habitat use by animals.** *Ecol Model* 2006, **197**:516–519.

33. R Development Core Team R: *A Language and Environment for Statistical Computing.* Vienna, Austria: R Foundation for Statistical Computing; http://www.R-project.org.

34. Seaman DE, Millspaugh JJ, Kernohan BJ, Brundige GC, Raedeke KJ, Gitzen RA: **Effects of sample size on kernel home range estimates.** *J Wildl Manage* 1999, **63**:739–747.

35. Hemson G, Johnson P, South A, Kenward R, Ripley R, Macdonald D: **Are kernels the mustard? Data from global positioning system (GPS) collars suggests problems for kernel home-range analyses with least-squares cross-validation.** *J Anim Ecol* 2005, **74**:455–463.

36. Fieberg J, Kochanny CO: **Quantifying home-range overlap: the importance of the utilization distribution.** *J Wildl Manage* 2005, **69**:1346–1359.

37. Latham ADM, Latham MC, Boyce MS: **Habitat selection and spatial relationships of black bears (*Ursus americanus*) with woodland caribou (*Rangifer tarandus caribou*) in northeastern Alberta.** *Can J Zool* 2011, **89**:267–277.

38. Peters W, Hebblewhite M, DeCesare N, Cagnacci F, Musiani M: **Resource separation analysis with moose indicates threats to caribou in human altered landscapes.** *Ecography* 2013, **36**:487–498.

39. Recio MR, Mathieu R, Denys P, Sirguey P, Seddon PJ: **Lightweight GPS-tags, one giant leap for wildlife tracking? An assessment approach.** *PLoS One* 2011, **6**:e28225.

40. Braza F, Alvarez F: **Habitat use by red deer and fallow deer in Doñana National Park.** *Miscel·lània Zoològica* 1987, **11**:363–367.

41. Consejería de Medio Ambiente y Ordenación del Territorio, Andalucía, España: *Red de Información Ambiental de Andalucía, REDIAM.* http://www.juntadeandalucia.es/medioambiente/site/rediam.

42. Tabachnick BG, Fidell LS: *Using Multivariate Statistics.* New York, USA: HarperCollins; 1996.

43. Hosmer DW, Lemeshow S: *Applied Logistic Regression.* New York, USA: John Wiley & Sons; 2000.

44. Frank E, Harrell J: *rms: Regression Modeling Strategies. R Package Version 4.0-0;* 2013. http://CRAN.R-project.org/package=rms.

45. Freedman DA: **On the so-called "Huber sandwich estimator" and "robust standard errors".** *Am Stat* 2006, **60**:299–302.

46. Boyce MS, Vernier PR, Nielsen SE, Schmiegelow FKA: **Evaluating resource selection functions.** *Ecol Model* 2002, **157**:281–300.

47. Akaike H: **A new look at the statistical model identification.** *IEEE Trans Automat Control* 1974, **19**:716–723.

48. Pearce J, Ferrier S: **Evaluating the predictive performance of habitat models developed using logistic regression.** *Ecol Model* 2000, **133**:225–245.

49. Acevedo P, González-Quirós P, Prieto JM, Etherington TR, Gortázar C, Balseiro A: **Generalizing and transferring spatial models: a case study to predict Eurasian badger abundance in Atlantic Spain.** *Ecol Model* 2014, **275**:1–8.

50. Vicente J, Höfle U, Garrido JM, Fernández-De-Mera IG, Juste R, Barral M, Gortazar C: **Wild boar and red deer display high prevalences of tuberculosis-like lesions in Spain.** *Vet Res* 2006, **37**:107–119.

51. Espacio Natural Doñana: *Spain: Plan de Aprovechamiento Ganadero Del Parque Nacional de Doñana;* 2000. http://www-rbd.ebd.csic.es/gestion/territorioyrecursos/ganaderia/PlanGanadero.pdf.

52. Boitani L, Mattei L, Nonis D, Corsi F: **Spatial and activity patterns of wild boars in Tuscany, Italy.** *J Mammal* 1994, **75**:600–612.

53. Massei G, Genov PV, Staines BW, Gorman ML: **Factors influencing home range and activity of wild boar (*Sus scrofa*) in a Mediterranean coastal area.** *J Zool* 1997, **242**:411–423.

54. Bugalho MN, Milne JA: **The composition of the diet of red deer (*Cervus elaphus*) in a Mediterranean environment: a case of summer nutritional constraint?** *Forest Ecol Manag* 2003, **181**:23–29.

55. Rodríguez-Prieto V, Martínez-López B, Barasona J, Acevedo P, Romero B, Rodriguez-Campos S, Gortázar C, Sánchez-Vizcaíno J, Vicente J: **A Bayesian approach to study the risk variables for tuberculosis occurrence in domestic and wild ungulates in South Central Spain.** *BMC Vet Res* 2012, **8**:148.

56. Barasona JA, Torres MJ, Armenteros JA, Diez-Delgado I, Gortázar C, Vicente J: **Environmental presence of M. bovis at aggregation points in the wild-life/livestock interface in Mediterranean areas.** In *Proceedings of the VI International M. bovis Conference: 16–19 June 2014; Cardiff, Wales.* Edited by Glyn Hewinson. Weybridge: British Cattle Veterinary Association; 2014:68.

57. Fine AE, Bolin CA, Gardiner JC, Kaneene JB: **A study of the persistence of *Mycobacterium bovis* in the environment under natural weather conditions in Michigan.** *USA Vet Med Int* 2011, **2011**:765430.

58. Munyeme M, Muma JB, Skjerve E, Nambota AM, Phiri IGK, Samui KL, Dorny P, Tryland M: **Risk factors associated with bovine tuberculosis in traditional cattle of the livestock/wildlife interface areas in the Kafue basin of Zambia.** *Prev Vet Med* 2008, **85**:317–328.

59. Vicente J, Höfle U, Garrido JM, Acevedo P, Juste R, Barral M, Gortazar C: **Risk factors associated with the prevalence of tuberculosis-like lesions in fenced wild boar and red deer in south central Spain.** *Vet Res* 2007, **38**:451–464.

60. Vicente J, Barasona JA, Acevedo P, Ruiz-Fons JF, Boadella M, Diez-Delgado I, Beltran-Beck B, González-Barrio D, Queirós J, Montoro V, de la Fuente J, Gortazar C: **Temporal trend of tuberculosis in wild ungulates from Mediterranean Spain.** *Transbound Emerg Dis* 2013, **60**:92–103.

61. Morris RS, Pfeiffer DU, Jackson R: **The epidemiology of M. bovis infections.** *Vet Microbiol* 1994, **40**:153–177.

62. Miguel E, Grosbois V, Caron A, Boulinier T, Fritz H, Cornélis D, de Garine-Wichatitsky M: **Contacts and foot and mouth disease transmission from wild to domestic bovines in Africa.** *Ecosphere* 2013, **4**:51.

63. Richomme C, Gauthier D, Fromont E: **Contact rates and exposure to inter-species disease transmission in mountain ungulates.** *Epidemiol Infect* 2006, **134**:21–30.

64. Drewe JA, Weber N, Carter SP, Bearhop S, Harrison XA, Dall SR, McDonald RA, Delahay RJ: **Performance of proximity loggers in recording intra-and inter-species interactions: a laboratory and field-based validation study.** *PLoS One* 2012, **7**:e39068.

65. Nishi JS, Shury T, Elkin BT: **Wildlife reservoirs for bovine tuberculosis (*Mycobacterium bovis*) in Canada: strategies for management and research.** *Vet Microbiol* 2006, **112**:325–338.

66. Reidy MM, Campbell TA, Hewitt DG: **Evaluation of electric fencing to inhibit feral pig movements.** *J Wildl Manage* 2008, **72**:1012–1018.

67. Beltrán-Beck B, Romero B, Sevilla IA, Barasona JA, Garrido JM, González-Barrio D, Díez-Delgado I, Minguijón E, Casal C, Vicente J, Gortázar C, Aranaz A: **Assessment of an oral Mycobacterium bovis BCG vaccine and an inactivated M. bovis preparation for wild boar in terms of adverse reactions, vaccine strain survival, and uptake by nontarget species.** *Clin Vaccine Immunol* 2014, **21**:12–20.

68. Boadella M, Vicente J, Ruiz-Fons F, de la Fuente J, Gortazar C: **Effects of culling Eurasian wild boar on the prevalence of *Mycobacterium bovis* and Aujeszky's disease virus.** *Prev Vet Med* 2012, **107**:214–221.

4

Pre-parturition staphylococcal mastitis in primiparous replacement goats: persistence over lactation and sources of infection

Iacome SC Jácome[1], Francisca GC Sousa[2], Candice MG De Leon[2], Denis A Spricigo[1], Mauro MS Saraiva[1], Patricia EN Givisiez[2], Wondwossen A Gebreyes[3,4], Rafael FC Vieira[1] and Celso JB Oliveira[2,4*]

Abstract

This investigation reported for the first time the occurrence of intramammary infections caused by *Staphylococcus* in primiparous replacement goats before parturition and the persistence of clinical *Staphylococcus aureus* infection during the lactation period. Subclinical infections, mainly caused by coagulase negative staphylococci (CoNS), did not persist during lactation. Genotyping analysis indicated that environment seems to play a moderate role as source of intramammary infections to goats before parturition, but causative agents of mastitis in lactating animals are not genotypically related to environmental staphylococci. The occurrence and persistence of intramammary infections in replacement goats demonstrate the need to consider those animals as potential sources of infections in dairy goat herds.

Introduction, methods, and results

In the past few years, studies demonstrating staphylococcal mastitis in replacement heifers have raised intriguing questions about the epidemiology of intramammary infection in dairy herds. This is mainly due to the fact that *Staphylococcus* has been considered a contagious agent basically transmitted among lactating animals during milking practices [1]. Recent findings suggested environment as a potential source of *Staphylococcus* causing mastitis in dairy cattle [2]. These reports clearly demonstrate that detailed knowledge on the epidemiology of intramammary infections is necessary for the establishment of control measures in order to reduce infections.

In goats, besides the fact that information about the epidemiology of mastitis is very scarce compared to dairy cattle, the occurrence of intramammary infections in replacement goats has not been reported before. Mastitis continues to be an important burden to the goat milk industry, especially in developing regions, where the goat milk production chain plays an important socio-economic role.

Therefore, this study aimed primarily to test the hypothesis that intramammary infection does not occur in replacement goats prior to parturition. Secondly, if infection does occur, the goal was to determine the persistence of infection over lactation and to identify possible contamination sources of the pathogens on herds.

In order to test the first hypothesis, primiparous replacement goats from two farms located in the municipalities of Areia (Farm A) and Bananeiras (Farm B), Paraiba State, Brazil, were examined for clinical and subclinical mastitis. Examination for clinical mastitis in those animals included visual inspection of the udder and colostrum in order to detect definitive abnormalities, such as blood clots. For subclinical mastitis investigation, bacteriological culture was performed in 26 colostrum samples from half (one teat) of the udders of seven animals in Farm A (AP 1–7) and six in Farm B (BP 1–6) within 15 days before parturition. Samples were aseptically collected and processed according to a reference protocol [3]. Before sampling procedures, teats were disinfected with iodine pre-milking solution, dried with disposable paper towels and disinfected using cotton balls moist with 70% ethyl alcohol. Samples were kept refrigerated and

---
* Correspondence: celso.bruno.oliveira@gmail.com
[2]Department of Animal Science, Federal University of Paraiba, Areia, PB 58397-000, Brazil
[4]Veterinary Public Health and Biotechnology Global Consortium (VPH-Biotec), The Ohio State University, Columbus, OH 43210, USA
Full list of author information is available at the end of the article

processed within 6 h after samplings. The identification of any mastitis agent by isolation approach in any of the animals was considered enough to accept or refute the initial hypothesis.

Persistence of pre-parturition infections over lactation was investigated using a follow-up approach by means of clinical examination and milk samplings performed in all primiparous goats two times after parturition (at 30 and 60 days after first sampling). As performed for colostrum samplings, pre-dipping using iodine solution, drying with disposable paper towel and disinfection with 70% ethyl alcohol were performed before milk samples were collected for microbiological analysis. Fore-milk was discarded and a strip-cup test was used to detect signs of clinical mastitis.

In order to detect potential sources of infection to primiparous replacement goats, three multiparous goats from Farm A (AM 1–3) and five from Farm B (BM 1–5) were included in the follow-up trial. Prepartum colostrum samples ($n = 16$) were collected from multiparous goats in the first sampling.

Swabs from teats ($n = 63$), and nostrils ($n = 63$) were collected from the primiparous and multiparous goats, as well as environmental samples, including milking restraint devices ($n = 6$), stalls ($n = 6$) and milking room wall ($n = 6$), and swabs from the hand of milkers ($n = 6$) from both farms in the three samplings. Samples were collected using Stuart agar gel medium transport swabs (product # 141C, Copan, USA), which were kept under refrigeration until microbiological analyses. Finally, milk samples ($n = 84$) were collected from the lactating primiparous and multiparous animals in the second and third samplings.

Bacteriological isolation was performed by streaking a loopful of milk samples onto blood agar (product # 7166A, Blood agar base no.2, Acumedia, USA, enriched with 5% sheep blood) and MacConkey agar (product # 212123, BD Difco, USA) plates. Positive cultures were identified by means of Gram staining, morphological characteristics and biochemical tests. Gram positive cocci were tested for catalase and oxidase production. Confirmed staphylococci were tested for production of coagulase in tubes. In the present study, we considered intramammary infections when milk or colostrum samples from half udders cultured positive for 4 or more non-hemolytic or one or more hemolytic colony forming units.

Staphylococcus species from milk and colostrum from primiparous and multiparous goats were identified by a microplate biochemical panel (Combo PC33, Siemens Healthcare, USA) using a semi-automated system (Autoscan 4, Siemens Healthcare).

Genotyping by Rep-PCR was performed to identify possible transmission routes of mastitis-causing agents in both farms. Genomic DNA was extracted [4] and 25-μL

reactions contained Taq DNA polymerase buffer (1X), MgCl$_2$ (3 mM), Taq DNA polymerase (1 U; Invitrogen, USA), dNTPs (200 μM each; Ludwing Biotec, Brazil), primer RW3A [5] (1 pMol; Invitrogen, USA), and DNA template (100 ng). Amplification cycles included 1 min at 94 °C, 1 min at 50 °C, and 2 min at 72 °C. Dendograms were built by an unweighted pair group method with arithmetic mean clustering algorithm (UPGMA) and the genetic similarity between isolates was calculated using the Dice coefficient (SD), using Bionumerics v. 7.1 (Applied Maths, Belgium). Clusters of isolates were assigned using 80% genetic similarity as a cutoff. The discriminatory index (DI value) of Rep-PCR was calculated as reported [6].

The frequency of staphylococci positive samples in the different sample sources collected from Farms A and B is presented in Table 1. The microbiological culture results of prepartum colostrum and milk samples collected in the three samplings performed in Farms A and B are shown in Table 2. Bacteria were recovered from 15 of the 126 (11.9%) milk and colostrum samples, from which five originated from Farm A and ten from Farm B. All isolates were staphylococci and the majority were CoNS. Amongst the five positive samples from Farm A, *S. haemolyticus* ($n = 5$) and *S. epidermidis* ($n = 1$) were identified. Positive samples for staphylococci included swabs of teats ($n = 25$), nostrils ($n = 26$), hands ($n = 2$), device ($n = 3$), stall ($n = 2$) and wall ($n = 3$). In Farm B, staphylococci were isolated from four primiparous goats and one multiparous goat, including *S. aureus* ($n = 5$), *S. hyicus* ($n = 2$), *S. epidermidis* ($n = 1$), *S. auricularis* ($n = 1$), *S. cohnii* ($n = 1$), *S. hominis* ($n = 1$), *S. xylosus* ($n = 1$). Positive samples for staphyloccoci were also identified in swabs of teats ($n = 27$), nostrils ($n = 26$), hands ($n = 3$), device ($n = 3$), stall ($n = 1$) and wall ($n = 3$).

Clinical mastitis was detected in one half udder of a primiparous goat (BP2) from Farm B in all three samplings. *S. aureus* was isolated from the prepartum colostrum and post-partum milk samplings. None of the other animals (12 primiparous and 8 multiparous goats) showed clinical mastitis. Subclinical intramammary infection (*S. haemolyticus*) was detected in the prepartum colostrum of both half udders of a replacement goat from Farm A (AP4). Interestingly, *S. epidermidis* was isolated in the second sampling from a half udder previously infected by *S. haemolyticus*. In Farm B, two prepartum colostrum samples from primiparous goats were positive for *S. hyicus* (BP3) and *S. cohnii* (BP6). Besides, *S. auricularis* was isolated from prepartum colostrum from a multiparous goat (BM4) in this herd. In this farm, different CoNS species were also cultured from the same half udder in consecutive samplings, such as *S. hyicus* and *S. epidermidis* isolated from the right half udder of a primiparous goat (BP3) in the second and

Table 1 Frequency of *Staphylococcus* sp. in different sample sources taken from two small-scale goat milk production systems in Paraiba, Northeastern Brazil

Sample source	Farm A				Farm B			
	1st (Prepartum)	2nd	3rd	Total	1st (Prepartum)	2nd	3rd	Total
Prepartum colostrum*	1/10	-	-	1/10	4/11	-	-	4/11
Milk	-	1/10	1/10	2/20	-	2/11	4/11	6/22
Teat swabs	9/10	7/10	9/10	25/30	9/11	8/11	10/11	27/33
Nostril swabs	9/10	8/10	9/10	26/30	8/11	8/11	10/11	26/33
Milkers' hand swabs	0/1	1/1	1/1	2/3	1/1	1/1	1/1	3/3
Milking restraint device	1/1	1/1	1/1	3/3	1/1	1/1	1/1	3/3
Stall	1/1	0/1	1/1	2/3	1/1	0/1	0/1	1/3
Wall of milking room	1/1	1/1	1/1	3/3	1/1	1/1	1/1	3/3

*Only prepartum animals were sampled.

Table 2 *Staphylococcus* spp. isolated from prepartum colostrum (1st sampling) and milk samples (2nd and 3rd samplings) collected from primiparous replacing goats (AP and BP) and multiparous goats (AM and BM) in Paraiba, Northeastern Brazil

Sampling source	Sampling order		
	1st (Prepartum)	2nd	3rd
Farm A			
AP1	-	-	-
AP2	-	-	-
AP3	-	-	-
AP4	*S. haemolyticus*[1]	*S. epidermidis*	-
AP5	-	-	-
AP6	-	-	-
AP7	-	-	-
AM1	-	-	*S. haemolyticus*[2]
AM2	-	-	-
AM3	-	-	-
Farm B			
BP1	-	-	-
BP2	*S. aureus; S. hyicus*[3]	*S. aureus*	*S. aureus*
BP3	*S. aureus*[2]	*S. hyicus*	*S. epidermidis*
BP4	-	-	-
BP5	-	-	*S. xylosus*
BP6	*S. cohnii*	-	-
BM1	-	-	-
BM2	-	-	-
BM3	-	-	-
BM4	*S. auricularis*	-	*S. hominis*
BM5	-	-	-

[1] *S. haemolyticus* isolated from right and left half udders; [2] One isolate from each half udder; [3] *S. aureus* from left half udder and *S. hyicus* from right half udder.

third samplings, respectively. *S. auricularis* and *S. hominis* were isolated from the same half udder in the first and third samplings of a multiparous goat (BM4).

Rep-PCR showed DI values of 0.99 (Farm A) and 0.98 (Farm B). Staphylococci isolates from Farm A were assigned to eight distinct clusters (A to H) and 12 non-clustered isolates (Figure 1). Interestingly, no clonal relatedness amongst *S. haemolyticus* from colostrum (AP4) and milk (AM1) was detected. Two *S. haemolyticus* isolated from prepartum colostrum (AP4) showed fingerprints similar to those staphylococci cultured from environment, teat surfaces and nostrils of other goats and hands (clusters C and D). In the majority of the clusters (B, C, D, F, G, and H), isolates from teat surface and nostrils were highly related to those from environment and in some instances showed indistinguishable patterns (clusters G and H).

In farm B, fifteen clusters (A to O) of staphylococci were identified (Figure 2). One half udder of BP2 was infected in the first and second samplings by *S. aureus* sharing indistinguishable genotypic patterns (Figure 2). Some staphylococci from environment sources and hands showed undistinguished fingerprints compared with isolates from nostrils and teat surfaces from primiparous and multiparous goats (clusters B, D, K, L and O). *S. auricularis* cultured from colostrum of a multiparous goat (BM4) was related to an isolate from the wall (cluster I). Interestingly, CoNS isolated from mastitic milk, such as *S. epidermidis* (BP3), *S. hominis* (BM4), and *S. xylosus* (BP5) were not clustered with isolates from environment sources. Cluster E was comprised exclusively by *S. aureus* with clonally related isolates infecting one half udder (BP2) in different samplings. This cluster included no isolates from environment.

Discussion

The recovery of *S. aureus* from the same clinically infected udder in primiparous replacement goats before and after parturition suggest that this agent can persist

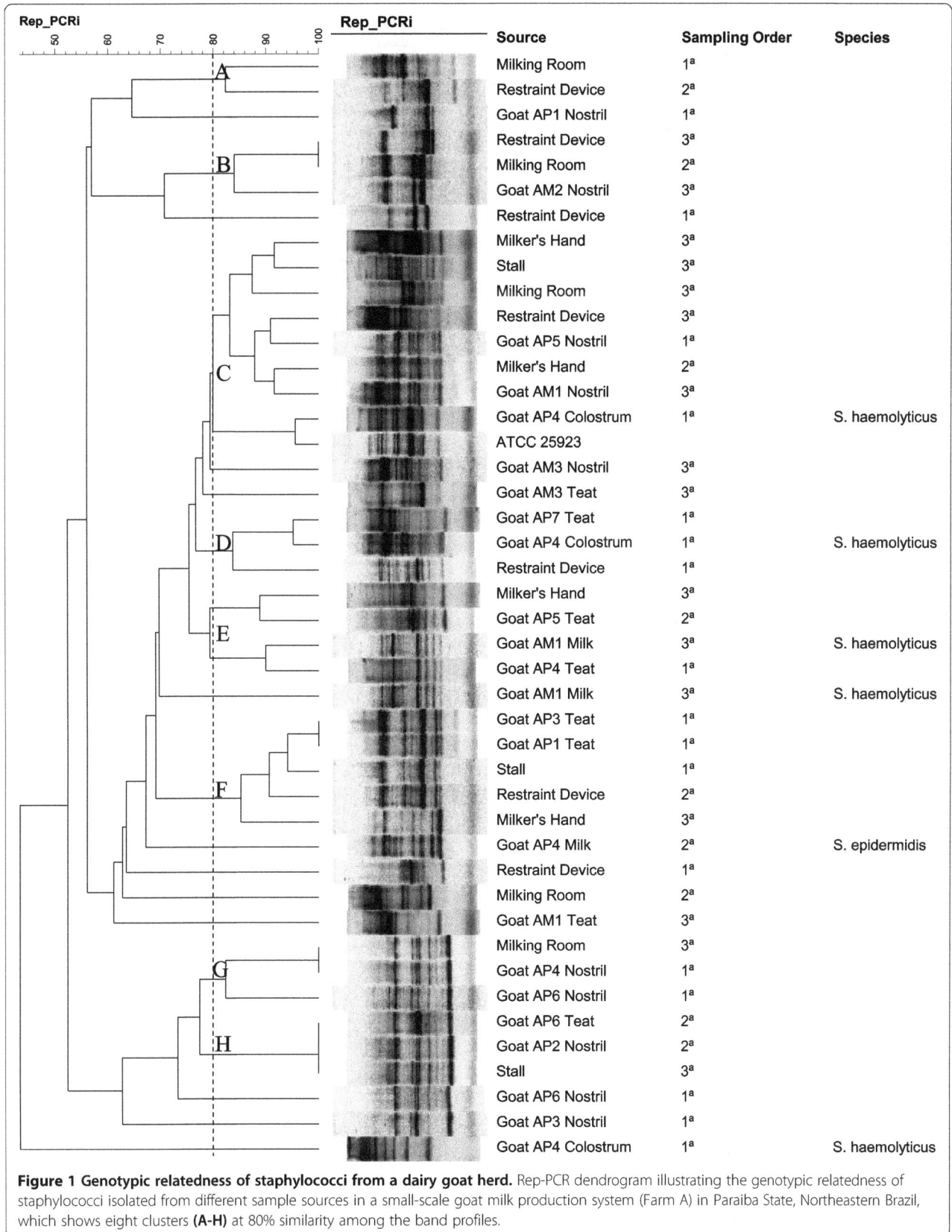

Figure 1 Genotypic relatedness of staphylococci from a dairy goat herd. Rep-PCR dendrogram illustrating the genotypic relatedness of staphylococci isolated from different sample sources in a small-scale goat milk production system (Farm A) in Paraiba State, Northeastern Brazil, which shows eight clusters **(A-H)** at 80% similarity among the band profiles.

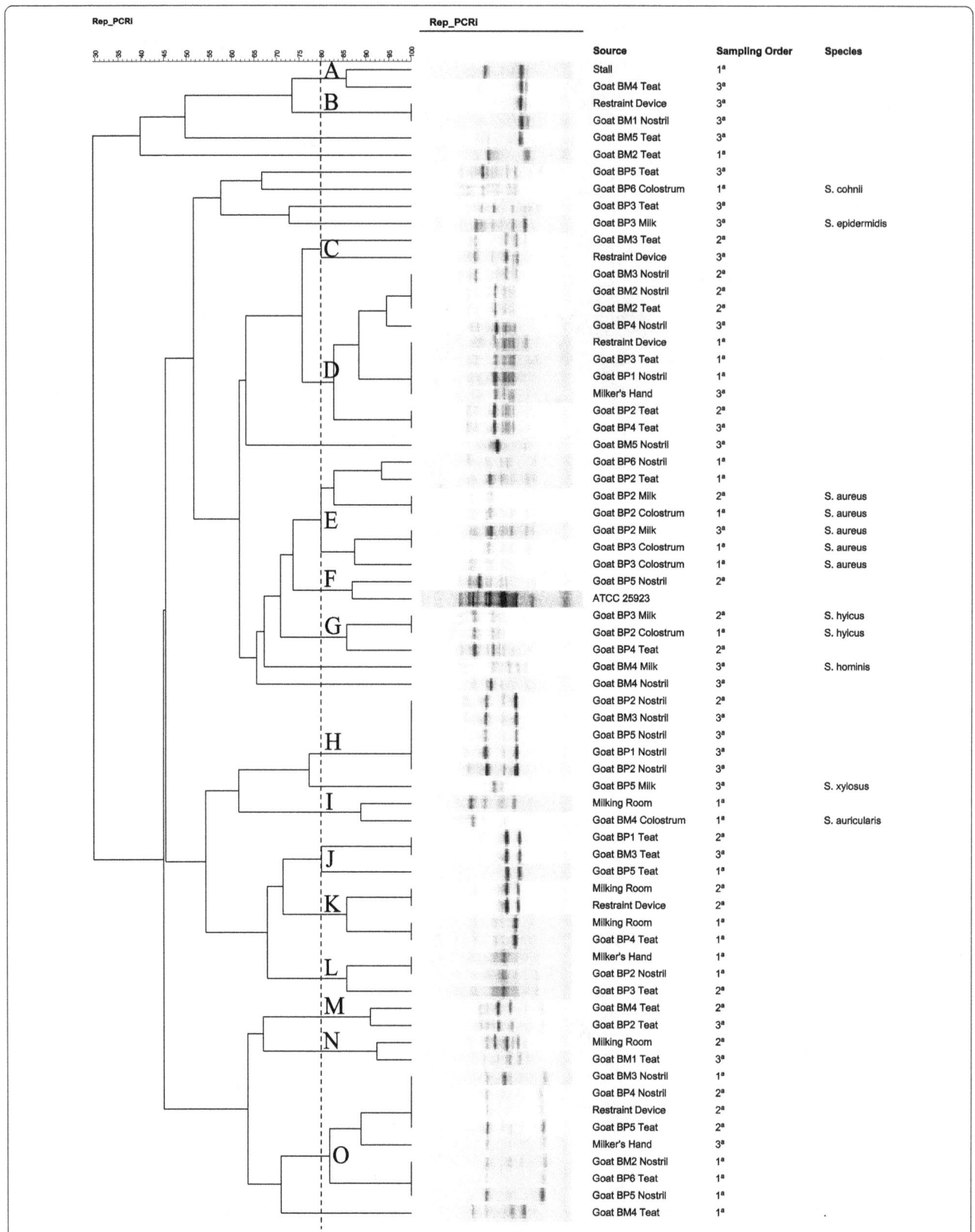

Figure 2 Genotypic relatedness of staphylococci from a dairy goat herd. Rep-PCR dendrogram illustrating the genotypic relatedness of staphylococci isolated from different sample sources in a small-scale goat milk production system (Farm B) in Paraiba State, Northeastern Brazil, which shows fifteen clusters **(A-O)** at 80% similarity among the band profiles.

over the lactation period. This assumption is reinforced since the isolates showed indistinguishable fingerprinting patterns. On the other hand, it seems not to be the case for subclinical intrammamary infections caused by the *S. aureus* (BP3) and CoNS species. This is because no species causing subclinical infections were cultured from a given infected udder in consecutive samplings. Moreover, the shift in the etiology of CoNS infections, as observed in AP4, suggests that subclinical infection caused by those organisms in primiparous replacement goats did not persist over the lactation period. Our results in goats corroborate previous findings observed in dairy cattle, suggesting that subclinical mastitis by CoNS is milder, has a shorter-term persistence and is associated to a higher spontaneous cure rate compared to *S. aureus* [7].

It is important to recognize the possible limitations of the semi-automated system used in the present study in identifying CoNS accurately, especially if we consider rare or infrequent species from animal origin. Therefore, assumptions on the putative transmission pathways of CoNS in the investigated farms were taken based on the findings of the Rep-PCR fingerprinting patterns. Rep-PCR was able to differentiate epidemiologically related isolates of the same *Staphylococcus* species. Besides, the high DI values indicate that Rep-PCR is a useful tool in typing staphylococci from goat farms. Rep-PCR using RW3A has been successfully used to discriminate epidemiologically related *S. aureus* of animal [5,8] and human origins [9].

The similar genotypic patterns of *S. haemolyticus* from prepartum colostrum (AP4) and environment in Farm A suggest that udder infections in the prepartum period might possibly be associated to environmental sources, even because no isolate from mastitis during lactation was related to environmental staphylococci. This assumption is reinforced by the fact that *S. haemolyticus* from prepartum colostrum of the same animal (AP4) showed a different DNA fingerprint pattern compared to *S. haemolyticus* cultured from milk from a multiparous goat in the same farm (AM1).

The fact that *S. auricularis* cultured from colostrum of a multiparous goat (BM4) was genotypically related to an isolate from the milking room (cluster I, Figure 2) suggest environment as the potential source of prepartum intramammary infection. Considering the similar results obtained for *S. haemolyticus* in Farm A, we believe that environment plays an important role as a source of intramammary infection for CoNS species in the prepartum period.

It is noteworthy that the genotypic patterns of some *Staphylococcus* isolated from nostrils and teat surface of primiparous goats in the prepartum period had indistinguishable DNA fingerprint patterns to isolates that originated from the wall of the milking room (cluster K). However, primiparous goats had no access to the milking room before lactation implying an independent source of contamination with the same strain. This finding corroborates with the earlier statement on *S. auricularis* isolated from a prepartum colostrum showing identical genotypic pattern with one isolated from the wall of the milking room (cluster I). The similar genotypic patterns of isolates from milkers' hand swabs, environment, and animals (nostrils and teat surface), as shown in clusters D, L, and O, might indicate the widespread dissemination of clonally related staphylococci in dairy goat milk production systems. Milkers could play a role on the dissemination of staphylococci, since isolates from the surface of teats of primiparous goats (non-lactating animals) were clonally related to isolates that originated from milkers' hand swabs (Figure 2, cluster D). Since primiparous and multiparous goats share the same environment in the prepartum period in dairy goat production systems in Northeastern Brazil, this continuous flow farming system facilitates the spread of microorganisms across the different groups. Recent reports in cows demonstrated a similar finding indicating higher risk of intramammary infections in heifers raised in contact to multiparous cows with the same mastitis causing agents involved [1,10].

Despite the high similarity amongst staphylococci from environmental sources and body surfaces of goats, our results indicated that those organisms were not the causal agents of intramammary infections in the primiparous lactating goats. The absence of environmental isolates clustered with *S. aureus* (Cluster E, Figure 2) strongly suggests *S. aureus*-associated intramammary infections to be contagious but environmental dissemination occurs rarely. Our study indicates that the epidemiology of mastitis caused by CoNS is complex in goats, which is expected, since this group is represented by a large range of species with different pathogenic traits. Indeed, CoNS are the most frequent mastitis-causing agents in lactating goats [8,11-13].

In conclusion, clinical and subclinical intramammary infections in primiparous replacement goats can occur in the prepartum period and can persist over the lactation if caused by *S. aureus* in the clinical form. While environment seems to play a role as source of intramammary infections to goats before parturition, causative agents of mastitis in lactating animals are not genotypically related to staphylococci of environmental origin. The occurrence and persistence of intramammary infections in replacement goats demonstrated herein indicate the need to consider testing the replacement animals and take necessary precaution and preventive measures to avoid spreading of mastitis-causing staphylococci as they remain potential sources of infections in goat dairy herds. Longitudinal studies investigating the extent of CoNS species as causative agents of intramammary infections in the goat species are recommended.

Competing interests
The authors declare that they have no competing interests.

Authors' contributions
CJBO and PENG conceived the hypothesis of the investigation and its design. ISCJ and MMSS coordinated and performed the study. DAS, CMGDL, and FGCS performed the microbial isolating and molecular analyses. WAG contributed to the genotyping analysis. ISCJ, CJBO, PENG, DAS and WAG wrote the manuscript. All authors read and approved the contents of this manuscript.

Acknowledgements
The authors are thankful to Coordination for the Improvement of Higher Education Personnel (CAPES) for scholarships and to National Council for Scientific and Technological Development (CNPq, proc. 483103/2007-1) for grants.

Author details
[1]Department of Veterinary Sciences, Federal University of Paraiba, Areia, PB 58397-000, Brazil. [2]Department of Animal Science, Federal University of Paraiba, Areia, PB 58397-000, Brazil. [3]Department of Veterinary Preventive Medicine, College of Veterinary Medicine, The Ohio State University, Columbus, OH 43210, USA. [4]Veterinary Public Health and Biotechnology Global Consortium (VPH-Biotec), The Ohio State University, Columbus, OH 43210, USA.

References
1. Castelani L, Santos AFS, Miranda MS, Zafalon LF, Pozzi CR, Arcaro JRP: **Molecular typing of mastitis-causing Staphylococcus aureus isolated from heifers and cows.** *Int J Mol Sci* 2013, **14**:4326–4333.
2. Anderson KL, Lyman R, Moury K, Ray D, Watson DW, Correa MT: **Molecular epidemiology of Staphylococcus aureus mastitis in dairy heifers.** *J Dairy Sci* 2012, **95**:4921–4930.
3. National Mastitis Council: *Laboratory Concepts of Bovine Mastitis.* Madison: National Mastitis Council; 1999.
4. Sambrook J, Fritsch EF, Maniatis T: *Molecular cloning: a laboratory manual.* 2nd edition. Cold Spring Harbor: Cold Spring Harbor Laboratory Press; 1989.
5. van der Zee A, Verbakel H, van Zon JC, Frenay I, van Belkum A, Peeters M, Buiting A, Bergmans A: **Molecular genotyping of Staphylococcus aureus strains: comparison of repetitive element sequence-based PCR with various typing methods and isolation of a novel epidemicity marker.** *J Clin Microbiol* 1999, **37**:342–349.
6. Hunter PR: **Reproducibility and indices of discriminatory power of microbial typing methods.** *J Clin Microbiol* 1990, **28**:1903–1905.
7. Taponen S, Pyörälä S: **Coagulase-negative staphylococci as cause of bovine mastitis - Not so different from Staphylococcus aureus?** *Vet Microbiol* 2009, **134**:29–36.
8. Peixoto RM, Peixoto RM, Lidan KCF, Costa MM: **Genotipificação de isolados de Staphylococcus epidermidis provenientes de casos de mastite caprina.** *Cien Rural* 2013, **43**:322–325.
9. Deplano A, Schuermans A, Van Eldere J, Witte W, Meugnier H, Etienne J, Grundmann H, Jonas D, Noordhoek GT, Dijkstra J, Van Belkum A, Van Leeuwen W, Tassios PT, Legakis NJ, Van Der Zee A, Bergmans A, Blanc DS, Tenover FC, Cookson BC, O'Neil G, Struelens MJ: **Multicenter evaluation of epidemiological typing of methicillin-resistant Staphylococcus aureus strains by repetitive-element PCR analysis.** *J Clin Microbiol* 2000, **38**:3527–3533.
10. De Vliegher S, Fox LK, Piepers S, Mcdougall S, Barkema HW: **Invited review: Mastitis in dairy heifers: nature of the disease, potential impact, prevention, and control.** *J Dairy Sci* 2012, **95**:1025–1040.
11. Aulrich K, Barth K: **Intramammary infections caused by coagulase-negative staphylococci and the effect on somatic cell counts in dairy goats.** *Agric Forest Res* 2008, **59**:59–64.
12. Koop G, van Werven T, Schuiling HJ, Nielen M: **The effect of subclinical mastitis on milk yield in dairy goats.** *J Dairy Sci* 2010, **93**:5809–5817.
13. Gebrewahid TT, Abera BH, Menghistu HT: **Prevalence and etiology of subclinical mastitis in small ruminants of Tigray regional State, north Ethiopia.** *Vet World* 2012, **5**:103–109.

5

Safety and immunogenicity of a delta inulin-adjuvanted inactivated Japanese encephalitis virus vaccine in pregnant mares and foals

Helle Bielefeldt-Ohmann[1,2*], Natalie A Prow[2,3], Wenqi Wang[1], Cindy SE Tan[2,3], Mitchell Coyle[4], Alysha Douma[4], Jody Hobson-Peters[2,3], Lisa Kidd[1], Roy A Hall[2,3] and Nikolai Petrovsky[5,6]

Abstract

In 2011, following severe flooding in Eastern Australia, an unprecedented epidemic of equine encephalitis occurred in South-Eastern Australia, caused by Murray Valley encephalitis virus (MVEV) and a new variant strain of Kunjin virus, a subtype of West Nile virus (WNV$_{KUN}$). This prompted us to assess whether a delta inulin-adjuvanted, inactivated cell culture-derived Japanese encephalitis virus (JEV) vaccine (JE-ADVAX™) could be used in horses, including pregnant mares and foals, to not only induce immunity to JEV, but also elicit cross-protective antibodies against MVEV and WNV$_{KUN}$. Foals, 74–152 days old, received two injections of JE-ADVAX™. The vaccine was safe and well-tolerated and induced a strong JEV-neutralizing antibody response in all foals. MVEV and WNV$_{KUN}$ antibody cross-reactivity was seen in 33% and 42% of the immunized foals, respectively. JE-ADVAX™ was also safe and well-tolerated in pregnant mares and induced high JEV-neutralizing titers. The neutralizing activity was passively transferred to their foals via colostrum. Foals that acquired passive immunity to JEV via maternal antibodies then were immunized with JE-ADVAX™ at 36–83 days of age, showed evidence of maternal antibody interference with low peak antibody titers post-immunization when compared to immunized foals of JEV-naïve dams. Nevertheless, when given a single JE-ADVAX™ booster immunization as yearlings, these animals developed a rapid and robust JEV-neutralizing antibody response, indicating that they were successfully primed to JEV when immunized as foals, despite the presence of maternal antibodies. Overall, JE-ADVAX™ appears safe and well-tolerated in pregnant mares and young foals and induces protective levels of JEV neutralizing antibodies with partial cross-neutralization of MVEV and WNV$_{KUN}$.

Introduction

Flaviviruses of the Japanese encephalitis virus (JEV) serocomplex are amongst the most important encephalitic viruses worldwide, affecting humans, wild birds, and several mammalian species, including domestic animal species such as horses. JEV is the leading cause of viral encephalitis in Asia, where 2–3 billion people are at risk of contracting the disease [1,2]. Annually, ~35 000 cases of JE are reported with a case fatality rate of nearly 30% and more than 50% of the survivors having neurological sequelae. Clinical manifestations vary and may include fever, headache, a change in mental status, seizures, tremors, generalised paresis, hypertonia and loss of coordination [3]. The clinical course in horses resembles that found in humans [4-7] with the majority of equine JEV infections being subclinical [8]. There is an estimated incidence of JE of 0.05% of JEV infections with a JE case fatality rate of ~50%. Treatment of JE patients, whether humans or horses, in the absence of availability of antiviral compounds, is supportive and the best means of preventing JE is immunization [9].

An inactivated JEV vaccine, developed in Japan in the 1960s (JE-VAX), dramatically reduced the number of human and equine cases of JE in that country [10]. However, this vaccine ceased to be manufactured in 2005, due to

* Correspondence: h.bielefeldtohmann1@uq.edu.au
[1]School of Veterinary Science, University of Queensland, Gatton Campus, Gatton, Qld 4343, Australia
[2]Australian Infectious Diseases Research Centre, University of Queensland, St. Lucia, Qld 4078, Australia
Full list of author information is available at the end of the article

perceived safety problems and excessive reactogenicity, with subsequent JEV vaccines being developed based on inactivated virus grown in cell culture [10,11].

Vaccination of thoroughbred horses against JEV is mandatory in several Asian countries. However, in many countries there is currently no widely available and approved equine JEV vaccine resulting in potential off-label human vaccine use in horses. For example, vaccine failure and fatal encephalitis due to naturally acquired JEV infection has been reported in a racing horse imported from Australia into Hong Kong [5]. Cases of equine JE have the potential to cause significant adverse economic effect on the horse industry, which is estimated to contribute greater than $6 billion to the GDP in Australia alone [12].

An inactivated Vero cell culture-derived JEV vaccine combined with delta inulin adjuvant (JE-ADVAX™) was previously tested in mice and adult horses and shown to have superior immunogenicity compared to the now-discontinued JE-VAX as well as a recently licensed, alum-adjuvanted cell culture-derived vaccine (JESPECT®, Novartis) [13]. The primary aim of the present study was to undertake vaccine efficacy and safety trials of the new JE-ADVAX™ vaccine in pregnant mares and in foals without or with passively acquired maternal antibodies. A second aim was to explore the potential ability of the JE-ADVAX™ vaccine to induce cross-reactivity and cross-protection against two related viruses, Murray Valley encephalitis virus (MVEV) and a new equine-virulent WNV$_{KUN}$ strain (strain NSW2011), which appeared in South-East Australia in early 2011 and caused a large epidemic of equine encephalitis [14,15]. Given the unlikely future development of equine vaccines specifically against MVEV and WNV$_{KUN}$, it would be useful if an adjuvanted JEV vaccine could provide cross-protection against these related flaviviruses.

In the present report we demonstrate safety and efficacy of the JE-ADVAX™ vaccine in young foals and pregnant mares. Foals born to unvaccinated mares responded to the vaccine with long-lasting humoral immunity, while foals with passively acquired maternal JEV antibodies had a blunted response to primary immunization, but after a vaccine booster as yearlings had a robust JEV-specific response indicating that memory B cells had been successfully primed during the primary immunization despite interference from maternal antibodies.

Materials and methods

Antigen and adjuvant

The Vero cell culture-grown inactivated JEV vaccine (Beijing-1 strain) [16] was obtained from the Kitasato Institute, Japan. The Advax™ adjuvant was described in detail in Lobigs et al. [13]. Briefly, Advax adjuvant is based on microparticulate delta inulin [17], and was obtained from Vaxine Pty Ltd, Adelaide, Australia. Advax™ is

supplied as a sterile, preservative-free, fine particulate suspension of delta inulin particles in a phosphate buffer. The vaccine antigen and Advax adjuvant were mixed together less than two hours prior to inoculation and the mixture kept on wet ice until injected.

Animals, vaccination protocol and sample collection

The studies were approved by the University of Queensland Animal Ethics Committee (AEC nos. SVS/306/11/VAXINE and SVS/298/13/VAXINE), and carried out in accordance with the ARC/NHMRC guidelines for ethical use of animals in research. A total of 53 thoroughbred and standard bred horses were enrolled in the studies (Tables 1, 2, 3 and 4). All horses were held in paddocks at the UQ Gatton Campus throughout the studies and received supplementary feed when needed. The first cohort of 19 foals, 74–152 days of age at first vaccination, were born to non-vaccinated mares and were all seronegative for flavivirus antibodies at entry into the trial (Table 3). Twelve foals were vaccinated with the Advax-adjuvanted JEV-vaccine, while seven foals received the adjuvant only. Seventeen mares in the second trimester of pregnancy were enrolled in the second phase, with 11 mares receiving the JEV-antigen plus Advax and six mares receiving adjuvant only. Two of the JEV-vaccinated mares had pre-existing antibodies specific for flaviviruses other than JEV, MVEV or WNV (data not shown; [18]). The foals born to the mares were subsequently enrolled in the third phase of the study (see below).

Vaccination was by subcutaneous inoculation on the rump (first foal cohort) or neck (mares and second foal cohort) in a volume of 150 µL. For both foals and mares the initial vaccine dose was 12 µg JEV-antigen plus 20 mg Advax™ and the booster vaccination, given four weeks later was 6 µg JEV-antigen and 20 mg Advax™. Blood samples were collected at each vaccination event and then at intervals of 4–36 weeks for up to 10 months post vaccination (Figure 1). The foals born to vaccinated mares were bled at birth, before colostrum uptake, and again 12 h after colostrum uptake, and a colostrum sample was obtained from the mares at foaling. This second cohort of foals was initially vaccinated at 36–83 days of age with a schedule similar to the first foal-cohort. They subsequently also received one additional vaccine booster (6 µg JEV-antigen and 20 mg Advax™) 10 months after the initial vaccination and blood samples were collected 2, 6, 12 and 18 weeks post vaccination. The six foals born to Advax™-only treated control mares were left untreated. Two of these unvaccinated foals were subsequently lost due to study-unrelated causes (birth complications and trauma, respectively).

Following each vaccine injection the animals were clinically assessed daily for 3–4 days while kept in small holding paddocks. The injection sites were inspected and

Table 1 Flavivirus specific antibody levels in foals born to flavivirus antibody-negative mares and vaccinated at 74–152 days of age[a]

Foal #	Age at Day 0	JEV neutralising antibodies			MVEV neutralising antibodies			WNV$_{KUN}$ neutralising antibodies		
		Day 28 (boost)	Day 56	Day 308	Day 28 (boost)	Day 56	Day 308	Day 28 (boost)	Day 56	Day 308
1 F11	74		80	20		<20	< 20		< 20	20
5 F11	115	40	160	160	< 20	<20	20	< 20	< 20	< 20
7 F11	108		160	40		<20	< 20		40	< 20
8 F11	132		160	< 20		20	< 20		40	< 20
11 F11	119		160	80		20	< 20		40	< 20
12 F11	81	40	1280	80	< 20	80	< 20	< 20	80	< 20
14 F11	123		320	20		<20	20		20	< 20
15 F11	125		320	< 20		<20	< 20		40	20
17 F11	111		320	20		<20	< 20		< 20	< 20
21 F11	97		320	< 20		20	< 20		< 20	20
26 F11	116	40	1280	80	20	80	20	< 20	< 20	20
30 F11	111		160	20		<20	< 20		< 20	20
Control A	115		< 20	< 20		<20	20		< 20	20
Control G	115		< 20	< 20		<20	< 20		< 20	< 20

[a]Samples negative in the flavivirus (4G2) blocking ELISA were not tested in the neutralization assays. This included five control foals (B-F), aged 125 to 152 days, which are not listed in the table.

any local reaction recorded. Body temperature and general demeanor were also recorded. With no adverse reactions recorded the animals were then returned to the main paddocks.

Flavivirus serology

Blood samples were collected by venepuncture into sterile vacutainers (BD Biosciences, Franklin Lakes, NJ, USA) and allowed to clot at room temperature, then centrifuged at 4 °C for 10 min at 3500 rpm. Procured sera were stored at –20 °C in sterile cryovials until assayed by ELISA and virus neutralization following heat inactivation at 56 °C for 30 min. Colostrum samples were centrifuged and the non-fat fraction collected and heat-treated as for serum before testing in the ELISA and neutralization assay.

All horse sera and colostrum samples were initially screened for flavivirus-specific antibodies using an epitope-blocking ELISA [19,20] with minor modifications as described in detail in Prow et al. [18]. Samples showing > 30% inhibition in this assay were subsequently tested for neutralizing antibody reactivity to JEV (strain Nakayama), MVEV (strain 1–51) and WNV$_{KUN}$ (strain NSW2011). The heat-inactivated test sera were titrated in doubling dilutions from 1:20 to 1:2560 and colostrum samples in dilutions from 1:40 to 1:5120 as previously described in detail [18].

Results

JE-ADVAX™ responses in foals born to naïve mares

In this trial, 19 foals, aged 74–152 days and born to non-vaccinated, flavivirus sero-negative mares, were enrolled. Twelve foals received two vaccinations four weeks apart with 12 μg and 6 μg JE-ADVAX™, respectively. Six control foals received ADVAX™ alone without antigen.

Table 2 Flavivirus antibody responses in mares vaccinated in second trimester of pregnancy

Time point	JEV neutralizing			MVEV neutralizing			WNV$_{KUN}$ neutralizing		
	Positive/total	Mean titre[≠]	Positive titre range	Positive/total	Mean titre[≠]	Positive titre range	Positive/total	Mean titre[≠]	Positive titre range
Day 0 (vaccination)	0/11	–	–	0/11	–	–	0/11	–	–
Day 28 (booster)	0/11	–	–	0/11	–	–	2/11	80	20-80
Days 56-183	8/11	180	20-320	4/11	100	20-160	3/11	560	20-1280
Day 230 (7.5 months)	11/11	47	20-80	9/11	31	20-80	2/11*	60	20-80
Day 331 (11 months)	7/11	26	20-40	4/11	40	20-80	2/11*	60	20-80

[≠]mean of titres ≥ 20.
*same two mares (# 10 & 33).

Table 3 Flavivirus-specific antibodies in colostrum and serum of JE + ADVAX™ vaccinated and unvaccinated mares at the time of foaling[a]

Mare #	Colostrum			Serum		
	JEV neutralizing antibody titres	MVEV neutralizing antibody titres	WNV$_{KUN}$ neutralizing antibody titres	JEV neutralizing antibody titres	MVEV neutralizing antibody titres	WNV$_{KUN}$ neutralizing antibody titres
2	2560	80	< 40	40	< 20	< 20
5	160	< 40	< 40	20	20	< 20
8	640	80	< 40	20	< 20	< 20
10	640	80	80	40	20	80
11	320	40	< 40	< 20	20	< 20
14	640	80	< 40	20	< 20	< 20
17	320	40	< 40	40	40	40
21	160	40	< 40	< 20	< 20	< 20
26	160	80	< 40	20	< 20	< 20
33	640	80	40	40	40	80
34	640	< 40	< 40	40	< 20	< 20
Control A[b]	160	40	< 40	< 20	< 20	< 20
Control B	40	40	< 40	< 20	< 20	< 20
Control C	320	40	< 40	< 20	< 20	< 20

[a]Samples negative in the flavivirus (4G2) blocking ELISA were not tested in the neutralization assays. This included three control mares (D-F), which are not shown in the Table.
[b]Entered trial at time of foaling, having received neither JEV + Advax nor Advax alone.

Only mild swelling at the inoculation site was noted in some of the foals 1–3 days following subcutaneous injection on the rump. No reaction was seen in the Advax-only treated foals. Three foals had flavivirus-specific antibodies at the time of vaccine-boosting (Table 1), though none had virus-neutralizing activity. However, four weeks after the booster 12/12 (100%) of JE-ADVAX™-vaccinated foals had high serum JEV-neutralizing antibody titres and this neutralizing activity was still present 8.5 months later in 9/12 (75%) foals (Table 1). In contrast, cross-reactivity to MVEV and WNV$_{KUN}$ was generally low or absent (Table 1). Two control foals had sero-converted to flaviviruses at the last sampling, 10 months after trial commencement, presumably due to natural exposure to flaviviruses circulating in South-East Queensland [18,22,23].

JE-ADVAX™ safety and immunogenicity in pregnant mares

The JE-ADVAX™ vaccine formulation was previously shown to be safe and immunogenic in adult horses [13], however, for licensing purposes it must also be shown to be safe in pregnant animals [21]. Therefore, 17 mares in second trimester of pregnancy were enrolled in a trial, where 11 mares received an initial dose of 12 µg of JEV antigen mixed with 20 mg of ADVAX™ subcutaneously in the neck and four weeks later were boosted with 6 µg of JEV antigen plus ADVAX™. No adverse reactions were noted, other than mild swelling at the inoculation site

of some mares 1–3 days following the booster vaccination. Four mares received ADVAX™ only at the two time points and no reactions to the adjuvant were recorded. The remaining two mares received neither antigen nor adjuvant. Pre-vaccination, two of the pregnant mares had flavivirus-specific antibodies, detected in the 4G2-blocking ELISA, however, these antibodies did not neutralize JEV, MVEV or WNV$_{KUN}$ (Table 2). At the time of vaccine boosting (four weeks after initial dose), an additional five mares had developed flavivirus specific antibodies, detected in the blocking ELISA (data not shown), although none had measurable JEV or MVEV neutralizing antibodies. At this time point one of the mares with pre-immunization flavivirus antibodies had developed a WNV$_{KUN}$-neutralizing titre of 80 (Table 2 and data not shown). Four weeks after the booster vaccination, 11/11 (100%) of mares had flavivirus-specific antibodies in the blocking ELISA and of these 8/11 (72%) had developed JEV-neutralizing antibodies, while only four (36%) and three (27%) had MVEV- and WNV$_{KUN}$-neutralizing antibodies, respectively (Table 2). Interestingly, 7.5 months following vaccination all 11 mares (100%) had JEV-neutralizing antibodies, while nine (82%) and two (18%) had neutralizing antibodies to MVEV and WNV$_{KUN}$, respectively (Table 2). This suggests that either some animals responded slowly to the vaccine or had been naturally exposed to flaviviruses, most likely MVEV or Alfuy virus [18,22], thereby providing a boost to the original vaccine response.

Table 4 Flavivirus specific antibody levels in foals born to vaccinated mares and vaccinated at 36–83 days of age, followed by booster vaccinations four weeks and approximately one year later

Time point	JEV neutralizing			MVEV neutralizing			WNV$_{KUN}$ neutralizing		
	Positive/total	Mean titre$^{\neq}$	Titre range	Positive/total	Mean titre$^{\neq}$	Titre range	Positive/total	Mean titre$^{\neq}$	Titre range
Pre-suckle	0/11	–	–	0/11	–	–	0/11	–	–
Post suckle	10/11	46	< 20-80	8/11	30	< 20-40	3/11	93	< 20-160
Age 13–49 days	3/10*	26	< 20-40	1/10*	40	< 20-40	2/10*	30	< 20-40
Vaccination Age 36–83 days	3/11	20	< 20-20	2/11	20	< 20-20	1/11	40	< 20-40
Booster 4 weeks post vaccination Age 64–111 days	2/11	20	< 20-20	3/11	20	< 20-20	2/11	20	< 20-20
4 weeks post booster Age 93–140 days	10/11	88	< 20-320	10/11	30	< 20-40	1/11	20	< 20-20
7 weeks post booster Age 114–161 days	3/11	53	< 20-80	6/11	26	< 20-40	3/11	20	< 20-20
10 weeks post booster Age 137–184 days	5/11	24	< 20-40	0/11	–	< 20	1/11	20	< 20-20
~9 months post 1st boost (2nd boost) Age 332–379 days	0/11	–	< 20	0/11	–	< 20	0/11	–	< 20
2 weeks post 2nd boost Age 346–393 days	11/11	> 902	160- > 2560	10/11	50	< 20-80	1/11	20	< 20-20
5.5 weeks post 2nd boost Age 370–417 days	11/11	465	160-1280	7/11	17	< 20-40	0/11	–	< 20
14 weeks post 2nd boost Age 454-501	8/11	150	< 20-640	0/11	–	< 20	9/11	31	< 20-80
20 weeks post 2nd boost Age 498–545 days	7/11	63	< 20-160	0/11	–	< 20	0/11	–	< 20

*one foal not yet born at this sampling point.
$^{\neq}$mean of titres ≥ 20.

The mares foaled 4.5-6 months after the initial vaccination and all had high JEV-neutralizing antibody titres in the colostrum, even though the serum-titres in two of the mares at the time of foaling were below the assay cut-off (Table 3). In 9/11 (82%) of the mares the colostrum antibodies also neutralized MVEV, while in only 2/11 (18%) mares did the colostrum antibodies neutralize WNV$_{KUN}$ (Table 3).

None of the control unvaccinated mares or mares injected with ADVAX™ alone had flavivirus-specific antibodies, based on the pre-vaccination blocking ELISA, however, three of these mares developed flavivirus specific antibodies during the trial period (Table 3). As none of these mares had neutralizing antibodies to JEV, MVEV or WNV$_{KUN}$, it is most likely they sero-converted to some of the other flaviviruses commonly circulating in the area [18]. Interestingly, the colostrum of these three control mares did have neutralizing activity towards JEV and MVEV, but not to WNV$_{KUN}$ (Table 3).

JE-ADVAX™ responses in foals born to JEV-immune mares
In the second foal trial, 11 foals born to the JE-ADVAX™ vaccinated mares (Tables 2 and 3) received a similar vaccine schedule to that described earlier for the first trial when they were between 36–83 days old. At vaccination, six (55%) foals still had measurable passively transferred maternal serum antibodies to flaviviruses, as detected by the blocking ELISA, although only three (27%) had measurable serum JEV neutralizing titres (Table 4). Nevertheless, all 11/11 (100%) foals responded to the JE-ADVAX vaccine with antibodies detectable by the 4G2-blocking ELISA four weeks after the booster vaccination (Table 4). Of these 10 (91%) had JEV- and 10 (91%) MVEV-neutralizing antibodies after the booster vaccination, but the titres rapidly decreased and by 10 weeks after the booster vaccination only 5/11 (45%) foals had low JEV-neutralizing antibody titres, none had MVEV-specific antibodies and only one had a low WNV$_{KUN}$-specific titre (Table 4). Four foals borne to non-vaccinated mares and left untreated

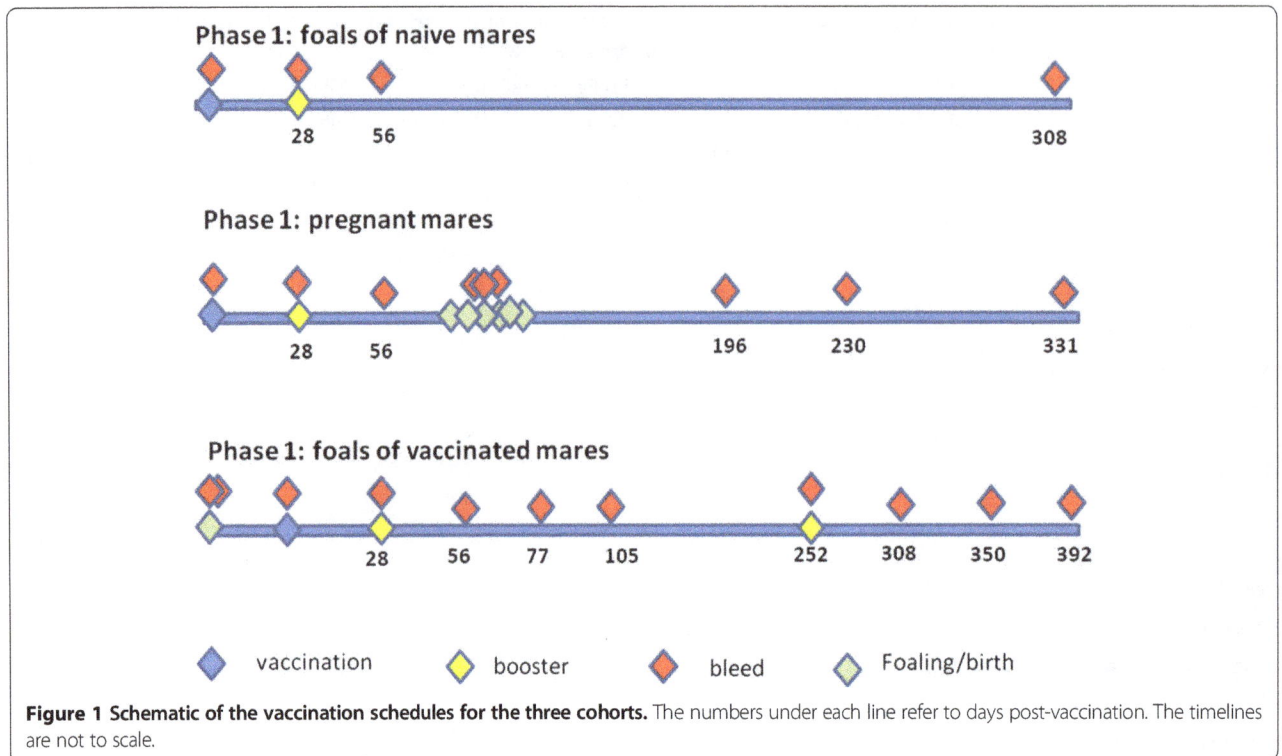

Figure 1 Schematic of the vaccination schedules for the three cohorts. The numbers under each line refer to days post-vaccination. The timelines are not to scale.

remained flavivirus sero-negative for the duration of the trial (data not shown).

When these 11 vaccinated foals were retested 10 months after the primary vaccination, only two (18%) had flavivirus-specific antibodies detectable in the blocking ELISA, but neither had virus-neutralizing activity (Table 4). The animals, now yearlings, then received a single booster vaccination with 6 μg of JE-ADVAX and were bled two, 5.5, 14 and 20 weeks post booster vaccination. All 11/11 animals were already strongly positive in the flavivirus blocking ELISA two weeks post vaccination, and 11/11 (100%) were confirmed to have JEV-neutralizing antibodies (Table 4), indicating that the original JE-ADVAX vaccination had primed them for a rapid B cell recall response despite interference of maternal antibodies. While the JEV-neutralizing antibody titres declined over the following 18 weeks, 7/11 horses (63%) still had JEV-neutralizing antibody titres > 20 at the last bleed (Table 4). None of the yearlings had MVEV- and WNV$_{KUN}$-neutralizing antibodies at the time of the second booster, but two weeks after the boost 10/11 (91%) horses had MVEV-neutralizing antibodies (Table 4). The yearlings remained negative for neutralizing antibodies to WNV$_{KUN}$ until three months after the booster, when 9/11 (82%) had a detectable titre. The cross-reactive antibody activity to MVEV and WNV$_{KUN}$ had declined below the assay cut-off of < 20 by 20 weeks post booster (Table 4).

Discussion

The results of this study corroborate and extend those of a previous study by Lobigs et al. [13] and show that the cell culture-derived, inactivated JE-vaccine is safe in horses of any age and when delivered with the novel polysaccharide adjuvant Advax elicits a strong JEV-specific neutralizing antibody response in both pregnant adult horses and in very young foals which lasts at least 10–11 months in the majority of the animals (Tables 1 and 2). While a 3rd booster vaccination was not given at that stage, the results of the vaccine trial in foals with passively acquired immunity suggest that the vaccine delivers robust priming of a memory B-cell response, which results in a strong humoral recall response despite serum antibodies having decreased to undetectable levels (Table 4).

In contrast to the high level of MVEV and WNV cross-protection seen in mice with JE-ADVAX™ vaccine [24] or the live Chimerivax-JE vaccine [25], cross-neutralization of WNV$_{KUN}$ was only present in serum of 27% (3/11) of mares and in 41% (5/12) of foals immunized with two doses of JE-ADVAX™ (Tables 1 and 2). In the foals the low WNV$_{KUN}$ titres detected at day 308 post primary vaccination may even be the result of boosting by natural exposure to JEV sero-complex flaviviruses, as MVEV, WNV$_{KUN}$ and Alfuy virus are known to circulate in the area where the horses were kept [18,22,23]. However, extensive JE-ADVAX dose ranging studies have not yet been performed in horses and hence with a larger vaccine dose higher levels of flavivirus cross-neutralization closer to the levels seen in mice may be achieved [24]. An alternative explanation might be that mice are not ideal models for equine vaccine responses [26].

As could be expected, the JEV-specific antibody titres in colostrum far exceeded those in the serum of the mares at the time of foaling (Table 3). This difference was even more notable for MVEV cross-reactive antibodies, with MVEV-neutralizing activity detectable in the colostrum of 82% (9/11) of immunized mares and in serum of 72% (8/11) of foals 12 h post colostrum uptake, despite being detectable in the serum of only 45% (5/11) of these mares (Tables 3 and 4). While this trial was not designed to assess the half-life of passively acquired immunity, it is nevertheless a notable finding, as it would suggest that vaccination of pregnant mares with the JE-ADVAX vaccine in areas of Australia where MVEV is endemic might confer protection of the foals against this almost invariably fatal infection [22,27-30]. In general, the cross-reactivity to MVEV was greater than that to WNV_{KUN}. Nevertheless, the results suggest that it might be possible to further enhance flavivirus cross-protection by additional vaccine boosters, as was seen in the study by Lobigs et al. [13], or increases in vaccine dose.

Two control mares, receiving Advax adjuvant only, were apparently naturally exposed to flavivirus(es) sometime between the start of the trial and foaling, giving rise to high cross-reactivity to JEV and MVEV in their colostrum (Table 3). Similarly, a control mare that received neither vaccine nor adjuvant, had high JEV- and MVEV-neutralizing antibody titres in its colostrum despite only having serum neutralizing activity to Kokobera virus (titre of 40 [18]), which normally does not confer cross-protection to JEV serocomplex viruses [18,31]. Two of the foals born to these three control mares were subsequently positive for flavivirus antibodies in the 4G2-blocking ELISA for a couple of months, but at no point was JEV- or MVEV-neutralizing activity detected in their serum (data not shown). This aspect was not further pursued, but it might be speculated that these were antibodies of low affinity and/or avidity and/or quickly catabolized in the foals.

The degree of interference with immune responses in young animals by passively acquired maternal antibodies may depend on the animal species, antigen type, route of vaccination and other variables [32-38]. While all the foals received flavivirus-specific antibodies in colostrum, resulting in detectable serum JEV-neutralizing antibodies in 91% of foals at 12 h post suckle, this neutralizing activity decreased to below detection level in all but the three youngest foals by the time of primary vaccination (Table 4), and all but one foal responded with moderately high to high JEV-neutralizing titres four weeks after the second vaccine dose. However, in the presence of maternal antibodies the antibody response to vaccination was shorter-lived, with only 5/11 (45%) foals still having JEV-neutralizing antibodies 10 weeks after the booster. Six months later all but two were negative for flavivirus antibodies in the 4G2-blocking ELISA, but all 11 animals, by then yearlings, responded to a second booster with a very rapid and robust antibody response. Thus, while vaccination at an age where passively acquired antibodies were still present prevented sustained serum neutralizing antibody responses, memory B cells were still induced in these foals immunized in the presence of passive antibodies, as reflected in their vigorous response to a single vaccine boost. This suggests that the apparent "window of susceptibility" created by vaccination in the presence of passively acquired antibodies, may not in reality be as much of a problem as generally thought [35,37-39], as even in the absence of pre-existing serum antibody, the primed memory B cell response is able to respond rapidly enough to control any infection. Arthropod-borne viruses initially replicate at the site of inoculation before spreading haematogenously or via the lymphatic system to local lymph nodes and beyond [40,41]. While the route and mechanisms of neuro-invasion by the encephalitic flaviviruses are still unknown [42], we recently described a case of MVEV-encephalitis in a horse, in which MVEV-neutralizing antibodies were present one week prior to clinical symptoms, but not two weeks prior to clinical disease [22]. This suggests that even in a primary infection the antibody response to JEV-serocomplex viruses may be relatively fast, and can be anticipated to be even faster in a recall response [43]. If this assumption is correct, then primed animals lacking detectable serum-neutralizing antibodies might still be protected by a rapid memory B cell recall response able to neutralize the virus before it spreads to the central nervous system. This is similar to the results obtained in JE-ADVAX-immunized beta-2-microglobulin knockout mice, which were still protected against JEV, despite having no detectable serum neutralizing antibody pre-challenge, thanks to a robust recall response and rapid rise in serum antibody titer in response to the challenge virus [44]. Future studies should aim to test this hypothesis in horses, since as discussed above, the murine immune response may not truly reflect that of equines [26], nor does the disease progression in mice reflect that seen in natural and experimental infections of horses with JEV, MVEV and WNV_{KUN} ([22,45-49]; Bielefeldt-Ohmann et al., unpublished data 2013).

In conclusion, JE-ADVAX™ was safe, well-tolerated and highly immunogenic in both young foals and in pregnant mares, in which it induced high titre JEV-specific antibodies in colostrum, thus ensuring passive transfer of protective antibodies to the newborn foals. Despite evidence of maternal antibody interference, foals of immune dams developed strong memory B cell responses to JEV, as reflected in a robust recall response to a single booster JE-ADVAX dose as yearlings. Although primarily designed to provide protection against JEV, some cross-neutralisation against MVEV and WNV was seen in some of the JE-ADVAX immunized horses. Future studies will test modifications to the vaccination protocol, including increasing the antigen or adjuvant dose, adding a further booster immunization, priming with JE-ADVAX and boosting with already licensed WNV vaccines [47,50] or with novel WNV vaccine candidates [48,51-54] to see whether it is possible to induce cross-protection against a wider spectrum of flaviviruses.

Competing interests

NP is affiliated with Vaxine Pty, Ltd, a company with commercial interests in Advax™, the adjuvant employed in the present studies. The authors declare that they have no competing interests.

Authors' contributions

Conceived and designed the experiments: HBO, NAP, LK, MC, RAH, NP. Performed the experiments: HBO, NAP, WW, CSET, JHP, LK, MC, AD. Analyzed the data: HBO, NAP, WW, CSET, JHP, RAH, NP. Drafted the manuscript: HBO, NAP, RAH, NP. All authors read and approved the final manuscript.

Acknowledgements

We thank Dr Mario Lobigs for constructive discussions on the study design, and Sharon Blum, Anita Barton, Dr Ristan Greer, and students at the UQ School of Veterinary Science and the UQ Gatton Campus Equine Unit for help with animal handling and sampling. The study was supported by grants from the UQ-CIEF program (RM20111110; HBO, RAH), the Australian Research Council (ARC-LP120100686; RAH, HBO et al.), and contract HHSN272200800039C from the National Institute of Allergy and Infectious Diseases, National Institutes of Health (NP). This paper's contents are solely the responsibility of the authors and do not necessarily represent the official views of the funders.

Author details

[1]School of Veterinary Science, University of Queensland, Gatton Campus, Gatton, Qld 4343, Australia. [2]Australian Infectious Diseases Research Centre, University of Queensland, St. Lucia, Qld 4078, Australia. [3]School of Chemistry & Molecular Biosciences, University of Queensland, St. Lucia, Australia. [4]Gatton Campus Equine Unit, University of Queensland, Gatton Campus, Gatton, Qld 4343, Australia. [5]Vaxine Pty., Ltd., Flinders Medical Centre, Adelaide, South Australia. [6]Flinders Medical Centre and Flinders University, Bedford Park, South Australia.

References

1. Mackenzie JS, Lindsay MD, Coelen RJ, Broom AK, Hall RA, Smith DW: **Arboviruses causing human disease in the Australasian zoogeographic region.** *Arch Virol* 1994, **136**:447-467.
2. Mackenzie JS, Johansen CA, Ritchie SA, van den Hurk AF, Hall RA: **Japanese encephalitis as an emerging virus: the emergence and spread of Japanese encephalitis virus in Australasia.** *Curr Top Microbiol Immunol* 2002, **267**:49-73.
3. Solomon T: **Flavivirus encephalitis.** *N Engl J Med* 2004, **351**:370-378.
4. Gould DJ, Byrne RJ, Hayes DE: **Experimental infection of horses with Japanese encephalitis virus by mosquito bits.** *Am J Trop Med Hyg* 1964, **13**:742-746.
5. Lam KH, Ellis TM, Williams DT, Lunt RA, Daniels PW, Watkins KL, Riggs CM: **Japanese encephalitis in a racing thoroughbred gelding in Hong Kong.** *Vet Rec* 2005, **157**:168-173.
6. Miyake M: **The pathology of Japanese encephalitis. A review.** *Bull World Hlth Organ* 1964, **30**:153-160.
7. Yamanaka T, Tsujimura K, Kondo T, Yasuda W, Okada A, Noda K, Okumura T, Matsumura T: **Isolation and genetic analysis of Japanese encephalitis virus from a diseased horse in Japan.** *J Vet Med Sci* 2006, **68**:293-295.
8. Konishi E, Shoda M, Kondo T: **Analysis of yearly changes in levels of antibodies to Japanese encephalitis virus nonstructural 1 protein in racehorses in central Japan shows high levels of natural virus activity still exist.** *Vaccine* 2006, **24**:516-524.
9. Monath TP: **Japanese encephalitis vaccines: current vaccines and future prospects.** *Curr Top Microbiol Immunol* 2002, **267**:105-138.
10. Tsai TF: **New initiatives for the control of Japanese encephalitis by vaccination: minutes of a WHO/CVI meeting, Bangkok, Thailand, 13-15 October 1998.** *Vaccine* 2000, **18**(Suppl 2):1-25.
11. Fischer M, Casey C, Chen RT: **Promise of new Japanese encephalitis vaccines.** *Lancet* 2007, **370**:1806-1808.
12. RIRDC 2006: **Rural Industries Research & Development Corporations – Horse R&D Plan 2006-2011.** [https://rirdc.infoservices.com.au/items/06-114]
13. Lobigs M, Pavy M, Hall RA, Lobigs P, Cooper P, Komiya T, Toriniwa H, Petrovsky N: **An inactivated Vero cell-grown Japanese encephalitis vaccine formulated with Advax, a novel inulin-based adjuvant, induces protective neutralizing antibody against homologous and heterologous flaviviruses.** *J Gen Virol* 2010, **91**:1407-1417.
14. Frost MJ, Zhang J, Edmonds JH, Prow NA, Gu X, Davis R, Hornitzky C, Arzey KE, Finlayson D, Hick P, Read A, Hobson-Peters J, May FJ, Doggett SL, Haniotis J, Russell RC, Hall RA, Khromykh AA, Kirkland PD: **Characterization of virulent West Nile virus Kunjin strain, Australia, 2011.** *Emerg Infect Dis* 2012, **18**:792-800.
15. Roche SE, Wicks R, Garner MG, East IJ, Paskin R, Moloney BJ, Carr M, Kirkland P: **Descriptive overview of the 2011 epidemic of arboviral disease in horses in Australia.** *Aust Vet J* 2012, **91**:5-13.
16. Toriniwa H, Komiya T: **Long-term stability of Vero cell-derived inactivated Japanese encephalitis vaccine prepared using serum-free medium.** *Vaccine* 2008, **26**:3680-3689.
17. Cooper P, Petrovsky N: **Delta inulin: a novel, immunologically-active, stable packing structure comprising β-D-[2 → 1] polyfructo-furanosyl α-D glucose polymers.** *Glycobiology* 2011, **21**:595-606.
18. Prow NA, Tan CSE, Wang W, Hobson-Peters J, Kidd L, Barton A, Hall RA, Bielefeldt-Ohmann H: **Natural exposure of horses to mosquito-borne flaviviruses in South-East Queensland, Australia.** *Int J Environ Res Public Health* 2013, **10**:4432-4443.
19. Hall RA, Broom AK, Hartnett AC, Howard MJ, Mackenzie JS: **Immunodominant epitopes on the NS1 protein of MVE and KUN viruses serve as targets for a blocking ELISA to detect virus specific antibodies in sentinel animal serum.** *J Virol Methods* 1995, **51**:201-210.
20. Blitvitch BJ, Bowen RA, Marlenee NL, Hall RA, Bunning ML, Beaty BJ: **Epitope-blocking enzyme-linked immunosorbent assays for detection of West Nile virus antibodies in domestic mammals.** *J Clin Microbiol* 2003, **41**:2676-2679.
21. APVMA. 2014. Australian Pesticides and Veterinary Medicines Authority – Guiidelines for registration of new veterinary vaccines [http://apvma.gov.au/node/1041]
22. Barton AJ, Prow NA, Hall RA, Kidd L, Bielefeldt-Ohmann H: **A case of Murray Valley encephalitis in a two-year old Australian stock horse in South-East Queensland.** *Aus Vet J*, in press.
23. Prow NA, Hewlett EK, Faddy HM, Coiacetto F, Wang W, Cox T, Hall RA, Bielefeldt-Ohmann H: **The Australian public is still vulnerable to emerging virulent strains of West Nile virus.** *Front Public Health* 2014, **2**:146.
24. Petrovsky N, Larena M, Siddharthan V, Prow NA, Hall RA, Lobigs M, Morrey J: **An inactivated cell culture Japanese encephalitis vaccine (JE-ADVAX) formulated with delta inulin adjuvant provides robust heterologous protection against West Nile encephalitis via cross-protective memory B cells and neutralizing antibody.** *J Virol* 2013, **87**:10324-10333.
25. Lobigs M, Larena M, Alsharifi M, Lee E, Pavy M: **Live chimeric and inactivated Japanese encephalitis virus vaccines differ in their cross-protective values against Murray Valley encephalitis virus.** *J Virol* 2009, **83**:2436-2445.
26. Karagianni AE, Kapetanovic R, McGorum BC, Hume DA, Pirie SR: **The equine alveolar macrophage: functional and phenotypic comparisons with peritoneal macrophages.** *Vet Immunol Immunopathol* 2013, **155**:219-228.
27. Gard GP, Marshall ID, Walker KH, Acland HM, Saren WG: **Association of Australian arboviruses with nervous disease in horses.** *Aust Vet J* 1977, **53**:61-66.
28. Gordon AN, Marbach CR, Oakey J, Edmunds G, Condon K, Diviney SM, Williams DT, Bingham J: **Confirmed case of encephalitis caused by Murray Valley encephalitis virus infection in a horse.** *J Vet Diagn Invest* 2012, **24**:431-436.
29. Holmes JM, Gilkerson JR, El Hage CM, Slocombe RF, Muurlink MA: **Murray Valley encephalomyelitis in a horse.** *Aust Vet J* 2012, **90**:252-254.

30. Selvey LA, Dailey L, Lindsay M, Armstrong P, Tobin S, Koehler AP, Markey PG, Smith DW: **The changing epidemiology of Murray Valley encephalitis in Australia: the 2011 outbreak and a review of the literature.** *PLoS Negl Trop Dis* 2014, **8**:e2556.

31. Poidinger M, Hall RA, Mackenzie JS: **Molecular characterization of the Japanese encephalitis serocomplex of the flavivirus genus.** *Virology* 1996, **218**:417–421.

32. Blasco E, Lambot M, Barrat J, Cliquet F, Brochier B, Renders C, Krafft N, Bailly J, Munier M, Pastoret P-P, Aubert MFA: **Kinetics of humoral immune response after rabies VR-G oral vaccination of captive fox cubs (*Vulpes vulpes*) with or without maternally derived antibodies against the vaccine.** *Vaccine* 2001, **19**:4805–4815.

33. Endsley JJ, Roth JA, Ridpath J, Neill J: **Maternal antibody blocks humoral but not T cell responses to BVDV.** *Biologicals* 2003, **31**:123–125.

34. Filho OA, Megid J, Geronutti L, Ratti J Jr, Almeida MFA, Kataoka APAG, Martorelli LFA: **Vaccine immune response and interference of colostral antibodies in calves vaccinated against rabies at 2, 4 and 6 months of age born from antirabies revaccinated females.** *Res Vet Sci* 2012, **92**:396–400.

35. Hodgins DC, Shewen PE: **Vaccination of neonates: problem and issues.** *Vaccine* 2012, **30**:1541–1559.

36. Oura CAL, Wood JLN, Floyd T, Sanders AJ, Bin-Tarif A, Henstock M, Edwards L, Simmons H, Batten CA: **Colostral antibody protection and interference with immunity in lambs born from sheep vaccinated with an inactivated Bluetongue serotype 8 vaccine.** *Vaccine* 2010, **28**:2749–2753.

37. Siegrist CA: **The challenges of vaccine responses in early life: selected examples.** *J Comp Pathol* 2007, **137**(Suppl 1):S4–S9.

38. Siegrist CA, Lambert PH: **Maternal immunity and infant responses to immunization: factors influencing infant responses.** *Dev Biol Stand* 1998, **95**:133–139.

39. Wilkins PA, Glasser AL, McDonnell SM: **Passive transfer of naturally acquired specific immunity against West Nile virus to foals in a semi-feral pony herd.** *J Vet Intern Med* 2006, **20**:1045–1047.

40. Brown AN, Kent KA, Bennett CJ, Bernard KA: **Tissue tropism and neuroinvasion of West Nile virus do not differ for two mouse strains with different survival rates.** *Virology* 2007, **368**:422–430.

41. Weiner LP, Cole GA, Nathanson N: **Experimental encephalitis following peripheral inoculation of West Nile virus in mice of different ages.** *J Hyg (Lond)* 1970, **68**:435–446.

42. Suen WW, Prow NA, Hall RA, Bielefeldt-Ohmann H: **Mechanism of West Nile virus neuroinvasion: a critical appraisal.** *Viruses* 2014, **6**:2796–2825.

43. Shirafuji H, Kanehira K, Kamio T, Kubo T, Shibahara T, Konishi M, Murakami K, Nakamura Y, Yamanaka T, Kondo T, Matsumura T, Muranaka M, Katayama Y: **Antibody responses induced by experimental West Nile virus infection with or without previous immunization with inactivated Japanese encephalitis vaccine in horses.** *J Vet Med Sci* 2009, **71**:969–974.

44. Larena M, Prow NA, Hall RA, Petrovsky N, Lobigs M: **JE-ADVAX vaccine protection against Japanese encephalitis virus mediated by memory B cells in the absence of CD8(+) T cells and pre-exposure neutralizing antibody.** *J Virol* 2013, **87**:4395–4402.

45. Angenvoort J, Brault AC, Bowen RA, Groschup MH: **West Nile viral infection of equids.** *Vet Microbiol* 2013, **167**:168–180.

46. Bowen RA, Nemeth NM: **Experimental infections with West Nile virus.** *Curr Opin Infect Dis* 2007, **20**:293–297.

47. Ellis PM, Daniels PW, Banks DJ: **Japanese encephalitis.** *Vet Clin North Am Equine Pract* 2000, **16**:565–578.

48. Long MT, Gibbs EPJ, Mellemcamp MW, Bowen RA, Seino KK, Zhang S, Beachboard SE, Humphrey PP: **Efficacy, duration, and onset of immunogenicity of a West Nile virus vaccine, live Flavivirus chimera, in horses with a clinical disease challenge model.** *Equine Vet J* 2007, **39**:491–497.

49. Kay BH, Pollitt CC, Fanning ID, Hall RA: **The experimental infection of horses with Murray Valley encephalitis and Ross River viruses.** *Aust Vet J* 1987, **64**:52–55.

50. Seino KK, Long MT, Gibbs EP, Bowen RA, Beachboard SE, Humphrey PP, Dixon MA, Bourgeois MA: **Comparative efficacies of three commercially available vaccines against West Nile Virus (WNV) in a short-duration challenge trial involving an equine WNV encephalitis model.** *Clin Vaccine Immunol* 2007, **14**:1465–1471.

51. Brandler S, Tangy F: **Vaccines in development against West Nile virus.** *Viruses* 2013, **5**:2384–2409.

52. Hall RA, Nisbet DJ, Pham KB, Pyke AT, Smith GA, Khromykh AA: **DNA vaccine coding for the full-length infectious Kunjin virus RNA protects mice against the New York strain of West Nile virus.** *Proc Natl Acad Sci U S A* 2003, **100**:10460–10464.

53. Roby JA, Bielefeldt-Ohmann H, Prow NA, Chang DC, Hall RA, Khromykh AA: **Increased expression of capsid protein in *trans* enhances production of single-round infectious particles by a West Nile virus DNA vaccine.** *J Gen Virol* 2014, **95**:2176–2191.

54. Siger L, Bowen RA, Karaca K, Murray MJ, Gordy PW, Loosmore SM, Audonnet JC, Nordgren RM, Minke JM: **Assessment of the efficacy of a single dose of a recombinant vaccine against West Nile virus in response to natural challenge with West Nile virus-infected mosquitoes in horses.** *Am J Vet Res* 2004, **65**:1459–1462.

6

Changes in leukocyte subsets of pregnant gilts experimentally infected with porcine reproductive and respiratory syndrome virus and relationships with viral load and fetal outcome

Andrea Ladinig[1,4*], Wilhelm Gerner[2], Armin Saalmüller[2], Joan K Lunney[3], Carolyn Ashley[1] and John CS Harding[1]

Abstract

In spite of more than two decades of extensive research, the understanding of porcine reproductive and respiratory syndrome virus (PRRSv) immunity is still incomplete. A PRRSv infection of the late term pregnant female can result in abortions, early farrowings, fetal death, and the birth of weak, congenitally infected piglets. The objectives of the present study were to investigate changes in peripheral blood mononuclear cell populations in third trimester pregnant females infected with type 2 PRRSv (NVSL 97–7895) and to analyze potential relationships with viral load and fetal mortality rate. PRRSv infection caused a massive, acute drop in total leukocyte counts affecting all PBMC populations by two days post infection. Except for B cells, cell counts started to rebound by day six post infection. Our data also show a greater decrease of naïve B cells, T-helper cells and cytolytic T cells than their respective effector or memory counterparts. Absolute numbers of T cells and γδ T cells were negatively associated with PRRSv RNA concentration in gilt serum over time. Additionally, absolute numbers of T helper cells may be predictive of fetal mortality rate. The preceding three leukocyte populations may therefore be predictive of PRRSv-related pathological outcomes in pregnant gilts. Although many questions regarding the immune responses remain unanswered, these findings provide insight and clues that may help reduce the impact of PRRSv in pregnant gilts.

Introduction

In spite of more than two decades of extensive research, understanding of porcine reproductive and respiratory syndrome virus (PRRSv) immunity is still incomplete. PRRSv is able to persist in infected pigs for several months [1,2] and uses different evasion strategies to circumvent innate and adaptive immune responses, summarized in several reviews [3-5]. Numerous reports have investigated immune responses against PRRSv in vivo including the measurement of cytokine production, the investigation of immune cells, or the measurement of antibody responses. However, a direct comparison of results across different experiments is complicated by several factors including the use of different virus isolates, age and genetics of animals, as well as criteria used to measure immune responses. For the investigation of immune cells by flow cytometry (FCM), additional factors complicating interpretation include methods of data presentation (absolute numbers versus percentages of different cell populations) as well as variation in marker selection used to define leukocyte subsets. In addition, investigations of peripheral blood mononuclear cells (PBMC) subsets in response to PRRSv infection have mainly used nursery or growing pigs in PRRSv respiratory models, whereas reports using pregnant females are sparse. Nielsen et al. [6] inoculated sows at 90 days of gestation to investigate leukocyte populations in piglets surviving in utero infection with PRRSv, but did not characterize leukocyte populations in sows. Christianson et al. [7] investigated peripheral blood leukocytes in sows experimentally infected with PRRSv in mid-gestation. A significant decrease in total leukocytes was found at 3 and 7 days post infection (dpi) and was

* Correspondence: andrea.ladinig@vetmeduni.ac.at
[1]Department of Large Animal Clinical Sciences, Western College of Veterinary Medicine, University of Saskatchewan, Saskatoon, SK, Canada
[4]Current address: University Clinic for Swine, Department for Farm Animals and Veterinary Public Health, University of Veterinary Medicine Vienna, Veterinaerplatz 1, 1210 Vienna, Austria
Full list of author information is available at the end of the article

most pronounced at 7 dpi. Absolute numbers of CD172a$^+$ cells, CD1$^+$ cells, CD4$^+$ and CD8α^+ T cells were significantly decreased compared to non-infected controls at 3 to 7 dpi; cell counts returned to control levels by 14 dpi [7].

As there are few reports describing changes in PBMC populations in late term pregnant sows or gilts following PRRSv infection, and no studies correlated changes in subpopulations with clinical outcome, the objectives of the present study were to: 1) characterize changes in the major PBMC subpopulations (monocytes, NK cells, B and T cells) of third trimester pregnant gilts following PRRSv infection; 2) analyze phenotypic changes of the major T cell populations ($\gamma\delta$ T cells, T helper cells and cytolytic T cells (CTL)) following PRRSv infection; 3) investigate relationships between PBMC subpopulations and viral load in gilt serum and tissues; 4) investigate relationships between PBMC subpopulations and fetal mortality rate defined at the level of the gilt as percent dead fetuses per litter.

Materials and methods
Experimental procedures and sample collection
The experimental protocol is described in detail in Ladinig et al. [8]. Briefly, on experimental day 0 (0 days post inoculation; dpi), 114 pregnant Landrace gilts (gestation day 85 ($\pm$1)) split over 12 replicates were inoculated (INOC) with PRRSv isolate NVSL 97–7895 (1×10^5 TCID$_{50}$; 2 mL intramuscularly and 1 mL into each nostril), while 19 control gilts were similarly sham inoculated (CTRL). Heparinized blood samples were collected on 0, 2, 6, and 19 dpi, and sera on 0, 2, 6, and 21 dpi. Automated white blood cell (WBC) counts (Z2 Coulter Particle Count and Size Analyzer, Beckman Coulter Inc., FL, USA) and manual differential counts were performed (300 cells total) on heparinized blood samples. On 21 dpi (gestation day 106 ± 1), gilts were humanely euthanized and necropsied. Fetal preservation status was recorded and the percent dead fetuses were calculated for each litter. Samples of lung, tonsil, reproductive (*Lnn. uterini*) and tracheobronchial lymph node from each gilt, as well as a sample of the uterus including adherent fetal placental layers adjacent to the umbilical stump of each fetus were collected and immediately frozen at –80 °C until further processing. The experiment was approved by the University of Saskatchewan's Animal Research Ethics Board, and adhered to the Canadian Council on Animal Care guidelines for humane animal use (permit #20110102).

Isolation of PBMC and FCM staining
PBMC were isolated from whole blood samples by gradient centrifugation using lymphocyte separation medium (Ficoll-Paque™ PLUS, GE Healthcare, Mississauga, ON,

Canada). Isolated PBMC were counted and transferred into staining buffer (PBS +0.2% gelatin +0.03% sodium azide).

For phenotypic analyses of PBMC, 5 sets of marker panels to detect surface antigens were used in two- or three-color labelling. Table 1 summarizes monoclonal antibodies (mAbs) used to characterize different PBMC subsets. Where commercially available, directly conjugated mAbs were used; otherwise, mAbs specific for CD8β, swine leukocyte antigen-DR (SLA-DR), and the $\gamma\delta$ T cell receptor (TCR), produced from hybridoma supernatants at the Institute of Immunology, University of Veterinary Medicine Vienna, Austria, were used in combination with fluorochrome-conjugated, isotype-specific secondary Abs (Table 1). Isotype-matched non-specific antibodies were used as negative controls. PBMC staining was performed in U-bottom 96-well microtiter plates (1×10^6 cells per well). All incubations were performed on ice in the dark. Mastermixes of primary Abs were prepared and 30 µL was added to each well prior to the first 20 min incubation step. After two washes in 200 µL of staining buffer, mastermixes of secondary Abs (10 µL per well) were added and cells were incubated for another 20 min. Finally, cells were washed twice in staining buffer and fixed by resuspension in 200 µL of 2% formaldehyde solution (PBS +2% formaldehyde solution (formaldehyde 37 wt % solution in water stabilized with 7-8% methanol, Alfar Aesar, Ward Hill, MA, USA)).

To stain the intracellular epitope recognized by the CD79α-specific mAb HM57, cells were fixed and permeabilized using a commercial kit (BD Cytofix/Cytoperm, BD Biosciences, Mississauga, ON, Canada) according to the manufacturer's instructions.

Prior to incubation and after each wash step, cells were resuspended using a plate shaker. For compensation controls, single-stain samples were prepared for each fluorochrome.

FCM analyses
Stained cells were analyzed using a FACSCalibur flow cytometer (BD Biosciences, Mississauga, ON) equipped with 2 lasers (488 and 635 nm). At least 5×10^4 cells were collected per sample. Results were analyzed using FlowJo, version 7.6.5 (Tree Star, Inc., Ashland, Oregon, USA). Gates were set according to isotype controls and fluorescence minus one (FMO) control samples [9]. The same gate position was used for all samples with a particular marker combination. Cell numbers for each population were corrected by subtracting the number of cells stained by isotype-matched non-specific antibodies. Automated WBC counts and manual differential counts (total number of lymphocytes plus total number of monocytes) were used to calculate the absolute numbers of different PBMC subsets.

Table 1 Antibodies used for flow cytometry analyses

Antigen	Clone	Isotype	Source	Fluorochrome	Secondary Ab
T-helper cells					
CD3	BB23-8E6-8C8	IgG2a	BD Biosciences	PerCP-Cy5.5	
CD4	74-12-4	IgG2b	BD Biosciences	FITC	
CD8α	76-2-11	IgG2a	BD Biosciences	Alexa647	
Cytolytic T cells					
CD3	BB23-8E6	IgG2b	Southern Biotech	FITC	
CD8β	PPT23	IgG1	In-house		goat anti-mouse IgG1, Alexa647 (Invitrogen)
SLA-DR	MSA3	IgG2a	In-house		goat anti-mouse IgG2a, PE (Southern Biotech)
γδ T cells					
Pan-γδ	PPT16	IgG2b	In-house		goat anti-mouse IgG2b, Alexa488 (Invitrogen)
CD2	RPA-2.10	IgG1	AbD Serotec	PE	
CD8α	76-2-11	IgG2a	BD Biosciences	Alexa647	
NK cells					
CD3	BB23-8E6-8C8	IgG2a	BD Biosciences	PerCP-Cy5.5	
CD8α	76-2-11	IgG2a	BD Biosciences	Alexa647	
B cells					
CD21	B-ly4	IgG1	BD	APC	
CD79α	HM57	IgG1	Dako	PE	
Monocytes					
CD172a	74-22-15	IgG1	Southern Biotech	PE	
CD4	74-12-4	IgG2b	BD Biosciences	Alexa647	
CD14	MIL-2	IgG2b	AbD Serotec	FITC	

Quantification of PRRSv RNA

PRRSv RNA concentrations were measured in gilt serum collected on 0, 2, 6 and 21 dpi (target $\log_{10}$ copies/μL), and in tissues collected at termination (21 dpi) (target $\log_{10}$ copies/mg), by strain-specific in-house quantitative reverse transcription polymerase chain reaction (qRT-PCR) as previously described [8].

Statistical analysis

Separate statistical analyses were conducted using Stata 13 (STATA Corp, College Station, Texas, USA) to address each of the objectives. To meet the key model assumptions, data were log-transformed ($\log$ base$_{10}$) as appropriate. Firstly, to determine if major PBMC subpopulations, including major T cell populations, differed between INOC and CTRL gilts over time, multilevel mixed-effects linear regression models were developed. These models used gilt as a random effect and accounted for repeated measures by day. All remaining analyses used data from INOC gilts only. Secondly, potential relationships between PBMC subsets (major PBMC subpopulations and major T cell populations) and PRRS viral load in serum and tissues were analyzed. For these analyses, multilevel

mixed-effects linear regression models controlling for experimental replicate were used. Area under the curve (AUC) from 0 to 19/21 dpi was calculated for PRRSv RNA concentration in serum (target copies/μL) and for the total number of each PBMC subset (cells $\times 10^9$/liter) using the formula AUC = $(t_1-t_0)(a_1 + a_0)/2 + (t_2-t_1)(a_1 + a_2)/2 + ... + (t_n-t_{n-1})(a_{n-1} + a_n)/2$. The final objective, to determine potential associations between the AUC of PBMC subsets and fetal mortality rate (represented as the percentage of dead fetuses per litter), was analysed using multilevel mixed-effects linear regression models controlling for experimental replicate. To account for multiple comparisons, all associations were considered statistically significant if $P < 0.01$. All final models were evaluated to ensure normality and homoscedasticity of residuals.

Results

Changes in total leukocytes and major PBMC subpopulations in response to PRRSv infection

One gilt died (11 dpi) and two gilts aborted (17 dpi, 20 dpi) after PRRSv inoculation; results from those three gilts were excluded from further analysis. Thus, data is presented on 111 INOC and 19 CTRL gilts. With the exception of reduced feed intake and increased rectal temperatures in individual gilts, no severe clinical signs were observed following infection.

Changes in total leukocyte numbers in INOC and CTRL gilts following PRRSv infection are displayed in Figure 1. Total leukocyte numbers in INOC gilts decreased 45% from 0 dpi ($11.0 \pm 1.8 \times 10^9$/L) to 2 dpi ($6.1 \pm 2.3 \times 10^9$/L) ($P < 0.001$). Values returned to pre-inoculation levels on 19 dpi. Neutrophil counts (data not displayed in figures) were also significantly decreased in INOC compared to CTRL on 6 dpi (INOC: $2.3 \pm 0.9 \times 10^9$/L, CTRL: $3.2 \pm 1.3 \times 10^9$/L, $P = 0.002$) and trended to increase on 19 dpi (INOC: $4.1 \pm 2.0 \times 10^9$/L, CTRL: $3.0 \pm 1.6 \times 10^9$/L, $P = 0.018$).

Monocytes were identified by a $CD172a^{high}CD4^-CD14^+$ phenotype (Figure 2A). Total numbers were significantly decreased in INOC gilts compared to CTRL on 2 dpi ($P < 0.001$) and 6 dpi ($P = 008$) (Figure 2B). Since there was a significant increase in the percentage of monocytes within PBMC from INOC gilts on D2 (Figure 2C), the drop in absolute numbers was less severe compared to other PBMC subpopulations (see below). Absolute numbers of monocytes on 19 dpi trended to increase in INOC compared to CTRL gilts ($P = 0.045$) (Figure 2B).

NK cells were identified by a $CD3^-CD8\alpha^+$ phenotype (Figure 3A). Their absolute numbers were highly variable in both INOC and CTRL groups. Compared to CTRL gilts, INOC gilts had significantly greater NK cells numbers on 0 dpi ($P = 0.005$), then showed a significant decrease on 2 dpi ($P < 0.001$) and 6 dpi ($P = 0.009$) followed by an increase on 19 dpi that trended towards significance ($P = 0.015$) (Figure 3B). The drop in NK cells from 0 dpi

($0.22 \pm 0.1 \times 10^9$/L) to 2 dpi ($0.05 \pm 0.04 \times 10^9$/L) represented a 73% decrease compared to 0 dpi counts, the most prominent drop of any major PBMC subpopulation.

Total B cells were identified by a $CD79\alpha^+$ phenotype (Figure 4A, turquois gate). Their absolute counts also decreased significantly on 2 dpi and 6 dpi ($P < 0.001$) in INOC gilts compared to CTRL (Figure 4B). In contrast to the remaining PBMC subpopulations, total B cells did not rebound on 6 dpi, but rather continued to decrease when compared to 2 dpi ($0.57 \pm 0.2 \times 10^9$/L on 2 dpi; $0.66 \pm 0.3 \times 10^9$/L on 6 dpi), before rebounding to pre-inoculation values on 19 dpi. CD21-defined B cell subpopulations, which can be used to distinguish naïve and activated from effector and memory B cells [10], were also studied (Figure 4A, purple and pink gates). Both B cell subpopulations, $CD21^-CD79\alpha^+$ (Figure 4C) and $CD21^+CD79\alpha^+$ (Figure 4D), were affected. $CD21^+$ B cells decreased more rapidly and severely than $CD21^-$ B cells, with their absolute numbers dropping to 35% of 0 dpi values by 2 dpi (Figure 4D). By contrast, the $CD21^-$ B cell subpopulation in INOC gilts decreased to only 91% and 70% of 0 dpi counts by 2 dpi and 6 dpi respectively, and trended higher than CTRL on 19 dpi ($P = 0.031$) (Figure 4C). In INOC gilts, the percentage of B cells expressing CD21 was significantly lower at all time points after infection compared to 0 dpi (Figure 4E).

Total T cells were identified by a $CD3^+$ phenotype (Figure 5A). Their absolute numbers decreased significantly in INOC compared to CTRL gilts on 2 dpi ($P < 0.001$), and trended lower on 6 dpi ($P = 0.013$) (Figure 5B). Three subpopulations of T cells, namely γδ T cells, T helper cells, and cytolytic T cells (CTLs), were analyzed in more detail.

γδ T cells

γδ T cells, identified by a mAb recognizing a CD3 molecule associated with the TCR-γδ (clone PPT16) [11], were analyzed for the expression of CD2 and CD8α. This lead to the identification of three distinct phenotypes: $CD2^-CD8\alpha^-$, $CD2^-CD8\alpha^+$, and $CD2^+CD8\alpha^+$ γδ T cells (Figure 6A). Absolute numbers of γδ T cells dropped 45% from 0 to 2 dpi in INOC gilts; 2 dpi counts were significantly lower than in CTRL gilts ($P < 0.001$) (Figure 6B). All three subpopulations showed a significant decrease on 2 dpi compared to CTRL gilts ($P < 0.001$) (Figure 6C to E). While absolute numbers of $CD2^-CD8\alpha^-$ γδ T (Figure 6C) and $CD2^-CD8\alpha^+$ (Figure 6D) γδ T cells did not differ significantly between INOC and CTRL on 6 and 19 dpi, $CD2^+CD8\alpha^+$ γδ T cells (Figure 6E) were significantly lower in INOC on 6 dpi ($P < 0.001$) and also trended lower on 19 dpi ($P = 0.028$). While the percentage of the $CD2^-CD8\alpha^-$ phenotype increased significantly in INOC gilts after infection (Figure 6F), the percentages of both $CD2^-CD8\alpha^+$ (Figure 6G) and $CD2^+CD8\alpha^+$

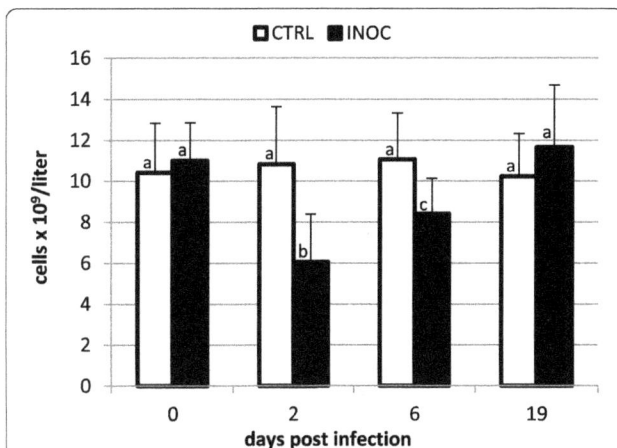

Figure 1 Changes in total leukocyte counts in response to PRRSv infection in pregnant gilts. Mean (+SD) total leukocyte counts are presented from 111 INOC and 19 CTRL gilts for the respective study days. Superscript letters indicate significant differences ($P < 0.001$) between INOC and CTRL gilts and between study days within each treatment group.

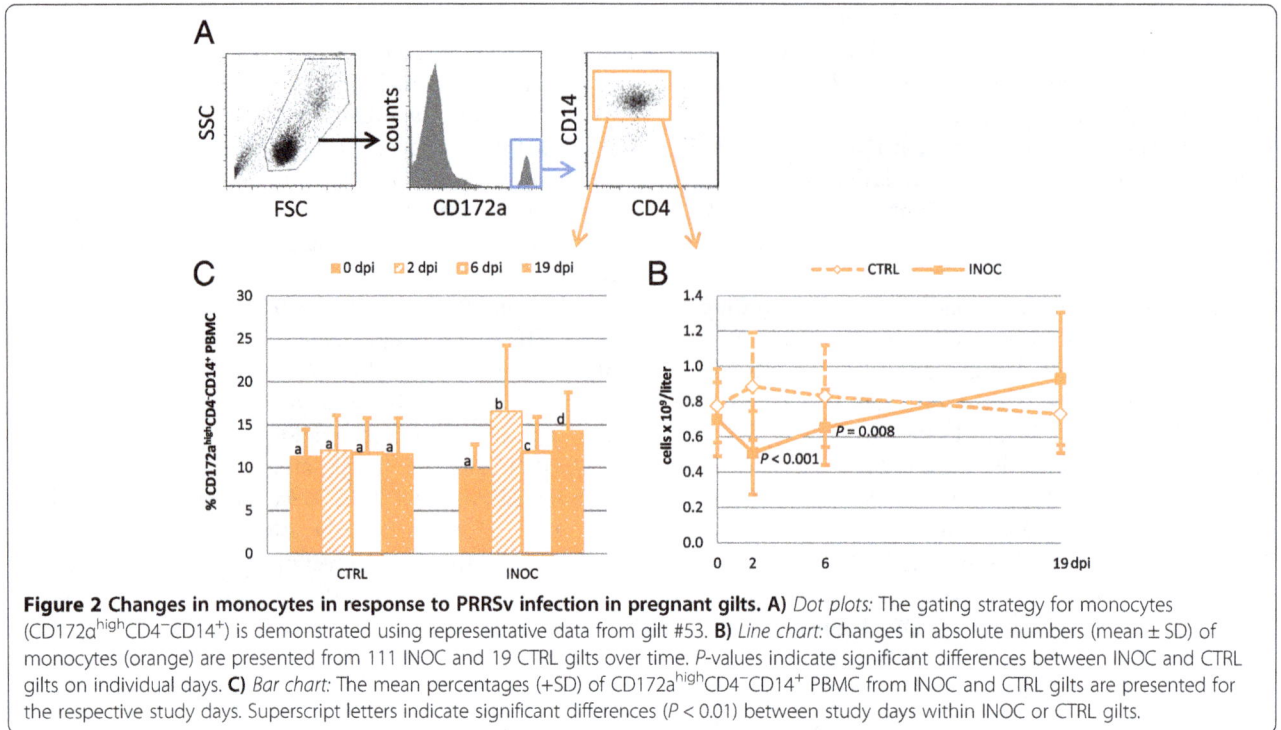

Figure 2 Changes in monocytes in response to PRRSv infection in pregnant gilts. A) *Dot plots:* The gating strategy for monocytes (CD172a^high CD4^−CD14^+) is demonstrated using representative data from gilt #53. **B)** *Line chart:* Changes in absolute numbers (mean ± SD) of monocytes (orange) are presented from 111 INOC and 19 CTRL gilts over time. *P*-values indicate significant differences between INOC and CTRL gilts on individual days. **C)** *Bar chart:* The mean percentages (+SD) of CD172a^high CD4^−CD14^+ PBMC from INOC and CTRL gilts are presented for the respective study days. Superscript letters indicate significant differences (*P* < 0.01) between study days within INOC or CTRL gilts.

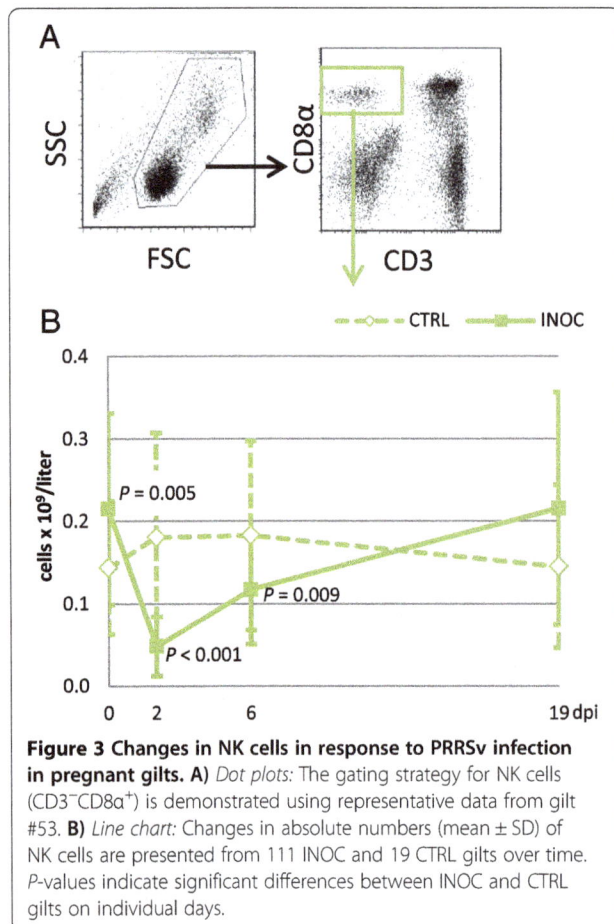

Figure 3 Changes in NK cells in response to PRRSv infection in pregnant gilts. A) *Dot plots:* The gating strategy for NK cells (CD3^−CD8α^+) is demonstrated using representative data from gilt #53. **B)** *Line chart:* Changes in absolute numbers (mean ± SD) of NK cells are presented from 111 INOC and 19 CTRL gilts over time. *P*-values indicate significant differences between INOC and CTRL gilts on individual days.

(Figure 6H) γδ T cells were significantly decreased in INOC gilts.

T helper cells

Absolute T helper cells, identified by a CD3^+CD4^+ phenotype (Figure 7A, yellow gate), were significantly decreased in INOC gilts on 2 dpi ($P < 0.001$) and trended lower on 6 dpi ($P = 0.044$) compared to CTRL (Figure 7B). To investigate their activation/memory status [11], expression of CD8α was analyzed (Figure 7A, brown and light blue gates). Compared to CRTL, INOC gilts had numerically increased numbers of CD8α^− T helper cells on 0 dpi ($P = 0.033$), but numbers decreased significantly on 2 dpi ($P < 0.001$) (Figure 7C). The decrease in CD8α^− T helper cells in INOC gilts was substantial with counts dropping to 22% ($0.22 \pm 0.1 \times 10^9$/L) of 0 dpi counts. Absolute numbers of CD8α^+ T helper cells were significantly lower in INOC gilts on 2 dpi ($P < 0.001$) and 6 dpi ($P = 0.003$), and trended lower on 19 dpi ($P = 0.021$) compared to CTRL gilts (Figure 7D). However, given the percentage of T helper cells expressing CD8α increased significantly on 2 dpi (Figure 7E), the drop in total T helper cells on 2 dpi to 42% of the 0 dpi counts was over represented by the CD8α^− phenotype, rather than the CD8α^+ phenotype.

CTLs

Absolute numbers of CTLs, defined as CD3^+CD8β^+ (Figure 8A, blue gate), were significantly decreased in

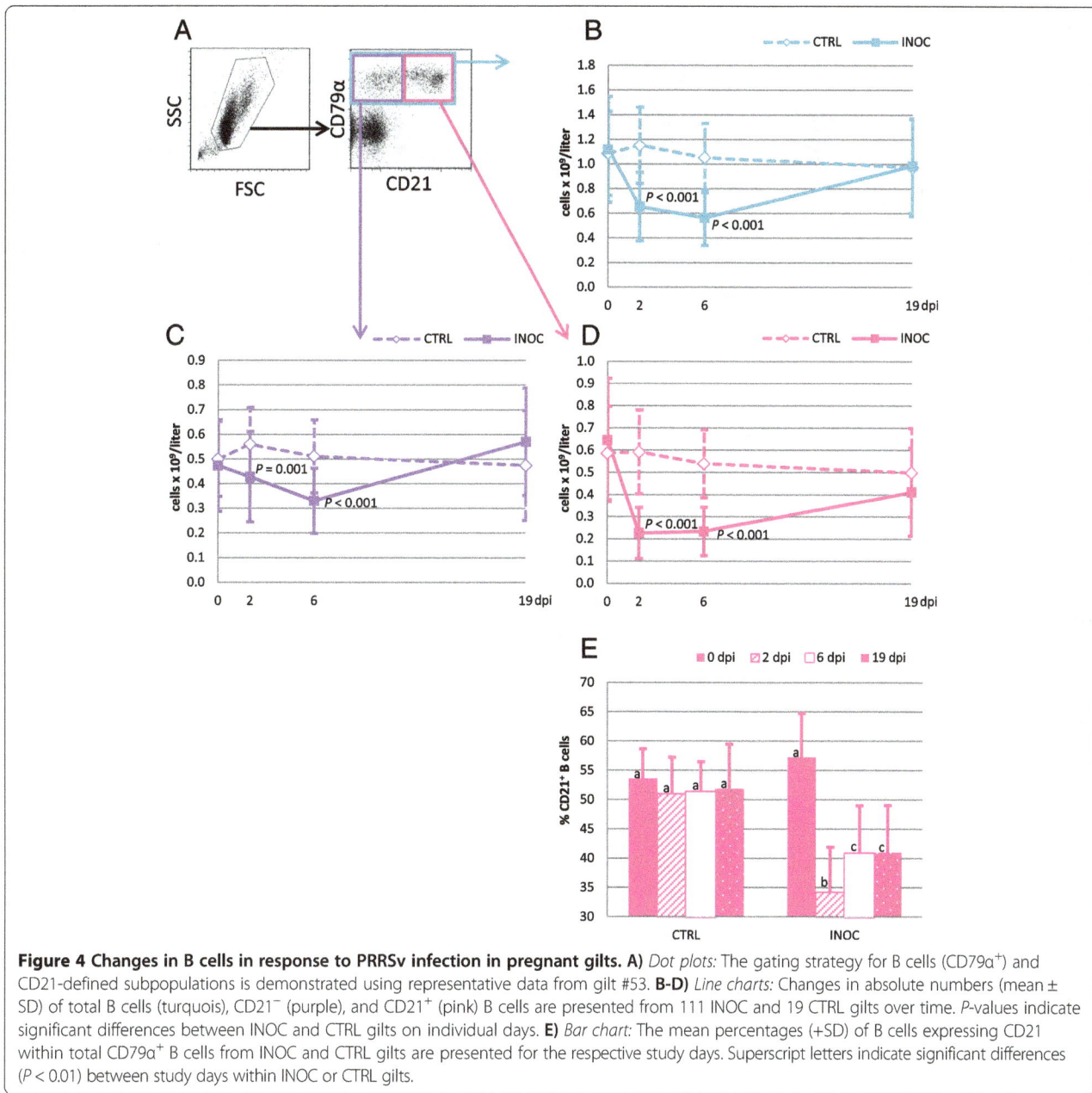

Figure 4 Changes in B cells in response to PRRSv infection in pregnant gilts. A) *Dot plots:* The gating strategy for B cells (CD79α⁺) and CD21-defined subpopulations is demonstrated using representative data from gilt #53. **B-D)** *Line charts:* Changes in absolute numbers (mean ± SD) of total B cells (turquois), CD21⁻ (purple), and CD21⁺ (pink) B cells are presented from 111 INOC and 19 CTRL gilts over time. *P*-values indicate significant differences between INOC and CTRL gilts on individual days. **E)** *Bar chart:* The mean percentages (+SD) of B cells expressing CD21 within total CD79α⁺ B cells from INOC and CTRL gilts are presented for the respective study days. Superscript letters indicate significant differences (*P* < 0.01) between study days within INOC or CTRL gilts.

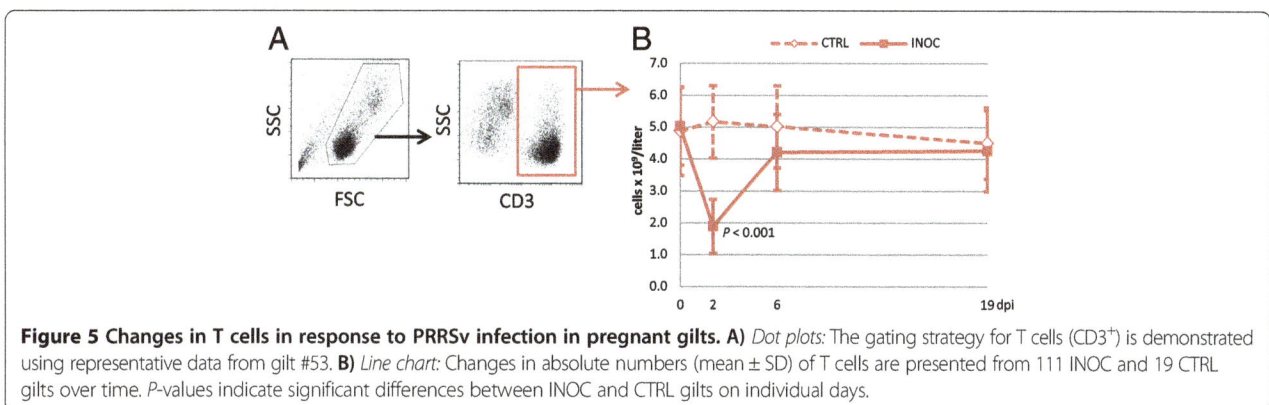

Figure 5 Changes in T cells in response to PRRSv infection in pregnant gilts. A) *Dot plots:* The gating strategy for T cells (CD3⁺) is demonstrated using representative data from gilt #53. **B)** *Line chart:* Changes in absolute numbers (mean ± SD) of T cells are presented from 111 INOC and 19 CTRL gilts over time. *P*-values indicate significant differences between INOC and CTRL gilts on individual days.

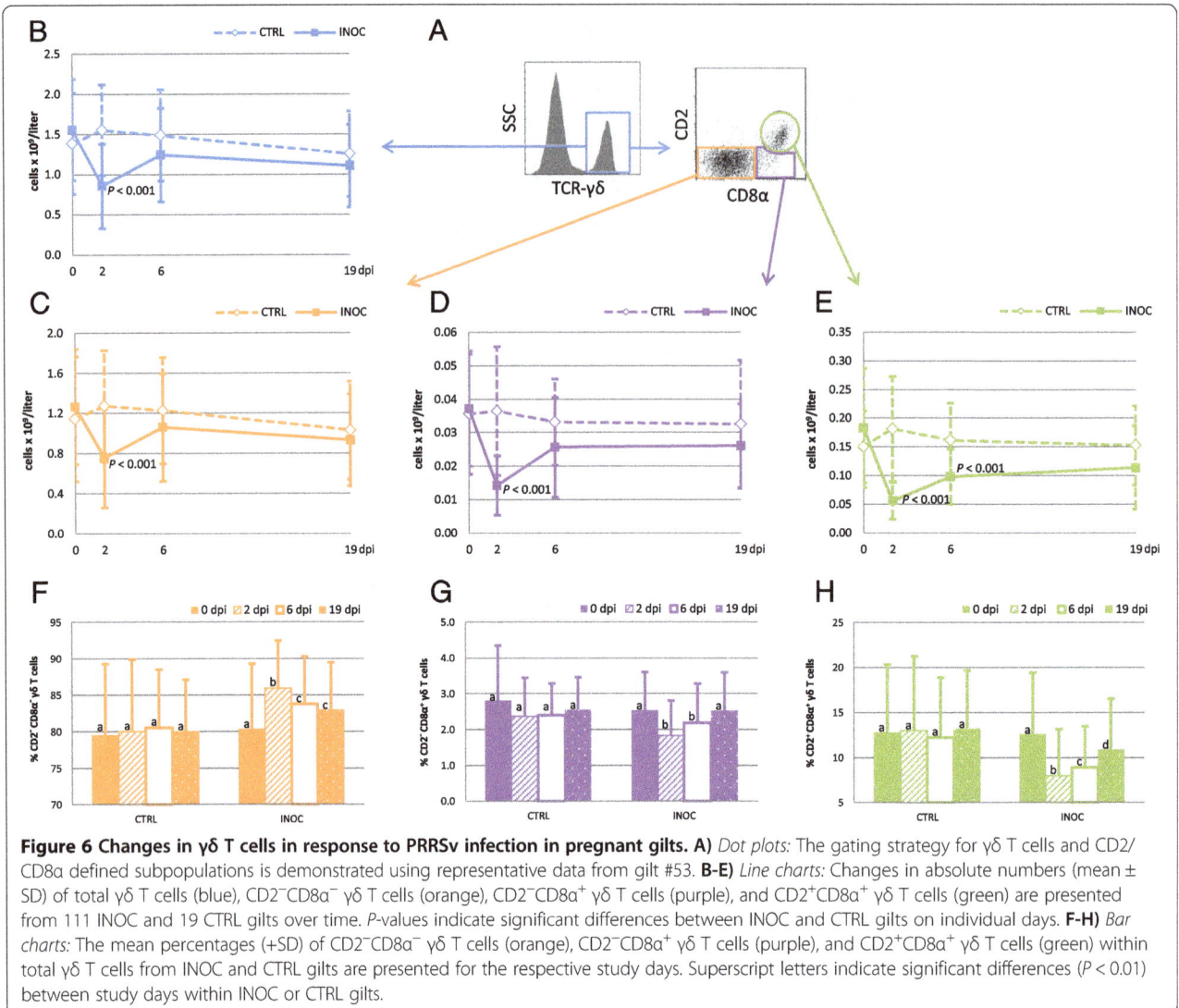

Figure 6 Changes in γδ T cells in response to PRRSv infection in pregnant gilts. **A)** *Dot plots:* The gating strategy for γδ T cells and CD2/CD8α defined subpopulations is demonstrated using representative data from gilt #53. **B-E)** *Line charts:* Changes in absolute numbers (mean ± SD) of total γδ T cells (blue), CD2⁻CD8α⁻ γδ T cells (orange), CD2⁻CD8α⁺ γδ T cells (purple), and CD2⁺CD8α⁺ γδ T cells (green) are presented from 111 INOC and 19 CTRL gilts over time. *P*-values indicate significant differences between INOC and CTRL gilts on individual days. **F-H)** *Bar charts:* The mean percentages (+SD) of CD2⁻CD8α⁻ γδ T cells (orange), CD2⁻CD8α⁺ γδ T cells (purple), and CD2⁺CD8α⁺ γδ T cells (green) within total γδ T cells from INOC and CTRL gilts are presented for the respective study days. Superscript letters indicate significant differences ($P < 0.01$) between study days within INOC or CTRL gilts.

INOC gilts compared to CTRL on 2 dpi ($P < 0.001$) and trended lower on 6 dpi ($P = 0.013$) (Figure 8B). 2 dpi CTL counts in INOC gilts were 77% lower ($0.30 \pm 0.2 \times 10^9$/L) compared to 0 dpi counts. CTLs were further analyzed for the expression of SLA-DR, suggested as a potential marker for activation and antigen encounter [11]. Absolute numbers of SLA-DR⁺ CTLs showed a similar trend and were significantly lower in INOC gilts on 2 dpi ($P < 0.001$) (Figure 8C). Although the percentage of CTLs expressing SLA-DR did not significantly change in CTRL gilts, in INOC gilts the percentage increased significantly to varying degrees on each study day following PRRS infection (Figure 8D). When analyzing the mean fluorescence intensity (MFI) of the three surface markers identified on CTLs, no changes were observed for CD3 (data not shown). The MFI of CD8β decreased significantly from 0 to 2 dpi in both INOC and CTRL gilts ($P < 0.001$), but the drop was more distinct in INOC

(Figure 8E). On the other hand, the MFI of SLA-DR significantly increased in INOC gilts on 2 and 6 dpi (Figure 8F), but decreased in CTRL.

Associations between PBMC subpopulations and PRRS outcome

Detailed results on viral loads (gilt serum and tissues) and on fetal preservation can be found in Ladinig et al. [8]. Briefly, all INOC gilts were viremic on 2 and 6 dpi, and 94/111 (84.7%) remained viremic until termination. The percentages of tissues that tested positive by PRRSv qRT-PCR at termination (21 dpi) in INOC gilts were 90, 99, 99, and 100 for lung, tonsil, tracheobronchial lymph node and reproductive lymph node, respectively. The mean viral loads of positive samples were 3.5 ± 1.2 $\log_{10}$ RNA copies/mg in lung, 5.6 ± 0.8 $\log_{10}$ RNA copies/mg in tonsil, 5.8 ± 0.8 $\log_{10}$ RNA copies/mg in reproductive lymph node, and 4.8 ± 0.9 $\log_{10}$ RNA copies/mg in

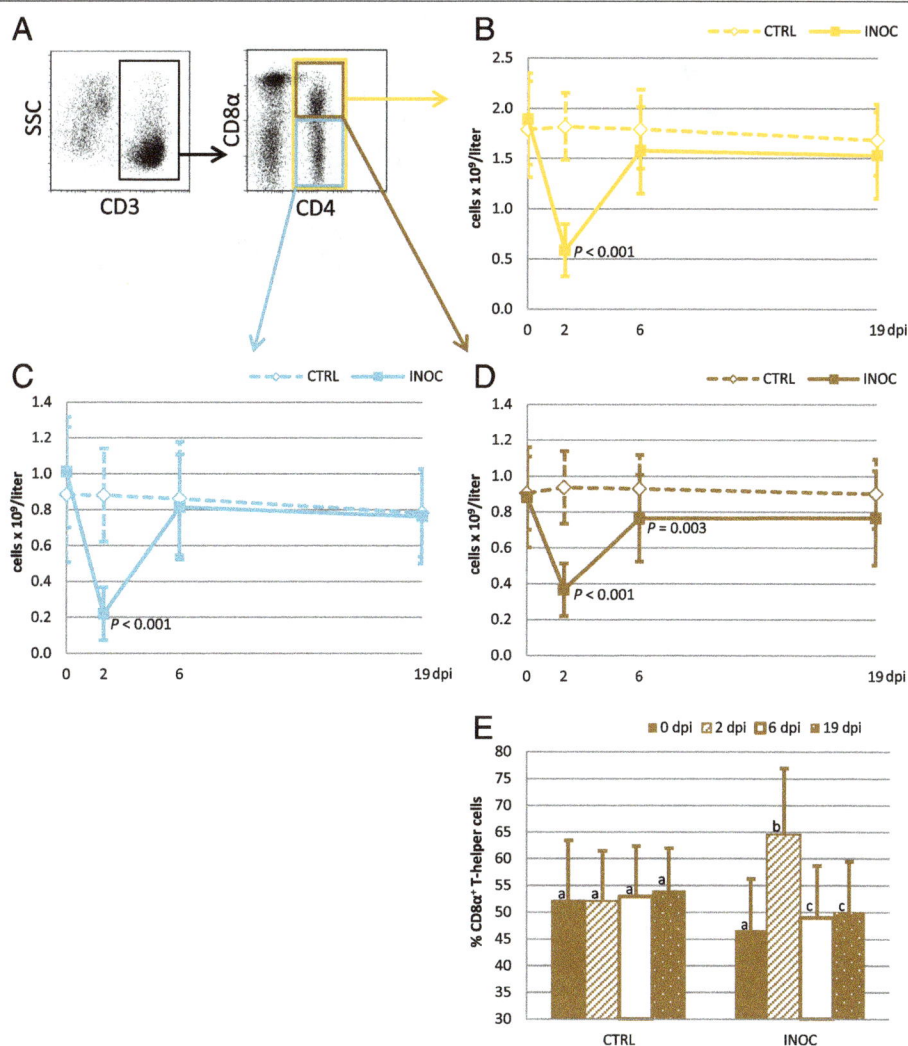

Figure 7 Changes in T helper cells in response to PRRSv infection in pregnant gilts. A) *Dot plots:* The gating strategy for T helper cells (CD4[+]) and CD8α-defined subpopulations is demonstrated using representative data from gilt #53. **B-D)** *Line charts:* Changes in absolute numbers (mean ± SD) of total T helper cells (yellow), CD8α[−] T helper cells (light blue), and CD8α[+] T helper cells (brown) are presented from 111 INOC and 19 CTRL gilts over time. *P*-values indicate significant differences between INOC and CTRL gilts on individual days. **E)** *Bar chart:* The mean percentages (+SD) of T helper cells expressing CD8α within total CD4[+] T cells from INOC and CTRL gilts are presented for the respective study days. Superscript letters indicate significant differences (*P* < 0.01) between study days within INOC or CTRL gilts.

tracheobronchial lymph node. In INOC gilts, the percentage of dead fetuses ranged from 0% to 94.4% (mean 41.0 ± 22.8%).

The total numbers (AUC) from 0 to 19 for monocytes, NK cells, B cells, total T cells, γδ T cells, T helper cells, and CTLs were used to test possible associations with viral load (AUC) and fetal mortality rate. None of the cell subsets were associated with viral load in any gilt tissue. Viral load (AUC) in gilt serum was negatively associated with total T cells ($\beta = -0.140$, $P = 0.007$) and total γδ T cells ($\beta = -0.236$, $P = 0.009$) over time. None of the analyzed PBMC populations were significantly associated with the percentage of dead fetuses per litter. Total T

helper cells (AUC) however, trended to be negatively associated with fetal mortality rate ($\beta = -0.743$, $P = 0.048$).

Discussion

The results presented are part of an extensive and complex dataset obtained in a large scale, multi-institutional project aimed at finding phenotypic and genotypic predictors of PRRSv resistance in pregnant gilts. To investigate genotypic variation in the severity of reproductive PRRS, a large number of gilts were experimentally inoculated in the third trimester of gestation. The number of CTRL gilts was reduced to the minimum to provide baseline data. The objectives of this present study were

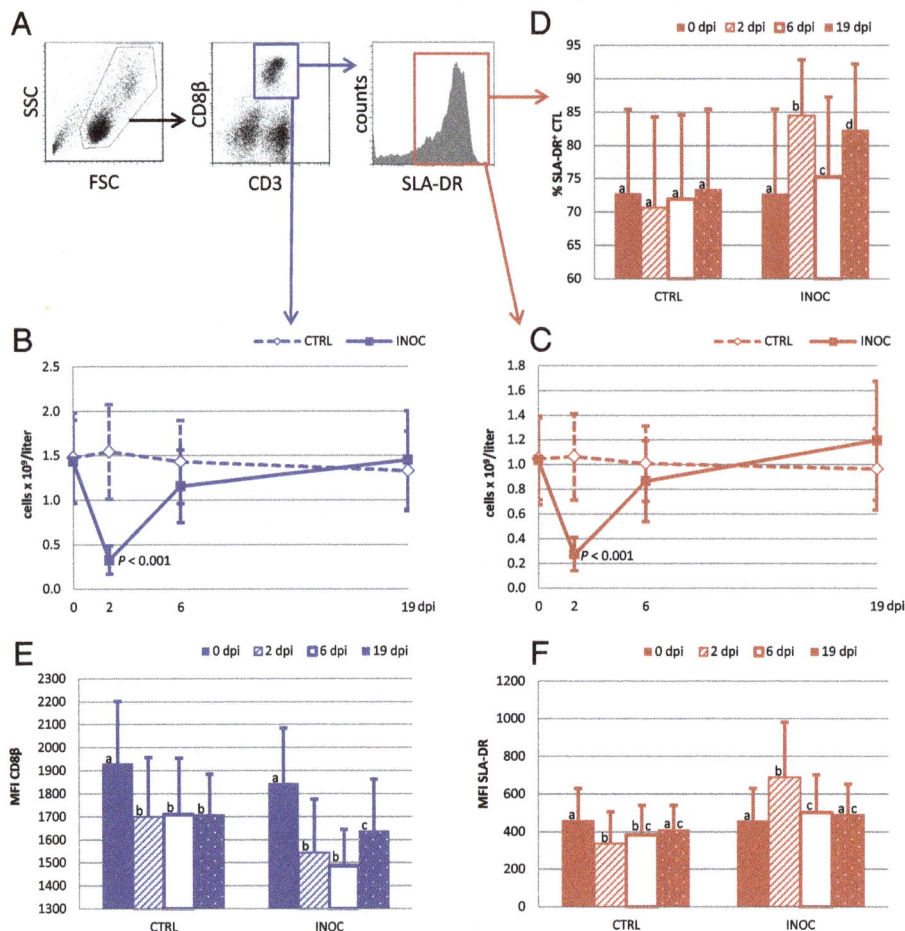

Figure 8 Changes in CTLs in response to PRRSv infection in pregnant gilts. A) *Dot plots:* The gating strategy for CTLs (CD3+CD8β+) and SLA-DR-defined subpopulations is demonstrated using representative data from gilt #53. **B-C)** *Line charts:* Changes in absolute numbers (mean ± SD) of total CTLs (blue) and SLA-DR+ CTLs (red) are presented from 111 INOC and 19 CTRL gilts over time. *P*-values indicate significant differences between INOC and CTRL gilts on individual days. **D)** *Bar chart:* The mean percentages (+SD) of CTLs expressing SLA-DR within total CTLs from INOC and CTRL gilts are presented for the respective study days. Superscript letters indicate significant differences (*P* < 0.01) between study days within INOC or CTRL gilts. **E-F)** *Bar charts:* The MFIs of CD8β and SLA-DR on CTLs from INOC and CTRL gilts are presented for the respective study days. Superscript letters indicate significant differences (*P* < 0.01) between study days within INOC or CTRL gilts.

to investigate temporal changes in the major PBMC and T cell populations and to determine possible associations with measures of PRRS outcome in a reproductive model.

A massive drop in total leukocyte counts was detected early after infection (2 dpi) in all INOC gilts to varying degrees. Leukocyte counts in INOC gilts started to rebound by 6 dpi. Leukopenia has been demonstrated in several other swine viral infections including African swine fever virus (ASFv) [12], classical swine fever virus (CSFv) [13], pseudorabies virus (PRv) [14], and porcine circovirus type 2 (PCV2) [15]. In both ASF and CSF the leukopenia which mainly involved lymphocytes, occurred during the first week after infection and was associated with necrosis and apoptosis of cells [12,13]. Similarly, a significant drop in lymphocytes between 3 and 7 dpi and probably due to apoptosis, was found in

pigs infected with H1N2 swine influenza virus. However, the lymphopenia was not accompanied by a drop in total leukocytes [16]. On the other hand, acute PRv infection induced leukopenia involved the loss of up to 40% of monocytes and up to 50% of lymphocytes; the authors hypothesized that besides the killing of infected cells, trafficking of effector cells from the circulation to sites of local infection also contributed to the observed leukopenia [14].

The specific mechanisms associated with the leukopenia observed in this study are speculative and cannot be answered with the current dataset; still this study provides several insightful findings. PRRSv induced apoptosis and necrosis of PRRSv-infected and non-infected bystander cells has previously been reported [17-21]. Cells affected by PRRSv induced apoptosis were mainly macrophages and mononuclear cells, as well as epithelial cells [17,20].

Recently, it was demonstrated that apoptotic cells in thymuses of PRRSv-infected fetuses were predominantly CD3$^+$ T cells [22]. Although apoptosis and necrosis might be one possible explanation for the observed leukopenia, in most studies apoptosis and necrosis were observed after 6 dpi [17,20,23]. Moreover, PRRSv was reported to activate anti-apoptotic pathways in macrophages early in in vitro infection models, while PRRSv-infected macrophages die by apoptosis late in infection [21]. For these reasons and given the acuteness of the response and rebound, the authors believe that apoptosis or necrosis of PBMC is unlikely. Moreover, there are no reports in the literature providing evidence of PRRSv replication within lymphocytes.

Therefore, another possible explanation for the leukopenia detected in the present study is an altered trafficking pattern of leukocyte subsets. Interestingly, the current immunological paradigm is that only effector and effector memory cells traffic into non-lymphoid tissue [24]. However, it also is conceivable that PRRSv infection affects entry and exit of lymphocytes from affected lymph nodes as was shown by early experiments in sheep treated with model antigens [25,26]. Obviously, sites of leukocyte migration in our infection model are currently speculative and need to be investigated in future experiments.

The primary sites of PRRSv replication are lung and lymphoid tissues [27]. PRRSv has a tropism to macrophages expressing the receptors sialoadhesin (Sn) and CD163 [28,29]. In the present study, monocytes significantly decreased in INOC gilts on 2 and 6 dpi. However, the drop in absolute numbers was less severe compared to other PBMC subsets. Similar to our findings, Dwivedi et al. [30] reported the frequency of CD172a$^+$ cells in PBMC to be significantly decreased 2 days after infection of 7 week-old piglets. A more recent study determined that changes in the absolute numbers of monocytes in PRRSv infected, 6 week-old piglets were virus strain dependent, particularly in the first 2 weeks post-infection. However, at 21 dpi piglets infected with all strains of PRRSv showed significantly increased numbers of monocytes compared to uninfected controls [31]. In the present study, a similar trend of increased monocytes on 19 dpi was observed in INOC gilts.

A prominent drop in NK cells was measured in inoculated gilts early after PRRSv infection. As members of the innate immune system, NK cells possess germ-line encoded, invariant receptors recognizing molecules on the surface of infected or malignantly transformed cells. This makes them particularly important in the early phase of viral infections [32,33]. In contrast to our findings, absolute numbers of NK cells were significantly increased at 2 dpi in 7 week-old piglets in direct contact with pen mates infected with type 2 PRRSv (strain MN 1-18-2). In the same experiment, NK cell numbers were not significantly increased in inoculated piglets [30]. An increase in absolute NK cell numbers was also detected at 10 and 35 dpi in 6 week-old piglets infected with certain European PRRSv isolates [31]. In contrast to European subtype 1 strains, the subtype 3 strain Lena did not induce an increase in NK cell numbers until 35 dpi, rather showing numerically decreased NK cell numbers until 10 dpi. This agrees with our findings. The differences in NK responses among these experiments might be caused by the different virus isolates used, since the results of Weesendorp et al. [31] clearly demonstrated that absolute numbers of NK cells vary between pigs infected with different virus strains.

We detected no association between viral load in gilt tissues and absolute numbers of major PBMC subpopulations or major T cell populations over time. However, increased absolute T cell and γδ T cell counts over time were associated with decreased viral load in gilt serum. This may be relevant for the control of PRRS by selection strategies for breeding programs.

B cells, T helper cells and CTLs with an effector or memory phenotype (CD21$^-$, CD8α$^+$, SLA-DR$^+$, respectively) were less affected by the drop in absolute counts after PRRSv infection. Studies investigating B cell responses towards PRRSv infection mainly measured Ab responses in serum of infected pigs. Only a few reports investigated B cells by FCM; results are somewhat difficult to compare due to differences in marker selection used to define B cells. Nevertheless, Christianson et al. [7] found absolute numbers of CD1$^+$ lymphocytes (which represent about 70% of CD79α$^+$ B cells; Gerner, unpublished findings) significantly decreased in PRRSv inoculated, mid-gestation sows 7 dpi, which is in accordance with our findings.

Similar to CD21$^-$ B cells, total numbers of CD4$^+$CD8α$^+$ T helper cells dropped less severely than CD4$^+$CD8α$^-$ T helper cells in INOC gilts on 2 dpi after PRRSv infection. It is well known that many porcine CD4$^+$ T helper cells in peripheral blood express CD8α [34] and that both activated and memory T helper cells belong to the CD4$^+$CD8α$^+$ population [35,36]. This may indicate stronger recruitment of naïve T helper cells from blood to the periphery. A PRRSv specific proliferation of CD4$^+$ T cells would likely not occur as early as 2 dpi, but a bystander proliferation of CD4$^+$CD8$^+$ memory cells may be a non-specific effect of PRRSv infection, and therefore cannot be excluded. From all investigated PBMC populations T helper cells seem to be most relevant for the fetal outcome after PRRSv infection. Although only a trend, absolute numbers of T helper cells over time were positively associated with fetal mortality rate. Therefore, T helper cell counts could be used as a possible indicator of susceptibility to reproductive PRRSv. This has to be confirmed in future experiments.

The fairly high percentage of CTLs expressing SLA-DR in this study agrees with previous data investigating the phenotypic maturation of porcine NK and T cell subsets from birth to six months of age. CTLs in newborn piglets are SLA-DR negative and the first phenotypic change occurs around 3 weeks of age with a massive appearance of SLA-DR$^+$ CTLs [36]. In our study, the percentage of SLA-DR$^+$ CTLs significantly increased in INOC gilts on 2 dpi. By assuming that SLA-DR expression in porcine CTL is a result of previous antigen contact, this points towards a higher loss of naïve (i.e. SLA-DR$^-$) CTLs from blood circulation. But again a non-specific bystander proliferation of antigen experienced CTLs cannot be excluded. A higher decrease of naïve CTLs further corroborated by the decrease in CD8β expression and increase in SLA-DR expression levels (Figure 8E and F) and as such, CD8β^{low}SLA-DR^{high} CTLs display the phenotype of terminally differentiated CTLs [37].

In conclusion, PRRSv infection with NVSL 97–7895 in pregnant gilts caused a massive, acute decrease in total leukocyte counts affecting all major PBMC populations, most severely NK cells and CTLs. For all PBMC subsets except B cells, counts started to rebound by 6 dpi indicating a well-functioning immune cell homeostasis, explaining the very mild to absent clinical signs following PRRSv infection in pregnant gilts. However, immune cells migrate extensively and only a very small proportion of immune cells are present in the blood [38], complicating the interpretation of PBMC analyses. That being said, three leukocyte populations may predict relevant biological outcomes in PRRS-infected pregnant gilts. Absolute numbers of total T cells and γδ T cells were negatively associated with PRRSv viral load (AUC of RNA concentration in serum over 21 dpi). Additionally, absolute numbers of T helper cells may predict fetal mortality rate. Although many questions regarding the immune responses remain unanswered, these findings provide insight and clues that may help reduce the impact of PRRSv in pregnant gilts.

Abbreviations
ASFv: African swine fever virus; AUC: Area under the curve; BVDv: Bovine viral diarrhea virus; CSFv: classical swine fever virus; CD: Cluster of differentiation; CTLs: Cytolytic T lymphocytes; dpi: Days post infection; FCM: Flow cytometry; FMO: Fluorescence minus one; INOC: Gilts inoculated with PRRSv; CTRL: gilts that were sham inoculated; ILL: Innate-like lymphocytes; SLA-DR: Major histocompatibility complex class II; MFI: Mean fluorescence intensity; mAbs: Monoclonal antibodies; NK cells: Natural killer cells; NKR: Natural killer receptor; PBMC: Peripheral blood mononuclear cells; PBS: Phosphate buffered saline; PCV2: Porcine circovirus type 2; PRRSv: Porcine reproductive and respiratory syndrome virus; PRv: Pseudorabies virus; qRT-PCR: Quantitative reverse transcription polymerase chain reaction; Sn: Sialoadhesin; SD: Standard deviation; TCR: T cell receptor; TLR: toll like receptor; WBCs: White blood cells.

Competing interests
The authors declare that they have no competing interests.

Authors' contributions
The animal experiment and laboratory work were conducted by AL, CA and JH. WG, AS, and JKL were involved in overall experimental design and interpretation of data. Statistical analyses were completed by JH and AL. JH

was the Principal Investigator. All authors read and approved the final manuscript.

Acknowledgements
The authors wish to acknowledge the numerous technicians and students from the Western College of Veterinary Medicine, Vaccine and Infectious Disease Organization, Prairie Diagnostic Services, Inc. and the University of Alberta who assisted with this project. We offer special thanks to Natasa Arsic and Philip Griebel for their greatly valued assistance with the flow cytometry, to Ian Dohoo for his guidance with statistical analyses, and to Graham Plastow for the overall coordination of the project. Pregnant gilts were provided and bred by Fast Genetics Inc., Spiritwood with management support of Dawn Friesen, Connie Heisler, Donell Wingerter and Benny Mote. Funding for the project was generously provided by grants from Genome Canada and Genome Prairie (grant number 2209-F), with administrative support from Genome Alberta.

Author details
[1]Department of Large Animal Clinical Sciences, Western College of Veterinary Medicine, University of Saskatchewan, Saskatoon, SK, Canada. [2]Institute of Immunology, Department of Pathobiology, University of Veterinary Medicine Vienna, Vienna, Austria. [3]Animal Parasitic Diseases Laboratory, Beltsville Agricultural Research Center, Agricultural Research Service, U.S. Department of Agriculture, Beltsville, MD, USA. [4]Current address: University Clinic for Swine, Department for Farm Animals and Veterinary Public Health, University of Veterinary Medicine Vienna, Veterinaerplatz 1, 1210 Vienna, Austria.

References
1. Allende R, Laegreid WW, Kutish GF, Galeota JA, Wills RW, Osorio FA: **Porcine reproductive and respiratory syndrome virus: description of persistence in individual pigs upon experimental infection.** *J Virol* 2000, **74**:10834–10837.
2. Wills RW, Doster AR, Galeota JA, Sur JH, Osorio FA: **Duration of infection and proportion of pigs persistently infected with porcine reproductive and respiratory syndrome virus.** *J Clin Microbiol* 2003, **41**:58–62.
3. Mateu E, Diaz I: **The challenge of PRRS immunology.** *Vet J* 2008, **177**:345–351.
4. Nauwynck HJ, Van Gorp H, Vanhee M, Karniychuk U, Geldhof M, Cao A, Verbeeck M, Van Breedam W: **Micro-dissecting the pathogenesis and immune response of PRRSV Infection paves the way for more efficient PRRSV vaccines.** *Transbound Emerg Dis* 2012, **59**:50–54.
5. Yoo D, Song C, Sun Y, Du Y, Kim O, Liu HC: **Modulation of host cell responses and evasion strategies for porcine reproductive and respiratory syndrome virus.** *Virus Res* 2010, **154**:48–60.
6. Nielsen J, Botner A, Tingstedt JE, Aasted B, Johnsen CK, Riber U, Lind P: **In utero infection with porcine reproductive and respiratory syndrome virus modulates leukocyte subpopulations in peripheral blood and bronchoalveolar fluid of surviving piglets.** *Vet Immunol Immunopathol* 2003, **93**:135–151.
7. Christianson WT, Choi CS, Collins JE, Molitor TW, Morrison RB, Joo HS: **Pathogenesis of porcine reproductive and respiratory syndrome virus infection in mid-gestation sows and fetuses.** *Can J Vet Res* 1993, **57**:262–268.
8. Ladinig A, Wilkinson J, Ashley C, Detmer SE, Lunney JK, Plastow G, Harding JC: **Variation in Fetal outcome, viral load and ORF5 sequence mutations in a large scale study of phenotypic responses to late gestation exposure to type 2 porcine reproductive and respiratory syndrome virus.** *PLoS One* 2014, **9**:e96104.
9. Roederer M: **Spectral compensation for flow cytometry: visualization artifacts, limitations, and caveats.** *Cytometry* 2001, **45**:194–205.
10. Sinkora M, Butler JE: **The ontogeny of the porcine immune system.** *Dev Comp Immunol* 2009, **33**:273–283.
11. Yang H, Parkhouse RM, Wileman T: **Monoclonal antibodies that identify the CD3 molecules expressed specifically at the surface of porcine gammadelta-T cells.** *Immunology* 2005, **115**:189–196.
12. Karalyan Z, Zakaryan H, Arzumanyan H, Sargsyan K, Voskanyan H, Hakobyan L, Abroyan L, Avetisyan A, Karalova E: **Pathology of porcine peripheral white blood cells during infection with African swine fever virus.** *BMC Vet Res* 2012, **8**:18.

13. Summerfield A, Knotig SM, McCullough KC: **Lymphocyte apoptosis during classical swine fever: implication of activation-induced cell death.** *J Virol* 1998, **72**:1853–1861.

14. Page GR, Wang FI, Hahn EC: **Interaction of pseudorabies virus with porcine peripheral blood lymphocytes.** *J Leukoc Biol* 1992, **52**:441–448.

15. Nielsen J, Vincent IE, Botner A, Ladekaer-Mikkelsen AS, Allan G, Summerfield A, McCullough KC: **Association of lymphopenia with porcine circovirus type 2 induced postweaning multisystemic wasting syndrome (PMWS).** *Vet Immunol Immunopathol* 2003, **92**:97–111.

16. Pomorska-Mol M, Markowska-Daniel I, Kwit K: **Immune and acute phase response in pigs experimentally infected with H1N2 swine influenza virus.** *FEMS Immunol Med Microbiol* 2012, **66**:334–342.

17. Labarque G, Van Gucht S, Nauwynck H, Van Reeth K, Pensaert M: **Apoptosis in the lungs of pigs infected with porcine reproductive and respiratory syndrome virus and associations with the production of apoptogenic cytokines.** *Vet Res* 2003, **34**:249–260.

18. Rossow KD, Bautista EM, Goyal SM, Molitor TW, Murtaugh MP, Morrison RB, Benfield DA, Collins JE: **Experimental porcine reproductive and respiratory syndrome virus infection in one-, four-, and 10-week-old pigs.** *J Vet Diagn Invest* 1994, **6**:3–12.

19. Rossow KD, Collins JE, Goyal SM, Nelson EA, Christopher-Hennings J, Benfield DA: **Pathogenesis of porcine reproductive and respiratory syndrome virus infection in gnotobiotic pigs.** *Vet Pathol* 1995, **32**:361–373.

20. Sur JH, Doster AR, Osorio FA: **Apoptosis induced in vivo during acute infection by porcine reproductive and respiratory syndrome virus.** *Vet Pathol* 1998, **35**:506–514.

21. Costers S, Lefebvre DJ, Delputte PL, Nauwynck HJ: **Porcine reproductive and respiratory syndrome virus modulates apoptosis during replication in alveolar macrophages.** *Arch Virol* 2008, **153**:1453–1465.

22. Li Y, Wang G, Liu Y, Tu Y, He Y, Wang Z, Han Z, Li L, Li A, Tao Y, Cai X: **Identification of apoptotic cells in the thymus of piglets infected with highly pathogenic porcine reproductive and respiratory syndrome virus.** *Virus Res* 2014, **189**:29–33.

23. Wang G, He Y, Tu Y, Liu Y, Zhou EM, Han Z, Jiang C, Wang S, Shi W, Cai X: **Comparative analysis of apoptotic changes in peripheral immune organs and lungs following experimental infection of piglets with highly pathogenic and classical porcine reproductive and respiratory syndrome virus.** *Virol J* 2014, **11**:2.

24. Mueller SN, Gebhardt T, Carbone FR, Heath WR: **Memory T cell subsets, migration patterns, and tissue residence.** *Annu Rev Immunol* 2013, **31**:137–161.

25. Cahill RN, Frost H, Trnka Z: **The effects of antigen on the migration of recirculating lymphocytes through single lymph nodes.** *J Exp Med* 1976, **143**:870–888.

26. Hall JG, Morris B: **The immediate effect of antigens on the cell output of a lymph node.** *Br J Exp Pathol* 1965, **46**:450–454.

27. Duan X, Nauwynck HJ, Pensaert MB: **Virus quantification and identification of cellular targets in the lungs and lymphoid tissues of pigs at different time intervals after inoculation with porcine reproductive and respiratory syndrome virus (PRRSV).** *Vet Microbiol* 1997, **56**:9–19.

28. Calvert JG, Slade DE, Shields SL, Jolie R, Mannan RM, Ankenbauer RG, Welch SK: **CD163 expression confers susceptibility to porcine reproductive and respiratory syndrome viruses.** *J Virol* 2007, **81**:7371–7379.

29. Nauwynck HJ, Duan X, Favoreel HW, Van Oostveldt P, Pensaert MB: **Entry of porcine reproductive and respiratory syndrome virus into porcine alveolar macrophages via receptor-mediated endocytosis.** *J Gen Virol* 1999, **80**:297–305.

30. Dwivedi V, Manickam C, Binjawadagi B, Linhares D, Murtaugh MP, Renukaradhya GJ: **Evaluation of immune responses to porcine reproductive and respiratory syndrome virus in pigs during early stage of infection under farm conditions.** *Virol J* 2012, **9**:45.

31. Weesendorp E, Morgan S, Stockhofe-Zurwieden N, Popma-De Graaf DJ, Graham SP, Rebel JM: **Comparative analysis of immune responses following experimental infection of pigs with European porcine reproductive and respiratory syndrome virus strains of differing virulence.** *Vet Microbiol* 2013, **163**:1–12.

32. Biron CA, Nguyen KB, Pien GC, Cousens LP, Salazar-Mather TP: **Natural killer cells in antiviral defense: function and regulation by innate cytokines.** *Annu Rev Immunol* 1999, **17**:189–220.

33. Murphy KP: *Janeway's Immunobiology.* Garland Science, Taylor & Francis Group, LLC: New York, USA; 2012.

34. Saalmuller A, Reddehase MJ, Buhring HJ, Jonjic S, Koszinowski UH: **Simultaneous expression of CD4 and CD8 antigens by a substantial proportion of resting porcine T lymphocytes.** *Eur J Immunol* 1987, **17**:1297–1301.

35. Saalmuller A, Werner T, Fachinger V: **T-helper cells from naive to committed.** *Vet Immunol Immunopathol* 2002, **87**:137–145.

36. Talker SC, Kaser T, Reutner K, Sedlak C, Mair KH, Koinig H, Graage R, Viehmann M, Klingler E, Ladinig A, Ritzmann M, Saalmüller A, Gerner W: **Phenotypic maturation of porcine NK- and T-cell subsets.** *Dev Comp Immunol* 2013, **40**:51–68.

37. Reutner K, Leitner J, Essler SE, Witter K, Patzl M, Steinberger P, Saalmuller A, Gerner W: **Porcine CD27: identification, expression and functional aspects in lymphocyte subsets in swine.** *Dev Comp Immunol* 2012, **38**:321–331.

38. Di Rosa F, Pabst R: **The bone marrow: a nest for migratory memory T cells.** *Trends Immunol* 2005, **26**:360–366.

7

Novel H5 clade 2.3.4.6 viruses with both α-2,3 and α-2,6 receptor binding properties may pose a pandemic threat

Qunhui Li[1], Xuan Wang[1], Min Gu[1,2], Jie Zhu[1], Xiaoli Hao[1], Zhao Gao[1], Zhongtao Sun[1], Jiao Hu[1,2], Shunlin Hu[1,2], Xiaoquan Wang[1,2], Xiaowen Liu[1,2] and Xiufan Liu[1,2]*

Abstract

The emerging H5 clade 2.3.4.6 viruses of different NA subtypes have been detected in different domestic poultry in China. We evaluated the receptor binding property and transmissibility of four novel H5 clade 2.3.4.6 subtype highly pathogenic avian influenza viruses. The results show that these viruses bound to both avian-type (α-2,3) and human-type (α-2,6) receptors. Furthermore, we found that one of these viruses, GS/EC/1112/11, not only replicated but also transmitted efficiently in guinea pigs. Therefore, such novel H5 subtype viruses have the potential of a pandemic threat.

Introduction, methods, and results

H5N1 subtype highly pathogenic avian influenza virus (HPAIV) was first isolated in sick geese in China in 1996,and has continued to evolve into over 10 distinct phylogenetic clades including different subclades based on the hemagglutinin (HA) gene [1]. Since 2010, H5 HPAIV subtypes which belong to the recommended novel clade 2.3.4.6 [2] with various neuraminidase (NA) subtypes (H5N1, H5N2, H5N6 and H5N8) have been detected in different domestic poultry in China [2-7]. Furthermore, the H5N8 virus-caused outbreaks have also been reported in wild birds and poultry in South Korea and Japan in January and April, 2014 respectively [8,9]. Here, we tested the receptor binding property of four novel clade 2.3.4.6 viruses, and guinea pigs were used as a mammalian model to examine the replication and transmission of these viruses. All animal experiments were approved by the Jiangsu Administrative Committee for Laboratory Animals (permission number SYXK-SU-2007-0005) and complied with the guidelines of the Jiangsu laboratory animal welfare and ethics of Jiangsu Administrative Committee of Laboratory Animals.

During surveillance of poultry for avian influenza viruses in live poultry markets in eastern China in 2013, one H5N8 avian influenza virus, A/duck/Shandong/Q1/2013 (DkQ1), was isolated from domestic ducks. The GenBank accession numbers for the DkQ1 segments are KM504098 to KM504105. Sequence analysis showed that all 8 genes of DkQ1 are closely related to those H5N8 viruses which have been reported in eastern China [4,5]. Furthermore, the HA gene of DkQ1 has high nucleotide identity with the H5N8 viruses circulating in South Korea and Japan in 2014 [8,9]. And all these H5N8 viruses belong to the recommended novel clade 2.3.4.6 [2]. In addition, one H5N8 virus A/duck/Jiangsu/k1203/2010 (Dkk1203) [4] and two H5N2 viruses A/duck/Eastern China/1111/2011 (DK/EC/1111/11) and A/goose/Eastern China/1112/2011 (GS/EC/1112/11) [3], which have been reported to circulate in eastern China, also possess HA genes belonging to the novel clade 2.3.4.6. Here, we investigated the receptor binding property and transmissibility of these four H5 (HPAIV) clade 2.3.4.6. All experiments with viruses were performed in a Biosafety Level 3 laboratory.

It is generally accepted that haemagglutinin-receptor-binding preference to α-2,6-linked sialylated glycans is the initial key step for a novel influenza-virus-causing pandemic [10]. First, we examined the receptor-binding specificity of these reassortant viruses by hemagglutination assays using goose red blood cells that were treated with a α-2,3-specific sialidase as previously described [11]. The A (H1N1)pdm2009 virus A/California/04/2009 (CA/04) and poultry H5N1 isolate A/mallard/Huadong/S/2005 (HD/05)

* Correspondence: xfliu@yzu.edu.cn
[1]Animal Infectious Disease Laboratory, College of Veterinary Medicine, Yangzhou University, Yangzhou, Jiangsu 225009, China
[2]Jiangsu Co-innovation Center for Prevention and Control of Important Animal Infectious Diseases and Zoonoses, Yangzhou, Jiangsu 225009, China

[12] were used as controls. Theoretically, the sialidase digestion should abolish hemagglutination by α-2,3-specific viruses, whereas viruses that can bind to α-2,6-receptors should maintain hemagglutination activity with the treated red blood cells. The sialidase treatment did not affect the hemagglutination titer of CA/04, as shown in Table 1. Compared to untreated GRBC, these reassortant viruses still show some lower HA activity with α-2,3-sialidase-treated GRBC, which had only α-2,6-receptors (Table 1).

To characterize the receptor-binding properties of these viruses further, we performed solid-phase binding assays with different glycans as previously described [13]. Briefly, the synthetic sialylglycopolymers Neu5Aca2-3Galb1-4GlcNAcb (3'SLN)-PAA-biotin and Neu5Aca2-3Galb1-4GlcNAcb (6'SLN)-PAA-biotin (GlycoTech) were serially diluted in PBS and added to the wells of 96-well streptavidin coated microtiter plates (Pierce). The plates were blocked with PBS containing 2% skim milk powder, and 128 HA units of live virus was added per well. Chicken antiserum against the virus was diluted in PBS and added to each well. Bound antibody was detected by sequential addition of HRP-conjugated rabbit anti-chicken IgG antibody and tetramethylbenzidine substrate solution. The reaction was stopped with 1 M H_2SO_4, and the absorbance was read at 450 nm. Each sample was measured in triplicate. Our results show these reassortant viruses were bound to both avian-type (α-2,3) and human-type (α-2,6) receptors, whereas HD/05 and CA/04 viruses were preferentially bound to α-2,3 and α-2,6 receptors respectively, as expected (Figure 1). These results indicate that the HA of these reassortant viruses binds to α-2,3 receptors as well as to α-2,6 receptors.

To investigate the replication of these reassortant viruses, groups of four animals were anesthetized with pentobarbital natricum (40–50 mg/Kg) and inoculated intranasally with 10^6EID_{50} of test virus in a 300 μL volume (150 μL per nostril). Two animals from each group were euthanized with CO2 on day 3 post inoculation (pi) and nasal washes, tracheas, lungs, kidneys, spleens, and brains were collected for virus titration in eggs. The remaining two animals were observed for two weeks for signs of disease and death. The A(H1N1)pdm2009 virus A/California/04/2009 (CA/04) and poultry H5N1 isolate A/mallard/Huadong/S/2005 (HD/05) were used as controls. As shown in Table 2, all reassortant viruses were detected in the nasal washes, tracheas and lungs of both inoculated animals, but only could be detected at lower titers in the trachea and lungs of infected guinea pigs. Virus was not detected in the brains, kidneys or spleens of any of the inoculated animals. We also infected two animals for each virus and observed them for two weeks for signs of pathogenicity. After two weeks pi, all of the animals seroconverted (Table 2). None of the animals showed disease signs during the observation period. These results indicate that replication of these reassortant viruses in guinea pigs is restricted to the respiratory system.

For the contact transmission studies, groups of three animals were inoculated intranasally with 10^6EID_{50} of test virus and housed in a cage placed inside an isolator. Three naïve animals were introduced into the same cage 24 h later. Nasal washes were collected at 2 day intervals, beginning on day 2 pi (1 day post contact) and titrated in eggs. Sera were collected from guinea pigs at 14 days post inoculation (dpi) for hemagglutinin inhibition (HI) antibody detection [14]. Evidence of transmission was based on the detection of virus in the nasal wash and on seroconversion at the end of the two-week observation period. The A/California/04/2009 (CA/04) virus was used as controls. As shown in Figure 2, reassortant virus was detected in the nasal washes of all three inoculated guinea pigs between days 2–6 pi, but not in any of the contact guinea pigs. In the GS/EC/1112/11-inoculated groups (Figure 2B), virus was detected in the nasal washes of all three inoculated guinea pigs between days 2–6 pi, respectively and was also detected in the nasal washes of all three contact animals between days 4–8 pi. Seroconversion occurred in all inoculated groups (Table 2). In the contact animal groups, seroconversion was only observed among animals placed with the GS/EC/1112/11-inoculated animals. These results indicate that the transmissibility of the reassortant viruses in guinea pigs varies among viral strains, and of the four test viruses, only GS/EC/1112/11 transmit efficiently in this mammalian host.

Discussion

Historically, changes in the receptor binding protein of influenza virus, HA, have been implicated in the initiation of a pandemic. It has been established for the H1N1 (1918), H2N2 (1957) and H3N2 (1968) pandemic

Table 1 Hemagglutination titers of viruses from humans and animals[a]

Virus stain	HA titers (log_2)	
	Untreated GRBCs	Treated GRBCs
CA/04	6	6
HD/05	8	0
DK/EC/1111/11	8	7
GS/EC/1112/11	7	6
Dkk1203	7	5
DkQ1	7	6

[a]Hemagglutination titers were determined using goose red blood cells treated with α-2, 3-sialidas.

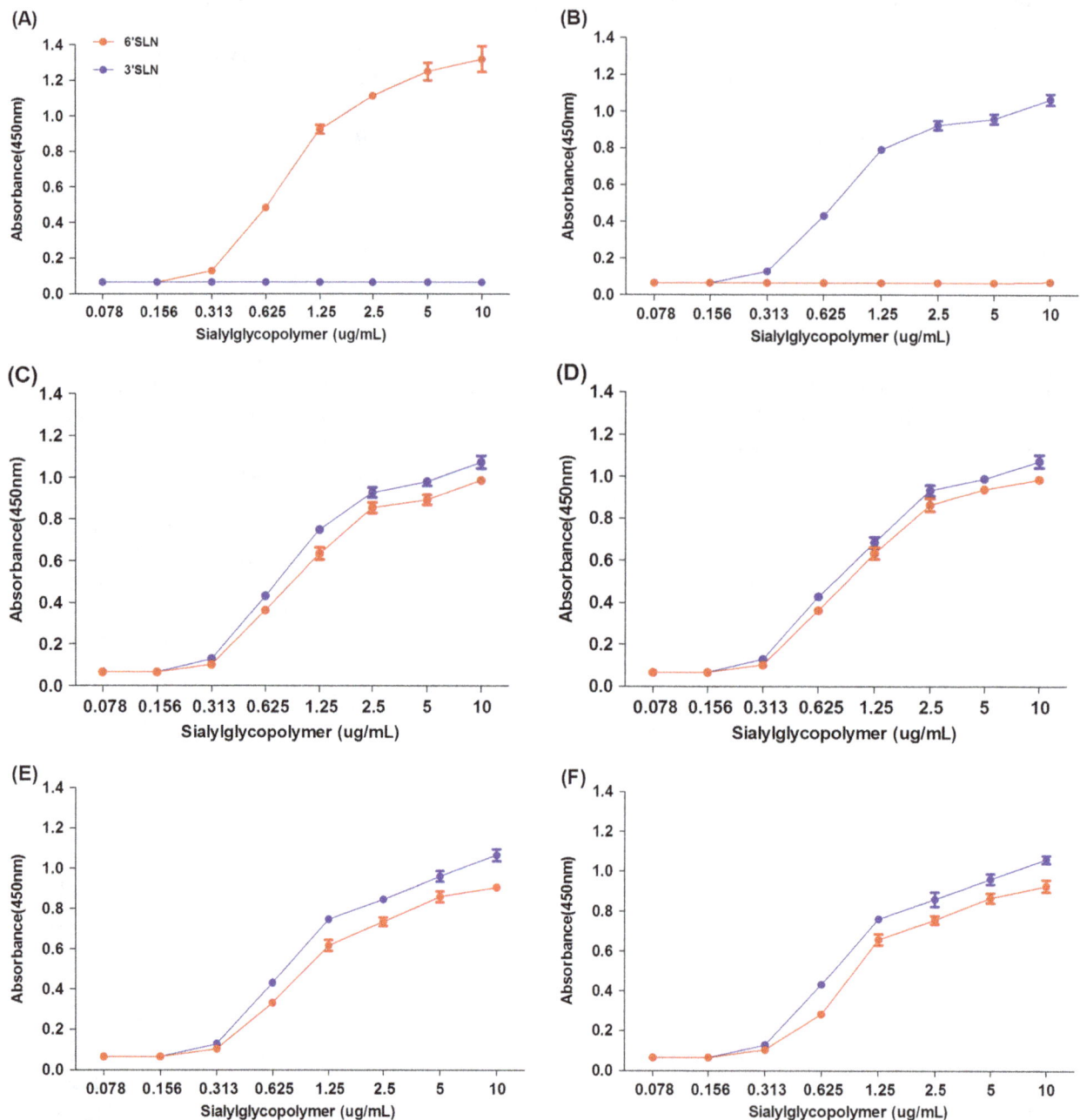

Figure 1 Solid-phase receptor-binding assay of the H5 (HPAIV) clades 2.3.4.6. Solid-phase receptor-binding assay of human isolate CA/04 **(A)**, poultry isolate HD/05 **(B)**, DK/EC/1111/11 virus **(C)**, GS/EC/1112/11 virus **(D)**, Dkk1203 virus **(E)** and DkQ1 virus **(F)**. Direct binding of viruses to sialylglycopolymers containing either 3'SLN-PAA or 6'SLN-PAA was measured. The data shown are representative of three independent binding experiments.

viruses that a change in HA protein from a preference for α-2,3-linked sialic acids (avian receptor) to a preference for α-2,6-linked sialic acids (human receptor) is a prerequisite for efficient transmission of avian viruses to humans [10]. H5 HPAIV pose a serious pandemic threat due to their virulence and high mortality in humans, and their increasingly expanding host reservoir and significant

ongoing evolution could enhance their human-to-human transmissibility. Recently, novel clade 2.3.4.6 H5 HPAIV with various NA subtypes (H5N1, H5N2, H5N6, and H5N8) were reported in Eastern China and South Korea [2-7,9,15]. Here, we evaluated their receptor specificity and transmission in guinea pigs. The results show that the viruses bound to both avian-type (α-2,3) and human-type

Table 2 Virus replication and seroconversion in guinea pigs

Virus stain	Replication in guinea pigs[a]							Seroconversion of the guinea pigs in transmission studies	
	Virus titers in organs(log$_{10}$EID$_{50}$/mL)						Seroconversion (positive/total)[d]	Seroconversion: positive/total (HI titers)[e]	
	Nasal wash[b]	Lung	trachea	spleen	kidney	brain		Inoculated	Contact
DK/EC/1111/11	4.8 ± 0.3	3.5 ± 0.2	1.2 ± 0.2	-[c]	-	-	2/2	3/3(40,40,40)	0/3
GS/EC/1112/11	4.4 ± 0.7	3.2 ± 0.4	1.0 ± 0.1	-	-	-	2/2	3/3(80,40,40)	3/3(20,20,20)
Dkk1203	4.2 ± 1.6	2.8 ± 0.5	0.8 ± 0.1	-	-	-	2/2	3/3(80,80,40)	0/3
DkQ1	4.3 ± 1.3	2.7 ± 0.3	0.8 ± 0.2	-	-	-	2/2	3/3(80,40,40)	0/3
HD/05	-	1.0 ± 0.2	-	-	-	-	0/2		
CA/04	5.4 ± 0.4	4.5 ± 0.3	2.8 ± 0.4	-	-	-	2/2	3/3(160,320,320)	3/3(80,160,160)

[a]Groups of four guinea pigs were slightly anesthetized and intranasally inoculated with 10^{6}EID$_{50}$ of test virus in a 300 μL volume, 150 μL per nostril. Two animals from each group were euthanized on day 3 pi and samples, including nasal wash, lung, trachea, spleen, kidney and brain, were collected for virus titration in eggs. The remaining two animals were observed for two weeks and sera were collected at the end of the observation period.
[b]Data shown are log$_{10}$EID$_{50}$/mL.
[c]virus was not detected in the undiluted sample.
[d]Seroconversion was confirmed by hemagglutination inhibition (HI) assay.
[e]Sera were collected from guinea pigs on day 14 pi and treated overnight with Vibrio cholera receptor-destroying enzyme. Seroconversion was confirmed by hemagglutination inhibition (HI) assay.

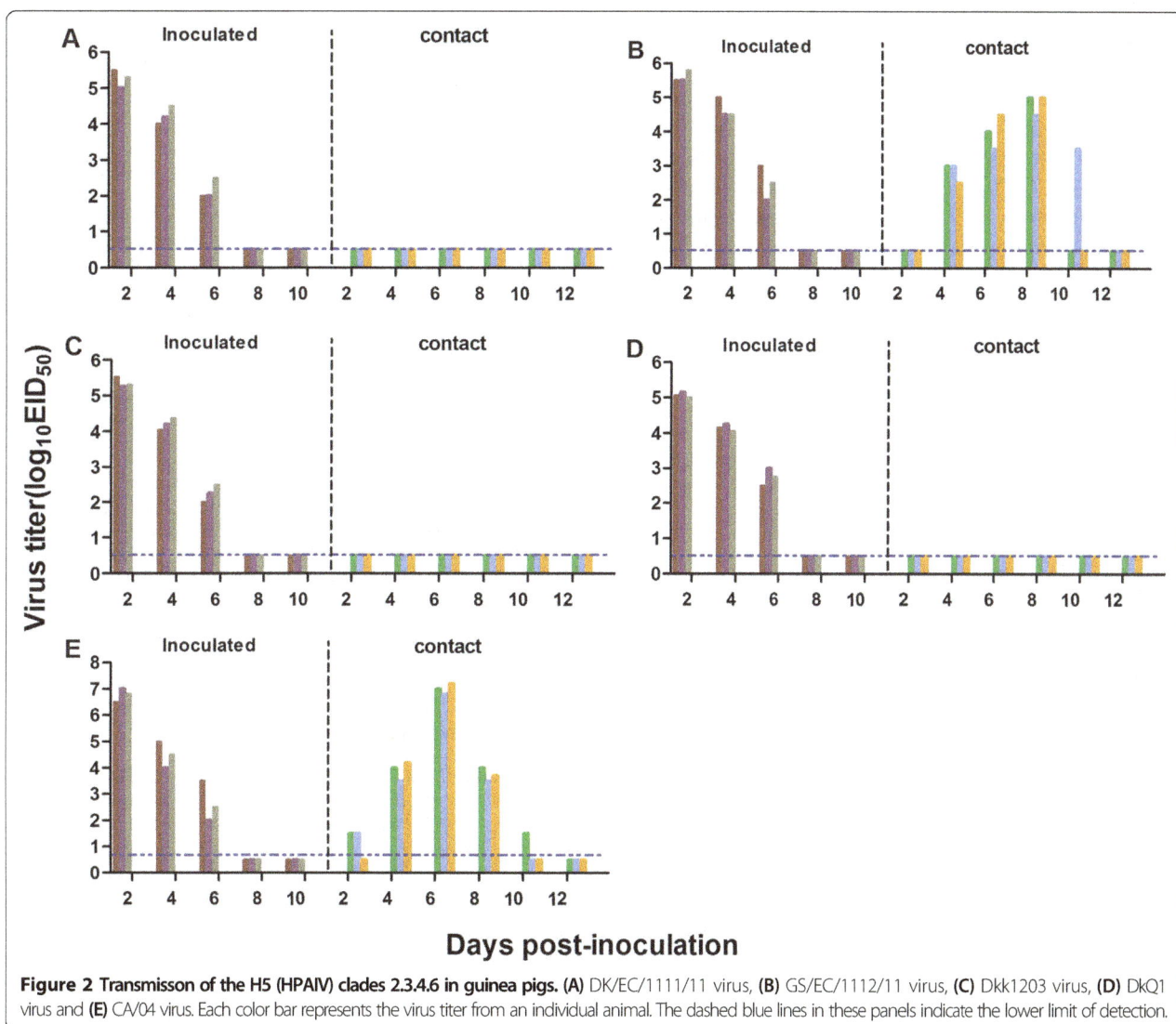

Figure 2 Transmisson of the H5 (HPAIV) clades 2.3.4.6 in guinea pigs. (A) DK/EC/1111/11 virus, **(B)** GS/EC/1112/11 virus, **(C)** Dkk1203 virus, **(D)** DkQ1 virus and **(E)** CA/04 virus. Each color bar represents the virus titer from an individual animal. The dashed blue lines in these panels indicate the lower limit of detection.

(α-2,6) receptors. In humans, the α-2,6 receptor is expressed mainly in the upper airway, while the α-2,3 receptor is expressed in alveoli and the terminal bronchiole [16]. A virus with good affinity to both α-2,3 and α-2,6 receptors may especially be harmful, as it could infect efficiently via its binding to α-2,6 receptors in the upper airway and simultaneously cause severe infection in the lung via its binding to α-2,3 receptors. And this hypothesis is supported by the fact that one of the two well-characterized HA genes from the H1N1 1918 pandemic virus binds efficiently to both α-2,3 and α-2,6 receptors [17]. In addition, previous studies showed that the human-infecting novel H7N9 and the latest reassortant H10N8 avian influenza viruses yet have substantial affinity to both avian-type (α-2,3) and human-type (α-2,6) receptors [18,19]. Sequence analysis showed that novel H5 (HPAIV) clade 2.3.4.6 simultaneously carry a T160A mutation which results in the lack of an oligosaccharide side chain at 158–160 of HA, and it is critical for the H5 subtype influenza viruses tested to bind to human-like receptors and to transmit among a mammalian host [20,21]. Whether this T160A variation affects the receptor-binding property deserves further investigation. Previous studies showed that some H5 subtype influenza viruses can transmit efficiently in guinea pigs [21]. In this study, we also found that one of these viruses, GS/EC/1112/11, not only replicated but also transmitted efficiently in guinea pigs. These findings emphasize that continued circulation of these viruses may pose health threats for humans. Therefore, we need to intensify our effort to detect such viruses as early as possible.

Abbreviations

HPAIV: Highly pathogenic avian influenza virus; HA: Hemagglutinin; NA: Neuraminidase; DkQ1: A/duck/Shandong/Q1/2013; Dkk1203: A/duck/Jiangsu/k1203/2010; DK/EC/1111/11: A/duck/Eastern China/1111/2011; GS/EC/1112/11: A/goose/Eastern China/1112/2011; CA/04: A/California/04/2009; HD/05: A/mallard/Huadong/S/2005; pi: Post inoculation; dpi: Days post inoculation; HI: Hemagglutinin inhibition.

Competing interests

The authors declare that they have no competing interests.

Authors' contributions

QL designed the study, drafted the manuscript and participated in all tests. XW verified design, participated in all tests. JZ participated in collecting samples. XH, ZS and ZG participated in testing samples. MG, JH, SH, XQW, XWL and XFL conceived the study, contributed to the analysis of the results and preparation of revised manuscript versions. All authors read and approved the final manuscript.

Acknowledgments

This work was supported by the Earmarked Fund for Modern Agro-Industry Technology Research System (grant no. nycytx-41-G07), the Jiangsu Provincial Natural Science Foundation of China (grant no. BK20130442), the Priority Academic Program Development of Jiangsu Higher Education Institutions (PAPD), the National Natural Science Foundation of China (grant no. 31101827), and the National High-Tech R&D Program of China (863 Program) (grant no. 2011AA10A200).

References

1. WHO/OIE/FAO H5N1 Evolution Working Group: **Toward a unified nomenclature system for highly pathogenic avian influenza virus (H5N1).** *Emerg Infect Dis* 2008, **14**:e1.
2. Gu M, Zhao G, Zhao K, Zhong L, Huang J, Wan H, Wang X, Liu W, Liu H, Peng D, Liu X: **Novel variants of clade 2.3.4 highly pathogenic avian influenza A(H5N1) viruses, China.** *Emerg Infect Dis* 2013, **19**:2021–2024.
3. Zhao G, Gu X, Lu X, Pan J, Duan Z, Zhao K, Gu M, Liu Q, He L, Chen J, Ge S, Wang Y, Chen S, Wang X, Peng D, Wan H, Liu X: **Novel reassortant highly pathogenic H5N2 avian influenza viruses in poultry in China.** *PLoS One* 2012, **7**:e46183.
4. Zhao K, Gu M, Zhong L, Duan Z, Zhang Y, Zhu Y, Zhao G, Zhao M, Chen Z, Hu S, Liu W, Liu X, Peng D, Liu X: **Characterization of three H5N5 and one H5N8 highly pathogenic avian influenza viruses in China.** *Vet Microbiol* 2013, **163**:351–357.
5. Wu H, Peng X, Xu L, Jin C, Cheng L, Lu X, Xie T, Yao H, Wu N: **Novel reassortant influenza A(H5N8) viruses in domestic ducks, eastern China.** *Emerg Infect Dis* 2014, **20**:1315–1318.
6. Wu H, Peng X, Xu L, Jin C, Cheng L, Lu X, Xie T, Yao H, Wu N: **Characterization of a novel highly pathogenic H5N2 avian influenza virus isolated from a duck in eastern China.** *Arch Virol* 2014, **159**:3377–3383.
7. World Organisation for Animal Health: *OIE 15698*; July 31, 2014, Country: China. [http://www.oie.int/wahis_2/public%5C..%5Ctemp%5Creports/en_fup_0000015698_20140731_162951.pdf]
8. World Organisation for Animal Health: *OIE 15127*; April 18, 2014, Country: Japan. [http://www.oie.int/wahis_2/public%5C..%5Ctemp%5Creports/en_fup_0000015127_20140423_175238.pdf]
9. Lee YJ, Kang HM, Lee EK, Song BM, Jeong J, Kwon YK, Kim HR, Lee KJ, Hong MS, Jang I, Choi KS, Kim JY, Lee HJ, Kang MS, Jeong OM, Baek JH, Joo YS, Park YH, Lee HS: **Novel reassortant influenza A(H5N8) viruses, South Korea, 2014.** *Emerg Infect Dis* 2014, **20**:1087–1089.
10. Matrosovich M, Tuzikov A, Bovin N, Gambaryan A, Klimov A, Castrucci MR, Donatelli I, Kawaoka Y: **Early alterations of the receptor-binding properties of H1, H2, and H3 avian influenza virus hemagglutinins after their introduction into mammals.** *J Virol* 2000, **74**:8502–8512.
11. Suptawiwat O, Kongchanagul A, Chan-It W, Thitithanyanont A, Wiriyarat W, Chaichuen K, Songserm T, Suzuki Y, Puthavathana P, Auewarakul P: **A simple screening assay for receptor switching of avian influenza viruses.** *J Clin Virol* 2008, **42**:186–189.
12. He L, Zhao G, Zhong L, Liu Q, Duan Z, Gu M, Wang X, Liu X: **Isolation and characterization of two H5N1 influenza viruses from swine in Jiangsu Province of China.** *Arch Virol* 2013, **158**:2531–2541.
13. Auewarakul P, Suptawiwat O, Kongchanagul A, Sangma C, Suzuki Y, Ungchusak K, Louisirirotchanakul S, Lerdsamran H, Pooruk P, Thitithanyanont A, Pittayawonganon C, Guo CT, Hiramatsu H, Jampangern W, Chunsutthiwat S, Puthavathana P: **An avian influenza H5N1 virus that binds to a human-type receptor.** *J Virol* 2007, **81**:9950–9955.
14. OIE: *Manual of diagnostic tests and vaccines for terrestrial animals. Chapter 2.3.4;* [http://www.oie.int/fileadmin/Home/eng/Health_standards/tahm/2008/pdf/2.03.04_AI.pdf]
15. Ku KB, Park EH, Yum J, Kim JA, Oh SK, Seo SH: **Highly pathogenic avian influenza A(H5N8) virus from waterfowl, South Korea, 2014.** *Emerg Infect Dis* 2014, **20**:1587–1588.
16. Shinya K, Ebina M, Yamada S, Ono M, Kasai N, Kawaoka Y: **Avian flu: influenza virus receptors in the human airway.** *Nature* 2006, **440**:435–436.
17. Glaser L, Stevens J, Zamarin D, Wilson IA, Garcia-Sastre A, Tumpey TM, Basler CF, Taubenberger JK, Palese P: **A single amino acid substitution in 1918 influenza virus hemagglutinin changes receptor binding specificity.** *J Virol* 2005, **79**:11533–11536.
18. Vachieri SG, Xiong X, Collins PJ, Walker PA, Martin SR, Haire LF, Zhang Y, McCauley JW, Gamblin SJ, Skehel JJ: **Receptor binding by H10 influenza viruses.** *Nature* 2014, **511**:475–477.
19. Zhou J, Wang D, Gao R, Zhao B, Song J, Qi X, Zhang Y, Shi Y, Yang L, Zhu W, Bai T, Qin K, Lan Y, Zou S, Guo J, Dong J, Dong L, Zhang Y, Wei H, Li X, Lu J, Liu L, Zhao X, Li X, Huang W, Wen L, Bo H, Xin L, Chen Y, Xu C, *et al*: **Biological features of novel avian influenza A (H7N9) virus.** *Nature* 2013, **499**:500–503.

20. Yen HL, Aldridge JR, Boon AC, Ilyushina NA, Salomon R, Hulse-Post DJ, Marjuki H, Franks J, Boltz DA, Bush D, Lipatov AS, Webby RJ, Rehg JE, Webster RG: **Changes in H5N1 influenza virus hemagglutinin receptor binding domain affect systemic spread.** *Proc Natl Acad Sci U S A* 2009, **106:**286–291.

21. Gao Y, Zhang Y, Shinya K, Deng G, Jiang Y, Li Z, Guan Y, Tian G, Li Y, Shi J, Liu L, Zeng X, Bu Z, Xia X, Kawaoka Y, Chen H: **Identification of amino acids in HA and PB2 critical for the transmission of H5N1 avian influenza viruses in a mammalian host.** *PLoS Pathog* 2009, **5:**e1000709.

8

Polymorphisms in the feline TNFA and CD209 genes are associated with the outcome of feline coronavirus infection

Ying-Ting Wang[1†], Li-En Hsieh[1†], Yu-Rou Dai[2] and Ling-Ling Chueh[1,2]*

Abstract

Feline infectious peritonitis (FIP), caused by feline coronavirus (FCoV) infection, is a highly lethal disease without effective therapy and prevention. With an immune-mediated disease entity, host genetic variant was suggested to influence the occurrence of FIP. This study aimed at evaluating cytokine-associated single nucleotide polymorphisms (SNPs), i.e., tumor necrosis factor alpha (TNF-α), receptor-associated SNPs, i.e., C-type lectin DC-SIGN (CD209), and the five FIP-associated SNPs identified from Birman cats of USA and Denmark origins and their associations with the outcome of FCoV infection in 71 FIP cats and 93 FCoV infected non-FIP cats in a genetically more diverse cat populations. A promoter variant, fTNFA - 421 T, was found to be a disease-resistance allele. One SNP was identified in the extracellular domain (ECD) of fCD209 at position +1900, a G to A substitution, and the A allele was associated with FIP susceptibility. Three SNPs located in the introns of fCD209, at positions +2276, +2392, and +2713, were identified to be associated with the outcome of FCoV infection, with statistical relevance. In contrast, among the five Birman FIP cat-associated SNPs, no genotype or allele showed significant differences between our FIP and non-FIP groups. As disease resistance is multifactorial and several other host genes could involve in the development of FIP, the five genetic traits identified in this study should facilitate in the future breeding of the disease-resistant animal to reduce the occurrence of cats succumbing to FIP.

Introduction

Feline infectious peritonitis (FIP), a highly lethal disease with nearly 100% mortality among ill cats once clinical signs appear, is caused by feline coronavirus (FCoV) infection [1]. Despite the ubiquitous existence of FCoV around the world, the prevalence of FIP is less than 5% [2]. There is currently no therapy proven to be effective for the treatment of FIP, and once diagnosis is confirmed, euthanasia is generally inevitable. Although this disease has been described for over fifty years [3], studies attempting to develop vaccines with different approaches have all failed due to the immunopathogenic features of infection by this virus [4]. However, among many FCoV experimental inoculations studies, some cats survived challenge with the virulent strain of FCoV [2,5-10], whereas certain

pedigreed cats were reported to be more likely to succumb to FIP than mixed bred cats [2,11,12]. All these findings indicate that genetic polymorphisms between cats might affect their susceptibility to FIP.

FIP is an immunopathological consequence of the abnormal production of various cytokines. Imbalanced Th1/Th2 immune responses with scarce or absent interferon-gamma (IFN-γ) is consistently found in FIP cases [4,8,10,13-15] and association of genetic polymorphisms in the IFN-γ gene with FIP occurrence has recently been identified [16]. In addition to IFN-γ, the upregulation of tumor necrosis factor-alpha (TNF-α) during the development of FIP has been reported to result in lymphopenia [17]. Feline dendritic cell (DC)-specific intercellular adhesion molecule-grabbing non-integrin (fDC-SIGN, encoded by fCD209), a key coreceptor during the infection of both type I and II FCoV [18], was found to affect binding and infection of type I FCoV. fDC-SIGN is also involved in the infection of type II FCoV, albeit not through the initial binding [19]. Despite the close relationship to FCoV

* Correspondence: linglingchueh@ntu.edu.tw
†Equal contributors
[1]Graduate institute of Veterinary Medicine, School of Veterinary Medicine, National Taiwan University, Taipei 10617, Taiwan
[2]Department of Veterinary Medicine, School of Veterinary Medicine, National Taiwan University, Taipei 10617, Taiwan

infection, polymorphisms in the *fCD209* and feline TNF-α (*fTNFA*) genes and their association with FIP occurrence have never been investigated.

Recently, the surveillance of FIP-associated single nucleotide polymorphisms (SNPs) in Birman cats from USA and Denmark was conducted using a commercialized feline SNP array [20], and five SNPs were found to be significantly associated with FIP occurrence. However, it is unclear whether these disease-associated SNPs are Birman cat specific or can also be applied to other purebred or mixed breed cat populations.

To elucidate the genetic traits that contribute to FIP susceptibility, the *fTNFA* and *fCD209* genes were screened to identify disease-associated SNPs. The five SNPs identified from Birman cats proposed to be genetically associated with the occurrence of FIP were further evaluated in populations with more variable genetic backgrounds. Among all the polymorphisms analyzed, SNPs located in the *fTNFA* and *fCD209* genes were found to be associated with the outcome of FCoV infection, with statistical relevance.

Materials and methods

Animals and specimens

Samples were collected from 71 FIP cats and 93 FCoV-infected asymptomatic cats from 2005 to 2014 at the National Taiwan University Animal Hospital for an association analysis. This study required no specific ethical approval, as the analysis was performed retrospectively from samples of diseased animals routinely submitted to our diagnostic laboratory.

Seventy-one FIP cats, including 35.2% (25/71) purebred and 64.8% (45/71) mixed breed, were confirmed by necropsy. Pedigree cats including Scottish Fold (6/25), American Shorthair (4/25), Chinchilla (3/25), Exotic Shorthair (3/25), Siamese (2/25), European Shorthair (1/25) and Russian Blue (1/25). Most of the FIP cats (46/71) were less than one years old, the other 19 FIP cats were between the ages of one and three. The rest six FIP cats elder than

three were from 3.5 to 10 years old. Also, FCoV detection by reverse transcription-nested polymerase chain reaction (RT-nPCR) [21] was confirmed in disease-associated tissue, including body effusions and/or internal organs with the typical lesions of FIP. Ninety-three asymptomatic healthy cats were included as a control group, including 75.3% (50/93) mixed breed and 24.7% (23/93) purebred, of an age of three years old or less and showing no FIP-related signs upon enrolment in this study. Pedigree cats including American Shorthair (8/23), Scottish Fold (7/23), Chinchilla (4/23), Persian (2/23), Abyssinian (1/23) and European Shorthair (1/23). All the asymptomatic cats were positive for FCoV detection in at least one sample collected, including whole blood, nasal/oral/conjunctival/rectal swabs, and feces. In addition, the detection of two feline retroviruses, i.e., feline leukemia virus and feline immunodeficiency virus, was performed [22,23]. FIP cats and FCoV infected non-FIP cats with a positive result for either of the feline retroviruses were excluded from the association study.

Identification of SNPs in target sequences

Genomic DNA was isolated from buccal swabs or whole blood samples from each cat using a genomic DNA mini kit (Geneaid Biotech, New Taipei City, Taiwan). Partial *fTNFA* and *fCD209* sequences and five FIP-associated SNPs identified in Birman cats, as reported by Golovko et al., namely, *A1.196617776*, *A1.206840008*, *Un.59861682*, *A2.191286425*, and *E2.65509996*, were amplified [20] using the polymerase chain reaction (PCR). The primers and conditions are listed in Tables 1 and 2. Briefly, each reaction contained 1 μL of template DNA, 500 nM of each primer, 200 μM dNTP, 1.5 mM MgCl$_2$, and 0.6 U Phusion DNA polymerase (Thermo Scientific, Waltham, USA) in a total volume of 30 μL with 1× Phusion HF buffer. The amplified products were subsequently sequenced using an auto-sequencer ABI 3730XL (Applied Biosystems, San Mateo, USA), and the obtained sequences were aligned by Geneious 4.8.5 (Biomatters, Auckland, New Zealand). The

Table 1 Primers used for SNP identification of *fTNFA* and *fCD209* gene

Target gene/region	Position[a]	Orientation[b]	Sequence (5' - 3')	T$_A$[c]	Amplicon size
fTNFA/5'-PRR[d]	−847 to −827	F	GAATTCCCAGGGTTGCTTTCA	65 °C	1018 bp
	+171 to +153	R	GCCGATCACTCCAAAGTGC		
fCD209/5'-PRR	−1057 to −1038	F	GAAGCGGGCTTCTTGTTGAC	65 °C	1076 bp
	+19 to +1	R	GCTCCTTGGGGTCACACAT		
fCD209/ECD[e]	+1818 to +1838	F	CCAAGATCTGATGCATCTGCT	67 °C	1350 bp
	+3168 to +3149	R	ATGAGCTCGTTGCCTGATCT		

[a]The nucleotide positions are numerated from the translation start point (+1).
[b]F: forward; R: reverse.
[c]Annealing temperature.
[d]5'-proximal regulatory region.
[e]Extracellular domain.

Table 2 Primers used for SNP identification of five suspected FIP-associated SNPs in Birman cats

SNP name	Chr-SNP position[a]	Orientation[b]	Sequence (5' - 3')	T_A[c]	Amplicon size
A1.196617776	A1-154265118	F	GGCAGTCAGAGAATGAGACAC	61 °C	337 bp
		R	TTGCCAGTTCTGCAGATTG		
A1.206840008	A1-164728174	F	AGGTGAAGTGTTGTGTGCAT	61 °C	388 bp
		R	ATGTTCTGCTAGATGAGCCG		
Un.59861682	A1-155715831	F	CTCATCCCAGTTGATCACAC	61 °C	230 bp
		R	TTCCTCCTGGAAAACCCT		
A2.191286425	A2-126618108	F	AGCGTATCAAGTGCCTGC	61 °C	299 bp
		R	CCTTCCTGTTTAGGTGCTTG		
E2.65509996	E2-54165589	F	CGCTTCAGTTTCCTTTCCAG	61 °C	417 bp
		R	TCTGAGCCTTGGTCTTCTG		

[a]Chr: chromosome.
[b]F: forward; R: reverse.
[c]Annealing temperature.

polymorphisms were further identified; the nucleotide positions of the SNPs are numerated from the translation start point (+1).

Association analysis

The association between the targeted SNPs and the occurrence of FIP was analyzed using Fisher's exact test, and a P value < 0.05 was considered to be a significant association.

Results

Polymorphism at fTNFA - 421 was found to be significantly associated with resistance to FIP

Because the overproduction of TNF-α is widely reported in FIP animals and is considered to contribute to the pathogenesis of FIP, we first screened the polymorphisms at the 5' terminus of the *fTNFA* gene, including the proximal regulatory region (PRR), the 5'-untranslated region (UTR), and part of exon 1, in 71 FIP and 93 control cats. Eight SNPs and three repeat regions were identified in the analyzed 1018 bp (Figure 1). One SNP located in exon

1 at position +23 results in the substitution of CGG to CAG, causing an amino acid change from Arg to Gly (R8G); the remaining SNPs were found in the PRR. The mean allele frequencies of the minor alleles ranged from 4.3% to 39.9%. To examine the association between the identified SNPs in *fTNFA* and the outcome of FCoV infection, the frequency of each genotype and allele was analyzed (Additional file 1). Only one allele (T allele) at position −421 appeared to be significantly associated with resistance to FIP ($P = 0.009$, OR = 3.925), whereas the others showed no significance to the disease (Table 3 and Additional file 1).

Polymorphisms in the extracellular domain and introns 6 and 7 of fCD209 were found to be significantly associated with the disease outcome

fCD209 is an important co-receptor for both type I and II FCoV infection. To demonstrate an association between polymorphisms and FIP, we sequenced polymorphisms of the PRR, 5'-UTR, and extracellular domain (ECD) of

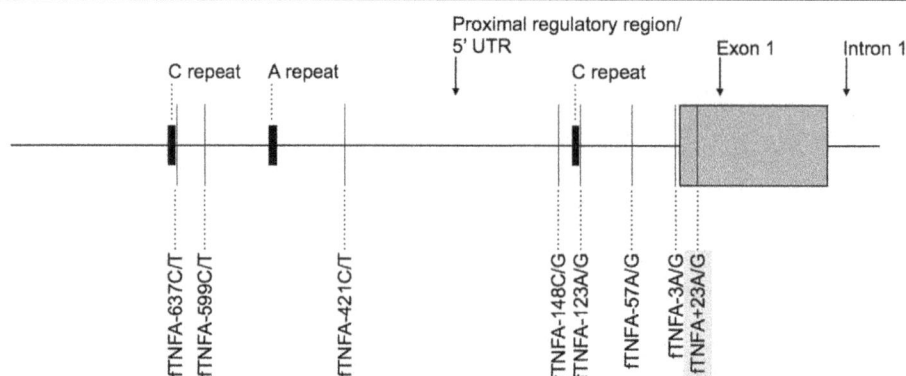

Figure 1 A schematic of the 5' terminal of the *fTNFA* gene analyzed in this study. A partial *fTNFA* sequence of 1018 bp was sequenced in this study, including the PRR, the 5'-UTR, and part of exon 1. All the SNPs and the corresponding positions are indicated with lines. Gray box: exon 1. Black boxes: repeat regions. SNPs located in the exon were shaded.

Table 3 FIP-associated genetic polymorphisms identified in the *fIFNG*, *fTNFA*, and *fCD209* gene and their associations with FIP

Target gene/position	Susceptible allele	Resistant allele	P value	OR[a]	Reference
fIFNG +428	C	T	0.03	3.4 (1.1-10.3)	[16]
fTNFA - 421	C	T	0.009	3.9 (1.3-11.8)	This study
fCD209 + 1900	A	G	0.014	3.7 (1.3-10.5)	This study
fCD209 + 2276	C	T	0.038	NA[b]	This study
fCD209 + 2392	G	A	0.016	2.6 (1.2-5.5)	This study
fCD209 + 2713	T	C	0.039	1.75 (1.1-2.9)	This study

[a]Odds Ratio.
[b]Not available.

fCD209 in 71 FIP and 93 control cats. Twenty-four SNPs and one AG repeat region were identified in the PRR, and one SNP was found in the 5′-UTR (Figure 2). Furthermore, polymorphism screening of ECD, revealed 25 SNPs and a G repeat in the 1350-bp region analyzed (Figure 2). Four SNPs were located in exons, including two SNPs in exon 6 at positions +1900 (TGG > TAG, W128*) and +1952 (AAC > AAA, N145K), one in exon 7 at position +2498 (ACG > ACT, T178T), and one in exon 8 at position +3070 (TTC > TCC, F241S). The remaining 21 SNPs were located in introns 6 and 7 (Figure 2). The mean allele frequencies of the minor alleles ranged from 0.6% to 47.6%.

To further demonstrate the association between the identified SNPs in *fCD209* and the outcome of FCoV infection, the frequency of each genotype and allele was analyzed. Among the 24 SNPs analyzed in the PRR and the 5′-UTR of the *fCD209* gene, no genotype or allele showed a significant association with the outcome of the infection (Additional file 2). In contrast, four SNPs, +1900 in the ECD of exon 6, +2276 and +2392 in intron 6, and +2713 in intron 7, identified in *fCD209* were found to be significantly associated with FIP. *fCD209 + 1900*, located in the ECD, which is characterized by a G-to-A substitution that

leads to a premature stop codon (TGG > TAG, W128*), had a significantly increased frequency in FIP animals (18.31%) compared with the control animals (5.38%) (*P* = 0.011, OR = 3.95), and the A allele was shown to be significantly associated with susceptibility to FIP (*P* = 0.014, OR = 3.65) (Table 3 and Additional file 2). Furthermore, three SNPs, +2276, +2392, and +2713, located in introns 6 and 7 were found to be associated with disease susceptibility. A higher frequency of the T allele at position +2276 in the control cats was significantly associated with resistance to FIP (*P* = 0.038). Similarly, the A allele at position +2392, with a higher frequency in FCoV-infected asymptomatic cats, showed a significant association with disease resistance (*P* = 0.016, OR = 2.57). Moreover, the T allele at position +2713 was identified with a higher frequency in FIP cats, showing a significant association with disease susceptibility (*P* = 0.039, OR = 1.75) (Table 3 and Additional file 2).

Evaluation of the association between the FIP-associated SNPs reported in Birman cats and disease susceptibility in a cat population with higher genetic variability

Five SNPs were reported to be associated with the occurrence of FIP in Birman cats in a recent study using

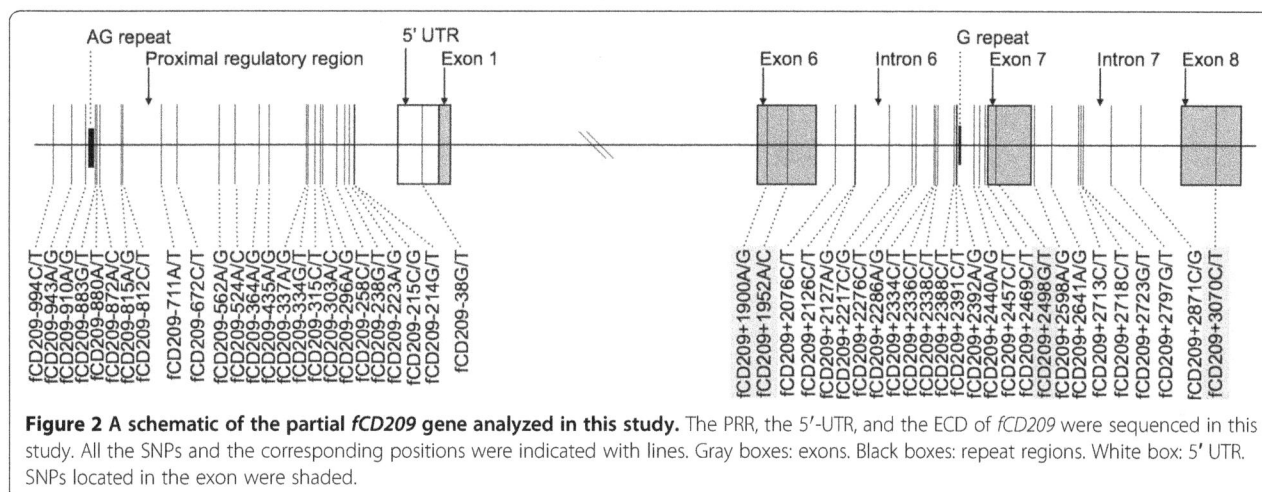

Figure 2 A schematic of the partial *fCD209* gene analyzed in this study. The PRR, the 5′-UTR, and the ECD of *fCD209* were sequenced in this study. All the SNPs and the corresponding positions were indicated with lines. Gray boxes: exons. Black boxes: repeat regions. White box: 5′ UTR. SNPs located in the exon were shaded.

genome-wide association analysis [20]. Due to the lack of information concerning the nucleotide sequence of the SNPs, the sequences were identified. The nucleotide sequences of *A1.196617776, A1.206840008, Un.59861682, A2.191286425,* and *E2.65509996* consisted of C/A, G/A, G/A, C/T, and C/T, respectively. To test for an association of these SNPs with the occurrence of FIP also applies to other breeds of cats, the frequency of each genotype and allele of the targeted SNPs was analyzed in all the FIP and control cats enrolled in this study, i.e., 29.3% purebred and 70.7% mixed breed. Among the five SNPs analyzed, neither the genotype nor allele percentage showed a significant association with the outcome of the disease (Additional file 3).

Association study

Among all the FIP animals analyzed in this study, 64 (64/ 71, 90.1%) cats were found to be effusive form (wet), and the rest seven of them (7/71, 9.9%) were non-effusive (dry). The association between the identified FIP-related SNPs (*fTNFA - 421, fCD209 + 1900, + 2276, + 2392* and *+2713*) and the form of FIP were analyzed. None of the SNPs was found to be associated with the biotype of FIP.

The number of the FIP-associated SNPs harbored is correlated to the disease outcome

This study attempted to distinguish multiple genetic traits associated with FIP susceptibility. The FIP-associated genetic polymorphisms identified in the *fIFNG* [16], *fTNFA,* and *fCD209* genes are summarized in Table 3. Moreover, the association between the number of FIP-associated SNPs harbored, including resistant or susceptible genotype/alleles identified at *fIFNG +428, fTNFA - 421,* and *fCD209 + 1900, + 2276, + 2392,* and *+2713,* and the occurrence of FIP, was analyzed in this study (Table 4). The number of FIP-resistant SNPs carried was found to be associated with the protection of cats from FIP ($P = 0.002$), and the odds ratios of FIP and non-FIP cats carrying one or more (≥ 2) resistance SNPs were 3.06 and 6.01, respectively; this result indicates that cats carrying more resistant SNPs appear to have a lower chance of developing FIP.

However, the FIP cats were identified with a higher frequency as carrying more than one FIP-susceptible SNP (50.7%) than the control cats (29.0%), showing a significant association with disease susceptibility ($P = 0.0059$, OR = 2.51) (Table 4).

Discussion

FIP is an important infectious disease in cats, with nearly 100% mortality. However, an understanding of the host determinants in the occurrence of FIP has been limited to date. An imbalance between cellular and humoral immunity - with excess antibodies contributing to disease progression [4,24] and a significant decrease in IFN-γ production [4,8,10,13-15] - has been consistently observed in FIP animals. We recently identified the first host gene – *fIFNG* – showing an association between host genetic polymorphisms and FIP [16]. A T allele at *fIFNG +428* was identified as a resistant allele, and the heterozygous genotypes (*CT*) at positions +401 and +408 were identified as associated with susceptibility to type I FCoV-induced FIP. In this study, five additional SNPs from *fTNFA* and *fCD209* were identified.

During the development of FIP, the upregulation of TNF-α, an important pro-inflammatory cytokine, has been consistently found [4,17,24,25]. The overproduction of TNF-α induces apoptosis in CD8+ T cells and is associated with the upregulation of a type II FCoV receptor, i.e., feline aminopeptidase N, which accelerates macrophage infection by the virus [26]. Moreover, TNF-α together with granulocyte monocyte-colony stimulating factor (GM-CSF), G-CSF, and other neutrophil survival factors are suggested to prolong the survival of neutrophils, activate monocytes/macrophages, and contribute to the formation of the pyogranulomatous lesions of FIP [25]. In several human diseases, the most commonly identified genetic polymorphisms are located at position −238 and −308 of the promoter region of *TNFA*, suggesting an effect on the binding of transcription factors [27], with susceptibility for the development of several viral diseases, including severe acute respiratory syndrome (SARS) [28], dengue hemorrhagic fever (DHF) [29], and hepatitis

Table 4 Association of the number of the disease-associated SNPs harbored, including *fIFNG +428, fTNFA - 421,* and *fCD209 + 1900, + 2276, + 2392,* and *+2713,* and the outcome of FIP

Genotypes/alleles harbored	FIP number (%)	Non-FIP number (%)	P value	OR (95% CI)
Resistant SNPs				
= 0	59 (83.1%)	54 (58.1%)	0.002	Reference
= 1	10 (14.1%)	28 (30.1%)		3.06 (1.36 - 6.88)
≥ 2	2 (3%)	11 (11.8%)		6.01 (1.27 - 28.35)
Susceptible SNPs				
= 0	35 (49.3%)	66 (71.0%)	0.0059	Reference
≥ 1	36 (50.7%)	27 (29.0%)		2.51 (1.32 - 4.80)

B virus (HBV) infection [30]. Compared to the human gene (*TNFA - 308*), SNP located in a slightly upstream region of the feline gene (*fTNFA - 421*) was found to be significantly associated with the occurrence of FIP. The variant *fTNFA - 421 T* allele was significantly associated with resistance to FIP. Through DNA transcriptional factor binding site prediction, we found that an *fTNFA - 421* C to T mutation might affect the binding of some transcription factors, such as myeloid zinc finger 1 (MZF1) [31], a transcriptional regulator [32]. Through promoter binding, MZF1 was identified to function as a transcription activator of hematopoietic cells in vitro [32]. Because macrophages are hematopoietic cells, the loss of the binding site for such transcription factors might decrease TNF-α production in macrophages, which might prevent the immunopathogenesis and result in a resistant phenotype.

DC-SIGN, which recognizes high-mannose oligosaccharides as its ligand, is a co-receptor augmenting many viral infections, including human immunodeficiency virus [33], dengue virus [34], HBV [35], and SARS-coronavirus [36]. In addition, feline DC-SIGN also serves as a co-receptor and is involved in infection by FCoV [19]. A human SNP in the promoter region of *CD209* (*−336 A/G*) was identified as related to disease prognosis [36]. A variant of *CD209 - 336* was reported to affect the binding of SP1-like transcription factor and might modulate transcriptional activities [34], indicating that *CD209 - 336* plays a crucial role in disease pathogenesis. However, in our study, none of the SNPs in the promoter region showed an association with the outcome of FCoV infection. The identified FIP-associated SNPs, +1900 G/A, +2276 C/T, +2392 G/A, and +2713 C/T, were all located at the 3′ end of *fCD209*. The polymorphism identified at *fCD209 + 1900* is located in the lectin binding domain of the ECD; a G to A substitution leads to a change from a tryptophan at amino acid 128 to a stop codon. This mutation might lead to an abortive mRNA [37] or a truncated protein if the mRNA is successfully translated. DC-SIGN serves as a pattern recognition receptor that interact with numerous pathogens, including FCoV, and mediates the clustering of DC with naive T cells [38]. Additionally, with a type II transmembrane domain, the truncated fDC-SIGN identified in this study (+1900) might still be expressed on the cell surface. However, it remains to be elucidated how the truncated protein, bearing only one half of the authentic protein, affect the normal function of DC-SIGN, i.e., pathogen recognition or T cell activation. The other three FIP-associated SNPs were located in introns 6 and 7. Although these polymorphisms are located in introns, which apparently would not affect the protein, a regulatory effect cannot be excluded. In humans, the SNP at *IFNG +874*, located in intron 1, was found to alter the binding activity of nuclear factor kappa-light-chain-enhancer of activated B cells and

influenced the production of IFN-γ [39]. In swine, an SNP (G3072A) in intron 3 of insulin-like growth factor 2 affected the binding of muscle growth regulator and was associated with the muscle content [40].

Several pedigreed cats, including Abyssinians, Himalayans, Birmans, Bengals, Ragdolls, and Rexes, were reported to have a higher incidence of FIP than other breed cats [2]. Recently, a genome-wide association study of Danish and American Birman cats populations identified five SNPs involved in FIP susceptibility [20]. However, none of these SNPs showed a similar correlation in the present study, concordant with the postulation by the authors that these associations might only be relevant to Birman breed or other breeds with similar genetic traits [24].

In addition to the three SNPs in *fIFNG*, we identified in this study five more SNPs from two genes - one in *fTNFA* and four in *fCD209* - that are associated with the occurrence of FIP. As the susceptibility or resistance to viral infections is a complex phenotype regulated by multiple interacting genes and gene networks, genes related to innate and adaptive immunity and other host genes remain to be pursued. The combination of all the FIP susceptibility genotypes into a single typing diagnosis assay should facilitate the screening of FIP-resistant cats in breeding and eventually decrease the loss of cats to this incurable disease.

Additional files

Additional file 1: Frequencies of the *fTNFA* genotypes and alleles and associations with the outcome of FCoV infection. The promoter variant, *fTNFA - 421 T*, was found to be a disease-resistance genotype.

Additional file 2: Frequencies of the *fCD209* genotypes and alleles and associations with the outcome of FCoV infection. Polymorphisms of *fCD209*, including *fCD209 + 1900*, *+ 2276*, *+ 2392* and *+2713*, were found to be significantly associated with the disease outcome.

Additional file 3: Frequencies of the genotypes and alleles of the proposed FIP-associated SNPs in Birman cats and associations with FIP. Neither the percentage of genotypes nor alleles was found to be associated with the outcome of FCoV infection in disease and non-disease group.

Competing interests
The authors declare that they have no competing interests.

Authors' contributions
YTW performed the sampling and preparation, DNA/RNA extraction, FCoV detection, the amplification and sequencing of fIFNG, fTNFA, fCD209 and five Birman FIP cat-associated SNPs and further analysis and prepared the manuscript. LEH participated in primers design, DNA extraction, fIFNG, fTNFA and fCD209 amplification, sequencing and further analysis and prepared the manuscript. YRD preformed DNA extraction and fIFNG, fTNFA and fCD209 amplification. LLC conceived of the study, participated in study design and coordination and contributed to the preparation of the manuscript. All authors read and approved the final manuscript.

Acknowledgements
We would like to thank Betty A. Wu-Hsieh from Graduate Institute of Immunology, National Taiwan University for the valuable suggestion in the selection of candidate genes. This work was supported by the grant MOST 103-2313-B-002-042 from the Ministry of Science and Technology, Taiwan.

References

1. Hartmann K: **Feline infectious peritonitis.** *Vet Clin North Am Small Anim Pract* 2005, **35**:39–79.

2. Pedersen NC: **A review of feline infectious peritonitis virus infection: 1963–2008.** *J Feline Med Surg* 2009, **11**:225–258.

3. Holzworth J: **Some important disorders of cats.** *Cornell Vet* 1963, **53**:157–160.

4. Kipar A, Meli ML: **Feline infectious peritonitis: still an enigma?** *Vet Pathol* 2014, **51**:505–526.

5. Satoh R, Furukawa T, Kotake M, Takano T, Motokawa K, Gemma T, Watanabe R, Arai S, Hohdatsu T: **Screening and identification of T helper 1 and linear immunodominant antibody-binding epitopes in the spike 2 domain and the nucleocapsid protein of feline infectious peritonitis virus.** *Vaccine* 2011, **29**:1791–1800.

6. de Groot-Mijnes JD, van Dun JM, van der Most RG, de Groot RJ: **Natural history of a recurrent feline coronavirus infection and the role of cellular immunity in survival and disease.** *J Virol* 2005, **79**:1036–1044.

7. Haijema BJ, Volders H, Rottier PJ: **Live, attenuated coronavirus vaccines through the directed deletion of group-specific genes provide protection against feline infectious peritonitis.** *J Virol* 2004, **78**:3863–3871.

8. Kiss I, Poland AM, Pedersen NC: **Disease outcome and cytokine responses in cats immunized with an avirulent feline infectious peritonitis virus (FIPV)-UCD1 and challenge-exposed with virulent FIPV-UCD8.** *J Feline Med Surg* 2004, **6**:89–97.

9. Hohdatsu T, Yamato H, Ohkawa T, Kaneko M, Motokawa K, Kusuhara H, Kaneshima T, Arai S, Koyama H: **Vaccine efficacy of a cell lysate with recombinant baculovirus-expressed feline infectious peritonitis (FIP) virus nucleocapsid protein against progression of FIP.** *Vet Microbiol* 2003, **97**:31–44.

10. Dean GA, Olivry T, Stanton C, Pedersen NC: **In vivo cytokine response to experimental feline infectious peritonitis virus infection.** *Vet Microbiol* 2003, **97**:1–12.

11. Pesteanu-Somogyi LD, Radzai C, Pressler BM: **Prevalence of feline infectious peritonitis in specific cat breeds.** *J Feline Med Surg* 2006, **8**:1–5.

12. Worthing KA, Wigney DI, Dhand NK, Fawcett A, McDonagh P, Malik R, Norris JM: **Risk factors for feline infectious peritonitis in Australian cats.** *J Feline Med Surg* 2012, **14**:405–412.

13. Giordano A, Paltrinieri S: **Interferon-gamma in the serum and effusions of cats with feline coronavirus infection.** *Vet J* 2009, **180**:396–398.

14. Gelain ME, Meli M, Paltrinieri S: **Whole blood cytokine profiles in cats infected by feline coronavirus and healthy non-FCoV infected specific pathogen-free cats.** *J Feline Med Surg* 2006, **8**:389–399.

15. Gunn-Moore DA, Caney SM, Gruffydd-Jones TJ, Helps CR, Harbour DA: **Antibody and cytokine responses in kittens during the development of feline infectious peritonitis (FIP).** *Vet Immunol Immunopathol* 1998, **65**:221–242.

16. Hsieh LE, Chueh LL: **Identification and genotyping of feline infectious peritonitis-associated single nucleotide polymorphisms in the feline interferon-gamma gene.** *Vet Res* 2014, **45**:57.

17. Takano T, Hohdatsu T, Hashida Y, Kaneko Y, Tanabe M, Koyama H: **A "possible" involvement of TNF-alpha in apoptosis induction in peripheral blood lymphocytes of cats with feline infectious peritonitis.** *Vet Microbiol* 2007, **119**:121–131.

18. Regan AD, Ousterout DG, Whittaker GR: **Feline lectin activity is critical for the cellular entry of feline infectious peritonitis virus.** *J Virol* 2010, **84**:7917–7921.

19. Van Hamme E, Desmarets L, Dewerchin HL, Nauwynck HJ: **Intriguing interplay between feline infectious peritonitis virus and its receptors during entry in primary feline monocytes.** *Virus Res* 2011, **160**:32–39.

20. Golovko L, Lyons LA, Liu H, Sorensen A, Wehnert S, Pedersen NC: **Genetic susceptibility to feline infectious peritonitis in Birman cats.** *Virus Res* 2013, **175**:58–63.

21. Herrewegh AA, de Groot RJ, Cepica A, Egberink HF, Horzinek MC, Rottier PJ: **Detection of feline coronavirus RNA in feces, tissues, and body fluids of naturally infected cats by reverse transcriptase PCR.** *J Clin Microbiol* 1995, **33**:684–689.

22. Nishimura Y, Goto Y, Pang H, Endo Y, Mizuno T, Momoi Y, Watari T, Tsujimoto H, Hasegawa A: **Genetic heterogeneity of env gene of feline immunodeficiency virus obtained from multiple districts in Japan.** *Virus Res* 1998, **57**:101–112.

23. Stiles J, Bienzle D, Render JA, Buyukmihci NC, Johnson EC: **Use of nested polymerase chain reaction (PCR) for detection of retroviruses from formalin-fixed, paraffin-embedded uveal melanomas in cats.** *Vet Ophthalmol* 1999, **2**:113–116.

24. Pedersen NC: **An update on feline infectious peritonitis: virology and immunopathogenesis.** *Vet J* 2014, **201**:123–132.

25. Takano T, Azuma N, Satoh M, Toda A, Hashida Y, Satoh R, Hohdatsu T: **Neutrophil survival factors (TNF-alpha, GM-CSF, and G-CSF) produced by macrophages in cats infected with feline infectious peritonitis virus contribute to the pathogenesis of granulomatous lesions.** *Arch Virol* 2009, **154**:775–781.

26. Takano T, Hohdatsu T, Toda A, Tanabe M, Koyama H: **TNF-alpha, produced by feline infectious peritonitis virus (FIPV)-infected macrophages, upregulates expression of type II FIPV receptor feline aminopeptidase N in feline macrophages.** *Virology* 2007, **364**:64–72.

27. Smith AJ, Humphries SE: **Cytokine and cytokine receptor gene polymorphisms and their functionality.** *Cytokine Growth Factor Rev* 2009, **20**:43–59.

28. Wang S, Wei M, Han Y, Zhang K, He L, Yang Z, Su B, Zhang Z, Hu Y, Hui W: **Roles of TNF-alpha gene polymorphisms in the occurrence and progress of SARS-Cov infection: a case–control study.** *BMC Infect Dis* 2008, **8**:27.

29. Perez AB, Sierra B, Garcia G, Aguirre E, Babel N, Alvarez M, Sanchez L, Valdes L, Volk HD, Guzman MG: **Tumor necrosis factor-alpha, transforming growth factor-beta1, and interleukin-10 gene polymorphisms: implication in protection or susceptibility to dengue hemorrhagic fever.** *Hum Immunol* 2010, **71**:1135–1140.

30. Xia Q, Zhou L, Liu D, Chen Z, Chen F: **Relationship between TNF-< alpha > gene promoter polymorphisms and outcomes of hepatitis B virus infections: a meta-analysis.** *PLoS One* 2011, **6**:e19606.

31. Heinemeyer T, Wingender E, Reuter I, Hermjakob H, Kel AE, Kel OV, Ignatieva EV, Ananko EA, Podkolodnaya OA, Kolpakov FA, Podkolodny NL, Kolchanov NA: **Databases on transcriptional regulation: TRANSFAC, TRRD and COMPEL.** *Nucleic Acids Res* 1998, **26**:362–367.

32. Morris JF, Rauscher FJ 3rd, Davis B, Klemsz M, Xu D, Tenen D, Hromas R: **The myeloid zinc finger gene, MZF-1, regulates the CD34 promoter in vitro.** *Blood* 1995, **86**:3640–3647.

33. Boily-Larouche G, Milev MP, Zijenah LS, Labbe AC, Zannou DM, Humphrey JH, Ward BJ, Poudrier J, Mouland AJ, Cohen EA, Roger M: **Naturally-occurring genetic variants in human DC-SIGN increase HIV-1 capture, cell-transfer and risk of mother-to-child transmission.** *PLoS One* 2012, **7**:e40706.

34. Sakuntabhai A, Turbpaiboon C, Casademont I, Chuansumrit A, Lowhnoo T, Kajaste-Rudnitski A, Kalayanarooj SM, Tangnararatchakit K, Tangthawornchaikul N, Vasanawathana S, Chaiyaratana W, Yenchitsomanus PT, Suriyaphol P, Avirutnan P, Chokephaibulkit K, Matsuda F, Yoksan S, Jacob Y, Lathrop GM, Malasit P, Despres P, Julier C: **A variant in the CD209 promoter is associated with severity of dengue disease.** *Nat Genet* 2005, **37**:507–513.

35. Rebbani K, Ezzikouri S, Marchio A, Ababou M, Kitab B, Dejean A, Kandil M, Pineau P, Benjelloun S: **Common polymorphic effectors of immunity against hepatitis B and C modulate susceptibility to infection and spontaneous clearance in a Moroccan population.** *Infect Genet Evol* 2014, **26**:1–7.

36. Chan KY, Xu MS, Ching JC, So TM, Lai ST, Chu CM, Yam LY, Wong AT, Chung PH, Chan VS, Lin CL, Sham PC, Leung GM, Peiris JS, Khoo US: **CD209 (DC-SIGN) -336A > G promoter polymorphism and severe acute respiratory syndrome in Hong Kong Chinese.** *Hum Immunol* 2010, **71**:702–707.

37. Waston JD, Baker TA, Bell SP, Gann A, Levine M, Losick R: **Translation.** In *Molecular Biology of the Gene*. Edited by W. B. New York: Cold harbor laboratory press; 2008:457–519.

38. den Dunnen J, Gringhuis SI, Geijtenbeek TB: **Innate signaling by the C-type lectin DC-SIGN dictates immune responses.** *Cancer Immunol Immunother* 2009, **58**:1149–1157.

39. Pravica V, Perrey C, Stevens A, Lee JH, Hutchinson IV: **A single nucleotide polymorphism in the first intron of the human IFN-gamma gene: absolute correlation with a polymorphic CA microsatellite marker of high IFN-gamma production.** *Hum Immunol* 2000, **61**:863–866.

40. Butter F, Kappei D, Buchholz F, Vermeulen M, Mann M: **A domesticated transposon mediates the effects of a single-nucleotide polymorphism responsible for enhanced muscle growth.** *EMBO Rep* 2010, **11**:305–311.

9

Modelling the spread of bovine viral diarrhea virus (BVDV) in a beef cattle herd and its impact on herd productivity

Alix Damman[1,2], Anne-France Viet[1,2], Sandie Arnoux[1,2], Marie-Claude Guerrier-Chatellet[3], Etienne Petit[3] and Pauline Ezanno[1,2]*

Abstract

Bovine viral diarrhea virus (BVDV) is a common pathogen of cattle herds that causes economic losses due to reproductive disorders in breeding cattle and increased morbidity and mortality amongst infected calves. Our objective was to evaluate the impact of BVDV spread on the productivity of a beef cow-calf herd using a stochastic model in discrete time that accounted for (1) the difference in transmission rates when animals are housed indoors versus grazing on pasture, (2) the external risk of disease introductions through fenceline contact with neighboring herds and the purchase of infected cattle, and (3) the risk of individual pregnant cattle generating persistently infected (PI) calves based on their stage in gestation. The model predicted the highest losses from BVDV during the first 3 years after disease was introduced into a naive herd. During the endemic phase, the impact of BVDV on the yearly herd productivity was much lower due to herd immunity. However, cumulative losses over 10 years in an endemic situation greatly surpassed the losses that occurred during the acute phase. A sensitivity analysis of key model parameters revealed that herd size, the duration of breeding, grazing, and selling periods, renewal rate of breeding females, and the level of numerical productivity expected by the farmer had a significant influence on the predicted losses. This model provides a valuable framework for evaluating the impact of BVDV and the efficacy of different control strategies in beef cow-calf herds.

Introduction

Bovine viral diarrhea virus (BVDV) affects most industrialized cattle farming systems by inducing reproductive disorders (abortion, delayed calving, reduced fertility) in breeding cattle and by lowering herd productivity through increased culling, morbidity, and mortality [1]. Introductions may occur through the direct purchase of infected animals when cattle are housed indoors as well as through fenceline contact with infected animals in neighboring herds when cattle are grazed outdoors on pasture. The likelihood of these introductions depends on the control measures that are implemented by individual farms. In some areas (e.g. Brittany, France: [2]), purchased animals are guaranteed not to be persistently infected based on knowledge of their dam status, previous diagnostic testing, or their source herd status. In other areas, although there are pre-purchase diagnostic tests available for BVDV, most farmers tend not to use them [3,4]. It is also difficult to determine whether pregnant females on pasture are at subsequent risk of delivering persistently infected (PI) calves since there are few reliable prenatal tests for BVDV. The severity of production losses following disease introduction is also related to several additional management factors, including (1) the level of herd immunity from previous natural exposure [5] or preventative vaccination [6], (2) the percentage of dams that are at risk for generating PI calves through vertical transmission, and (3) the ability for BVDV to spread within and between different production subgroups within a herd [7]. In the absence of a calf surveillance scheme, it may be difficult for farmers to detect the presence of BVDV in the herd leading to the establishment of an endemic disease state and long term production losses.

* Correspondence: pauline.ezanno@oniris-nantes.fr
[1]INRA, UMR1300 BioEpAR, CS 40706, F-44307 Nantes, France
[2]Oniris, LUNAM Université, UMR BioEpAR, F-44307 Nantes, France
Full list of author information is available at the end of the article

Modelling is a pertinent approach to predict pathogen spread and persistence in a herd and to evaluate its impact on herd dynamics and productivity for a large range of management scenarios [8]. Many of the modelling studies conducted to date have concerned dairy cattle herds, both at the herd [7,9,10] and regional scales [11-13]. However, beef cow-calf herds have a unique demographic structure that has not been captured by previously published models. First, beef cattle are frequently grazed outside for long periods, particularly at the time when pregnant dams have the greatest risk of generating PI calves following exposure to BVDV through fenceline contacts. Second, the calving period is concentrated over a few months and calves are raised with cows until weaning. This increases the duration and intensity of exposure to BVDV as PI animals mainly are observed in young stock due to a shortened life expectancy [14]. Therefore, conclusions drawn for dairy herds cannot be directly transferred to beef farming systems. Models of BVDV spread in a beef herd have been proposed to evaluate the costs associated with epidemics in naive herds [15] or to compare control [16] and testing [17] strategies. Two recent models account for BVDV introduction due to animal purchases or fenceline contacts [5,18], representing an endemic situation. However, none of these models simultaneously account for the within-herd contact structure, the difference between the indoor and outdoor periods in within-herd virus transmission, and the risk of continuous virus introduction due to the purchase of animals and contacts with neighboring infected herds. All of these processes are expected to greatly influence BVDV spread and persistence in a beef cow-calf herd and, consequently, impact the associated losses.

Our objective was to evaluate the impact of BVDV spread on the productivity of a beef cow-calf herd across a large range of management scenarios. A stochastic epidemiological model was proposed that accounted for different transmission rates between separately managed production groups during the outdoor grazing period versus a homogeneous population structure during the indoor period. The model also incorporated an external risk of BVDV introduction through fenceline contacts with neighboring herds as well as through animal purchases. A sensitivity analysis was conducted to determine the relative importance of management factors such as herd size, the length of breeding, grazing, and selling periods, the replacement rate of breeding females, and level of numerical productivity expected by the farmer. Comparisons of production losses in acute outbreaks and endemic situations were also performed.

Materials and methods

A stochastic compartmental model in discrete time was developed to simulate the spread of BVDV. A time interval of 7 days was chosen as the longest as possible to properly represent transiently-infected animals in the infection process. The model was fully implemented in C++, allowing the model to be run rapidly.

Herd dynamics

The farming system modelled and used for simulations in this work was based on the characteristics of beef cow-calf herds in Bourgogne, one of the main beef production regions in France. In this area, animals are indoors during the winter and most of them are outdoors from spring to autumn (Figure 1). Purchases are limited over time and consist of replacement calves, pregnant females, and bulls for replacement. The herd dynamics presented here was based on that presented in [19].

The number of females kept for breeding was fixed according to the target number of calves weaned per year, adjusted according to the anticipated losses from routine infertility and calf mortality. Anticipated losses varied according to the level of numerical productivity expected by the farmer, stated by the adjustment factor ε (Table 1).

The herd was structured into 7 groups: calves from birth until weaning, male and female weaned calves for selling (grassers), heifers under the age of two kept for renewal, bred heifers, cows from the first pregnancy diagnosis until fattening decision, cows from fattening decision until culling, and bulls. The herd dynamics relies on specific dates when animals change groups (Figure 1, Table 1).

At weaning, some female calves were grouped with young heifers for renewal while others were fattened for sale during the year. The gender of calves was determined stochastically according to the sex ratio ρ_{sex} (Table 1). The number of females selected for renewal was fixed. In case of unexpectedly high calf mortality, replacement calves could be purchased. The replacement of a dead calf was allowed from the beginning of the calving period until three months after its end. Purchase occurred if the number of calves present and to be born in the herd fell below the production objective.

At the beginning of the indoor period, all pregnant heifers and cows were merged to be raised together while non-pregnant ones were fattened for 100 days before being sold. The model determines the expected number of calvings according to the production objective. If the expected number of pregnant animals was below the target number of calvings to meet production objectives, pregnant females were purchased at the beginning of the indoor period to reach this number.

At the beginning of the breeding period, a fixed number of females was selected among the 2-year-old heifers to form the group of bred heifers. The remaining 2-year-old heifers were sold. Cows were split into two groups. A fixed

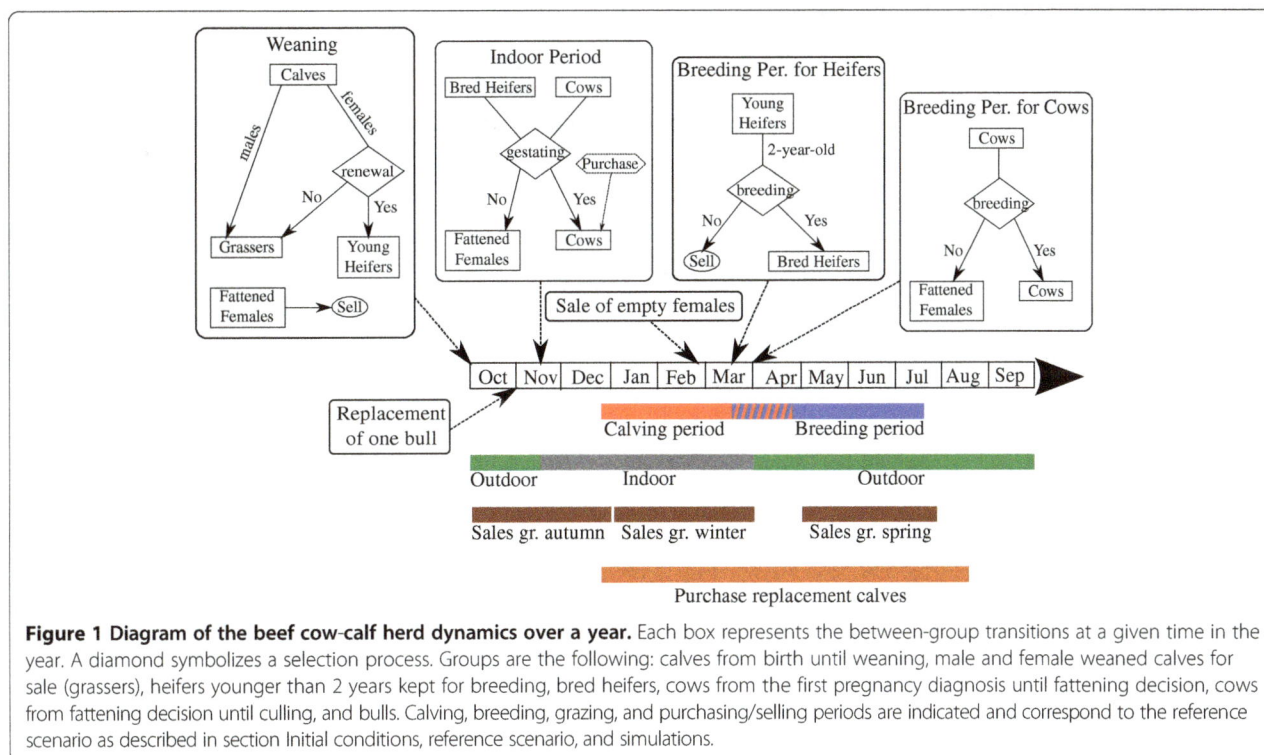

Figure 1 Diagram of the beef cow-calf herd dynamics over a year. Each box represents the between-group transitions at a given time in the year. A diamond symbolizes a selection process. Groups are the following: calves from birth until weaning, male and female weaned calves for sale (grassers), heifers younger than 2 years kept for breeding, bred heifers, cows from the first pregnancy diagnosis until fattening decision, cows from fattening decision until culling, and bulls. Calving, breeding, grazing, and purchasing/selling periods are indicated and correspond to the reference scenario as described in section Initial conditions, reference scenario, and simulations.

number of cows formed the breeding stock while the others were fattened until their calves were weaned. Then, they were culled. The period began 2 weeks earlier for heifers than for cows, and ended when bulls were separated from breeding females. We integrated in the compartmental model an individual-based monitoring of pregnant females. From the start of pregnancy until calving, each female is represented individually to precisely predict her stage of pregnancy over time.

Calving occurred 285 days after the beginning of gestation and the mother was then not available for breeding for a period of 20 days. Twins were born with probability δ (Table 1). During the breeding period, the delay between the moment when a cow was available for breeding and the start of a new pregnancy was determined by a gamma distribution with parameters a and b. The values of these parameters (Table 1) were chosen to reproduce the observed calving-to-calving intervals as presented in [19]. The same gamma distribution with the same parameter values was used regardless of whether breeding females were indoors or at pasture. The date of a new pregnancy was calculated if the animal was not declared infertile. The probability of infertility of heifers and cows is given by parameters τ_{He} and τ_{Co}, respectively (Table 1). The calculated new pregnancy date must be before the end of the breeding period otherwise the animal was considered as non-pregnant.

The simulated average date of calving was 60 days after the beginning of the calving period. The indoor

and breeding periods can be chosen within a certain range. It was assumed that both the calving and the breeding periods started during the indoor period. The date of weaning was chosen so that calves were weaned at the average age of 6 up to 8 months on the field.

All animals placed in the group of grassers after weaning were sold over the course of the year. The model simulates various periods for sales. These periods were specifically considered because they impact the duration that potentially infected animals are present in the herd. Indeed, animals can be sold at one, two or three periods in the year. Dates of selling were randomly chosen each year using triangular distributions for the three periods: (23/10, 15/11, 07/12), (23/01, 15/02, 07/03) and (23/05, 15/06, 07/07). The proportion of animals sold at each period was fixed at the beginning of each simulation.

The number of bulls present in the herd was assumed to be constant. The model assigns one bull per 20 bred heifers or cows. Each year, on November 1st, a bull was randomly selected for replacement.

Within-herd infection dynamics

Animals were classified into mutually exclusive BVDV health states (Figure 2): susceptible (S), transiently-infected (T), recovered, i.e. immune (R), protected by maternal antibodies (M) or persistently infected (PI; P). The M to S and T to R transitions depend on transition rates ϕ_{MS} and ϕ_{TR} (Table 1). Since maternal protection generally lasts 4-6 months [31], we assumed that the M to S transition

Table 1 Definitions and values of model parameters

Parameters	Values	Definitions	Sources
ρ_{sex}	0.5	Sex ratio	
a, b	8.7, 6	Parameters of the gamma distribution used to calculate the next start of pregnancy	
δ	0.035	Probability of twin birth	
τ_{He}	0.02	Probability of infertility for heifers	
τ_{Co}	0.08	Probability of infertility for cows	
breeding_start	15th of March	Date of start of the breeding period	
breeding_dur	[16 **18** 20]	Duration of the breeding period (in weeks)	
weaning	1st October	Date of weaning	
pasture_start	1st April	Date of start of the pasture period	
pasture_dur	[29 **32** 35]	Duration of the pasture period (in weeks)	
renewal_rate	[0.286 **0.317** 0.349]	Ratio heifers/cows	
sell_period	[autumn **winter** spring]	Sell period of grassers[1]	
size	[42 **83** 125]	Number of bred females[2]	
$\mu_{Ca,bi}$	0.0225	Probability of mortality at birth of calves	
μ_{Ca}	0.000333	Mortality rate of calves (d^{-1})	
intro_week	[(20 25 30) **27** 40]	Week of introduction of PI animal(s)[3].	
ε	[0.95 **1** 1.05]	Level of numerical productivity expected by the farmer	
$\mu_{P,bi}$	[0.06 **0.0667** 0.0733]	Probability of mortality at birth of PI calves	
μ_P	[0.0017 **0.0019** 0.0021]	Mortity of PI animals per day	[20]
φ_{MS}	[0.006 **0.00667** 0.00733]	Trantion rate from state M to state S (d^{-1})	[21]
φ_{TR}	[0.18 **0.2** 0.22]	Transition rate from state T to state R (d^{-1})	[22]
β^T	[0.027 **0.03** 0.033]	Daily transmission rate for T animals	[9,23]
β^P	[0.45 **0.5** 0.55]	Daily transmission rate for PI animals	[9,24]
β^P_b	[0.09 **0.1** 0.11]	Daily between-group transmission rate for PI animals	[9,25,26]
a_{Ra}	[0.72 **0.8** 0.88]	Abortion rate due to infection in early pregnancy	[22,27]
a_{Rb}	[0.18 **0.2** 0.22]	Abortion rate due to infection in mid-pregnancy	[28,29]
η_X		Probability of giving birth to a calf in state X if infection in mid-pregnancy and no abortion	[24,28-30]
η_P	[0.875 **0.9375** 1]		
η_M	[0.0625 **0.03125** 0]		
η_R	[0.0625 **0.03125** 0]		
K_{ext}	0	Risk of virus introduction on pasture	

Nominal values are in bold. Other values are the ones tested in the model sensitivity analysis.
[1]In the reference scenario, grassers were sold at the three periods: 45% in autumn, 45% in winter, and 10% in spring.
[2]Bred females are heifers and cows, with: 42 = 10 heifers + 32 cows, 83 = 20 heifers + 63 cows, 125 = 30 heifers + 95 cows.
[3]In the first case, 3 PI animals were introduced successively in weeks 20, 25, and 30. In the two other cases, a single PI animal was introduced.

occurred only in the Calf group. The S to T transition represents horizontal transmission. It depends on the repartition of the shedding animals (T, PI) in the herd.

During the indoor winter period, the risk of infection is assumed to be equally distributed among all animals. In that case, the transmission rate f is given by

$$f = \beta^P \frac{N^P}{N} + \beta^T \frac{N^T}{N}, \qquad (1)$$

where N^P and N^T are the total numbers of PI and T animals in the herd, respectively; N the herd size, and β^P

and β^T the transmission rates per day associated with the PI and T animals, respectively (see Table 1).

During the outdoor period, animals were split into separate pastures except remaining grassers which remain indoors until they were sold. Three groups were considered to be raised on different pastures: young heifers, bred heifers plus part of the bulls, and cows (with their calves) plus remaining bulls. We assumed this latter group to be homogeneously mixed. Virus transmission outdoors was due to transmission within each group (with the same formulation as indoors) and between pairs of groups (as in [7], accounting for the

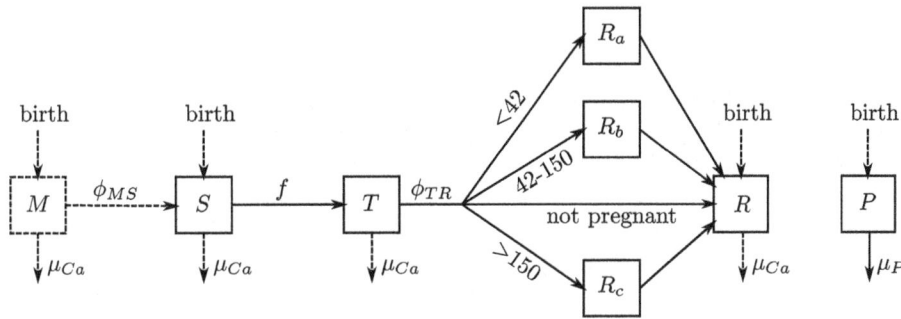

Figure 2 Diagram of the transitions between health states. S: susceptible; T: transiently-infected; P: persistently infected; M: protected by maternal antibodies; R: immune; R_a, R_b, R_c: immune which have been infected in early, mid and late pregnancy, respectively. Dotted lines concern only calves. The values of the transition rates φ_{MS} and φ_{TR} are given in Table 1. The value of the transition rate f is derived from eq. 1 and eq. 2.

size of both groups in contact and for PI animals only as virus sources). Contacts with PI animals from neighboring farms may also occur. Since this risk is unknown, we assumed here a constant risk K_{ext}. Hence, transmission rate f_k associated with animals in pasture k reads:

$$f_k = \beta^P \frac{N_k^P}{N_k} + \beta^T \frac{N_k^T}{N_k} + \beta_b^P \left(\frac{K_{ext}}{N_k} + \sum_{k' \neq k} \frac{N_{k'}^P}{N_{k'} N_k} \right), \quad (2)$$

with N_k^P and N_k^T the numbers of PI and T animals in pasture k, respectively, N_k the number of animals in pasture k, k' all the pastures in contact with pasture k, and β_b^P the between-group transmission rate per day associated with PI animals.

Immune cows (R) gave birth to calves protected by maternal antibodies (M) acquired via colostrum. Susceptible (S) or PI (P) cows gave birth to calves in the same state. If mothers were infected during pregnancy, consequences differed depending on the stage of the pregnancy at the time of infection. As females are individually monitored during pregnancy, their stages are known precisely. The pregnancy period was divided into three stages: early pregnancy (0-41 days; R_a), mid pregnancy (42-150 days; R_b), and late pregnancy (151-285 days; R_c). Infection during the first stage led to either embryonic or fetal death with probability α_{Ra} (Table 1), or the birth of a calf protected by maternal antibodies (M). Different consequences of infection during mid-pregnancy are possible [22,24,27-30]. The pregnant female may abort with probability α_{Rb} (Table 1). If not, the calf can be born in states M, R, or P with probabilities η_M, η_R, or η_P respectively. Finally, if infection occurs during late pregnancy, the mother gives birth to an immune calf (R). In case of abortion, a delay of 60 days is applied between the end of infection and abortion. The female is then unavailable for breeding for 20 days. If abortion occurs not too late, i.e. at least 20 days before the end of the breeding period, the female may return to

the pregnancy state using the algorithm explained in the previous section.

All transitions between health states as well as births and deaths are schematically represented in Figure 2. Transition rates per day are given in Table 1. Transfers between health states were performed using binomials. The probability of transition from compartment i to j is given by

$$p_{ij} = 1 - exp(-\Delta t \tau_{ij}), \quad (3)$$

where Δt is the time step (7 days) and τ_{ij} the daily transition rate between compartments i and j. The transition ΔN_{ij} is then calculated as

$$\Delta N_{ij} = Bin(N_i, p_{ij}), \quad (4)$$

where N_i represents the number of individuals present in compartment i. In the case of multiple transfers, we used multinomials instead [32]. The transfers between groups were made by randomly selecting animals from all health states.

Females in the group of young heifers stayed two years in that group. For this group, all compartments were doubled to differentiate one-year and two-year-old heifers. At the beginning of the reproduction period, only two-year-old heifers were either selected for breeding and transferred in the bred heifer group, or sold.

At birth, PI and non-PI calves had a probability of dying of $\mu_{P,bi}$ and $\mu_{Ca,bi}$, respectively (Table 1). The proportion of deaths at birth for PI calves encompassed the deaths of abnormal calves. The model associates a mortality rate μ_{Ca} with non-PI calves between calving and weaning and μ_P with all PI animals (Table 1). Finally, 9% of all calves died before weaning and PI animals had a half-life of 1 year.

Purchased animals (calves, pregnant females, and bulls) can be of any health state in the model (S, T, P, RP).

Initial conditions, reference scenario, and simulations

A simulation year started after weaning (1st October), corresponding to week 0 (Figure 1). In the reference scenario, the indoor period ranged from week 6 to 26 (mid-November to March). The breeding period started during the indoor period on week 23 (mid-March) for bred heifers and on week 25 (end of March) for cows. It finished on week 41 (mid-July) when bulls were separated from breeding females. The calving period ranged from week 12 to 29. It corresponds to the indoor period plus one week. The initial herd was obtained by running the model for 4 years without BVDV introduction. The fourth year was used to obtained mean reference values for purchases, sales, and number of weaned calves. Then, the birth of a PI calf was simulated at the beginning of the cow breeding period (week 27) in an average herd representative of herds in the Bourgogne region (France). The number of bred heifers and cows are 20 and 63, respectively. We assumed a basic level of numerical productivity expected by the farmer, i.e. the farmer does not expect losses to differ from usual infertility of breeding females and calf mortality ($\varepsilon = 1$). In such a situation, the production objective was equal to 73 weaned calves per year (for 83 bred females). After introducing a PI animal, the simulation continued for 15 years, the first three years being representative of an acute phase (infection arising in a naive herd), whereas years 6 to 15 were representative of an endemic phase (when infection persists in the herd). In the reference scenario, we assumed that all the purchased animals were susceptible and that no infection due to neighboring contacts occurred ($K_{ext} = 0$). For each scenario considered thereafter, 3000 repetitions were performed.

Outputs

Outputs were selected to represent infection dynamics and the impact of BVDV on herd productivity. Outputs associated with infection dynamics are the probability of virus persistence in the herd (infected herds having ≥ 1 PI or T animal, or ≥ 1 immune dam carrying a PI fetus), and the prevalence of PI and T animals and of immune dams carrying a PI fetus (state RP). Prevalence of PI and T animals represents the proportion of PI and T animals in the whole herd while prevalence of immune dams carrying a PI fetus is restricted to breeding females only. Outputs related to herd productivity are the number of losses (abortions and deaths of PI animals), purchases (replacement calves, pregnant females and bulls), weaned calves, sales of grassers and young heifers, and sales of empty and fattened females. To evaluate the impact of BVDV on herd productivity, we subtracted the contribution of the reference year (the last year before the first BVDV introduction) from these last outputs, considering only the relative change with and without BVDV circulating. Losses

and purchases were also evaluated per bred female to remove the direct impact of herd size on such outputs.

For all outputs except virus persistence, we calculated the annual median value with an 80% credible interval (P10-P90) for each year after BVDV introduction by selecting only repetitions in which the virus was still present in the herd at the end of the year, i.e. at weaning. Virus persistence was calculated weekly.

Impact of the herd structure outdoors on BVDV spread

To test the effect of our assumptions regarding the structure of herds during the indoor and outdoor periods, two options were compared with the reference scenario: (1) no structure is considered, assuming all animals are homogeneously mixed as indoors; (2) three groups are considered as in the reference case but with no contact between them ($\beta_b^P = 0$).

Sensitivity analysis

To identify the parameters which influence BVDV spread and its impact on herd productivity, we carried out a sensitivity analysis of the model, assuming here the outdoor reference structure (3 groups with between-group contacts). The selected input parameters were the following:

- parameters related to the herd management: level of numerical productivity expected by the farmer ε, duration of both the breeding (*breeding_dur*) and outdoor (*pasture_dur*) periods, renewal rate of breeding females (*renewal_rate*), herd size (*size*), and period of selling (*sell_period*);
- parameters related to the infection dynamics: mortality at birth of PI animals ($\mu_{P,bi}$), mortality of PI animals (μ_P), transition rates (ϕ_{MS}) and (ϕ_{TR}), transmission rates (β^P, β^T, β_b^P), abortion probabilities in early (α_{Ra}) and mid-pregnancy (α_{Rb}), probability of giving birth to a PI calf for a dam infected during mid-pregnancy (η_P), and type of virus introduction (*intro_week*).

Three values were tested per parameter (Table 1). For continuous parameters (rates and proportions), we tested variations of 90%, 100%, and 110% of their nominal value (except for ε for which the variation was ± 5% to remain within a plausible range, and for η_P which cannot be above 1). For other parameters (periods, herd size, and virus introduction), we tested for plausible values. Three selling periods are possible in the field, animals (including PI) being kept longer or shorter accordingly. We tested for selling all of the sold animals at each of these 3 periods. Durations of the breeding and the pasture periods varied by ± 2 and 3 weeks, respectively. To cover the variety of herd sizes in the Bourgogne region, we tested three numbers of females kept for breeding: 42 (10 heifers - 32 cows), 83 (20 heifers - 63 cows, reference scenario), and 125 (30 heifers - 95 cows). Finally, BVDV introduction may occur through different ways in a naive beef cattle herd. In addition to the birth of a single PI (week 27, reference scenario), we tested the case of multiple births of PI calves (weeks 20, 25, and 30 successively, i.e. at the start, in mid, and at the end of the calving period), and the case where a PI replacement calf is purchased during the outdoor period (week 40). Other purchased animals could also be infected and therefore introduce BVDV in the herd. However, pregnant females are purchased at the start of the building period, thus when most of the females are in late gestation. Introducing a transiently infected female will barely have any effect. Introducing an immune dam carrying a PI fetus will have the same influence as introducing a PI calf at birth. Introducing a PI pregnant female is quite rare. Lastly introducing a PI bull could have a large effect but only if introduced directly in a group of bred females among which some are already pregnant, which also corresponds to the period of purchase of replacement calves. Therefore, we chose to present here the most probable cases that are the birth of PI calves and the purchase of a PI replacement calf.

Since herd size and the type of virus introduction in the herd were expected to largely impact model outputs, 9 (3 herd sizes × 3 types of introduction) sensitivity analyses were carried out to evaluate the effect of other model parameters. We used a fractional factorial design to sample parameter values [33]. A factorial design is appropriate when the levels of some input variables are discrete (such as periods). In such a design, all the combinations between variable levels are considered, leading to p^n scenarios when n parameters with p levels are considered. Using a fractional design (using the *proc factex*, SAS) enabled us to considerably reduce the number of scenarios and is appropriate when sensitivity indices for principal effects and first-order interactions only are estimated. Two thousand one-hundred and eighty-seven scenarios were run for each analysis.

We analyzed aggregated outputs calculated as the mean values over the first 5 years after BVDV introduction of *losses* (mortality and abortion) and of the prevalence of T (*prevT*) and PI (*prevP*) animals, and of immune dams carrying a PI fetus (*prevRP*), in an infected herd.

For each output k, a linear regression model (ANOVA) was run with all model parameters: $k_{ij...} = \mu + f(i, j, ...) + \epsilon$, with μ a constant, f the relation between factors $(i, j, ...)$, and ϵ the residual. The total sum of squares then writes: S

$$S_{tot}^k = \sum_{i,j,...} \left(k_{ij...} - k'...\right)^2 = SS_i^k + SS_j^k + SS_{i:j}^k + SS_\epsilon^k \quad \text{(here}$$

for two factors i and j), with SS_i^k and $SS_{i:j}^k$ the sum of

squares related to factor i and to the first-order interaction between factors i and j for output k, respectively. The contribution of factor i to variations in output k is $C_i^k = \frac{SS_i^k + \frac{1}{2}\sum_{j \neq i} SS_{i:j}^k}{SS_{tot}^k}$. The sum of the contributions was equal to model R^2.

Impact of BVDV spread in an endemic situation

Five years after BVDV first introduction, if the virus is still present in the herd then an endemic state has been reached. To evaluate the impact of BVDV spread in such an endemic situation, cumulated outputs over 10 years (year 6 to 15 after virus introduction) were calculated to enable a comparison between the endemic situation and the acute one (based on the first 3 years). Only repetitions for which virus was present at least one week were included. Moreover, cumulated outputs were normalized to account for the proportion of time the herd truly was infected. Outputs thus were multiplied by the ratio of the number of weeks the virus was present in the herd over the total duration in weeks of the acute and the endemic periods, respectively. The comparison between the acute and the endemic periods was initially evaluated without allowing virus reintroduction through purchases of infected animals or fenceline contacts with infected neighboring herds during the outdoor period. As these factors can significantly influence disease persistence, we also simulated BVDV reintroduction in the herd accounting for a probability of purchasing infected animals (TI, P or immune dam carrying a PI fetus) and for a probability of fenceline contacts with neighboring infected herds during the outdoor period (K_{ext}). As no information was available on observed within-herd prevalence of BVDV infection in infected herds, we assumed a risk of purchasing infected animals on our best knowledge (1% for TI, 1% for P, and 0.5% for immune dams carrying a PI fetus) and assuming two levels of regional prevalence of infected herds: weak (10%) and strong (50%). For fenceline contacts, we evaluated three levels of external risk: nil ($K_{ext} = 0$), weak ($K_{ext} = 0.0025$), and strong ($K_{ext} = 0.01$). Each case was tested for each of the three herd sizes and type of initial virus introduction which is expected to impact the acute phase.

Results
BVDV spread in a naive cow-calf herd
Herd size and the type of initial BVDV introduction in the herd impacted the spread and persistence of BVDV in a naive cow-calf herd.

Regardless of herd size, introducing the BVDV through multiple births of PI calves (weeks 20, 25, and 30) or through the purchase of a PI replacement calf (week 40) gave rise to virus persistence in almost all of the repetitions for 1 to 3 years, whereas the birth of a single PI (week 27) was followed quickly by a 10% drop in persistence (in 10% of the repetitions, the infection had faded out; Figure 3A). Two years after the initial virus introduction, the persistence reached almost the same level in the three scenarios. Persistence increased with herd size. To reach a 50% probability of BVDV extinction, 3.1 to 3.7 years were needed in small herds, 4 to 4.3 in medium ones, and 4.7 to 5 in large ones. Without reintroduction, the virus persisted for more than 3 years in 55-75%, 78-88%, and 85-96% of the repetitions in small, medium, and large herds, respectively. It

persisted for 8 years in 2-4% of the repetitions in small herds vs. 9-11% in large ones.

Regardless of herd size, the annual prevalence of PI animals and immune dams carrying a PI fetus in an infected herd reached a maximum the year after the year of virus introduction (i.e. year 2). The prevalence of transiently infected animals was the highest during the year of virus introduction (year 1) when 3 PI were successively introduced. In the other scenarios, it was the highest the second year. In medium herds, after the birth of a single PI calf, the prevalence on year 2 of T, PI and dams carrying a PI fetus in 80% of the repetitions ranged from 1.6 to 2.0%, 1.0 to 3.6%, and 2.8 to 6.6%,

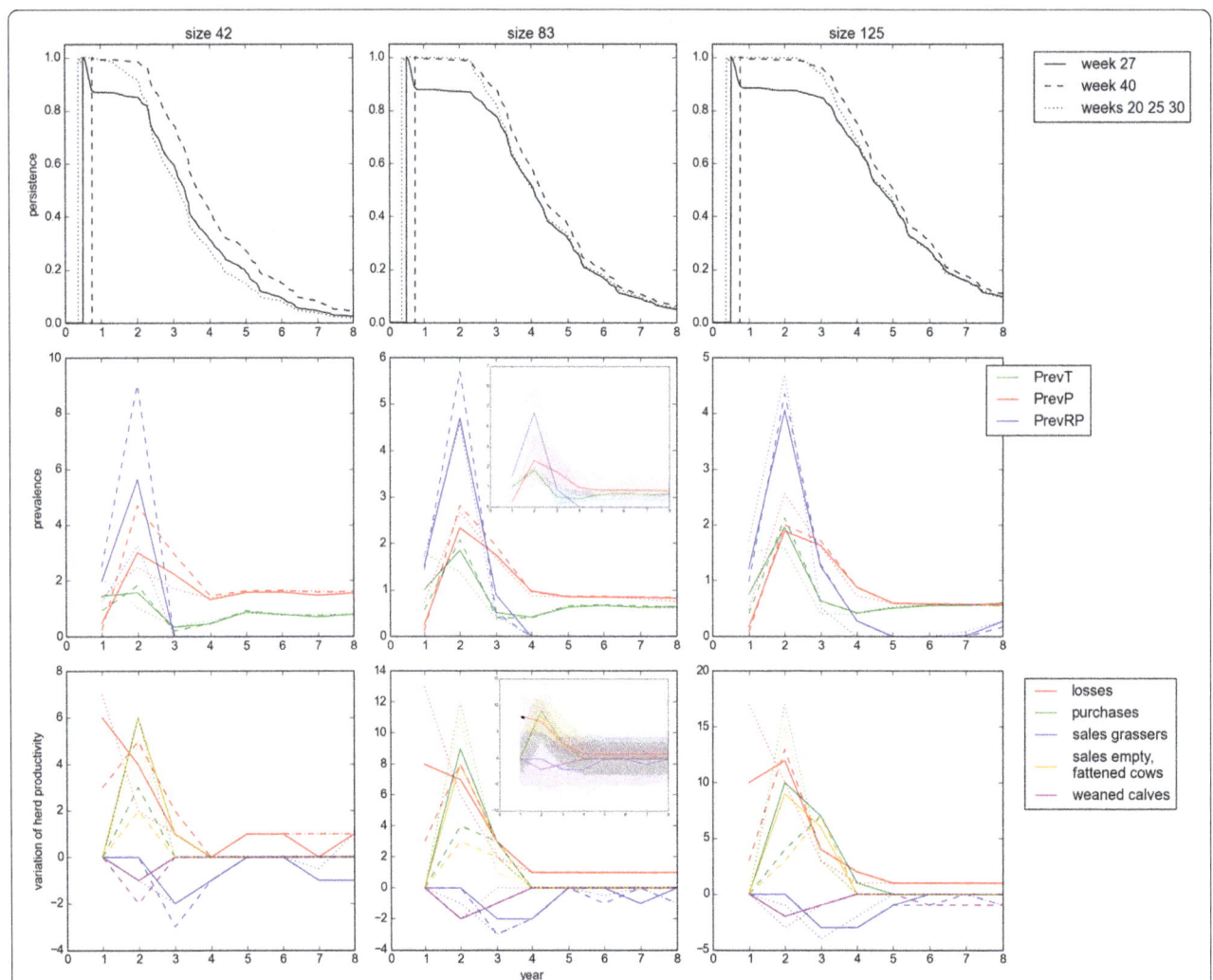

Figure 3 BVDV spread in a beef cow-calf herd according to virus introduction and herd size. Three types of initial virus introduction were considered: in week 27 (solid line), in week 40 (dashed line), in weeks 20, 25 and 30 (dotted line). Three herd sizes were considered: 42 (on the left), 83 (on the middle), 125 bred females (on the right). The first row shows the probability of virus persistence in the herd over time. The second row shows the median values (with for medium herds an 80% credible interval shown for *intro_week* = 27 on the small figure) of the prevalence of transiently (*T*) and persistently infected (PI) animals in the herd, and of immune dams carrying a PI fetus (*RP*) among bred females. The third row shows the median values (with for medium herds an 80% credible interval shown for *intro_week* = 27 on the small figure) of productivity outputs: losses (red), purchases (green), sales of grassers and heifers (blue), sales of empty and fattened females (orange), and number of weaned calves (purple). Annual prevalence and productivity outputs were estimated each year considering only repetitions with the virus still present at the end of the year.

respectively (Figure 3B). The prevalences slightly decreased with herd size. In small herds only, the median prevalences were higher if a PI calf was introduced outdoors (1.8%, 4.7%, 9.0%, respectively) than during the calving period (1.6%, 3.0%, 5.6%, respectively). For other herd sizes, the prevalences were mostly similar among types of virus introduction. Three to four years after BVDV introduction, the prevalences tended to stable values, denoting that an endemic state had been reached which was not affected by the initial virus introduction. An endemically infected herd was predicted to have from 0.3 to 1.1% of T animals, from 0.3 to 2.4% of PI animals, and from none to 0.9% of its dams carrying a PI fetus.

Regardless of herd size and type of virus introduction, the highest impact of BVDV spread on herd productivity occurred during the second year (Figure 3C). Losses associated with abortions and PI mortality were the highest the first two years, ranging from 0.16 to 0.26 per bred female. Losses per bred female were slightly lower in large herds. Additional purchases and sales of empty and fattened females, and losses in weaned calves that were due to BVDV spread were the highest the second year and then rapidly decreased. Purchases and sales of empty and fattened females per bred female were closely related and ranged from 0.05 to 0.17, with no effect of herd size. In more than half the repetitions (median), less than 2 weaned calves were lost due to BVDV spread over 3 years. The number of grassers and heifers sold was not impacted the first two years, a decrease occurring only in the third and fourth years. If the virus was introduced outdoors, losses were later and lower. Without any subsequent virus introduction, the productivity outputs tended to be barely affected 5 years after the first BVDV introduction.

Impact on BVDV spread of the herd structure outdoors
Assuming a heterogeneous mixing outdoors modified the predicted model outputs compared with assuming a homogeneous mixing. On the contrary, in the case of a heterogeneous mixing outdoors, assuming no contact between groups did not change model predictions compared with assuming the occurrence of between-group contacts (reference scenario).

The predicted virus persistence slightly increased when assuming a homogeneous mixing compared with a heterogeneous one, especially for large herds and for risky types of virus introduction (a PI replacement calf purchased during the outdoor period or 3 PI calves born successively; Figure 4). In the reference scenario, the impact of herd structure can hardly be seen. However, in the largest herds (125 bred females), the virus persisted 8 years after its introduction in 16-18% of the repetitions in the homogeneous mixing scenario compared with 9-12% of the repetitions in the heterogeneous mixing scenario.

The predicted prevalences of PI animals and immune dams carrying a PI fetus in infected herds were higher during the acute phase when assuming a homogeneous vs. heterogeneous mixing outdoors, regardless of herd size and type of virus introduction. In a herd of 83 bred females, the predicted median prevalence of PI animals on year 2 varied with the type of BVDV introduction and ranged from 3.1 to 3.8% in the homogeneous mixing scenario compared with 2.3 to 2.8% in the heterogeneous mixing scenario. The median prevalence of dams carrying a PI fetus on year 2 ranged from 6.0 to 6.7% in the homogeneous mixing scenario compared with 4.6 to 5.7% in the heterogeneous mixing scenario. Herd structure on pasture had no effect of the prevalence of T animals.

Predicted losses (abortion and PI mortality), purchases, and sales of empty and fattened females were slightly higher during the acute phase when assuming a homogeneous mixing outdoors, regardless of herd size and type of virus introduction.

Impact of herd management and infection characteristics on BVDV spread
Herd management and infection characteristics both influenced losses over the first five years of infection, as well as the prevalence of T animals, PI animals, and dams carrying a PI fetus (Figure 5). The type of virus introduction impacted parameters identified as key in the sensitivity analyses, especially in small herds. Otherwise, key parameters were nearly the same regardless of herd size.

Losses varied among scenarios of the sensitivity analysis in the ranges 8-15, 13-30, and 18-42 animals in small, medium, and large herds, respectively. The prevalence of T animals varied among scenarios between 0.8 and 1.6%, the prevalence of PI animals varied between 0.9 and 3.0%, and the prevalence of dams carrying a PI fetus varied from 1.4 and 4.8%, irrespective of herd size.

Losses variations were mainly explained by pasture duration (*pasture_dur*) and the choice of the selling period (*sell_period*) for parameters related to herd management, and by the abortion rate due to infection in early pregnancy (α_{Ra}) and the transmission rate by PI animals (β^P) for parameters related to infection characteristics (Figure 5A). Introducing a PI replacement calf (week 40) in small herds led to a decrease in the contributions of these key parameters except *sell_period*, and led to an additional contribution of the probability of given birth to a PI calf for dams infected in mid-pregnancy (η_P) and of PI mortality (μ_P).

The variations in the prevalence of T animals in an infected herd (Figure 5B) were mainly explained by the choice of the selling period (*sell_period*), the transient infection duration (ϕ_{TR}), and slightly by pasture duration (*pasture_dur*), the transmission rate by PI animals (β^P),

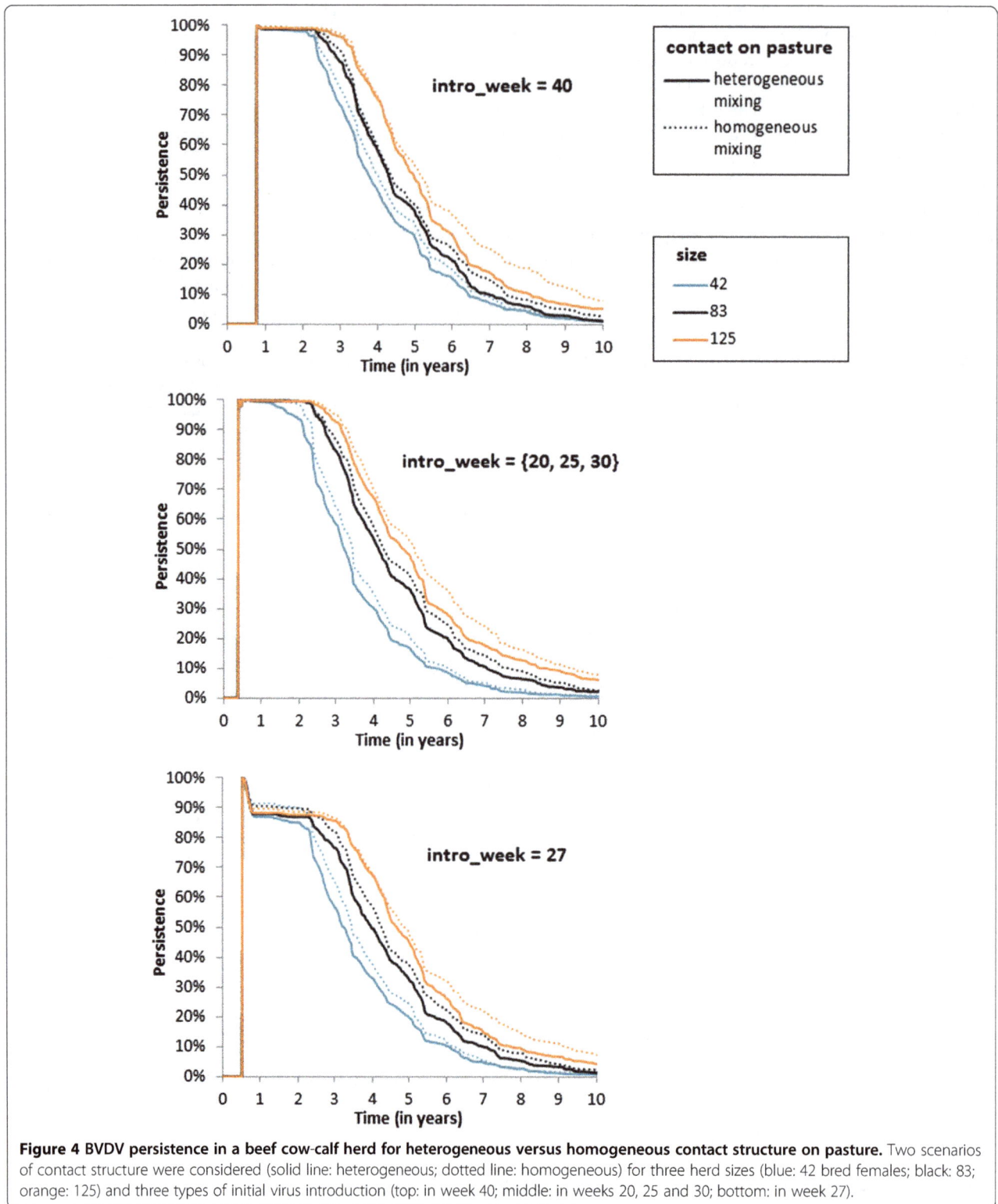

Figure 4 BVDV persistence in a beef cow-calf herd for heterogeneous versus homogeneous contact structure on pasture. Two scenarios of contact structure were considered (solid line: heterogeneous; dotted line: homogeneous) for three herd sizes (blue: 42 bred females; black: 83; orange: 125) and three types of initial virus introduction (top: in week 40; middle: in weeks 20, 25 and 30; bottom: in week 27).

and PI mortality (μ_P). The variations in the prevalence of PI animals (Figure 5C) were mainly explained by *sell_period* and the renewal rate (*renewal_rate*), and in some cases *pasture_dur*, as well as by the probability of given birth to a PI calf for dams infected in mid-pregnancy (η_P), μ_P, and in some cases β^P. The variations in the prevalence of dams carrying a PI fetus (Figure 5D) were mainly explained by the same parameters as the variations in the

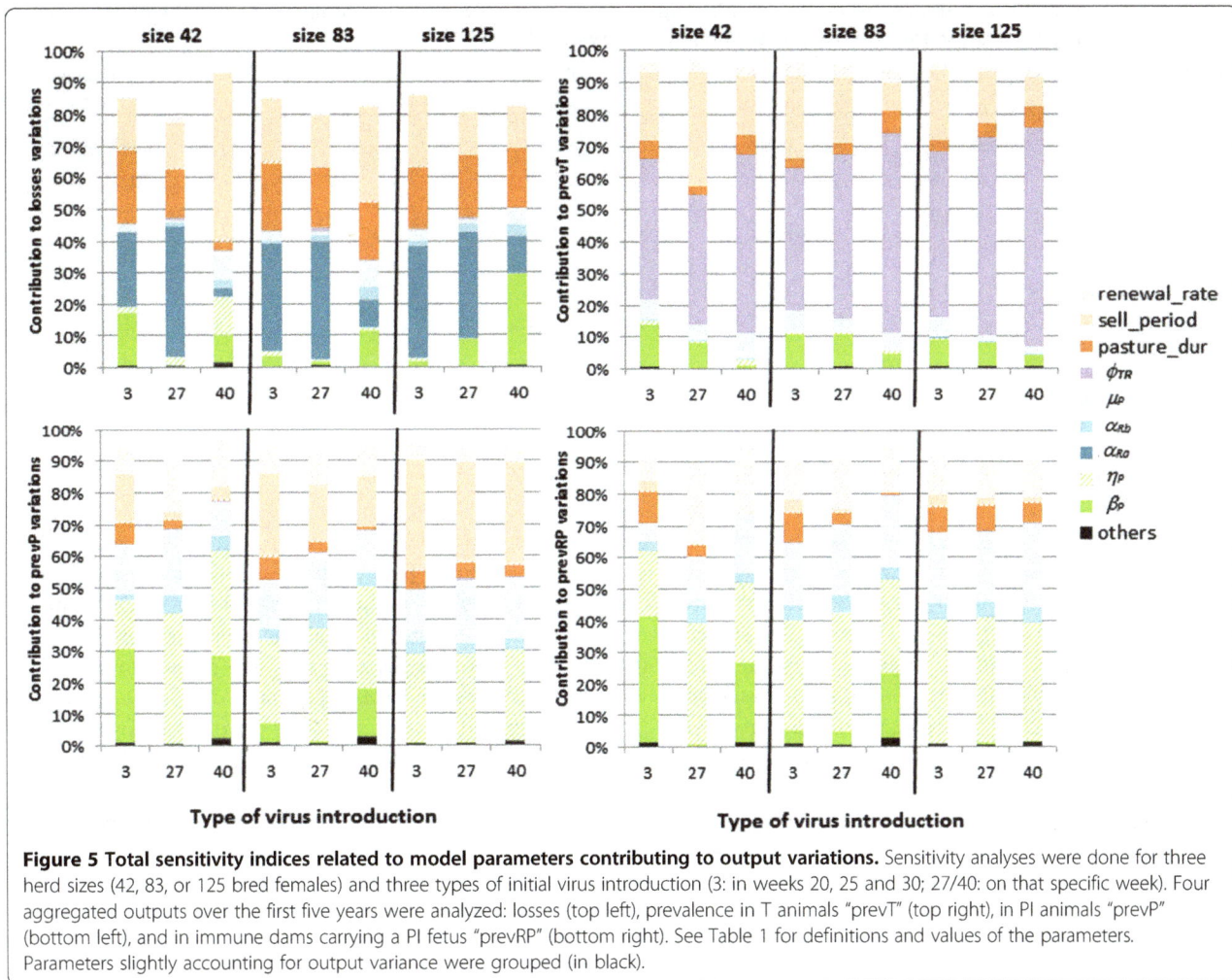

Figure 5 Total sensitivity indices related to model parameters contributing to output variations. Sensitivity analyses were done for three herd sizes (42, 83, or 125 bred females) and three types of initial virus introduction (3: in weeks 20, 25 and 30; 27/40: on that specific week). Four aggregated outputs over the first five years were analyzed: losses (top left), prevalence in T animals "prevT" (top right), in PI animals "prevP" (bottom left), and in immune dams carrying a PI fetus "prevRP" (bottom right). See Table 1 for definitions and values of the parameters. Parameters slightly accounting for output variance were grouped (in black).

prevalence of PI animals, except *sell_period* which barely contributed.

BVDV spread in an endemic situation

The risk of buying infected animals was low. Even when half of the source herds for replacement animals were assumed to be infected with BVDV, the model predicted that BVDV would be reintroduced to medium herds only once every 20 years during the endemic period. Indeed, only 1 to 5 animals were purchased per year per herd irrespective of the BVDV herd status, with a low risk that these animals were infected due to the low within-herd prevalence of infection.

The tested levels for an external risk of infection on pasture (K_{ext}) corresponded to BVDV reintroductions during the endemic phase once every 6-7 years for the low level, and once every 2-3 years for the high level (Table 2). During the acute phase, as herds were mainly already infected, herd reinfection barely occurred. Median prevalence of infection in infected herds was twice as high during the acute phase as during the endemic phase

(Table 2). However, cumulative losses, purchases, sales and variations in weaned calves over 10 years per bred female in an endemic situation greatly surpassed the ones occurring during the acute phase (Table 2). Moreover, when BVDV was reintroduced once every 2-3 years, losses per bred females during the endemic phase in an infected herd were twice as high as when BVDV was not reintroduced or was reintroduced only once every 6-7 years (with for example 36% vs. 15% of losses per bred female in medium herds).

Discussion

We propose a stochastic model of BVDV spread in a structured beef cow-calf cattle herd. Originally, we accounted for a variation in exposure of animals (especially adults) between the indoor period, during which a homogeneous contact structure is assumed, and the outdoor period, during which groups are formed and raised on different pastures. Moreover, we accounted for a risk of continuous virus introduction in the herd through animal purchases and contacts with neighboring infected herds. This enabled

Table 2 Comparison of the outputs of the model of BVDV spread in a beef cow-calf herd cumulated over the acute (years 1 to 3 after initial introduction) versus the endemic phase (years 6 to 15)

Output definition	Acute phase	Endemic phase
Average probability of virus presence[1]	0.75-0.76-0.76	0.14-0.17-0.25
Average frequency of herd reinfection[1] (yr^{-1})	0-0.02-0.08	0-0.14-0.38
Median prevT (when the virus is present) (%)	1.3-1.5	0.5-1.0
Median prevP (when the virus is present) (%)	1.4-3.5	0-1.2
Median prevRP (when the virus is present) (%)	2.1-5.5	0-1.3
Median losses/100 bred females	23-37	12-53
Median purchases/100 bred females	13-26	34-125
Median sales of grassers & heifers/100 bred females	-7--2	-1-29
Median sales of fattened females/100 bred females	10-23	23-108
Median weaned calves/100 bred females	-5--2	2-39

Ranges came from variations in herd size, type of initial virus introduction, and external risk of reintroduction.
[1]For three levels of $K_{ext} = \{0, 0.0025, 0.01\}$ (per day).

the model to represent a large range of possible situations, from a single introduction into a naive herd to endemic situations potentially maintained by an external risk of virus reintroduction. Lastly, the model was flexible enough to represent beef herds of different sizes and management types, as illustrated by the different types of herds observed in Bourgogne, one of the main beef cattle farming regions in France. Such a model was pertinent to investigate the impact of BVDV spread on the productivity of a herd for a large range of scenarios.

To precisely represent the infection process, several modelling choices had to be made. The model was stochastic to enable an estimation of the probability of virus persistence. The variability in model outputs if the virus persisted was not very large. However, the prevalence in PI animals and in immune dams carrying a PI fetus in infected herds was low and therefore better estimated using a stochastic model. A discrete time step of 1 week was used as the longest permitting to precisely estimate the morbidity related to transiently infected animals (transient infection being quite short). We chose to implement a combination of compartmental and individual-based models - instead of using a fully individual-based approach as used in [34,35] – with the anticipation of using this within-herd model as part of a more complex simulation framework where computational efficiency is paramount, to represent between-herd BVDV spread and control at a regional scale. Indeed, representing individually each animal all its lifetime was not necessary, except during pregnancy to precisely predict when infection will occur relative to the stage of pregnancy of the dam, and which consequence it will have for the calf to be born. Hence, we integrated in the compartmental model an individual-based monitoring of pregnant females (from the start of pregnancy until calving). To account for the seasonality of breeding and outdoor contacts, discrete periods were designed for

reproduction and grazing. Such an approach is suitable when the continuous epidemic process (infection occurring possibly each day) is influenced by seasonal population dynamics (and therefore seasonal contacts) occurring on a discrete basis (with for instance only two periods in a year with different types or levels of contact). All of the model parameters related to herd size (number of bred cows and heifers) and management (target number of weaned calves, occurrence and intensity of purchases and of neighboring relationships, within herd contact structure, breeding/calving and indoor/outdoor periods) are user-defined. Hence, our model is highly flexible and may also be used to represent beef cattle herds in other regions.

The simulation results show that failing to account for the separation of cattle into different management groups on pasture could lead to overestimations of the predicted disease prevalence and persistence in affected herds. In our study, we assumed that there were three management groups and that these management groups remained fixed over the entire grazing period. However, in the real world, herd structure is often dictated by complex management constraints such as herd size, pasture availability, and labor resources. Furthermore, the management groups of bred females with bulls may be reformed several times during the grazing period, which may lead towards more homogeneous mixing dynamics. There is a need for further research into the effects of herd structure on BVDV spread using empirically derived data.

When introduced into a naive herd, BVDV spread was shown to have a large impact on herd productivity, especially the first 3 years after the initial introduction of the virus, during which yearly losses may be up to 6 times higher than in subsequent years when herd immunity has developed. The impact expressed per bred female was slightly lower in larger herds. Moreover, in the absence of control measures, BVDV may persist for years, which is currently observed in some regions [3,4,36,37]. We found that the virus was more likely to persist over time in larger herds. Virus persistence may increase with herd size because self-clearance may be more frequent in small herds due to stochastic events [38,39]. In such an endemic situation, our model predicted that yearly losses will be limited and that the production objective in weaned calves will be reached most of the time, in good agreement with the results obtained for Scottish beef herds [5]. However, the low yearly losses have to be balanced by the duration of virus persistence. Cumulated over several years, losses occurring during the endemic phase cannot be neglected, especially when virus reintroduction is frequent.

The sensitivity analysis shows that herd management (through pasture duration, selling period, and renewal rate) and the infection dynamics (though the transmission rate from PI, the duration of transient infection, the vertical transmission, PI mortality, and abortion rates) were very influential processes on at least some of the model outputs (prevalence of T and PI animals and of immune dams carrying a PI fetus, losses), regardless of herd size and type of virus introduction. As for dairy herds [10], it suggests that control of PI animals is the key for preventing BVDV spread in beef herds. PI animals may be introduced via either purchases or births to immune dams infected during mid-pregnancy. In Bourgogne, the breeding period occurs essentially during the outdoor period. Hence, it is an at-risk period for breeding females since they can become infected from contact with neighboring herds.

Among the available strategies to control BVDV spread in beef herds, vaccination is one of the main current options. According to our findings, female vaccination before breeding seems to be a valuable strategy to limit losses due to BVDV spread and persistence [40-43]. Vaccination has been used largely in the US [44], but much less in the EU [43], except in Germany where it has been used in combination with eradication [45]. Such a strategy could become efficient and should be further evaluated in a context where herds may be regularly reinfected through neighboring contact. In the present study, the impact of BVDV on herd productivity was evaluated by measuring biological outputs (losses, variations in weaned calves, etc.). For the model to be useful in evaluating control strategies, it would be important to assign economic values to variations in herd productivity [5,18] and to account for farmer's decisions [46,47]. Indeed, farmers may be unwilling to implement control measures if the economic impact of BVDV on their herd is perceived to be low. Farmers of endemically infected herds may also become unaware of their own BVDV status [3,4,36] and of the risk they pose of transmitting the virus through animal movements and neighboring contact with other herds [48]. Moreover, if the risk of disease reintroduction is high, farmers may not perceive the value of controlling it even if they are aware it is present. Our model then can be used to estimate the expected prevalence of PI animals as well as of immune dams carrying a PI fetus in such endemically infected herds, therefore providing a prior for the risk of infection for (potentially naive) contact herds. Several groups are identified in the modelled herd based on age/physiological stages and health statuses, enabling the model to be used in the future to evaluate targeted control strategies at the herd scale in either naive or endemic situations.

Competing interests
The authors declare that they have no competing interests.

Authors' contributions
AD and PE conceived the study and were involved in all aspects of the work; AFV and SA contributed to developing the model; all authors were involved in the model parameterization, contributed to the result interpretation, and read and approved the final manuscript.

Acknowledgements
This work was carried out with the financial support of the French Research Agency (ANR), Program Investments for the Future, project ANR-10-BINF-07 (MIHMES), by the European fund for the regional development (FEDER Pays-de-la-Loire), and by INRA. The authors thank J. Devun (Institut de l'Elevage) and R. Vermesse (GDS35) for their help in defining the assumptions on the herd demography. The authors also thank two anonymous referees for their helpful comments on a previous version of the manuscript.

Author details
[1]INRA, UMR1300 BioEpAR, CS 40706, F-44307 Nantes, France. [2]Oniris, LUNAM Université, UMR BioEpAR, F-44307 Nantes, France. [3]FRGDS Bourgogne, F-21000 Dijon, France.

References
1. Stott AW, Humphry RW, Gunn GJ (2010) Modelling the effects of previous infection and re-infection on the costs of bovine viral diarrhoea outbreaks in beef herds. Vet J 185:138–143
2. Joly A, Fourichon C, Beaudeau F (2005) Description and first results of a BVDV control scheme in Brittany (western France). Prev Vet Med 72:209–213
3. Gates MC, Woolhouse MEJ, Gunn GJ, Humphry RW (2013) Relative associations of cattle movements, local spread, and biosecurity with bovine viral diarrhoea virus (BVDV) seropositivity in beef and dairy herds. Prev Vet Med 112:285–295
4. Gates MC, Humphry RW, Gunn GJ (2013) Associations between bovine viral diarrhoea virus (BVDV) seropositivity and performance indicators in beef suckler and dairy herds. Vet J 198:631–637
5. McCormick B, Stott A, Brülisauer F, Vosough Ahmadi B, Gunn G (2010) An integrated approach to assessing the viability of eradicating BVD in Scottish beef suckler herds. Vet Microbiol 142:129–136
6. Bennett RM (1992) Case-study of a simple decision support system to aid livestock disease control decisions. Agr Syst 38:111–129
7. Ezanno P, Fourichon C, Seegers H (2008) Influence of herd structure and type of virus introduction on the spread of bovine viral diarrhoea virus (BVDV) within a dairy herd. Vet Res 39:39
8. Ezanno P, Vergu E, Langlais M, Gilot-Fromont E (2012) Modelling the dynamics of host-parasite interactions: basic principles. In New Frontiers of Molecular Epidemiology of Infectious Diseases. Edited by Morand S, Beaudeau F, Cabaret J: Springer; pp 79–101.
9. Viet A-F, Fourichon C, Seegers H (2007) Review and critical discussion of assumptions and modelling options to study the spread of the bovine viral diarrhoea virus (BVDV) within a cattle herd. Epidemiol Infect 135:706–721
10. Ezanno P, Fourichon C, Viet A-F, Seegers H (2007) Sensitivity analysis to identify key-parameters in modelling the spread of bovine viral diarrhoea virus in a dairy herd. Prev Vet Med 80:49–64

11. Courcoul A, Ezanno P (2010) Modelling the spread of Bovine Viral Diarrhoea Virus (BVDV) in a managed metapopulation of cattle herds. Vet Microbiol 142:119–128

12. Ersbøll AK, Ersbøll BK, Houe H, Alban L, Kjeldsen A (2010) Spatial modelling of the between-herd infection dynamics of bovine virus diarrhoea virus (BVDV) in dairy herds in Denmark. Prev Vet Med 97:83–89

13. Tinsley M, Lewis FI, Brülisauer F (2012) Network modeling of BVD transmission. Vet Res 43:11

14. Houe H (1993) Survivorship of animals persistently infected with bovine virus diarrhoea virus (BVDV). Prev Vet Med 15:275–283

15. Gunn GJ, Stott AW, Humphry RW (2004) Modelling and costing BVD outbreaks in beef herds. Vet J 167:143–149

16. Smith RL, Sanderson MW, Renter DG, Larson R, White B (2010) A stochastic risk-analysis model for the spread of bovine viral diarrhea virus after introduction to naive cow-calf herds. Prev Vet Med 95:86–98

17. Nickell JS, White BJ, Larson RL, Renter DG, Sanderson MW (2011) A simulation model to quantify the value of implementing whole-herd Bovine viral diarrhea virus testing strategies in beef cow-calf herds. J Vet Diagn Invest 23:194–205

18. Smith RL, Sanderson MW, Jones R, N'Guessan Y, Renter D, Larson R, White BJ (2013) Economic risk analysis model for bovine viral diarrhea virus biosecurity in cow-calf herds. Prev Vet Med 113:492–503

19. Viet A-F, Ezanno P, Petit E, Devun J, Vermesse R, Fourichon C (2012) Resilience of a beef cow-calf farming system to variations in demographic parameters. J Anim Sci 91:413–424

20. Lindberg ALE (2003) Bovine viral diarrhoea virus infections and its control. A review. Vet Q 25:1–16

21. Kendrick JW (1971) Bovine viral diarrhea-mucosal disease virus infection in pregnant cows. Am J Vet Res 32:533–544

22. Done J, Terlecki S, Richardson C, Harkness J, Sands J, Patterson D, Sweasey D, Shaw I, Winkler C, Duffell S (1980) Bovine virus diarrhoea-mucosal disease virus: pathogenicity for the fetal calf following maternal infection. Vet Rec 106:473–479

23. McClurkin AW, Littledike ET, Cutlip RC, Frank GH, Coria MF, Bolin SR (1984) Production of cattle immunotolerant to bovine viral diarrhea virus. Can J Comp Med 48:156–161

24. Carlsson U, Fredriksson G, Alenius S, Kindahl H (1989) Bovine virus diarrhea virus, a cause of early pregnancy failure in the cow. Zentralbl Veterinarmed A 36:15–23

25. McGowan M, Kirkland P, Richards S, Littlejohns I (1993) Increased reproductive losses in cattle infected with bovine pestivirus around the time of insemination. Vet Rec 133:39–43

26. Moerman A, Straver P, de Jong M, Quak J, Baanvinger T, van Oirschot J (1993) A long term epidemiological study of bovine viral diarrhoea infections in a large herd of dairy cattle. Vet Rec 132:622–626

27. Breto C, He D, Ionides EL, King AA (2009) Time series analysis via mechanistic models. Ann Appl Stat 3:319–348

28. Saltelli A, Chan K, Scott EM (2000) Sensitivity Analysis. Wiley, New York

29. Viet A-F, Fourichon C, Seegers H, Jacob C, Guihenneuc-Jouyaux C (2004) A model of the spread of the bovine viral-diarrhoea virus within a dairy herd. Prev Vet Med 63:211–236

30. Carslake D, Grant W, Green LE, Cave J, Greaves J, Keeling M, McEldowney J, Weldegebriel H, Medley GF (2011) Endemic cattle diseases: comparative epidemiology and governance. Philos Trans R Soc Lond B Biol Sci 366:1975–1986

31. Sarrazin S, Veldhuis A, Méroc E, Vangeel I, Laureyns J, Dewulf J, Van Der Stede Y (2013) Serological and virological BVDV prevalence and risk factor analysis for herds to be BVDV seropositive in Belgian cattle herds. Prev Vet Med 108:28–37

32. Moennig V, Houe H, Lindberg A (2005) BVD control in Europe: current status and perspectives. Anim Health Res Rev 6:63–74

33. Ståhl K, Lindberg A, Rivera H, Ortiz C, Moreno-López J (2008) Self-clearance from BVDV infections—a frequent finding in dairy herds in an endemically infected region in Peru. Prev Vet Med 83:285–296

34. Lindberg AL, Alenius S (1999) Principles for eradication of bovine viral diarrhoea virus (BVDV) infections in cattle populations. Vet Microbiol 64:197–222

35. Greiser-Wilke I, Grummer B, Moennig V (2003) Bovine viral diarrhoea eradication and control programmes in Europe. Biologicals 31:113–118

36. Moennig V, Brownlie J: Vaccines and vaccination strategies. In EU Thematic network on control of bovine viral diarrhoea virus: position paper (QLRT – 2001-01573). Edited online (http://www.afbini.gov.uk/chs-thematic-network-position-paper-on-bvd-control.pdf); 2006:73-98.

37. Lindberg A, Brownlie J, Gunn G, Houe H, Moennig V, Saatkamp H, Sandvik T, Valle P (2006) The control of bovine viral diarrhea virus in Europe: today and in the future. Rev Sci Tech 25:961–979

38. Ståhl K, Alenius S (2012) BVDV control and eradication in Europe - an update. Jpn J Vet Res 60:S31–S39

39. Fulton RW (2013) Host response to bovine viral diarrhea virus and interactions with infectious agents in the feedlot and breeding herd. Biologicals 41:31–38

40. Moennig V, Eicken K, Flebbe U, Frey HR, Grummer B, Haas L, Greiser-Wilke I, Liess B (2005) Implementation of two-step vaccination in the control of bovine viral diarrhoea (BVD). Prev Vet Med 72:109–114

41. Rat-Aspert O, Fourichon C (2010) Modelling collective effectiveness of voluntary vaccination with and without incentives. Prev Vet Med 93:265–275

42. Santarossa J, Stott A, Humphry R, Gunn G (2005) Optimal risk management versus willingness to pay for BVDV control options. Prev Vet Med 72:183–187

43. Bitsch V, Hansen KE, Rønsholt L (2000) Experiences from the Danish programme for eradication of bovine virus diarrhoea (BVD) 1994–1998 with special reference to legislation and causes of infection. Vet Microbiol 77:137–143

44. Duffell S, Harkness J (1985) Bovine virus diarrhoea-mucosal disease infection in cattle. Vet Rec 117:240–245

45. Kendrick JW, Franti CE (1974) Bovine viral diarrhea: decay of colostrum-conferred antibody in the calf. Am J Vet Res 35:589–592

46. Baker JC (1987) Bovine viral diarrhoea virus: a review. J Am Vet Med Assoc 190:1449–1458

47. Mars MH, Bruschke CJM, van Oirschot JT (1999) Airborne transmission of BHV1, BRSV, and BVDV among cattle is possible under experimental conditions. Vet Microbiol 66:197–207

48. Niskanen R, Lindberg A (2003) Transmission of bovine viral diarrhoea virus by unhygienic vaccination procedures, ambient air, and from contaminated pens. Vet J 165:125–130

10

Bovine Neonatal Pancytopenia is a heritable trait of the dam rather than the calf and correlates with the magnitude of vaccine induced maternal alloantibodies not the MHC haplotype

Lindert Benedictus[1*], Henny G Otten[2], Gerdien van Schaik[3], Walter GJ van Ginkel[2], Henri CM Heuven[4,5], Mirjam Nielen[6], Victor PMG Rutten[1,7] and Ad P Koets[1,6]

Abstract

Bovine Neonatal Pancytopenia (BNP), a bleeding syndrome of neonatal calves, is caused by alloantibodies absorbed from the colostrum of particular cows. A commercial BVD vaccine is the likely source of alloantigens eliciting BNP associated alloantibodies. We hypothesized that the rare occurrence of BNP in calves born to vaccinated dams could be associated with genetic differences within dams and calves. We found that the development of BNP within calves was a heritable trait for dams, not for calves and had a high heritability of 19%. To elucidate which genes play a role in the development of BNP we sequenced candidate genes and characterized BNP alloantibodies. Alloantigens present in the vaccine have to be presented to the dam's immune system via MHC class II, however sequencing of DRB3 showed no differences in MHC class II haplotype between BNP and non-BNP dams. MHC class I, a highly polymorphic alloantigen, is an important target of BNP alloantibodies. Using a novel sequence based MHC class I typing method, we found no association of BNP with MHC class I haplotype distribution in dams or calves. Alloantibodies were detected in both vaccinated BNP and non-BNP dams and we found no differences in alloantibody characteristics between these groups, but alloantibody levels were significantly higher in BNP dams. We concluded that the development of BNP in calves is a heritable trait of the dam rather than the calf and genetic differences between BNP and non-BNP dams are likely due to genes controlling the quantitative alloantibody response following vaccination.

Introduction

Since 2007 an increase in newborn calves with the bleeding syndrome Bovine Neonatal Pancytopenia (BNP) was observed all over Europe [1-3]. Epidemiological studies showed a strong association between the occurrence of BNP in calves and vaccination of their dams with the PregSure© BVD vaccine (Pfizer Animal Health) [2]. Symptoms of BNP are severe internal and external bleeding, first seen around 10–20 days of age. Hematological signs are severe leukopenia and thrombocytopenia. In addition, trilineage hypoplasia of the bone marrow can be observed upon post-mortem examination [3-5].

Colostrum of dams that had previously given birth to a calf which developed BNP contained alloantibodies recognizing bovine leukocytes [6-9]. Feeding this colostrum to healthy neonatal calves induced the symptoms of BNP [4,8,10]. Proteins from the bovine kidney cell line MDBK [11], used to grow the BVD type 1 virus present in PregSure© BVD, are the likely source of alloantigens that induce alloantibody production in vaccinated dams. The alloantibodies bind MDBK cells and it was shown that an important target of these antibodies were MHC class I proteins [7,9,12]. Moreover, MDBK derived MHC class I proteins were detected in the PregSure© BVD vaccine [9,12] and immunization of calves with PregSure© BVD induced alloantibodies recognizing MDBK cells [7,13].

* Correspondence: l.benedictus1@uu.nl
[1]Department of Infectious Diseases and Immunology, Faculty of Veterinary Medicine, Utrecht University, Utrecht, The Netherlands
Full list of author information is available at the end of the article

Since the incidence of BNP calves born to PregSure© BVD vaccinated dams was estimated to be lower than 0.3% [7,9,13], it was hypothesized that factors other than vaccination per sé play a role in the etiology of BNP. The prevailing hypothesis is that the pathogenesis of BNP resembles a histocompatibility (mis)match between dam and calf and is based on immunization of the dam with MDBK derived MHC class I [9,12]. First, in the dam MDBK cell derived proteins, present in the Pregsure© BVD vaccine, are presented in the context of MHC class II. The resulting T cell help to B cells recognizing allogeneic differences between MDBK cells and the dam will result in the generation of alloantibodies which are also present in the colostrum. Due to tolerance to self-antigens, dams do not exhibit adverse effects after vaccination, i.e. the vaccine induced alloantibodies do not recognize alloantigens expressed in the dam. The maternal alloantibodies transferred to the calf via the colostrum will recognize alloantigens in case of a partial alloantigen match between MDBK cells and the calf. We hypothesized that the rare occurrence of BNP after Pregsure© BVD vaccination may depend both on the capability of the dam's immune system to present the MDBK alloantigens via MHC class II, as well as the degree of alloantigen (mis)match between the dam and the MDBK cell line (and the calf and the MDBK cell line, respectively) and the ensuing immune response of the dam. Since alloantigens (including MHC I and MHC class I associated B2M) and MHC class II are genetically determined and therefore heritable, we studied whether differences in these genes between dams and/or calves may explain why BNP only occurs in part of the calves born to PregSure© BVD vaccinated dams. First we studied the heritability of the development of BNP in the calf as a potential dam or calf trait. Next, to elucidate if these genes genes play a role in the development of BNP we sequenced and compared the MHC and B2M candidate genes and characterized BNP associated alloantibodies.

Materials and methods
Heritability study
The data used for the heritability study were a subset of data from a large multi country epidemiological study on BNP [2] and concerned Dutch farms that participated in this study. Data on herd matched BNP and non-BNP calves were collected by on farm questionnaires. We looked at the heritability of the development of BNP within the calf as a trait of Pregsure© BVD vaccinated dams as well as of calves born to these dams. The definitions for BNP and non-BNP calves used, were according to Jones et al. [2]. A BNP calf was defined as a calf that showed one or more BNP clinical signs on or before 28 days of age; bone marrow depletion as assessed by

histopathology and/or thrombocytopenia ($<150 \times 10^9$/litre) and leucopenia ($<5 \times 10^9$/litre). A non-BNP calf was defined as a calf on the same farm as a case, aged 10–28 days at the time of case reporting, no clinical signs of BNP up to 28 days of age, and normal blood parameters (thrombocytes $\geq 300 \times 10^9$/litre, leucocytes $\geq 5 \times 10^9$/litre). To ensure that the correct phenotype, BNP or non-BNP, was assigned to the dam, only calves that were fed colostrum from their own dam were included. Furthermore, dam-calf combinations without pedigree information were excluded. Pedigrees of calves and dams were provided by the Dutch Cattle Improvement Organization (CRV, Arnhem, the Netherlands). The pedigree of dam-calf combinations meeting the inclusion criteria were traced back up to 21 generations and the final pedigree included 12 586 records. The first generation of the pedigree was a 100% complete for calves and 95% complete for dams. The data were analyzed using the software package ASReml [14], a statistical package that fits generalized linear mixed models using Residual Maximum Likelihood. The heritability of the development of BNP within the calf as a dam and calf trait was estimated from the dam and sire variance components of a sire-dam model. Only alloantigens inherited from the sire can be recognized by maternal alloantibodies and therefore the heritability of the development of BNP as a calf trait was estimated by calculating BNP as a sire trait. Variables included in the data set were:

- Vaccination history of the dam (Yes or No) with other BVD vaccines, Blue Tongue Virus, Rota/Corona virus, Infectious Bovine Rhinotracheitis virus or other.
- The number of Pregsure© BVD vaccinations (1, 2, 3, ≥ 4).
- Time since the last Pregsure© BVD vaccination of the dam (divided in classes of three months).
- Lactation number of the dam (1, 2, 3, 4, ≥ 5).

BNP was fitted as a binomial variable using the logistic link function to relate binomial outcome of BNP to the linear predictor used for the generalized linear mixed model. The following general model was used:

$$\text{Logit(BNP)} = \mu + (X_i)_n + \text{sire}_j + \text{dam}_k + e_{(i)n\,jk,}$$

where BNP is the outcome of BNP, μ is the general mean, $(X_i)_n$ is one or more of the aforementioned variables, sire_j is the random effect of the jth sire; dam_k is the random effect of the kth dam and $e_{(i)n\,jk}$ is the vector of residuals. Heritability was calculated using the variance components of the model, as follows: BNP as dam trait $h^2 = \sigma_{\text{dam}}^2/\sigma_p^2$; BNP as a sire trait $h^2 = \sigma_{\text{sire}}^2/\sigma_p^2$; $\sigma_p^2 = \sigma_{\text{dam}}^2 + \sigma_{\text{sire}}^2 + (\pi^2)/3$, where σ_p^2 is the phenotypic variance, σ_{dam}^2 is the dam variance, σ_{sire}^2 is the sire variance and the residual variance was fixed at $(\pi^2)/3$.

First we looked at the effect of each individual variable on BNP in a sire-dam model. Next all variables with a P-value < 0.2 were included in the final sire-dam model. Immune responses normally decline with time and to test if the incidence of BNP after the last Pregsure© BVD vaccination also declines with time, the variable *Time since last Pregsure© BVD vaccination* was forced into the final model despite having a P-value higher than 0.2 in the univariate model. Because the estimates for *Time since last Pregsure© BVD vaccination* appear to have a linear effect on BNP, the variable was added as a linear covariable in the final model. There were only eight dams with one Pregsure© BVD vaccination and because the vaccination scheme consists of an initial prime and subsequent boost vaccination which may have been interpreted as one vaccination by the farmer, in the final model animals with one or with two Pregsure© BVD vaccinations were grouped.

Animals

Blood of calves was drawn as part of the multi country epidemiological study on BNP [2]. Farms with more than one living BNP dam were revisited in 2013 to collect blood- and colostrum-samples from dams.

Throughout our study we used the following definitions for dams and calves:

- non-BNP dam – Dam that had been vaccinated with Pregsure© BVD and had not given birth to a calf that developed BNP following colostrum feeding.
- BNP dam – Dam that had been vaccinated with Pregsure© BVD and had given birth to a calf which developed BNP following colostrum feeding.
- Non-BNP calf – Calf born to a Pregsure© BVD vaccinated dam, that upon receiving colostrum from its dam did not show signs of BNP, confirmed via hematology and/or pathology.
- BNP calf – Calf born to a Pregsure© BVD vaccinated dam, that upon receiving colostrum from its dam showed clear signs of BNP, confirmed via hematology and/or pathology.

This study was approved by the Animal Ethical Committee of Utrecht University and conducted according to their regulations.

Sequence based typing of MHC class I, B2M and DRB3

Madin Darby Bovine Kidney cells (MDBK; ATCC-CCL22) were cultured in DMEM (Gibco, Life Technologies, Logan, USA), supplemented with Glutamax™, 50 IU/mL Penicillin, 50 ug/mL Streptomycin and 10% FCS. DNA was isolated from whole blood of animals and MDBK cells using the MagNA Pure Compact Instrument (Roche Diagnostics, Indianapolis, USA) according to manufacturer instructions.

Sequence based typing of MHC class I was done using gene specific primers aligning with intron 1 and intron 3 of MHC class I genes 1,2,3 and 6 [15] (Additional file 1). These primers amplify exon 2 and 3, which encode the most polymorphic regions of the MHC class I gene. For genes 1,2 and 3 PCR was carried out in 25 µL containing 1.4U Expand High fidelity Taq (Roche Diagnostics, Indianapolis, USA), 2.5 mM $MgCl_2$, 0.5 mM each dNTP and 0.4 µM, or 0.2uM in the case of primers with ambiguous nucleotide, of each primer. The thermal cycling profile was 95 °C for 5 min, 35 cycles of 95 °C for 30 s, 63 °C for 20 s, 72 °C for 60 s followed by 72 °C for 5 min. For gene 6 PCR conditions were similar, except 1.25U of AmpliTaq® 360 (Applied Biosystems, Life Technologies) was added, the $MgCl_2$ concentration was 1 mM and the annealing temperature was 56 °C. Sequencing of PCR's resulting in a product were performed on the 3730 DNA Analyzer (Applied Biosystems) using the same primers used for the PCR and the BigDye® Terminator v1.1 Cycle Sequencing Kit (Applied Biosystems). Sequence products were analyzed using SeqScape© (v2.5, Applied Biosystems). Forward and reverse sequences were aligned to a reference sequence to produce a consensus sequence. Using the IPD MHC database [16] a library of the exon 2 and 3 sequences of known MHC class I alleles was constructed using Seqscape©. Seqscape© is able to cope with ambiguous nucleotides and, in the case of heterozygous PCR products, matches the consensus read to the best combinations of alleles from the library. Consensus read basecalling of the amplified genomic DNA and library matches to known full length MHC class I cDNA sequences were checked. Using the assigned MHC class I alleles, MHC class I haplotypes were determined using haplotypes defined in Codner et al. [17] and this study (Additional file 2).

MHC class I haplotypes define a set of MHC class I alleles that are inherited together and haplotype differences between animals do not give information on differences in MHC class I as an alloantigen. To better estimate allogeneic differences between MDBK cells and dams/calves we looked at MHC class I protein differences between MDBK cells and dams/calves. Alloantibodies recognize the extracellular part of expressed proteins and we therefore looked at protein differences within the extracellular part of MHC class I (Exon 2–4). DNA sequences of exon 2–4 were translated into protein sequences and the difference in protein sequence between two MHC class I alleles was calculated, expressed as percentage of the protein sequence that was different. Dams can recognize MDBK alleles (listed in Additional file 2) as non-self if there are differences between the dam and MDBK MHC class I and for dams we calculated the difference between the MDBK allele that was most different to the dam MHC class I alleles. For alloantibodies to recognize MHC class I in the calf, there has to be a (partial) match between the MDBK and paternally inherited calf MHC class I and for calves we calculated the difference between the most similar MDBK and paternally inherited calf MHC class I allele.

Beta-2-microglobulin (B2M) primers (Additional file 1) flanking exon 2 were designed using the bovine whole genome assembly UMD3.1. PCR was carried out in 50 μL containing 2.5U PfuTurbo Cx Hotstart DNA Polymeras (Agilent, Santa Clara, USA), 2 mM MgCl$_2$, 0.2 mM each dNTP and 0.5 μM each primer. The thermal cycling profile was 95 °C for 2 min, 30 cycles of 95 °C for 30 s, 63 °C for 30 s, 72 °C for 60 s followed by 72 °C for 10 min. Sequencing was performed as described for MHC class I. Forward and reverse sequences were aligned to the UMD3.1 reference sequence using SeqScape©.

DRB3 sequence based typing was based on the method described by Miltiadou et al. [18]. Primers aligning with intron 1 and 3 of the DRB3 locus (Additional file 1) amplify exon 2, the most polymorphic region of the DRB3 gene. PCR was carried out in 25 μL containing 0.6U AmpliTaq Gold (Applied Biosystems), 1.5 mM MgCl$_2$, 0.4 mM each dNTP and 0.4 μM each primer. The thermal cycling profile was 95 °C for 10 min, 30 cycles of 94 °C for 30 s, 62 °C for 30 s, 72 °C for 30 s followed by 72 °C for 5 min. Sequencing was performed as described for MHC class I. Sequence reads were analysed using SeqScape© as described for MHC class I.

Flow cytometry

Total alloantibody levels were assessed as serum antibody levels specific for MDBK cells. The latter were suspended in serum diluted 1:20 in PBS supplemented with 2% FCS and 0.1% sodium azide. Bovine IgG binding was detected using polyclonal biotinylated sheep anti-bovine IgG antibodies (Abd Serotec, Bio-Rad Laboratories Inc, Hercules, USA) and Streptavidin-Phycoerythrin (BD biosciences, Franklin Lakes, USA). Isotype specific alloantibodies were measured in a similar way. MDBK cells were suspended in serum or colostrum diluted 1:10 and alloantibody binding was detected by bovine isotype specific mouse monoclonal antibodies [19] and FITC conjugated polyclonal goat anti-mouse antibodies (BD Biosciences). Total leukocytes were isolated from blood collected from ten healthy randomly selected dams at the slaughterhouse by hypotonic lysis of erythrocytes. Whole blood was suspended in 9 parts of distilled water, after lysis of erythrocytes isotonicity was restored using 1 volume of 10x PBS. Total leukocytes, used to detect alloantibody binding to Peripheral Blood Mononuclear Cells (PBMC), were suspended in serum or colostrum diluted 1:10. Alloantibody binding was detected by anti-bovine IgG1 mouse

monoclonal antibodies and FITC conjugated polyclonal goat anti-mouse antibodies.

In all alloantibody binding experiments serum from non Pregsure© BVD vaccinated dams were used as (isotype) controls. Flow cytometry (BD FACSCanto™, BD biosciences) was used to measure alloantibody binding and data was analyzed using Flowjo software (Tree Star Inc., Ashland, USA). PBMC were selected based on Forward and Sideward scatter. Data are depicted as Geometric Mean Fluorescent Intensity (GMFI). In the case of alloantibody binding to PBMC depicted GMFI values are GMFI values subtracted by the GMFI of the isotype controls. In order to be able to compare alloantibody binding of PBMC irrespective of total alloantibody levels in serum or colostrum, relative alloantibody binding was calculated by dividing the GMFI of each sample by the GMFI of alloantibody staining of MDBK cells, representing total alloantibody binding. A positive PBMC sample was defined as a sample that had a higher geometric mean fluorescent intensity (GMFI) than the average of all measured samples or in the case of alloantibody level compensated values defined as having a higher relative signal than the average of the relative signal of all samples.

Statistics

The Wald test was used to test whether a variable improved the fit of the sire-dam model. Haplotype/allele frequencies were analyzed using Fisher's Exact test. Alloantibody binding levels were compared by two tailed simple T-tests for unequal variance. To adjust for multiple comparisons the false discovery rate (FDR) was controlled using the method by Benjamini and Hochberg [20]. This method controls the chance of falsely declaring the result of a statistical test as significant. The largest P-value lower than its FDR-derived significance threshold and all P-values smaller were considered to be significant. The number of significant P-values that are false positive was controlled at 5%. Correlation was tested with Pearsons correlation. Normality was tested with D'Agostino and Pearsons omnibus normality test.

Effects were considered significant at $P < 0.05$. When applicable, values were given as mean ± the standard error of the mean, with the latter between brackets.

Results

Heritability of the development of BNP within the calf as a trait for Pregsure© BVD vaccinated dams and for calves

Based on the inclusion criteria 411 dam-calf combinations were selected for the heritability analysis. The 411 calves were born from 405 dams, fathered by 192 sires and comprised 102 BNP cases. The effect of each individual variable on BNP is summarized in Additional file 3.

The parameter estimates and odds ratios for the final model are shown in Table 1. For Pregsure© BVD vaccinated dams the heritability estimate for *the development of BNP within the calf* was 0.19 (0.08) and for sires it was 0.00 (0.00). The odds of BNP increased with an increased number of Pregsure© BVD vaccinations. The odds of BNP increased up to the third lactation and was lower for the fourth and fifth lactation. The effect of *Time since last Pregsure© BVD vaccination* on BNP was not significant.

Sequence based typing of MHC class I

MHC class I of Pregsure© BVD vaccinated dams

Sequence based typing was used to determine MHC class I haplotypes in vaccinated non-BNP and BNP dams (Table 2). The largest frequency differences between dams were seen for variants of the A19 MHC class I haplotype, but with a *P*-value of 0.053, which was much higher than the FDR-threshold of 0.003, this was not significant. Assuming an incidence of BNP of 0.3% for Pregsure© BVD vaccinated dams [9], the positive predictive value of the A19 haplotypes was 0.007. Implying that BNP only occurred in 0.7% of calves born to Pregsure© BVD vaccinated dams with the A19 MHC class I haplotype.

The difference in protein sequence between the extracellular parts of the MDBK and dam MHC class I alleles was 13.6% (0.35%) for vaccinated non-BNP dams and 12.9% (0.40%) for BNP dams, with a *P*-value of 0.266 this was not significantly different between both groups (Additional file 4).

Table 1 Summarizing results of the multivariable analysis of BNP using a sire-dam model (n = 411)

	Heritability estimate (SE)			
Sire	0.00 (0.00)			
Dam	0.19 (0.08)			
Variable	**Category (n)**	**β (SE)**	**Odds ratio**	**Wald test P-value**
Lactation number	1 (67)	Referent	1	0.021
	2 (106)	0.49 (0.57)	1.63	
	3 (96)	1.10 (0.60)	3.00	
	4 (70)	0.77 (0.63)	2.17	
	5 ≥ (72)	−0.14 (0.68)	0.87	
Number of Pregsure© BVD vaccinations	≤2 (118)	Referent	1	0.014
	3 (134)	0.35 (0.42)	1.42	
	4 ≥ (159)	1.17 (0.45)	3.21	
Time since last Pregsure© BVD vaccination	Per month	0.03 (0.02)	1.03	0.214

The data included 102 BNP and 309 non-BNP dam-calf combinations.

Table 2 Comparison of MHC class I haplotype frequencies in Pregsure© BVD vaccinated non-BNP and BNP dams

MHC class I Haplotype[a]	Non-BNP dams (n = 27)	BNP dams (n = 22)	P-value[b]	FDR-derived significance thresholds[c]
A19 variants	5	11	0.053	0.003
H2	4	0	0.125	0.006
A13	2	6	0.135	0.009
UU6	0	2	0.199	0.012
UU5	0	1	0.449	0.015
A20v3 (UU)	5	2	0.454	0.018
UU1	2	0	0.500	0.021
A11	3	1	0.625	0.024
A10	4	2	0.688	0.026
H5v2 (UU)	4	2	0.688	0.029
A14	9	6	0.782	0.032
A15v1	9	8	1.000	0.035
A12vUU	3	2	1.000	0.038
UU3	1	0	1.000	0.041
A18v2	1	0	1.000	0.044
UU4	1	0	1.000	0.047
UU7	1	1	1.000	0.050

[a]Bovine MHC class I haplotypes are based on Codner et al. [17] and results from this study (detailed in Additional file 2).
[b]Ordered *P*-values from Fisher's exact test.
[c]To adjust for multiple comparisons the False Discovery Rate (FDR) was controlled at 5% using the principle from Benjamini and Hochberg [19]. The largest *P*-value lower than its FDR-derived significance threshold and all *P*-values smaller are significant.

MHC class I of calves born to Pregsure© BVD vaccinated dams

The paternal MHC class I haplotype frequencies of Non-BNP and BNP calves are shown in Table 3. Based on the Fisher's exact test the frequency of the A11 haplotype was significantly higher in BNP calves, however with a *P*-value of 0.008 this value was higher than the FDR threshold of 0.004. Assuming an incidence of BNP of 0.3% for Pregsure© BVD vaccinated dams [9], the positive predictive value of the A11 haplotype was 0.014. Which implies that only 1.4% of calves with a paternally inherited A11 MHC class I haplotype born to Pregsure© BVD vaccinated dams get BNP.

In five non-BNP and three BNP calves fathered by the same sire, the MHC class I haplotypes were also typed (Additional file 5). Since all eight calves had the A11 MHC class I haplotype, it is likely that the sire was A11 homozygous. In that case both non-BNP and BNP calves inherited the A11 haplotype from their father and for these calves there was no association between the paternally inherited A11 haplotype and the development of BNP.

The protein difference between the extracellular part of the MDBK MHC class I alleles and paternally inherited

Table 3 Paternal MHC class I haplotype frequencies of non-BNP and BNP calves born from Pregsure© BVD vaccinated dams

Paternal MHC class I Haplotype[a]	Non-BNP calves ($n = 21$)	BNP calves ($n = 9$)	P-value[b]	FDR-derived significance thresholds[c]
A11	3	6	0.008	0.004
A14	0	1	0.300	0.007
UU3	0	1	0.300	0.011
UU9	3	0	0.535	0.014
UU8	2	1	1.000	0.018
A13	1	0	1.000	0.021
UU1	2	0	1.000	0.025
A18v2 (UU)	1	0	1.000	0.029
A12 (UU)	2	0	1.000	0.032
A15v1	1	0	1.000	0.036
A19variants	2	0	1.000	0.039
A20variant	1	0	1.000	0.043
H2	1	0	1.000	0.046
H5v2(UU)	2	0	1.000	0.050

[a,b,c]As in Table 2.

Table 4 Comparison of DRB3 allele frequencies within Pregsure© BVD vaccinated dams and BNP dams

DRB3 allele frequencies	Non-BNP dams ($n = 21$)	BNP dams ($n = 21$)	P-value[a]	FDR-derived significance thresholds[b]
1001	7	1	0.0574	0.004
14011	7	1	0.0574	0.008
2703	2	7	0.1555	0.013
0902	2	6	0.2646	0.017
1601	1	4	0.3597	0.021
0201	4	1	0.3597	0.025
0101	3	6	0.4827	0.029
0601	2	0	0.494	0.033
1101	9	11	0.7983	0.038
1201	3	4	1.000	0.042
0701	1	0	1.000	0.046
UU01[c]	1	1	1.000	0.050

[a]Ordered P-values from Fisher's exact test.
[b]To adjust for multiple comparisons the False Discovery Rate (FDR) was controlled at 5% using the principle from Benjamini and Hochberg [19]. The largest P-value lower than its FDR-derived significance threshold and all P-values smaller are significant.
[c]Denotes a local name and is not included in the IPD Bovine MHC class II database.

calf MHC class I alleles was 9.44% (0.84%) for non-BNP calves and 9.37% (0.29%) for BNP calves, with a P-value of 0.938 this was not significantly different between both groups (Additional file 6).

Sequence based typing of beta-2-microglobulin in Pregsure© BVD vaccinated dams and MDBK cells

Exon 2 of the beta-2-microglobulin (B2M) gene, encoding 97% of the mature protein, was sequenced in MDBK cells and in five vaccinated non-BNP dams and five BNP dams that were farm matched. The B2M sequences of all vaccinated non-BNP dams, BNP dams and MDBK cells were identical.

Sequence based typing of DRB3 in Pregsure© BVD vaccinated dams

Results of the DRB3 typing of vaccinated non-BNP dams and BNP dams are shown in Table 4. The largest frequency differences were seen for the DRB3 alleles 1001 and 14011 both with a higher frequency in vaccinated non-BNP dams. However, the P-values were well above the FDR threshold and not significant.

Characterization of alloantibodies from Pregsure© BVD vaccinated dams

Total alloantibody levels in dams not vaccinated with Pregsure© BVD and in Pregsure© BVD vaccinated non-BNP and BNP dams were assessed as serum antibody levels specific for MDBK cells using flow cytometry (Figure 1). Alloantibody levels in BNP dams were

significantly higher than in both non-BNP dams and dams not vaccinated with Pregsure© BVD, levels in vaccinated non-BNP dams are significantly higher than in dams not vaccinated with Pregsure© BVD.

Isotype specific alloantibody binding of MDBK cells is shown in Figure 2. IgG1 alloantibodies were most abundant and the levels were significantly higher in serum of non-BNP dams and in serum and colostrum of BNP dams compared to dams not vaccinated with Pregsure© BVD. IgG2 alloantibody levels were significantly higher in serum and colostrum of BNP dams compared to dams not vaccinated with Pregsure© BVD. IgG2 alloantibody levels tended to be higher in non-BNP dams as well, but due to higher variation among dams, did not differ significantly from that in dams not vaccinated with Pregsure© BVD. For IgM and IgA there were no significant differences between groups.

Antibodies present in serum and colostrum from non-BNP and BNP dams bind PBMC (Figure 3A). Alloantibody binding of PBMC was significantly higher for both serum and colostrum of BNP dams compared to non-BNP dams. The number of PBMC samples that were positive were also higher for both serum and colostrum of BNP dams. However, average alloantibody binding of PBMC and alloantibody binding of MDBK cells had a high correlation (Figure 3B) and when alloantibody binding of PBMC was compensated for MDBK specific alloantibody levels to enable comparison of the binding of PBMC irrespective of total alloantibody levels, the relative signal was

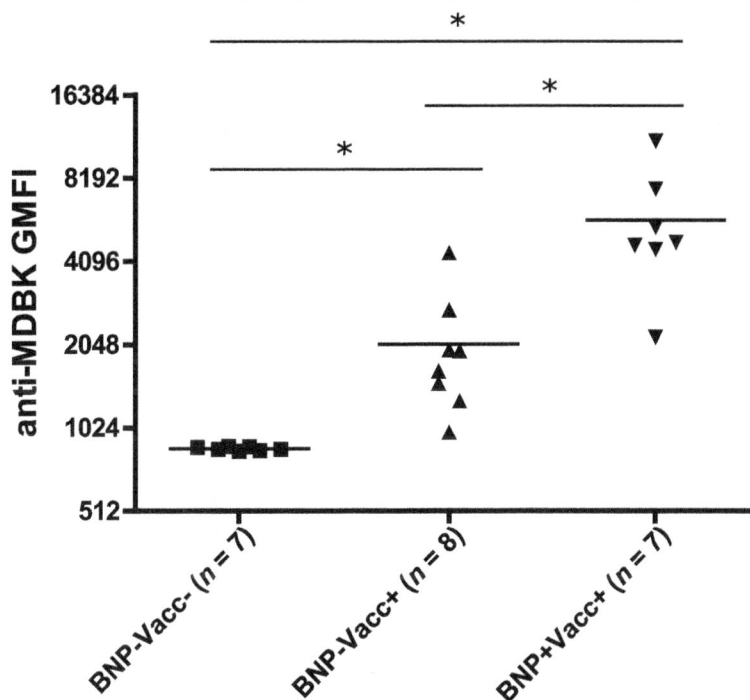

Figure 1 Serum of Pregsure© BVD vaccinated dams contain alloantibodies. Total IgG alloantibody binding of MDBK cells was measured in serum of i) dams not vaccinated with Pregsure© BVD (BNP-VAcc-) ii) Pregsure© BVD vaccinated non-BNP dams (BNP-Vacc+) and iii) Pregsure© BVD vaccinated BNP dams (BNP + Vacc+) using flow cytometry. The black bars denote the mean Geometric Mean Fluorescent Intensity (GMFI). Results were compared by two tailed simple T-tests for unequal variance. To adjust for multiple comparisons, the False Discovery Rate (FDR) was controlled at 5% using the principle from Benjamini and Hochberg [19]. The largest P-value lower than its FDR-derived significance threshold and all P-values smaller are significant and are depicted by an asterisk (*).

the same for BNP dams and non-BNP dams for serum as well as colostrum (Figure 3C). Also, the number of PBMC samples that were positive were similar in both groups for serum as well as colostrum. Results of individual serum and colostrum samples are shown in Additional file 7.

Discussion

We hypothesized that the rare occurrence of BNP after Pregsure© BVD vaccination depends both on the capability of the dam's immune system to present the MDBK alloantigens via MHC class II, as well as the degree of alloantigen (mis)match between the dam and the MDBK cell line (and the calf and the MDBK cell line, respectively) and the ensuing immune response of the dam. As a corollary we hypothesized that genetic differences in MHC class II in dams and alloantigens in dams and calves (e.g. MHC I and MHC class I associated B2M) would then explain why BNP only occurs in part of the calves born to PregSure© BVD vaccinated dams. The present study demonstrates that the development of BNP in calves is a heritable trait for Pregsure© BVD vaccinated dams with the high heritability estimate of 19%, which shows that genetic differences between dams explain in part why only the colostrum of some Pregsure© BVD vaccinated dams cause BNP in the calf. Genetic variation in the paternal

haplotype of the calves is not related to the development of BNP in the calf, since the heritability of the development of BNP in calves born to Pregsure© BVD vaccinated dams is 0%. Demasius et al. [21] found that in an experimental German Holstein x Charolois crossbred herd with a limited number of sire lines, all BNP cases were restricted to a single maternal grandsire, also indicating the importance of the genetic background of the dam. In addition from a limited number of BNP dams was shown to induce BNP in randomly selected healthy calves [8-10] which supports the notion that the genetic background of the calf is not critical. The phenotype of the calf was based on very strict objective criteria, whereas the phenotype of the dam was based on the phenotype of the calf. BNP is caused by alloantibodies present in the colostrum and the phenotype of the calf therefore depends on the quality, quantity and source (own dam or other dam) of the ingested colostrum. This means that the phenotype of the calf, may not always be the proper phenotype of the dam. Much of this information was farmer reported and although we have tried to control for these aspects, the possibility exists that non-differential misclassification of the phenotype of the dam occurred in this study and implies that the heritability for the development of BNP within calves of 19% for dams is potentially underestimated.

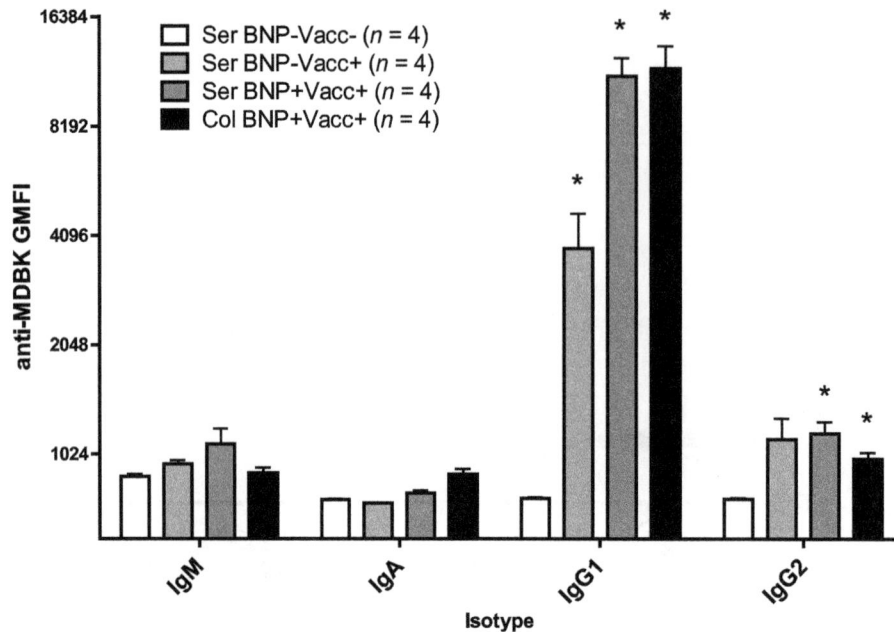

Figure 2 Isotype characterization of alloantibodies from Pregsure© BVD vaccinated dams. Flow cytometry was used to measure the isotype of alloantibodies binding to MDBK cells in serum (Ser) or colostrum (Col) from i) dams not vaccinated with Pregsure© BVD (BNP-VAcc-) ii) Pregsure© BVD vaccinated non-BNP dams (BNP-Vacc+) and iii) Pregsure© BVD vaccinated BNP dams (BNP + Vacc+). All results were compared by two tailed simple T-tests for unequal variance. Within each isotype, all groups are compared to the non Pregsure© BVD vaccinated dams (Ser BNP-Vacc-). To adjust for multiple comparison, the False Discovery Rate (FDR) was controlled at 5% using the principle from Benjamini and Hochberg [19]. The largest P-value lower than its FDR-derived significance threshold and all P-values smaller are significant and are depicted by an asterisk (*). GMFI = Geometric Mean Fluorescent Intensity.

In our more in depth analyses of the genetic differences between Pregsure© BVD vaccinated non-BNP and BNP dams we sequenced a number of specific candidate genes. An important target of BNP alloantibodies is MHC class I [9,12], a highly polymorphic alloantigen [17]. Hence MHC class I was genotyped to see if differences in MHC class I alloantigen repertoire of dams and/or calves were associated with the development of BNP in the calf. We did not find an association between the MHC class I of the Pregsure© BVD vaccinated dams and the occurrence of BNP. Although the number of BNP calves in the MHC class I haplotyping analysis was limited, it showed that BNP calves do not have a single paternal MHC class I haplotype and that most of the paternal haplotypes are shared between BNP and non-BNP calves (Table 3, Additional file 5), together indicating that the paternally inherited MHC class I of calves is not associated with the occurrence of BNP. This result supports our finding that the heritability of the development of BNP in calves is zero and shows that BNP and non-BNP calves do not have a different allogeneic background. Ballingall et al. [22] found no differences in DRB3 allele frequencies between BNP and non-BNP calves. Since DRB3 and MHC class I are in linkage disequilibrium, this corroborates our MHC class I typing result in calves.

The binding of certain monoclonal antibodies to the B2M-MHC class I heavy chain heterodimer can depend on the associated B2M allele [23] or MHC class I allele [24]. Although polymorphisms within the bovine B2M gene are known, none lead to changes in the amino acid sequence [25]. Nevertheless we wanted to exclude the possibility that an unknown rare allelic variant of B2M influences the recognition and immune response to MDBK MHC class I proteins present in the vaccine. Since sequences of B2M were identical in the MDBK cell line and all typed Pregsure© BVD vaccinated non-BNP and BNP dams, it is highly unlikely that allelic variations of B2M play a role in the etiology of BNP.

Another aspect of immune recognition of MDBK alloantigens present in the Pregsure© BVD vaccine is their presentation to the dam's immune system via MHC class II. MHC class II haplotypes have been associated with disease resistance and susceptibility [26,27] and influence antibody responses after vaccination [28,29]. We found no association between MHC class II haplotypes, as assessed by sequencing the highly polymorphic DRB3 locus, and the occurrence of BNP in Pregsure© BVD vaccinated dams.

Pregsure© BVD vaccinated BNP dams had significantly higher serum alloantibody levels compared to Pregsure© BVD vaccinated non-BNP dams. Nonetheless

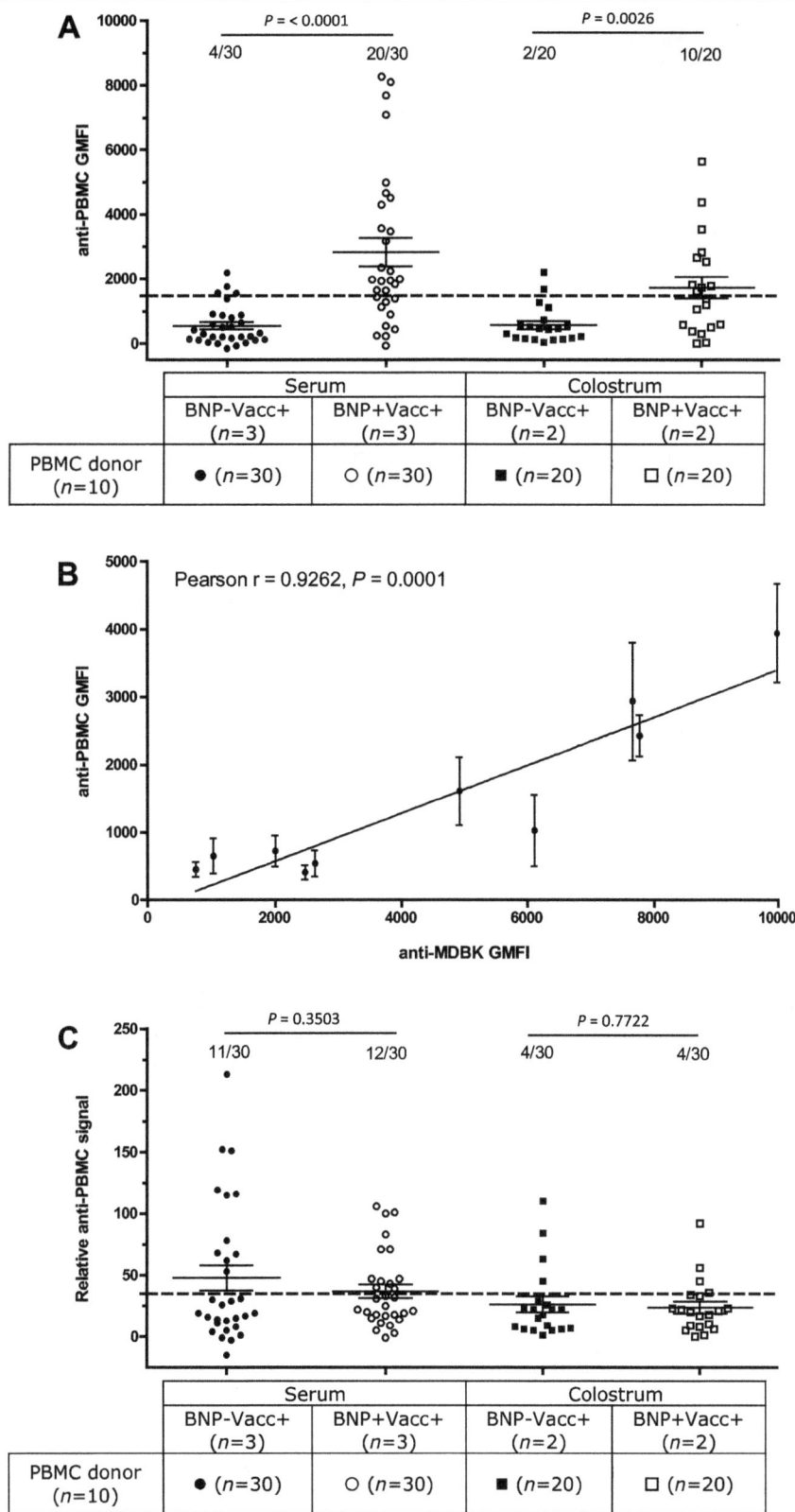

Figure 3 (See legend on next page.)

Figure 3 **Binding of peripheral blood mononuclear cells by alloantibodies from Pregsure© BVD vaccinated dams. A**: Peripheral Blood Mononuclear Cells (PBMC) from ten random dams were stained with serum (n = 3) and colostrum (n = 2) of different Pregsure© BVD vaccinated non-BNP dams (BNP-Vacc+, n = 5) and with serum (n = 3) and colostrum (n = 2) of Pregsure© BVD vaccinated BNP dams (BNP + Vacc+, n = 5). IgG1 alloantibody binding was measured by flow cytometry. GMFI subtracted by isotype control is plotted on the y-axis. The horizontal dotted line depicts the overall average geometric mean fluorescent intensity (GMFI) and the number above the plots describes the number of samples with a signal above the horizontal line. **B**: Correlation between the average IgG1 alloantibody binding of PBMC's from ten dams to IgG1 alloantibody binding of MDBK cells by serum or colostrum samples as in Figure 3A. **C**: The data from Figure 3A were divided by the GMFI signal of the alloantibody staining of MDBK cells by the respective serum or colostrum. The horizontal dotted line depicts the overall average relative signal and the number above the plots describes the number of samples with a signal above the horizontal line. Mean ± standard error of the mean is depicted in all graphs. Two tailed simple T-tests for unequal variance was used to compare serum or colostrum alloantibody binding of PBMC's between Pregsure© BVD vaccinated non-BNP and BNP dams. Correlation was tested with Pearsons correlation. Normality was tested with D'Agostino and Pearsons omnibus normality test.

alloantibodies were produced both in Pregsure© BVD vaccinated non-BNP and BNP dams, confirming results from a previous study [7]. Alloantibody production by all Pregsure© BVD vaccinated dams indicated there were allogeneic differences between the bovine MDBK proteins and both Pregsure© BVD vaccinated non-BNP and BNP dams. This corroborated the sequencing results, where we did not find a difference between MHC class I or B2M between Pregsure© BVD vaccinated non-BNP and BNP dams. It also indicated that all dams were able to present alloantigens from the Pregsure© BVD vaccine in the context of MHC class II and fitted with the lack of an association between DRB3 and the occurrence of BNP within Pregsure© vaccinated dams.

The antibody isotype produced by B-cells depends on the cytokines that are produced during an (vaccine induced) immune response [30,31]. The type of vaccine induced immune response may therefore influence the quality of the ensuing antibody response. As different antibody isotypes induce different biological effector functions, such as complement activation and neutralization, we studied the quality of the antibody response in Pregsure© BVD vaccinated non-BNP and BNP dams to determine if BNP dams only differ in alloantibody levels or also in the isotype and specificity of alloantibodies produced. BNP is caused by alloantibodies from colostrum and for BNP dams serum and colostrum alloantibodies were compared to see if results for serum alloantibodies can be extrapolated to colostrum derived alloantibodies. Alloantibody isotypes were similar in serum of Pregsure© BVD vaccinated non-BNP dams and serum and colostrum of BNP dams, indicating a similar response to vaccination in both groups. Likewise, studying cattle responding with high or low antibody levels after vaccination with hen-egg white lysozyme or Candida albicans extract Heriazon et al. [32] also did not find any differences in IgG1 and IgG2 levels between animals, whereas antibody levels following vaccination varied significantly.

When stained with serum or colostrum from Pregsure© BVD vaccinated BNP dams higher numbers of (random) PBMC samples were positive for alloantibody binding and on average staining intensity was higher than when stained with serum or colostrum from Pregsure© BVD vaccinated non-BNP dams. However, when compensated for alloantibody binding of MDBK cells to enable comparison of binding to PBMC irrespective of total alloantibody levels, numbers of positive PBMC samples and the relative staining intensity with alloantibodies were comparable between Pregsure© BVD vaccinated BNP and non-BNP dams, indicating that the specificity for allogeneic cells was also comparable. Based on the similar antibody isotypes and relative staining of PBMC we argue that alloantibodies from Pregsure© BVD vaccinated non-BNP and BNP dams are qualitatively similar and that only the level of alloantibodies is higher in Pregsure© vaccinated BNP dams. The high correlation between binding of alloantibodies to MDBK cells and PBMC corroborates the notion that the most important alloantigens in the Pregsure© BVD vaccine are derived from the producer cell line. Bastian et al. [7] found that BNP dams also had higher BVD neutralizing antibody levels than Pregsure© BVD vaccinated non-BNP dams, showing that BNP dams generally respond with higher antibody levels to components in the Pregsure© BVD vaccine. In combination with the high heritability estimate for the development of BNP in calves for Pregsure© BVD vaccinated dams, it is likely that genetic differences between vaccinated non-BNP and BNP dams are due to genes that determine the level of antibody production after Pregsure© BVD vaccination. In cattle high heritability estimates have been found for antibody production after vaccination, these ranged from 13% to 88% [33,34]. High antibody production after BRSV vaccination was associated with single nucleotide variants of TLR4 and TLR 8 [28]. Likewise, differences in responsiveness of the innate immune system of BNP dams to the adjuvant of the Pregsure© BVD vaccine may have led to higher antibody production to antigens in the vaccine. The occurrence of BNP shows that in an outbred population some individuals may respond very differently to vaccination than the general population. This emphasizes the importance of monitoring adverse effects of both existing and new vaccines, but may on the other hand also provide opportunities for selective breeding for an increased humoral immune response.

Bovine MHC class I has an unusual organization, with six putative genes of which a variable number of genes are functionally present per haplotype [17], making MHC class I typing in cattle difficult. Several techniques with different (dis)advantages have been used to type MHC class I in cattle, including serology [35], cloning and sequencing of full length cDNA [36] and next generation sequencing of polymorphic regions [37]. In this study we use gene specific primers for four of the six MHC class I genes to amplify exon 2 and 3 [15], encoding the most polymorphic region of the MHC class I. Alleles are distinguished based on exon 2 and 3 sequence and full length sequences are imputed from the IPD bovine MHC class I database [16], a method commonly used for HLA typing (e.g. [38]). Advantages of this typing method are that the amplified gene specific sequence normally only contains two alleles, allowing the use of traditional sanger sequencing, and that a relatively large number of samples can be typed, as was necessary for the present study. However, there are also some limitations to this method. The gene specific primers are only validated for Holsteins, which was not a problem in this study as all dams were of Holstein origin, and alleles from MHC class I gene 4 and 5 are not directly typed. However, genes 4 and 5 are the least polymorphic of the bovine MHC class I genes with only seven documented alleles of which only two have been reported in Holsteins [16]. One of these alleles (4*02401) can be imputed based on haplotype and the other (5*03901) is amplified by gene 3 specific primers. MHC class I haplotypes define a set of MHC class I alleles that are inherited together and because different haplotypes can define very similar MHC class I alleles, haplotype differences between animals do not accurately represent allogeneic or immunological differences between animals. It has been hypothesized that the occurrence of BNP depends on allogeneic (mis)matches between the dam, the MDBK cell line and the calf [9,12]. The likelihood of an alloimmune response is directly related to the number of epitope mismatches between the foreign alloantigen and the host [39] and in order to better estimate allogeneic (mis)matches between animals and MDBK cells, we analyzed protein differences in the extracellular domain of the MHC class I protein between MDBK cells and dams/calves. Although this method is potentially a better estimate of allogeneic differences between animals than only relying on MHC class I haplotypes, accurate prediction of antibody epitopes is much more complicated and depends on many other factors, such as conformation, non-linear epitopes and flanking residues [40]. Since genes 4 and 5 are not directly typed in the MHC class I method used in this paper, in some animals the presence of certain alleles

was imputed from the defined haplotype for that animal and for newly defined haplotypes the presence of additional alleles cannot be excluded, giving an extra level of uncertainty to the analysis of the MHC class I protein differences. However, previously published haplotypes comprise the majority of the haplotypes typed in this study and the results from the MHC class I halpotyping corroborates the results from other experiments in this study. Together, the results indicate that the occurrence of BNP is not associate with a specific allogeneic background of BNP dams or calves. The only difference we found between Pregsure© BVD vaccinated non-BNP and BNP dams were in the alloantibody levels and this would imply that the development of BNP in the calf primarily depends on the alloantibody dose the calf absorbs. The finding by Jones et al. [2] that the odds of BNP increases with increased colostrum intake, and thus alloantibody intake, strengthens this hypothesis. The risk of BNP increases with increased number of Pregsure© BVD vaccinations and this can be explained by boosting of antibody production, increasing the alloantibody levels in the colostrum and thus increasing the alloantibody dose of the calf after colostrum ingestion. Furthermore, our findings that the heritability for the development of BNP in the calf was 0% for calves, whereas as a dam trait the heritability was 19% and the observation that BNP can be induced in unrelated healthy calves by alloantibodies/colostrum from BNP dams [8-10] show that the dam and not the calf plays a pivotal role in determining whether a calf gets BNP or not. We conclude that the development of BNP in calves is a heritable trait of the dam rather than the calf and that genetic differences between BNP and non-BNP dams are likely due to genes controlling the quantitative alloantibody response following vaccination.

Additional files

Additional file 1: Primers used for the amplification of MHC class I genes, Bèta-2-Microglobulin and DRB3. The table lists the sequences and the location of the forward and reverse primers used to amplify the MHC class I genes, Bèta-2-Microglobulin and DRB3 genes.

Additional file 2: List of MHC class I haplotypes and MHC class I typing results of the MDBK cell line. List of MHC class I haplotype definitions used in this article and the MHC class I typing results of the MDBK cell line. The newly defined haplotypes, containing an UU prefix or suffix, are provisional haplotypes. These haplotypes have not been confirmed using different MHC class I typing methods and because the gene specific primers used in this study do not amplify gene 4 and 5 and have not been validated for all known MHC class I alleles, the presence of additional alleles cannot be excluded. In some cases previously defined haplotypes [17] have been renamed to accommodate for additional haplotype variants within a group. Allele nomenclature refers to the IPD Bovine MHC class I database [16].

Additional file 3: Summarizing results of the univariable analysis of the effect of independent variables on BNP, including sire and dam heritability estimates ($n = 411$). The table provides results from the univariable analysis of the effect of independent variables on BNP. The number of records per category, the estimate (β), the odds ratio and the P-value from the Wald test are given. The heritability estimates for BNP as a sire trait and BNP as a dam trait are also depicted.

Additional file 4: Comparison of the difference in protein sequence of the extracellular part of the MHC class I protein (Exon 2–4) between the the MDBK MHC class I allele that is most different to the MHC class I alleles of Pregsure© BVD vaccinated non-BNP and BNP dams. DNA sequences of the extracellular part of MHC class I, exon 2–4, were translated into protein sequences and the percentage of sequence difference between the MDBK MHC class I allele that was most different to the dam MHC class I alleles was calculated. Results for Pregsure© BVD vaccinated non-BNP and BNP dams were compared using an Unpaired t-test for unequal variance.

Additional file 5: MHC class I haplotypes of calves (n = 8) fathered by the same sire. The table lists sequence based MHC class I haplotyping results for three BNP and five non-BNP calves fathered by the same sire.

Additional file 6: Comparison of the difference in protein sequence of the extracellular part of the MHC class I protein (Exon 2–4) between the most similar MDBK and paternally inherited MHC class I allele from non BNP and BNP calves. DNA sequences of the extracellular part of MHC class I, exon 2–4, were translated into protein sequences and the percentage of sequence difference between the most similar MDBK and paternally inherited calf MHC class I allele was calculated. Results for non-BNP and BNP calves were compared using an Unpaired t-test for unequal variance.

Additional file 7: Binding of peripheral blood mononuclear cells by alloantibodies from Pregsure© BVD vaccinated dams. A: Peripheral Blood Mononuclear Cells (PBMC) from ten random dams were stained with serum (Ser, n = 3) and colostrum (Col, n = 2) of different Pregsure© BVD vaccinated non-BNP dams (BNP-Vacc+, n = 5) and with serum (n = 3) and colostrum (n = 2) of Pregsure© BVD vaccinated BNP dams (BNP + Vacc+, n = 5). IgG1 alloantibody binding was measured by flow cytometry. GMFI subtracted by isotype control is plotted on the y-axis. The horizontal dotted line depicts the overall average geometric mean fluorescent intensity (GMFI) and the number above the plots describes the number of samples with a signal above the horizontal line. B: The data from Additional file 7A were divided by the GMFI signal of the alloantibody staining of MDBK cells by the respective serum or colostrum. The horizontal dotted line depicts the overall average relative signal and the number above the plots describes the number of samples with a signal above the horizontal line. Mean ± standard error of the mean is depicted in all graphs. Two tailed simple T-tests for unequal variance was used to compare alloantibody binding of PBMC's between Pregsure© BVD vaccinated non-BNP and BNP dams.

Competing interests
This study was funded by Zoetis.

Authors' contributions
LB participated in the design of the study, carried out the experiments, the data collection and analysis and prepared the manuscript. HGO and WGJvG participated in the design, the experiments, the data collection and analysis of the sequencing experiments and revised the manuscript. HCMH, MN and GvS participated in the design, the experiments, the data collection and analysis of the heritability study and revised the manuscript. VPMGR and APK participated in the design of the study, the experiments, the data collection and analysis and prepared the manuscript. All authors read and approved the final manuscript.

Acknowledgements
We thank the Dutch dairy farmers and veterinary practitioners who enabled the sample collection. We also thank Matthijs Schouten for taking the on farm questionnaires, CRV (Arnhem, the Netherlands) for supplying the pedigrees and GD Animal Health Service (Deventer, the Netherlands), especially Ingrid den Uijl and Iwan Kristens, for help with processing the serum samples and data of the calves.

Author details
[1]Department of Infectious Diseases and Immunology, Faculty of Veterinary Medicine, Utrecht University, Utrecht, The Netherlands. [2]Laboratory of Translational Immunology, University Medical Center Utrecht, Utrecht, The Netherlands. [3]GD Animal Health Service, Deventer, The Netherlands. [4]Department of Clinical Sciences of Companion Animals, Faculty of Veterinary Medicine, Utrecht University, Utrecht, the Netherlands. [5]Animal Breeding and Genomics Centre, Wageningen University, Wageningen, the Netherlands. [6]Department of Farm Animal Health, Faculty of Veterinary Medicine, Utrecht University, Utrecht, The Netherlands. [7]Department of Veterinary Tropical Diseases, Faculty of Veterinary Science, University of Pretoria, Onderstepoort, South Africa.

References
1. Friedrich A, Rademacher G, Weber BK, Kappe E, Carlin A, Assad A, Sauter-Louis CM, Hafner-Marx A, Buttner M, Böttcher J, Klee W: **Gehäuftes Auftreten von hämorrhagischer Diathese infolge Knochenmarkschädigung bei jungen Kälbern.** Tierärztl Umschau 2009, **64:**423–431 (in German).
2. Jones BA, Sauter-Louis C, Henning J, Stoll A, Nielen M, Van Schaik G, Smolenaars A, Schouten M, den Uijl I, Fourichon C, Guatteo R, Madouasse A, Nusinovici S, Deprez P, De Vliegher S, Laureyns J, Booth R, Cardwell JM, Pfeiffer DU: **Calf-level factors associated with bovine neonatal pancytopenia - a multi-country case–control study.** PLoS ONE 2013, **8:**e80619.
3. Pardon B, Steukers L, Dierick J, Ducatelle R, Saey V, Maes S, Vercauteren G, De Clercq K, Callens J, De Bleecker K, Deprez P: **Haemorrhagic diathesis in neonatal calves: an emerging syndrome in Europe.** Transbound Emerg Dis 2010, **57:**135–146.
4. Bell CR, Rocchi MS, Dagleish MP, Melzi E, Ballingall KT, Connelly M, Kerr MG, Scholes SF, Willoughby K: **Reproduction of bovine neonatal pancytopenia (BNP) by feeding pooled colostrum reveals variable alloantibody damage to different haematopoietic lineages.** Vet Immunol Immunopathol 2013, **151:**303–314.
5. Kappe EC, Halami MY, Schade B, Alex M, Hoffmann D, Gangl A, Meyer K, Dekant W, Schwarz BA, Johne R, Buitkamp J, Böttcher J, Müller H: **Bone marrow depletion with haemorrhagic diathesis in calves in Germany: characterization of the disease and preliminary investigations on its aetiology.** Berl Munch Tierarztl Wochenschr 2010, **123:**31–41.
6. Assad A, Amann B, Friedrich A, Deeg CA: **Immunophenotyping and characterization of BNP colostra revealed pathogenic alloantibodies of IgG1 subclass with specifity to platelets, granulocytes and monocytes of all maturation stages.** Vet Immunol Immunopathol 2012, **147:**25–34.
7. Bastian M, Holsteg M, Hanke-Robinson H, Duchow K, Cussler K: **Bovine Neonatal Pancytopenia: is this alloimmune syndrome caused by vaccine-induced alloreactive antibodies?** Vaccine 2011, **29:**5267–5275.
8. Bridger PS, Bauerfeind R, Wenzel L, Bauer N, Menge C, Thiel HJ, Reinacher M, Doll K: **Detection of colostrum-derived alloantibodies in calves with bovine neonatal pancytopenia.** Vet Immunol Immunopathol 2011, **141:**1–10.
9. Foucras G, Corbiere F, Tasca C, Pichereaux C, Caubet C, Trumel C, Lacroux C, Franchi C, Burlet-Schiltz O, Schelcher F: **Alloantibodies against MHC Class I: a novel mechanism of neonatal pancytopenia linked to vaccination.** J Immunol 2011, **187:**6564–6570.
10. Friedrich A, Buttner M, Rademacher G, Klee W, Weber BK, Muller M, Carlin A, Assad A, Hafner-Marx A, Sauter-Louis CM: **Ingestion of colostrum from specific cows induces Bovine Neonatal Pancytopenia (BNP) in some calves.** BMC Vet Res 2011, **7:**10.
11. Madin SH, Darby NB: **Established kidney cell lines of normal adult bovine and ovine origin.** Proc Soc Exp Biol Med 1958, **98:**574–576.
12. Deutskens F, Lamp B, Riedel CM, Wentz E, Lochnit G, Doll K, Thiel HJ, Rumenapf T: **Vaccine-induced antibodies linked to bovine neonatal pancytopenia (BNP) recognize cattle major histocompatibility complex class I (MHC I).** Vet Res 2011, **42:**97.
13. Kasonta R, Sauter-Louis C, Holsteg M, Duchow K, Cussler K, Bastian M: **Effect of the vaccination scheme on PregSure (R) BVD induced alloreactivity and the incidence of Bovine Neonatal Pancytopenia.** Vaccine 2012, **30:**6649–6655.
14. Gilmour AR, Gogel BJ, Cullis BR, Thompson R: ASReml User Guide. Release 3.0. Hemel Hempstead, UK: VSN International Ltd; 2009.

15. Birch J, Murphy L, MacHugh ND, Ellis SA: Generation and maintenance of diversity in the cattle MHC class I region. *Immunogenetics* 2006, 58:670–679.

16. IPD-MHC Database [http://www.ebi.ac.uk/ipd/mhc/bola/index.html]

17. Codner GF, Birch J, Hammond JA, Ellis SA: Constraints on haplotype structure and variable gene frequencies suggest a functional hierarchy within cattle MHC class I. *Immunogenetics* 2012, 64:435–445.

18. Miltiadou D, Law AS, Russell GC: Establishment of a sequence-based typing system for BoLA-DRB3 exon 2. *Tissue Antigens* 2003, 62:55–65.

19. Vanzaane D, Ijzerman J: Monoclonal-antibodies against bovine immunoglobulins and their use in isotype-specific ELISAs for rotavirus antibody. *J Immunol Methods* 1984, 72:427–441.

20. Benjamini Y, Hochberg Y: Controlling the false discovery rate - a practical and powerful approach to multiple testing. *J R Stat Soc B* 1995, 57:289–300.

21. Demasius W, Weikard R, Kromik A, Wolf C, Muller K, Kuhn C: Bovine neonatal pancytopenia (BNP): novel insights into the incidence, vaccination-associated epidemiological factors and a potential genetic predisposition for clinical and subclinical cases. *Res Vet Sci* 2014, 96:537–542.

22. Ballingall KT, Nath M, Holliman A, Laming E, Steele P, Willoughby K: Lack of evidence for an association between MHC diversity and the development of bovine neonatal pancytopenia in Holstein dairy cattle. *Vet Immunol Immunopathol* 2011, 141:128–132.

23. Kahn-Perles B, Boyer C, Arnold B, Sanderson AR, Ferrier P, Lemonnier FA: Acquisition of HLA class I W6/32 defined antigenic determinant by heavy-chains from different species following association with bovine beta-2-microglobulin. *J Immunol* 1987, 138:2190–2196.

24. Bensaid A, Kaushal A, MacHugh ND, Shapiro SZ, Teale AJ: Biochemical characterization of activation-associated bovine class I major histocompatibility complex antigens. *Anim Genet* 1989, 20:241–255.

25. Clawson ML, Heaton MP, Chitko-McKown CG, Fox JM, Smith TPL, Snelling WM, Keele JW, Laegreid WW: Beta-2-microglobulin haplotypes in US beef cattle and association with failure of passive transfer in newborn calves. *Mamm Genome* 2004, 15:227–236.

26. Juliarena MA, Poli M, Sala L, Ceriani C, Gutierrez S, Dolcini G, Rodriguez EM, Marino B, Rodriguez-Dubra C, Esteban EN: Association of BLV infection profiles with alleles of the BoLA-DRB3.2 gene. *Anim Genet* 2008, 39:432–438.

27. Park YH, Joo YS, Park JY, Moon JS, Kim SH, Kwon NH, Ahn JS, Davis WC, Davies CJ: Characterization of lymphocyte subpopulations and major histocompatibility complex haplotypes of mastitis-resistant and susceptible cows. *J Vet Sci* 2004, 5:29–39.

28. Glass EJ, Baxter R, Leach RJ, Jann OC: Genes controlling vaccine responses and disease resistance to respiratory viral pathogens in cattle. *Vet Immunol Immunopathol* 2012, 148:90–99.

29. Sitte K, Brinkworth R, East IJ, Jazwinska EC: A single amino acid deletion in the antigen binding site of BoLA-DRB3 is predicted to affect peptide binding. *Vet Immunol Immunopathol* 2002, 85:129–135.

30. Estes DM, Brown WC: Type 1 and type 2 responses in regulation of Ig isotype expression in cattle. *Vet Immunol Immunopathol* 2002, 90:1–10.

31. House JK, Smith BP, O'Connell K, VanMetre DC: Isotype-specific antibody responses of cattle to Salmonella Dublin lipopolysaccharide and porin following Salmonella Dublin vaccination and acute and chronic infection. *J Vet Diagn Invest* 2001, 13:213–218.

32. Heriazon A, Hamilton K, Huffman J, Wilkie BN, Sears W, Quinton M, Mallard BA: Immunoglobulin isotypes of lactating Holstein cows classified as high, average, and low type-1 or-2 immune responders. *Vet Immunol Immunopathol* 2011, 144:259–269.

33. O'Neill RG, Woolliams JA, Glass EJ, Williams JL, Fitzpatrick JL: Quantitative evaluation of genetic and environmental parameters determining antibody response induced by vaccination against bovine respiratory syncytial virus. *Vaccine* 2006, 24:4007–4016.

34. Wagter LC, Mallard BA, Wilkie BN, Leslie KE, Boettcher PJ, Dekkers JCM: A quantitative approach to classifying Holstein cows based on antibody responsiveness and its relationship to peripartum mastitis occurrence. *J Dairy Sci* 2000, 83:488–498.

35. Davies CJ, Joosten I, Bernoco D, Arriens MA, Bester J, Ceriotti G, Ellis S, Hensen EJ, Hines HC, Horin P, Kristensen B, Lewin HA, Meggiolaro D, Morgan AL, Morita M, Nilsson PR, Oliver RA, Orlova A, Ostergard H, Park CA, Schuberth HJ, Simon M, Spooner RL, Stewart JA: Polymorphism of bovine MHC class I genes. Joint report of the Fifth International Bovine Lymphocyte Antigen (BoLA) Workshop, Interlaken, Switzerland, 1 August 1992. *Eur J Immunogenet* 1994, 21:239–258.

36. Ellis SA, Staines KA, Morrison WI: cDNA sequence of cattle MHC class I genes transcribed in serologically defined haplotypes A18 and A31. *Immunogenetics* 1996, 43:156–159.

37. Benedictus L, Thomas AJ, Jorritsma R, Davies CJ, Koets AP: Two-way calf to dam major histocompatibility class I compatibility increases risk for retained placenta in cattle. *Am J Reprod Immunol* 2012, 67:224–230.

38. Cotton LA, Rahman MA, Ng C, Le AQ, Milloy MJ, Mo T, Brumme ZL: HLA class I sequence-based typing using DNA recovered from frozen plasma. *J Immunol Methods* 2012, 382:40–47.

39. Dankers MKA, Witvlied MD, Roelen DL, Lange de P, Korfage N, Persijn GG, Duquesnoy R, Doxiadis IIN, Claas FHJ: The number of amino acid triplet differences between patient and donor is predictive for the antibody reactivity against mismatched human leukocyte antigens. *Transplantation* 2004, 77:1236–1239.

40. Duquesnoy RJ, Askar M: HLAMatchmaker: a molecularly based algorithm for histocompatibility determination. V. Eplet matching for HLA-DR, HLA-DQ, and HLA-DP. *Hum Immunol* 2007, 68:12–25.

11

Natural and experimental hepatitis E virus genotype 3 - infection in European wild boar is transmissible to domestic pigs

Josephine Schlosser[1], Martin Eiden[1], Ariel Vina-Rodriguez[1], Christine Fast[1], Paul Dremsek[1], Elke Lange[2], Rainer G Ulrich[1] and Martin H Groschup[1*]

Abstract

Hepatitis E virus (HEV) is the causative agent of acute hepatitis E in humans in developing countries, but sporadic and autochthonous cases do also occur in industrialised countries. In Europe, food-borne zoonotic transmission of genotype 3 (gt3) has been associated with domestic pig and wild boar. However, little is known about the course of HEV infection in European wild boar and their role in HEV transmission to domestic pigs. To investigate the transmissibility and pathogenesis of wild boar-derived HEVgt3, we inoculated four wild boar and four miniature pigs intravenously. Using quantitative real-time RT-PCR viral RNA was detected in serum, faeces and in liver, spleen and lymph nodes. The antibody response evolved after fourteen days post inoculation. Histopathological findings included mild to moderate lymphoplasmacytic hepatitis which was more prominent in wild boar than in miniature pigs. By immunohistochemical methods, viral antigens were detected mainly in Kupffer cells and liver sinusoidal endothelial cells, partially associated with hepatic lesions, but also in spleen and lymph nodes. While clinical symptoms were subtle and gross pathology was inconspicuous, increased liver enzyme levels in serum indicated hepatocellular injury. As the faecal-oral route is supposed to be the most likely transmission route, we included four contact animals to prove horizontal transmission. Interestingly, HEVgt3-infection was also detected in wild boar and miniature pigs kept in contact to intravenously inoculated wild boar. Given the high virus loads and long duration of viral shedding, wild boar has to be considered as an important HEV reservoir and transmission host in Europe.

Introduction

Hepatitis E virus (HEV) is the causative agent of hepatitis E in humans and the sole member of the genus *Hepevirus* in the family *Hepeviridae*. It is a small, non-enveloped virus with a single-stranded RNA genome of positive polarity [1,2]. In many developing countries where sanitary conditions are suboptimal, hepatitis E is an important public health problem, with the virus being primarily transmitted via the fecal-oral route through contaminated food or water [3]. However, emerging cases of sporadic and autochthonous hepatitis E also occur in industrialised countries, including Japan and European countries [4-6]. HEV infections are known to

be responsible for acute hepatitis, however, HEV genotype 3 was recently also identified in Europe in severely immunocompromised patients as a new causative agent of chronic hepatitis [7,8]. Four genotypes (gt) of HEV (gt1 to gt4) infecting humans have been identified. Gt1 and gt2 are restricted to humans, and gt3 and gt4 are zoonotic with wild boar, domestic pig and deer representing reservoirs [9,10]. Although a consensus classification system for HEV genotypes is currently unavailable, HEV variants from Japanese wild boar (*Scrofa scrofa leucomystax*) have provisionally been classified into two novel genotypes (gt5 and gt6) [11]. The identification and characterization of additional HEV strains in chicken, rabbit, different rat species, and mongoose have significantly broadened the host range and diversity of HEV [12,13]. Recently, novel HEV-related viruses were identified in carnivores such as ferret [14] and fox [15], different bat species [16], moose

* Correspondence: Martin.Groschup@fli.bund.de
[1]Institute for Novel and Emerging Infectious Diseases, Friedrich-Loeffler-Institut, Südufer 10, 17493 Greifswald-Insel Riems, Germany
Full list of author information is available at the end of the article

[17] and cutthroat trout [18]. Cross-species transmission to non-human primates and pigs have been shown experimentally for gt3 and gt4 [19]. Severe human HEV infection after ingestion of uncooked liver from wild boar S. scrofa leucomystax) was reported in Japan, whereas food-borne zoonotic transmissions in Europe have been primarily associated with domestic pigs [4,20]. Furthermore, individuals with direct contact to pigs are at higher risk of HEV infection and as previously shown, forestry workers have a higher HEV seroprevalence rate compared to blood donors [21-23]. Recent studies in Asia and Europe revealed high HEV seroprevalences and molecular evidence for HEV infection in wild boar [24-31]. In Germany, wild boar is discussed as one of the main sources of human autochthonous infections [32,33]. Moreover, phylogenetic analyses of Japanese HEV isolates indicated former transmission events from domestic pig to wild boar [34].

Until now several studies in domestic pigs have been performed by intravenous or contact transmission of domestic pig-derived HEV [35-40], showing histopathological signs of a hepatitis but no clinical symptoms [37,41,42]. Conversely, little is known about the course of HEV infection in European wild boar and their role in HEV transmission to domestic pigs to date. Experimental challenge studies have not been carried out yet. Therefore, the aim of this study was to investigate the pathogenesis of a wild boar-derived HEV gt3 strain after experimental inoculation and to reveal possible horizontal transmissions to miniature pigs (S. scrofa domestica) and European wild boar (S. scrofa scrofa).

Materials and methods

Inoculum

The HEV gt3 strain used in this study originated from a liver sample of a naturally infected wild boar hunted in Northern Germany (Mecklenburg-Western Pomerania) in 2010. The liver was frozen immediately at −20 °C and stored at −70 °C. For preparation of the inoculum, the liver was ground in phosphate-buffered saline (PBS) with a mortar and pestle (10%, w/v). The suspension was transferred to a 15 mL tube and mixed for 1 min using a vortex mixer. After centrifugation (20 min at 4000 × g at 4 °C) the supernatant was transferred to a new tube and filtered (0.22 µm MILLEX®GP filter unit, Millipore, Ireland). The suspension was aliquoted in volumes of 2.5 mL and stored at −70 °C. The inoculum contained about 2×10^4 HEV RNA copies per µL RNA.

Experimental design

Seven sub-adult miniature pigs of three months age, three wild boar piglets of three months age and two adult wild boar of six month age were used in the experiment under biosafety level 3** conditions. Prior to the start of the experiment all animals were tested to be negative for anti-HEV antibodies in serum and HEV RNA in faeces, respectively. The wild boar piglets used in the study were obtained from a local farmer. Miniature pigs and adult wild boar were bred in the quarantine facilities at the Friedrich-Loeffler-Institut, Insel Riems, Germany. Following an initial clinical examination, including rectal body temperature, wild boar were allowed to accustom themselves to new surroundings for approximately 1–2 weeks prior to the initiation of experiments. The animals were fed with commercial pig feed and had access to water ad libitum. Two additional miniature pigs and one additional wild boar served as negative controls and were housed separately. Control animals remained negative for the whole experiment and were not considered further on in this manuscript. All animals were observed daily during the entire period of the experiment. In Group 1 and Group 2, four wild boar (wb93, wb95, wb10 and wb11) and four miniature pigs (mp30, mp37, mp39 and mp40) were inoculated intravenously via the vena cava cranialis with 2.0 mL liver suspension each. For the direct contact infection experiment (Group 3), one non-inoculated wild boar piglet (wb87) was kept together with the intravenously inoculated wild boar piglets (wb93 and wb95). For animal welfare reasons three miniature pigs (mp63, mp68 and mp79) were kept in an adjacent compartment. To facilitate an indirect transmission, excrements of intravenously inoculated wild boar (wb93 and wb95) were placed daily into stable of miniature pigs. Conveniently, time points of the experiment were designated as days post inoculation (dpi). An overview of the animal experiment is shown in Table 1.

Measurements of the body weight and rectal temperature as well as collection of blood and faecal samples were done at time points 0, 1, 3, 5, 8, 11, 14, 17, 21, 24, 27, 29 dpi in Group 2 and 0, 3, 7, 10, 14, 17, 21, 25, 28 dpi in Group 1 and 3. Fever was defined as a body temperature ≥40.0 °C for at least two consecutive days. Aliquots of serum samples were stored at −20 °C for antibody detection and clinical chemistry, and at −70 °C for RNA extraction. Faecal samples were diluted in isotonic saline solution (10%, w/v) and stored at −70 °C for RNA extraction. The experiment was finished after 29 dpi (Group 2) or after 28 dpi (Group 1 and 3). At necropsy, tissue samples (liver, liver lymph node, mesenteric and mandibular lymph nodes, gall bladder, small and large intestine, pancreas, kidney, spleen, tonsil, heart, brain, gonads, uterus or prostate, and quadriceps femoris muscle) were collected for virological, histopathological and immunohistochemical investigations. One part of each tissue sample was fixed immediately in 4% neutral buffered formalin for histological examination and the other part was stored at −70 °C for RNA extraction.

Table 1 Overview of the animal experiment

Group no.	Animal	Sex	Age (in months)	Clinical signs and blood chemistry*	Gross lesions	Liver histopathology	Viral antigens in liver by IHC Grading	Distribution
Group 1. Intravenous inoculation of wild boar	wb93**	♀	3	both with reduced feed intake, mild diarrhea, BA, ALT and γGT ↑	in all animals mild hyperplasia of liver lymph nodes and lymphoid tissue in large intestine	both with panlobular hepatocellular swelling, vacuolation and single cell necrosis of hepatocytes	+++	diffuse mainly in Kupffer cells and LSEC
	wb95	♀	3				++	
	wb10	♂	6	both with γGT ↑		both with multifocal lymphoplasmacytic infiltrates and hepatocellular degeneration (mainly centrilobular)	+++	mainly centrilobular in Kupffer cells associated with degenerated hepatocytes
	wb11	♀	6				+++	
Group 2. Intravenous inoculation of miniature pigs	mp30**	♀	3	γGT ↑ (not in mp30)	nematodes in gut and milk spots in liver (mp39)	multifocal lymphoplasmacytic infiltrates and single cell necrosis of hepatocytes (mp37 and mp39)	0	diffuse mainly in Kupffer cells and LSEC
	mp37	♀	3				+	
	mp39	♀	3				++	
	mp40	♀	3				0	
Group 3. Contact infection of wild boar and miniature pigs	wb87	♂	3	reduced feed intake, mild diarrhea, BA, ALT and γGT ↑	mild hyperplasia of liver and intestinal lymph nodes, altered liver consistency and milk spots, moderate splenomegaly	intralobular lymphohistiocytic infiltrates and single cell necrosis of hepatocytes	++	mainly centrilobular in Kupffer cells and LSEC
	mp63	♀	3	all with γGT ↑	mild hyperplasia of lymphoid tissue in large intestine, nematodes in gut and renal cyst (mp68)	all with mild lymphohistiocytic infiltrates within liver lobules	0	-
	mp68	♂	3				0	
	mp79	♀	3				0	

Tissues were taken on days 29 (Group 2) and 28 (Group 1, Group 3). Grades are formulated on a result of viral antigen density throughout a uniform tissue type. Sections were graded on two separate occasions, without referring to previous recorded results to help standardize the classification. Definition of immunolabelling grades as: 0 = no antigen staining seen, + = mild immunolabelling, ++ = moderate antigen staining, +++ = marked immunolabelling. LSEC = liver sinusoidal endothelial cells. *For details see Figure 1. **Sudden death at 1 dpi (after blood collection). ↑ = elevated biochemical parameter.

The experiments were approved by the competent authority of the Federal State of Mecklenburg-Western Pomerania, Germany, on the basis of national and European legislation, namely the EU council directive 86/609/EEC for the protection of animals used for experiments (LALLF M-V/TSD/7221.3-2.1.-014/10).

Clinical chemistry

Serum samples were analysed longitudinally by a spectrophotometric method in an automated analyzer (VetScan Chemistry Analyzer, Abaxis, Union City, USA) using special rotors (VetScan Mammalian Liver Profile reagent rotor, Abaxis) to provide quantitative determinations for alanine aminotransferase (ALT), albumin (ALB), alkaline phosphatase (ALP), bile acids (BA), total bilirubin (TBIL), total cholesterol (CHOL), gamma-glutamyl transferase (γGT) and blood urea nitrogen (BUN) in serum. For the evaluation of the results, upper reference value ranges for the tested biochemical parameters were calculated. Therefore, different serum samples of the negative control wild boar and miniature pigs were analysed (for each subspecies n =13).

Antibody and RNA detection

Sera were tested for the presence of total anti-HEV antibodies with a species independent HEV-Ab ELISA kit (Axiom, Bürstadt, Germany) according to the manufacturer's instructions. The ELISA uses recombinant HEV gt1 antigens for the detection of anti-HEV antibodies in serum or plasma. Values of the optical density at 450 nm (OD450) equal to or greater than 1 are prescribed as seropositive.

Manual extraction of viral RNA from all serum samples and faecal suspensions was performed using the QIAamp® Viral RNA Mini Kit (QIAGEN GmbH, Hilden, Germany) according to manufacturer's recommendations. From all tissue samples, viral RNA was extracted using the RNeasy Mini Kit (QIAGEN GmbH). For both extraction methods, an internal control RNA (IC2) was added as described previously [43]. HEV RNA was detected by a novel diagnostic quantitative real-time RT-PCR assay (RT-qPCR) using the CFX96™ Real-Time System (Bio-Rad Laboratories GmbH, München, Germany). All primer and probes used in this study are listed in Table 2. The RT-qPCR was performed using the Quanti-Tec Probe RT-PCR kit (QIAGEN GmbH) in 25 µL reaction volume with final concentrations of each primer with 0.8 µM, and of the probe with 0.1 µM. A volume of 5 µL RNA was added. Reverse transcription (RT) was carried out at 50 °C for 30 min, followed by denaturation/activation at 95 °C for 15 min. DNA was amplified immediately with 45 cycles at 95 °C (10 s), 55 °C (25 s) and 72 °C (25 s). The determination of the HEV copy number was carried out using a standard curve according to a synthetic

Table 2 Primers and probe used in this study

Region	Primers and probe	Position	Sequence	Product length
ORF 3	Forward primer1 (HEV.Fa)	5278-5294	GTGCCGGC GGTGGTTTC	81 bp
	Forward primer2 (HEV.Fb)	5278-5296	GTGCCGGCG GTGGTTTCTG	
	Reverse primer (HEV.R)	5340-5359	GCGAAGGGGT TGGTTGGATG	
	Probe (HEV.P)	5300-5320	FAM-TGACMG GGTTGATTCTC AGCC-BHQ1	

ORF = open reading frame.

external calibrator encompassing the 81 bp sequence of the RT-qPCR amplicon.

Histopathology and immunohistochemistry

For histopathological examinations formalin fixed tissue samples were stained with hematoxylin and eosin (HE) according to standard protocols. For immunohistochemistry (IHC) 3 µm sections were cut, deparaffinised and rehydrated. The pretreatment included a blocking step for the endogenous peroxidase using 3% H_2O_2/methanol for 30 min, followed by an antigen retrieval step in the microwave for 10 min at 600 W. A 1:200 diluted commercially available polyclonal rabbit anti-human CD3 antibody (Dako Deutschland GmbH, Hamburg, Germany), which is also binding to porcine CD3 antigen, was used to characterise the inflammatory response in the liver. Viral antigens were detected using a rabbit anti-HEV gt3 hyper-immune serum (rHEVgt3-HIS) in a 1:1000 dilution. For the production of this serum, a rabbit was immunised with an *Escherichia coli* expressed and purified His-tagged C-terminal segment of HEV gt3 capsid protein [21]. The slides were incubated with biotinylated goat anti-rabbit immunoglobulin (Vector Laboratories, LINARIS, Dossenheim, Germany) and an avidin/biotinylated enzyme complex (VECTASTAIN®ABC Reagent, Vector Laboratories, Burlingame, United States of America) followed by visualisation with 3,3-Diaminobenzidine (DAB, Sigma-Aldrich Chemie GmbH, Steinheim, Germany). The viral antigen density was graded as follows: 0 = no antigen staining seen; + = mild immunolabelling (<20% positive cells); ++ = moderate antigen staining (20 − 40% positive cells); +++ = marked immunolabelling (>40% positive cells). The sections were examined independently on two separate occasions.

Results

Experiments were carried out to determine i.) the pathogenesis of wild boar-derived HEV gt3 in wild boar and miniature pigs (Groups 1 and 2), and ii.) the horizontal transmissibility following such infections (Group 3).

i.) Intravenous inoculation of wild boar (Group 1) and miniature pigs (Group 2) with HEV gt3 of wild boar origin:

Clinical and biochemical parameters

Intravenously inoculated wild boar did not develop a significant rise in their body temperatures. Only wb93 and wb95 developed moderate clinical signs such as mild depression, slight diarrhea and mild anorexia, and displayed an increase in the BA and γGT serum levels. An elevated ALT level was only observed in wb93. Increase of γGT levels were observed in all intravenously infected wild boar after 21 dpi. Interestingly, ALT and γGT serum levels returned to normal in wb93 after day 25. None of the intravenously inoculated miniature pigs showed febrile temperatures or any other clinical signs, and none of these animals had altered BA serum levels. Increased γGT levels were observed in mp39 and mp40 at 29 dpi, whereas an elevation of the ALT level was only seen in mp39. An overview of the clinical signs is given in Table 1. Figure 1 depicts the time line of serum levels of BA, ALT and γGT. Other biochemical parameters remained within normal limits (data not shown).

Serology and HEV RNA detection

Two of the four intravenously inoculated wild boar (wb10 and wb11) seroconverted after 17 dpi, whereas the other two (wb93 and wb93) showed no seroconversion during the observation period (28 days). In the intravenously inoculated miniature pigs antibodies were detected first time in mp37 and mp40 at 14 dpi, whereas mp39 seroconverted thirteen days later. The serological results regarding HEV antibodies are shown in Figure 2A. HEV RNA with copy numbers exceeding 10 copies per µL RNA was found in the sera of two intravenously inoculated wild boar (wb93 at 17, 25, 28 dpi and wb95 at 21 dpi). Viral RNA was detectable in faeces of all wild boar within 3 to 5 dpi at levels of up to 10^5 copies per µL RNA (wb93, wb95 and wb11). In the two wild boar without seroconversion (wb93 and wb95), RNA copy numbers in faeces persisted until to the end of the experiment, albeit at slightly reduced levels. The two animals which seroconverted (wb10 and wb11) showed a marked reduction of faecal HEV shedding (< 10^1 copies per µL RNA) eventually. Viral RNAs were detected in liver, gall bladder, caecum, colon and spleen of all intravenously inoculated wild boar. In wb95 positive signals (>20 copies per µL RNA) were also found in brain, muscle and uterus. In general, comparable RNA copy numbers in serum and faeces were found in the miniature pigs. A marked decrease of faecal HEV shedding was also observed in two miniature pigs which seroconverted within 14 dpi (mp37 and mp40). In most of the intravenously infected miniature pigs viral RNAs were also detected in liver, gall bladder, caecum, colon and spleen. Already at 1 dpi, relatively high viral RNA copy numbers were found in the liver of mp30. The results of HEV RNA in serum and faeces are shown in Figure 2B. Table 3 summarises the viral loads of selected tissue samples. Additionally, HEV RNA was found in bile of wb93, wb95, wb11 and mp39.

Pathology

No gross pathological changes specific for viral hepatitis were seen in the livers of any of the pigs. However, macroscopic signs like mild to moderate follicular hyperplasia of lymphoid tissues in large intestine and mild hyperplasia of liver lymph nodes in intravenously inoculated wild boar were seen in some animals. Necropsy revealed also moderate intestinal nematode infestations and multifocal white spots ("milk spots") in the liver characteristic for chronic infection with Ascaris suum. Intralobular lesions of different sizes, patterns and frequencies associated with varying distribution of viral antigens were observed in the liver of intravenously inoculated pigs, but not in the negative control animals. Mild to moderate periportal lymphoplasmacytic infiltrates and Kupffer cell proliferations were also found in the liver of all intravenously inoculated pigs. However, no viral antigens were detected in periportal fields. By immunohistochemistry, viral antigens within hepatic lobules were found mainly in Kupffer cells and liver sinusoidal endothelial cells, and to a lesser extent in hepatocytes. Partially, hepatic lesions and infiltrates of CD3-positive cells were associated with viral antigens in Kupffer cells and liver sinusoidal endothelial cells. In detail, the liver of intravenously inoculated wild boar showed a more heterogeneous pattern in comparison to the miniature pigs. Two animals (wb93 and wb95) revealed a mild to moderate multifocal intralobular lymphohistiocytic infiltration with multifocal hepatocellular swelling and vacuolation, and a diffuse viral antigen distribution (Figure 3A-D). However, more severe liver lesions were observed in the two other intravenously inoculated wild boar (wb10 and wb11), with a pronounced mainly centrilobular hepatocellular degeneration associated with infiltrates of lymphocytes, plasma cells and Kupffer cells (Figure 3E and F). These lesions were clearly associated with a marked immunolabelling of viral antigens (Figure 3G and H). The liver of intravenously inoculated miniature pigs displayed diffuse mild intralobular lymphoplasmacytic infiltrations with single cell necrosis of hepatocytes and small to moderate amounts of diffusely distributed viral antigens (Figure 3I-L). In some animals, viral antigens were also found in the sub-capsular layer and follicles of distinct lymph nodes and in the germinal centre of lymphoid follicles in spleen (Figure 4A and B). In none of the other tested tissues viral antigens were found. An overview of gross lesions, histopathology and immunohistochemistry is given in Table 1. All IHC

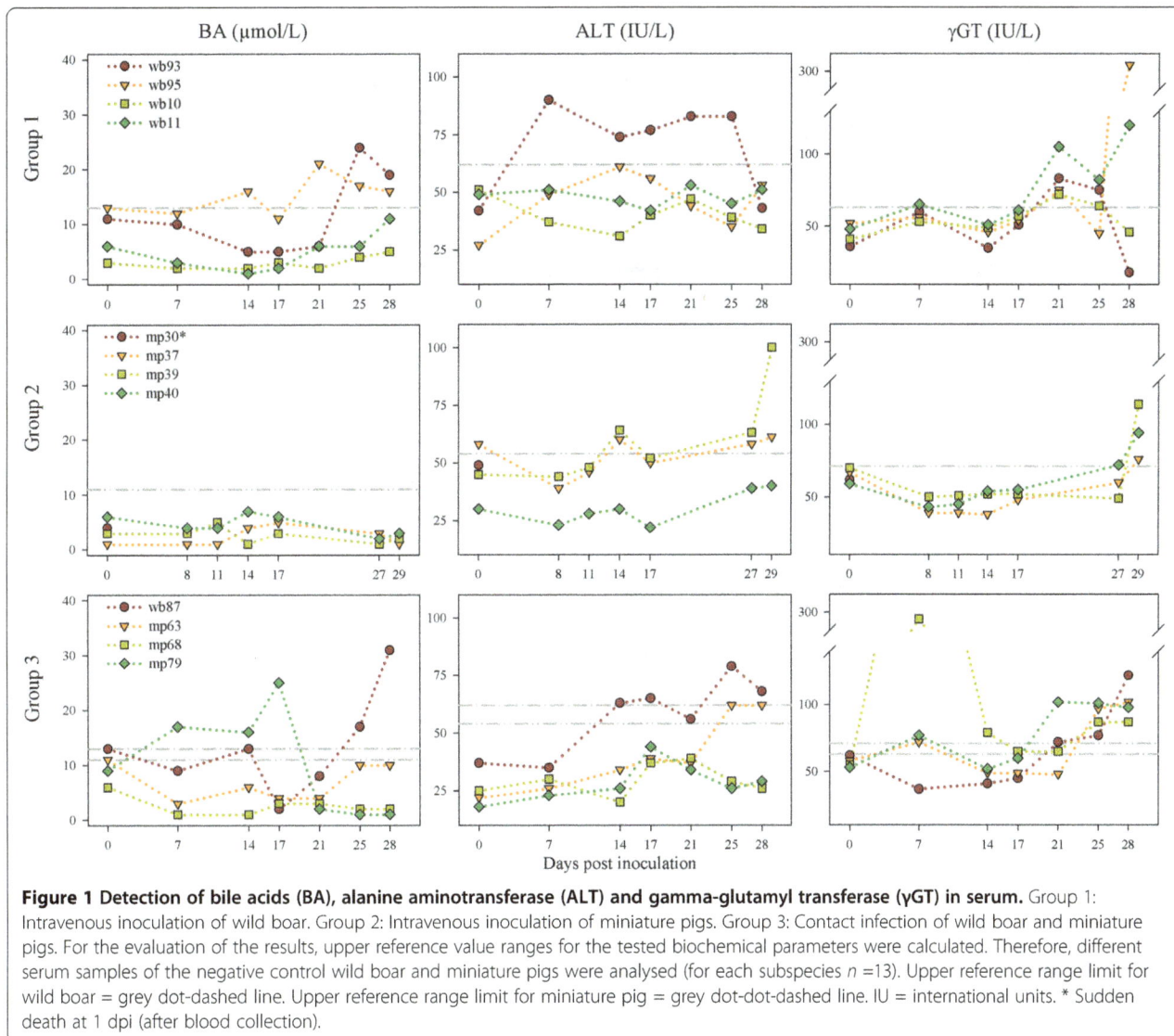

Figure 1 Detection of bile acids (BA), alanine aminotransferase (ALT) and gamma-glutamyl transferase (γGT) in serum. Group 1: Intravenous inoculation of wild boar. Group 2: Intravenous inoculation of miniature pigs. Group 3: Contact infection of wild boar and miniature pigs. For the evaluation of the results, upper reference value ranges for the tested biochemical parameters were calculated. Therefore, different serum samples of the negative control wild boar and miniature pigs were analysed (for each subspecies n =13). Upper reference range limit for wild boar = grey dot-dashed line. Upper reference range limit for miniature pig = grey dot-dot-dashed line. IU = international units. * Sudden death at 1 dpi (after blood collection).

results of viral antigen detection are summarised in the Additional file 1.

ii.) Transmission of HEV gt3 from intravenously inoculated wild boar to contact wild boar and miniature pigs (Group 3).

Clinical and biochemical parameters

None of the contact animals became pyrexic. Only wb87 showed moderate clinical signs characterized by mild depression, slight diarrhea and reduced feed intake in combination with elevated BA and ALT serum levels after 25 dpi. In the contact miniature pig mp79 a slight increase of BA in serum was also observed (7 to 17 dpi). All contact animals had increased γGT serum levels at different time points, most strikingly in mp68 at 7 dpi. An overview of the clinical signs is given in Table 1.

Figure 1 depicts the time lines of serum levels of BA, ALT and γGT. Other tested biochemical parameters remained within normal limits (data not shown).

Serology and HEV RNA detection

Two out of four contact pigs seroconverted during the observation period (wb87 at 25 dpi and mp63 at 28 dpi), while the other two contact animals (mp68 and mp79) developed no detectable HEV antibodies during this time. Serological results are shown in Figure 2A. Only wb87 was tested positive for viral RNA in serum with over 10 copies per µL RNA at 28 dpi. Viral RNA in faecal samples was detectable in all contact pigs with over 10 copies per µL RNA after 7 dpi in wb87, and after 10 to 17 dpi in the miniature pigs. The results of HEV RNA in serum and faeces are shown in Figure 2B. Viral RNA was detected in liver, gall bladder, small and large

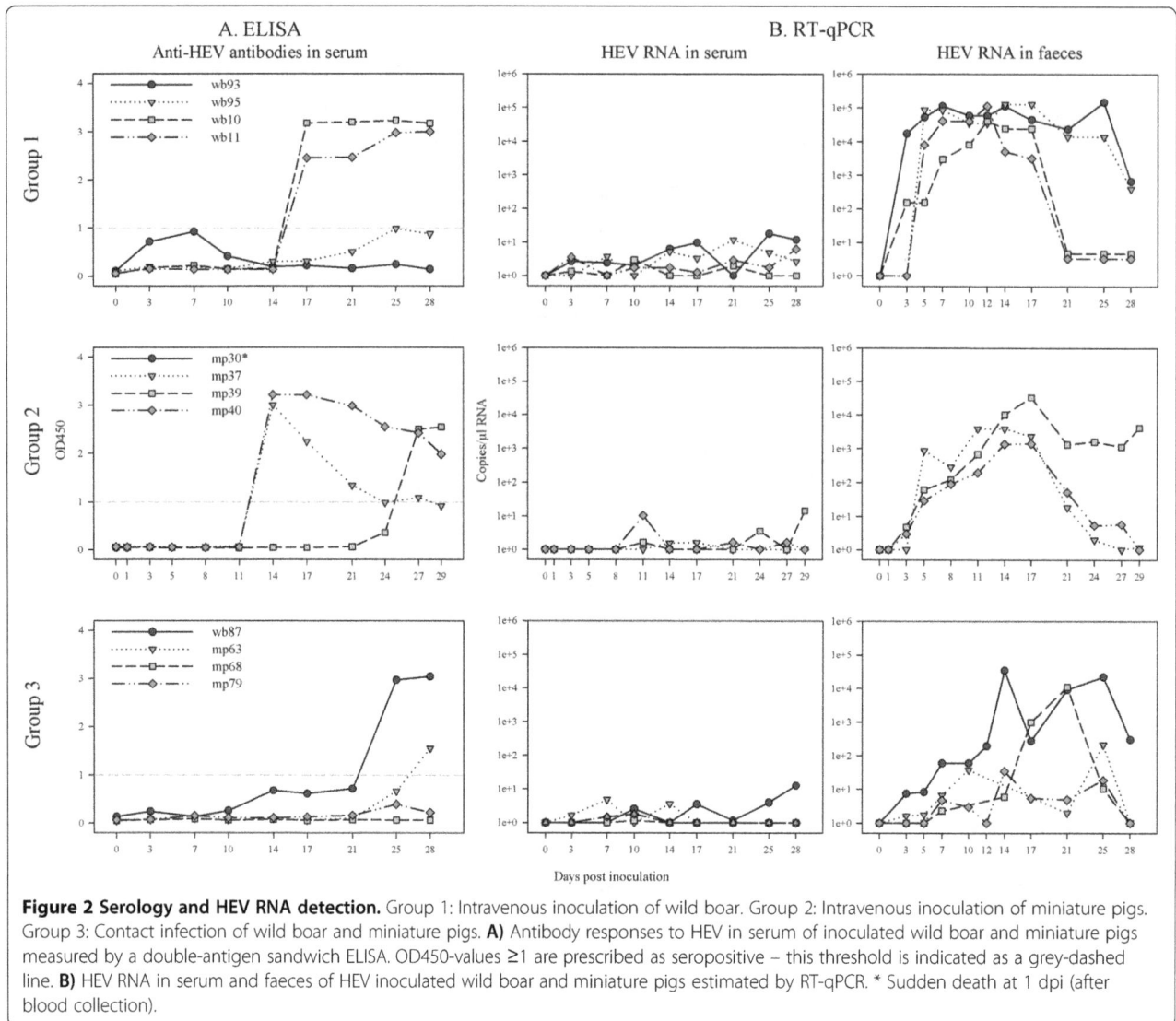

Figure 2 Serology and HEV RNA detection. Group 1: Intravenous inoculation of wild boar. Group 2: Intravenous inoculation of miniature pigs. Group 3: Contact infection of wild boar and miniature pigs. **A)** Antibody responses to HEV in serum of inoculated wild boar and miniature pigs measured by a double-antigen sandwich ELISA. OD450-values ≥1 are prescribed as seropositive – this threshold is indicated as a grey-dashed line. **B)** HEV RNA in serum and faeces of HEV inoculated wild boar and miniature pigs estimated by RT-qPCR. * Sudden death at 1 dpi (after blood collection).

intestine, and spleen of wb87. The livers of the contact miniature pigs were tested positive for HEV RNA as well, except for mp68. Compared to the contact miniature pigs, higher viral copy numbers were detectable in wb87. Table 3 summarises the viral loads of selected tissue samples. Viral RNA was also found in bile of mp163 and wb87.

Pathology

No gross pathological changes specific for viral hepatitis were seen in the livers of any of the contact animals, but a mild follicular hyperplasia of lymphoid tissues in intestine and of liver lymph nodes were frequently seen. Additionally, moderate splenomegaly was found in the infected contact wild boar. All contact animals showed a randomly distributed multifocal mild lymphohistiocytic infiltration in the liver associated with single cell necrosis (Figure 5A). However, viral antigens were only found in the liver of the

contact wild boar (Figure 5B). In the miniature pigs, viral antigens were demonstrated exclusively in the follicles of the mandibular lymph nodes. An overview of gross lesions, histopathology and immunohistochemistry is given in Table 1. All IHC results of viral antigen detection are summarised in the Additional file 1.

Discussion

To date, the food-borne zoonotic transmission of HEV gt3 in Europe is primarily associated with domestic pigs [4], while data on the pathogenicity of HEV in wild boar and their role in HEV transmission to domestic pigs are missing. HEV prevalence studies in hunted wild boar and serological studies in humans being in contact with them suggest zoonotic transmissions [21,22,27,29-31]. Several HEV transmission studies in domestic pigs were performed [35,36,38,40], but none involving wild boar. Therefore, the current study was carried out to elucidate

Table 3 Results of RT-qPCR analysis of selected tissue samples from wild boar (wb) and miniature pigs (mp)

Tissue	CT-value / copies/µL RNA	Goup 1. Intravenous inoculation of wb				Group 2. Intravenous inoculation of mp				Group 3. Contact infection of wb and mp			
		wb93	wb95	wb10	wb11	mp30*	mp37	mp39	mp40	wb87	mp63	mp68	mp79
Liver		20.7	22.6	24.1	24.6	28.1	32.3	24.3	No CT	23.0	24.2	No CT	35.3
		6521.0	*2259.6*	*952.4*	*685.8*	*94.6*	*8.4*	*834.2*		*1763.9*	*888.8*		*1.5*
Gall bladder		24.0	22.0	32.0	31.0	32.5	No CT	27.0	No CT	30.0	No CT	No CT	35.9
		991.5	*3137.8*	*9.9*	*17.6*	*7.3*		*175.1*		*31.3*			*1.0*
Duodenum		27.6	27.2	31.4	No CT	34.5	No CT	29.1	No CT	31.1	No CT	No CT	No CT
		124.0	*157.0*	*13.8*		*2.3*		*51.3*		*16.9*			
Jejunum		31.6	24.9	No CT	No CT	34.1	No CT	31.8	No CT	29.6	No CT	No CT	No CT
		12.3	*577.0*			*3.0*		*11.0*		*40.3*			
Ileum		33.3	30.0	34.4	No CT	35.4	No CT	33.8	No CT	29.9	No CT	No CT	No CT
		4.8	*31.7*	*2.6*		*1.4*		*3.5*		*33.1*			
Caecum		25.9	32.3	35.3	34.8	35.5	No CT	26.5	No CT	25.0	35.9	No CT	35.0
		337.7	*8.4*	*1.5*	*2.0*	*1.3*		*23.,9*		*557.4*	*1.0*		*1.8*
Colon		34.4	23.7	31.8	34.4	No CT	No CT	28.9	33.8	25.0	34.2	No CT	No CT
		2.6	*1171.8*	*10.8*	*2.4*			*60.7*	*3.6*	*557.4*	*2.7*		
Rectum		24.9	30.2	No CT	No CT	N. d.	No CT	32.6	No CT	33.0	No CT	No CT	No CT
		607.7	*28.2*					*7.2*		*5.5*			
Pancreas		No CT	34.7	No CT	No CT	N. d.	No CT	No CT	No CT	No CT	No CT	No CT	No CT
			2.1										
Mandibular LN		No CT	No CT	No CT	33.6	No CT	No CT	No CT	No CT	No CT	No CT	No CT	No CT
					3.9								
Kidney		34.7	33.2	No CT	No CT	No CT	No CT	31.7	No CT	No CT	No CT	No CT	No CT
		2.0	*5.0*					*11.6*					
Spleen		31.0	31.7	34.1	34.0	35.8	No CT	32.5	No CT	34.0	No CT	No CT	No CT
		17.6	*11.7*	*3.0*	*3.1*	*1.1*		*7.4*		*3.1*			
Heart		No CT	33.9	32.6	No CT	N. d.	No CT	No CT	No CT	34.6	No CT	No CT	No CT
			3.3	*6.9*						*2.2*			
Brain		32.3	28.9	No CT	No CT	N. d.	No CT	No CT	No CT	No CT	No CT	No CT	No CT
		8.2	*59.3*										
Muscle		No CT	30.7	No CT	No CT	No CT	No CT	No CT	No CT	No CT	No CT	No CT	No CT
			20.7										
Ovary/Testicle		No CT	30.9	No CT	No CT	N. d.	No CT	No CT	No CT	No CT	No CT	No CT	No CT
			19.1										
Uterus/Prostate		No CT	30.6	No CT	No CT	N. d.	No CT	35.0	No CT	No CT	No CT	No CT	No CT
			22.3					*1.8*					

Tissues were taken on days 29 (Group 2) and 28 (Group 1, Group 3). No CT ≥36.0 (= negative). Viral copy numbers in tissues were calculated from CT values determined by RT-qPCR. LN = lymph node. N. d. = not determined. *Sudden death at 1 dpi (after blood collection).

the transmission and pathogenesis of wild boar-derived HEV gt3 in European wild boar and in miniature pigs. Compared to common domesticated swine breeds, the miniature pig offers several breeding and handling advantages. Miniature pigs have been used extensively already in several fields of biomedical research [44], but HEV infection studies have never been carried out in this pig breed.

The experimental inoculation of wild boar and miniature pigs reveals an efficient HEV replication with substantial virus shedding. Following intravenous challenge of wild boar, HEV infection was successfully transmitted to contact animals. These contact animal infections resemble the natural course of the disease. Wild boar-derived HEV gt3 was detected in serum, faeces and different tissues of all intravenously inoculated pigs. Moreover,

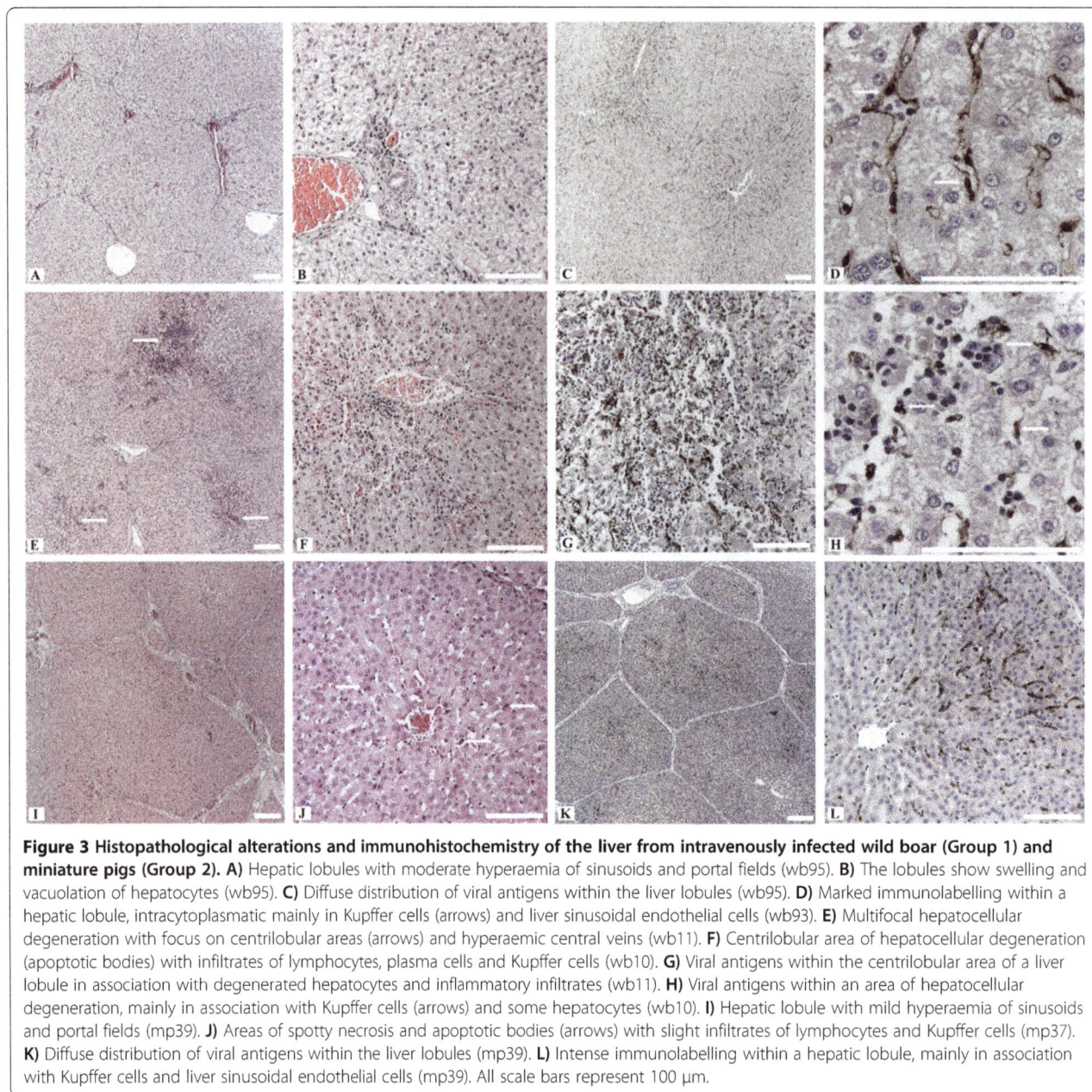

Figure 3 Histopathological alterations and immunohistochemistry of the liver from intravenously infected wild boar (Group 1) and miniature pigs (Group 2). **A)** Hepatic lobules with moderate hyperaemia of sinusoids and portal fields (wb95). **B)** The lobules show swelling and vacuolation of hepatocytes (wb95). **C)** Diffuse distribution of viral antigens within the liver lobules (wb95). **D)** Marked immunolabelling within a hepatic lobule, intracytoplasmatic mainly in Kupffer cells (arrows) and liver sinusoidal endothelial cells (wb93). **E)** Multifocal hepatocellular degeneration with focus on centrilobular areas (arrows) and hyperaemic central veins (wb11). **F)** Centrilobular area of hepatocellular degeneration (apoptotic bodies) with infiltrates of lymphocytes, plasma cells and Kupffer cells (wb10). **G)** Viral antigens within the centrilobular area of a liver lobule in association with degenerated hepatocytes and inflammatory infiltrates (wb11). **H)** Viral antigens within an area of hepatocellular degeneration, mainly in association with Kupffer cells (arrows) and some hepatocytes (wb10). **I)** Hepatic lobule with mild hyperaemia of sinusoids and portal fields (mp39). **J)** Areas of spotty necrosis and apoptotic bodies (arrows) with slight infiltrates of lymphocytes and Kupffer cells (mp37). **K)** Diffuse distribution of viral antigens within the liver lobules (mp39). **L)** Intense immunolabelling within a hepatic lobule, mainly in association with Kupffer cells and liver sinusoidal endothelial cells (mp39). All scale bars represent 100 µm.

an early virus replication in the liver was observed in one intravenously infected animal already at 1 dpi. Our findings confirm that the liver is the primary location of HEV replication. Extra-hepatic replication sites have been reported [45] and in this study, HEV RNA or viral antigens were also observed in liver, spleen and different lymph nodes. Interestingly, HEV RNA was detected in the brain of two out of four intravenously inoculated wild boar. Neurotropic HEV gt3 variants in humans are under discussion and HEV RNA was detected recently in the cerebrospinal fluid of patients with chronic HEV infection and neurological symptoms [46]. Of course a contamination of tissue specimens with HEV containing blood cannot be

excluded completely, but is rather unlikely as the viral loads of all collected serum samples were mostly below those detected in different tissue samples. The duration of faecal HEV shedding in most intravenously inoculated pigs was similar, but higher viral loads were found in faeces of wild boar. In intravenously inoculated animals anti-HEV antibodies were first time detected 14 dpi which is in line with results obtained in previous studies [37,47]. However, seroconversion between three and eight weeks post infection were more often reported [40,48]. The ELISA system used in this study detects all classes of antibodies to HEV in serum. Therefore, the rise of antibody titres observed in the current experiment cannot be associated with a single

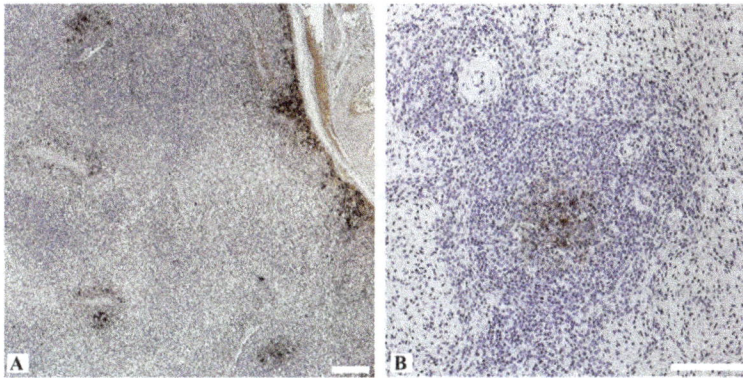

Figure 4 Immunohistochemistry of liver lymph node and spleen from intravenously HEV inoculated wild boar (Group 1). A) Viral antigens in the subcapsular layer and in the germinal centre of secondary follicles of a liver lymph node (wb93). **B)** Splenic immunolabelling of viral antigens in the germinal centre of a lymphoid follicle (wb11). All scale bars represent 100 µm.

Ig class. HEV total antibody levels might be also influenced by HEV-specific immunoglobulin (Ig) A in serum, as IgA can be detected in serum of patients with hepatitis E [49,50]. Moreover, a reduction of virus shedding in faeces was observed in the intravenously inoculated pigs which seroconverted after 14 to 17 dpi. Our findings support the hypothesis that adaptive immune responses are crucial to control HEV infection [51].

The faecal-oral transmission of HEV is considered to be the main transmission route among pigs [48]. Based on a study in non-human primates, the infectious dose of HEV required for oral infection is assumed to be higher than for intravenous infection [52]. In our study, the infectious dose of the contact animals remains unknown. It can be assumed that the contact wild boar might have had a higher exposure to HEV because of their direct and permanent contact to excreta of the infected animals than the miniature pigs which were only exposed to collected faeces. As HEV RNA was detected in urine of experimentally infected domestic pigs [35],

HEV might be also transmitted via urine. The reason for the lacking antibody response in two contact miniature pigs, despite elevated enzyme levels and viral shedding via faeces, remains unclear. Most probably the duration of the experiment was not long enough or the HEV infection was not systemic, as described before [39]. In a previous study it could be demonstrated that domestic pigs could be infected orally, nevertheless, not each contact pig was infected and the antibody response was less efficient as compared to the intravenous inoculation route [45].

In former studies only subclinical HEV infections have been described in domestic pigs [35-37]. In the present study a clinical course of HEV infection in pigs could be proven, based on elevated γGT-levels in serum. Increased γGT-levels have also been reported for experimentally HEV-infected non-human primates [53], but not described for pigs before. Moreover, increased ALT and BA serum levels were also observed, especially in wild boar and to a lesser extent in miniature pigs. In the

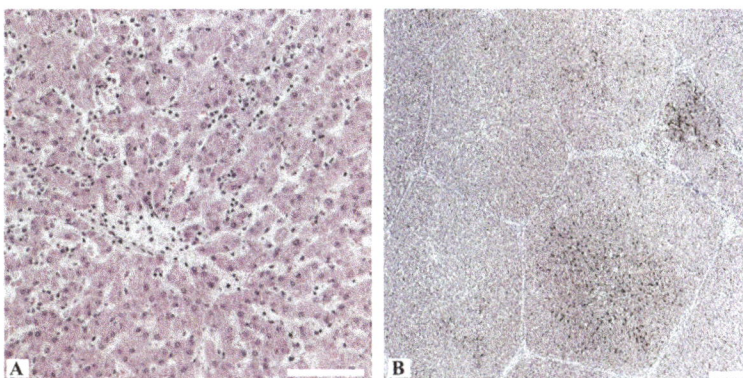

Figure 5 Histopathological alterations and immunohistochemistry of the liver from the contact wild boar (Group 3). A) Intralobular area with inflammatory infiltrates mostly lymphocytes and histiocytes. **B)** Multifocal distribution of viral antigens especially in centrilobular areas (arrows). All scale bars represent 100 µm.

infected wild boar piglets the moderate clinical signs were concomitant with increasing serum levels of BA and liver enzymes. Obviously these results support laboratory findings in humans with HEV infection which are similar to other forms of viral hepatitis and characterised also by elevated serum levels of ALT and γGT [54] due to marked hepatic necrosis and cellular exhaustion of enzymes [55]. Also elevated levels of BA in serum are found in viral hepatitis in humans [56]. The inter-individual variations in these parameters may have resulted from factors such as age, sex, physical condition and unrelated co-infections.

Swelling of hepatocytes with vacuolation of the cytoplasm was seen in acute liver injury of domestic pigs as a result of the HEV infection as described before [35]. Non-lipid hepatocellular vacuolation is attributed to alterations in the injured cell as a result of hydropic change, but may also reflect a beneficial cellular adaptation rather than degenerative change [51]. Especially in wild boar mild to moderate intralobular lymphoplasmacytic or lymphohistiocytic infiltrates with variable degree of hepatocellular degeneration were found histopathologically. In previous studies microscopic liver lesions with multifocal lymphoplasmacytic viral hepatitis were observed in both experimentally [35,37] and naturally [42] HEV infected domestic pigs. Our histopathological findings for hepatic lesions in the miniature pigs were comparable, but varied for wild boar ranging from diffuse moderate lesions with swelling, vacuolation and single cell necrosis of hepatocytes and multifocal moderate to severe hepatocellular degenerations.

Only few immunohistochemical studies on HEV infected animals and humans have been published before [57-60]. HEV has been shown to replicate in hepatocytes and in extra-hepatic tissues such as small intestine, colon, spleen, bile duct and lymph nodes [45,61]. By immunohistochemistry, we were able to detect viral antigens mainly in Kupffer cells and liver sinusoidal endothelial cells, partially associated with hepatic lesions and infiltrates of CD3-positive cells. Since Kupffer cells and liver sinusoidal endothelial cells have antigen presenting functions [62], they may also play a role in the host defense mechanisms and immunopathogenesis. Anyhow, a virus proliferation in these cells is possible, if not essential. Lymphatic tissue might also represent extra-hepatic HEV replication sites, as viral antigens were found in spleen, hepatic and mandibular lymph nodes. Interestingly, no viral antigens were detected by immunohistochemistry in intestine as described in a previous HEV infection study in gerbils [63].

Host cell injury in a viral infection may be mediated by either a direct effect of the infectious agent or indirectly through the antiviral host response, or a combination of both. In this study, different patterns in the immunohistochemical detection of HEV antigens and varying lesions were seen in the liver. HEV antigens were either diffusely distributed without association to liver lesions or associated with hepatocellular degeneration, especially in centrilobular areas. As HEV itself appears to be non-cytopathic [64], an immunopathogenesis is assumed for hepatitis E in humans [65]. Previous immunohistochemical studies in liver biopsies of patients with acute hepatitis E revealed that lymphocyte infiltrates consisted mainly of CD3-positive T cells containing a predominantly cytotoxic CD8-positive cell subpopulation which probably is playing an important role in HEV-induced liver injury [66]. Interestingly, CD3-positive T cell infiltrations within liver lesions were also observed in this study. The consistent coincidence of infiltrates of lymphocytes, plasma cells and histiocytes with hepatocellular degenerations and viral antigens supports the assumption that liver damage in pigs might also be immune-mediated.

Two different patterns within the course of HEV infection were observed: Animals with early anti-HEV seroconversion are able to clear the virus, while animals with lacking antibody responses suffered from prolonged HEV persistence until the end of the investigation period. Perhaps a weak cytotoxic response in pigs leads to viral persistence, yet without obvious liver damage, whereas a sufficient immune response may lead to an effective HEV clearance that is accompanied by a variable degree of hepatic damage, however. In humans the course of HEV infection can vary substantially between different individuals and chronic hepatitis E cases have been described in immunosuppressed patients [65]. Recent studies in humans were able to associate the activation of the interferon system and viral evolution with severity or chronicity of hepatitis E [37]. Studies in humans also revealed that chronic hepatitis E might be associated with impaired HEV-specific T-cell responses and enhancing adaptive cellular immunity against HEV might prevent persistent HEV infections [36]. In swine factors like virus titer, ratio of infectious to defective particles, route of infection and host factors like the immune status, age of exposure and the presence of co-infections have been discussed to modulate the clinical outcome of HEV infection [27,28]. In the study presented here, some of the experimental animals were carrying also nematodes and showed mild gastrointestinal symptoms possibly caused by other infectious agents affecting swine, but also by stress or a modified feeding regime. Wild boar piglets used in this study were obtained from a local farmer, therefore pre-existing infections with other pathogens cannot be excluded. Liver homogenates given to the experimental animals were sterile filtered to prevent parasitic and bacterial superinfections. Moreover, clinical and pathological examinations showed no indication of other infections. However, future studies should clarify the impact of co-infections on the HEV pathogenesis. Moreover, the pathomechanisms for the development of persistent HEV infections in pigs should be further assessed as this may provide an animal model for the chronic hepatitis E infection in humans.

Taken together, our data underline the importance of wild boar as reservoir host and for transmission of HEV gt3 to domestic swine and reveal Kupffer cells, liver sinusoidal endothelial cells and extra-hepatic lymphatic cells as potential virus replication sites. Since large amounts of virus particles are excreted in faeces of wild boar, droppings can contaminate the environment and pose a particular risk to susceptible species. Actually, in most industrialised countries the HEV infected population of domestic swine is far larger than those of the wild boar. Accordingly, wild boar and other wildlife also can be at infection risk by using pig manure as fertilizer on agricultural land.

Additional file

> **Additional file 1: HEV-antigen detection within post mortem tissues of wild boar (wb) and miniature pigs (mp) assessed by immunohistochemistry.** All results of viral antigen detection in examined tissues were summarised in this overview. The viral antigen density was graded as follows: 0 = no antigen staining seen; + = mild immunolabelling (<20% positive cells); ++ = moderate antigen staining (20 – 40% positive cells); +++ = marked immunolabelling (>40% positive cells). The sections were examined independently on two separate occasions.

Competing interests
The authors declare that they have no competing interests.

Authors' contributions
Conceived and designed the experiments: JS, ME, MHG. Performed the experiments and necropsy: JS, EL, CF. Analyzed the data: JS, ME, AV, CF, MHG. Contributed to reagents/materials/analysis tools: JS, ME, AV, CF, PD, RGU, MHG. Wrote the paper: JS, ME, MHG. All authors read and approved the final manuscript.

Acknowledgements
We thank Birke Boettcher and Gina Lucht for excellent technical assistance. This study was partly funded by the EU commission (project NADIR).

Author details
[1]Institute for Novel and Emerging Infectious Diseases, Friedrich-Loeffler-Institut, Südufer 10, 17493 Greifswald-Insel Riems, Germany. [2]Department of Experimental Animal Facilities and Biorisk Management, Friedrich-Loeffler-Institut, Südufer 10, 17493 Greifswald-Insel Riems, Germany.

References
1. Tam AW, Smith MM, Guerra ME, Huang CC, Bradley DW, Fry KE, Reyes GR: **Hepatitis E virus (HEV): molecular cloning and sequencing of the full-length viral genome.** *Virology* 1991, **185**:120–131.
2. Emerson SU, Purcell RH: **Hepatitis E virus.** *Rev Med Virol* 2003, **13**:145–154.
3. Emerson SU, Purcell RH: **Hepatitis E virus.** In *Fields Virology*, Volume 2. 2nd edition. Philadelphia: Wolters Kluwer Health/Lippincott Williams and Wilkins; 2013:2242–2258.
4. Colson P, Borentain P, Queyriaux B, Kaba M, Moal V, Gallian P, Heyries L, Raoult D, Gerolami R: **Pig liver sausage as a source of hepatitis E virus transmission to humans.** *J Infect Dis* 2010, **202**:825–834.
5. Tei S, Kitajima N, Takahashi K, Mishiro S: **Zoonotic transmission of hepatitis E virus from deer to human beings.** *Lancet* 2003, **362**:371–373.
6. Yazaki Y, Mizuo H, Takahashi M, Nishizawa T, Sasaki N, Gotanda Y, Okamoto H: **Sporadic acute or fulminant hepatitis E in Hokkaido, Japan, may be food-borne, as suggested by the presence of hepatitis E virus in pig liver as food.** *J Gen Virol* 2003, **84**:2351–2357.
7. Kamar N, Selves J, Mansuy JM, Ouezzani L, Peron JM, Guitard J, Cointault O, Esposito L, Abravanel F, Danjoux M, Durand D, Vinel JP, Izopet J, Rostaing L: **Hepatitis E virus and chronic hepatitis in organ-transplant recipients.** *New Engl J Med* 2008, **358**:811–817.
8. Gerolami R, Moal V, Colson P: **Chronic hepatitis E with cirrhosis in a kidney-transplant recipient.** *New Engl J Med* 2008, **358**:859–860.
9. Lu L, Li C, Hagedorn C: **Phylogenetic analysis of global hepatitis E virus sequences: genetic diversity, subtypes and zoonosis.** *Rev Med Virol* 2006, **16**:5–36.
10. Okamoto H: **Genetic variability and evolution of hepatitis E virus.** *Virus Res* 2007, **127**:216–228.
11. Takahashi M, Nishizawa T, Nagashima S, Jirintai S, Kawakami M, Sonoda Y, Suzuki T, Yamamoto S, Shigemoto K, Ashida K, Sato Y, Okamoto H: **Molecular characterization of a novel hepatitis E virus (HEV) strain obtained from a wild boar in Japan that is highly divergent from the previously recognized HEV strains.** *Virus Res* 2014, **180**:59–69.
12. Meng XJ: **From barnyard to food table: the omnipresence of hepatitis E virus and risk for zoonotic infection and food safety.** *Virus Res* 2011, **161**:23–30.
13. Johne R, Plenge-Bonig A, Hess M, Ulrich RG, Reetz J, Schielke A: **Detection of a novel hepatitis E-like virus in faeces of wild rats using a nested broad-spectrum RT-PCR.** *J Gen Virol* 2010, **91**:750–758.
14. Raj VS, Smits SL, Pas SD, Provacia LB, Moorman-Roest H, Osterhaus AD, Haagmans BL: **Novel hepatitis E virus in ferrets, the Netherlands.** *Emerg Infect Dis* 2012, **18**:1369–1370.
15. Bodewes R, van der Giessen J, Haagmans BL, Osterhaus AD, Smits SL: **Identification of multiple novel viruses, including a parvovirus and a hepevirus, in feces of red foxes.** *J Virol* 2013, **87**:7758–7764.
16. Drexler JF, Seelen A, Corman VM, Fumie Tateno A, Cottontail V, Melim Zerbinati R, Gloza-Rausch F, Klose SM, Adu-Sarkodie Y, Oppong SK, Kalko EK, Osterman A, Rasche A, Adam A, Muller MA, Ulrich RG, Leroy EM, Lukashev AN, Drosten C: **Bats worldwide carry hepatitis E virus-related viruses that form a putative novel genus within the family Hepeviridae.** *J Virol* 2012, **86**:9134–9147.
17. Lin J, Norder H, Uhlhorn H, Belák S, Widén F: **Novel hepatitis E like virus found in Swedish moose.** *J Gen Virol* 2014, **95**:557–570.
18. Batts W, Yun S, Hedrick R, Winton J: **A novel member of the family Hepeviridae from cutthroat trout (Oncorhynchus clarkii).** *Virus Res* 2011, **158**:116–123.
19. Pavio N, Meng XJ, Renou C: **Zoonotic hepatitis E: animal reservoirs and emerging risks.** *Vet Res* 2010, **41**:46.
20. Matsuda H, Okada K, Takahashi K, Mishiro S: **Severe hepatitis E virus infection after ingestion of uncooked liver from a wild boar.** *J Infect Dis* 2003, **188**:944.
21. Dremsek P, Wenzel J, Johne R, Ziller M, Hofmann J, Groschup M, Werdermann S, Mohn U, Dorn S, Motz M, Mertens M, Jilg W, Ulrich R: **Seroprevalence study in forestry workers from eastern Germany using novel genotype 3- and rat hepatitis E virus-specific immunoglobulin G ELISAs.** *Med Microbiol Immunol* 2012, **201**:189–200.
22. Chaussade H, Rigaud E, Allix A, Carpentier A, Touzé A, Delzescaux D, Choutet P, Garcia-Bonnet N, Coursaget P: **Hepatitis E virus seroprevalence and risk factors for individuals in working contact with animals.** *J Clin Virol* 2013, **58**:504–508.
23. Krumbholz A, Mohn U, Lange J, Motz M, Wenzel JJ, Jilg W, Walther M, Straube E, Wutzler P, Zell R: **Prevalence of hepatitis E virus-specific antibodies in humans with occupational exposure to pigs.** *Med Microbiol Immunol* 2012, **201**:239–244.
24. Hara Y, Terada Y, Yonemitsu K, Shimoda H, Noguchi K, Suzuki K, Maeda K: **High prevalence of hepatitis E virus in wild boar (Sus scrofa) in Yamaguchi Prefecture, Japan.** *J Wildl Dis* 2014, **50**:378–383.
25. Martinelli N, Pavoni E, Filogari D, Ferrari N, Chiari M, Canelli E, Lombardi G: **Hepatitis E virus in wild boar in the Central Northern part of Italy.** *Transbound Emerg Dis* in press.
26. Denzin N, Borgwardt J: **Occurrence and geographical distribution of antibodies to hepatitis E virus in wild boars of Saxony-Anhalt, Germany (2011).** *Berl Munch Tierarztl Wochenschr* 2013, **126**:230–235 (in German).
27. Carpentier A, Chaussade H, Rigaud E, Rodriguez J, Berthault C, Boue F, Tognon M, Touze A, Garcia-Bonnet N, Choutet P, Coursaget P: **High hepatitis E virus seroprevalence in forestry workers and in wild boars in France.** *J Clin Microbiol* 2012, **50**:2888–2893.
28. Boadella M, Ruiz-Fons JF, Vicente J, Martin M, Segales J, Gortazar C: **Seroprevalence evolution of selected pathogens in Iberian wild boar.** *Transbound Emerg Dis* 2012, **59**:395–404.

29. Rutjes SA, Lodder-Verschoor F, Lodder WJ, van der Giessen J, Reesink H, Bouwknegt M, de Roda Husman AM: **Seroprevalence and molecular detection of hepatitis E virus in wild boar and red deer in The Netherlands.** *J Virol Methods* 2010, **168**:197–206.

30. Adlhoch C, Wolf A, Meisel H, Kaiser M, Ellerbrok H, Pauli G: **High HEV presence in four different wild boar populations in East and West Germany.** *Vet Microbiol* 2009, **139**:270–278.

31. Kaba M, Davoust B, Marié J-L, Colson P: **Detection of hepatitis E virus in wild boar (Sus scrofa) livers.** *Vet J* 2010, **186**:259–261.

32. Wichmann O, Schimanski S, Koch J, Kohler M, Rothe C, Plentz A, Jilg W, Stark K: **Phylogenetic and case-control study on hepatitis E virus infection in Germany.** *J Infect Dis* 2008, **198**:1732–1741.

33. Schielke A, Sachs K, Lierz M, Appel B, Jansen A, Johne R: **Detection of hepatitis E virus in wild boars of rural and urban regions in Germany and whole genome characterization of an endemic strain.** *Virol J* 2009, **6**:58.

34. Nakano T, Takahashi K, Arai M, Okano H, Kato H, Ayada M, Okamoto H, Mishiro S: **Identification of European-type hepatitis E virus subtype 3e isolates in Japanese wild boars: molecular tracing of HEV from swine to wild boars.** *Infect Genet Evol* 2013, **18**:287–298.

35. Bouwknegt M, Rutjes S, Reusken C, Stockhofe-Zurwieden N, Frankena K, de Jong M, de Roda Husman AM, van der Poel W: **The course of hepatitis E virus infection in pigs after contact-infection and intravenous inoculation.** *BMC Vet Res* 2009, **5**:7.

36. Casas M, Pina S, de Deus N, Peralta B, Martín M, Segalés J: **Pigs orally inoculated with swine hepatitis E virus are able to infect contact sentinels.** *Vet Microbiol* 2009, **138**:78–84.

37. Halbur P, Kasorndorkbua C, Gilbert C, Guenette D, Potters M, Purcell R, Emerson S, Toth T, Meng X: **Comparative pathogenesis of infection of pigs with hepatitis E viruses recovered from a pig and a human.** *J Clin Microbiol* 2001, **39**:918–923.

38. Kasorndorkbua C, Thacker B, Halbur P, Guenette D, Buitenwerf R, Royer R, Meng X: **Experimental infection of pregnant gilts with swine hepatitis E virus.** *Can J Vet Res* 2003, **67**:303–306.

39. Kasorndorkbua C, Guenette DK, Huang FF, Thomas PJ, Meng XJ, Halbur PG: **Routes of transmission of swine hepatitis E virus in pigs.** *J Clin Microbiol* 2004, **42**:5047–5052.

40. Meng X, Halbur P, Haynes J, Tsareva T, Bruna J, Royer R, Purcell R, Emerson S: **Experimental infection of pigs with the newly identified swine hepatitis E virus (swine HEV), but not with human strains of HEV.** *Arch Virol* 1998, **143**:1405–1415.

41. Martin M, Segales J, Huang F, Guenette D, Mateu E, de Deus N, Meng X: **Association of hepatitis E virus (HEV) and postweaning multisystemic wasting syndrome (PMWS) with lesions of hepatitis in pigs.** *Vet Microbiol* 2007, **122**:16–24.

42. Meng XJ, Purcell RH, Halbur PG, Lehman JR, Webb DM, Tsareva TS, Haynes JS, Thacker BJ, Emerson SU: **A novel virus in swine is closely related to the human hepatitis E virus.** *Proc Natl Acad Sci U S A* 1997, **94**:9860–9865.

43. Hoffmann B, Depner K, Schirrmeier H, Beer M: **A universal heterologous internal control system for duplex real-time RT-PCR assays used in a detection system for pestiviruses.** *J Virol Methods* 2006, **136**:200–209.

44. Vodicka P, Smetana K Jr, Dvorankova B, Emerick T, Xu YZ, Ourednik J, Ourednik V, Motlik J: **The miniature pig as an animal model in biomedical research.** *Ann N Y Acad Sci* 2005, **1049**:161–171.

45. Williams TP, Kasorndorkbua C, Halbur PG, Haqshenas G, Guenette DK, Toth TE, Meng XJ: **Evidence of extrahepatic sites of replication of the hepatitis E virus in a swine model.** *J Clin Microbiol* 2001, **39**:3040–3046.

46. Kamar N, Bendall RP, Peron JM, Cintas P, Prudhomme L, Mansuy JM, Rostaing L, Keane F, Ijaz S, Izopet J, Dalton HR: **Hepatitis E virus and neurologic disorders.** *Emerg Infect Dis* 2011, **17**:173–179.

47. Meng XJ, Halbur PG, Shapiro MS, Govindarajan S, Bruna JD, Mushahwar IK, Purcell RH, Emerson SU: **Genetic and experimental evidence for cross-species infection by swine hepatitis E virus.** *J Virol* 1998, **72**:9714–9721.

48. Kasorndorkbua C, Halbur PG, Thomas PJ, Guenette DK, Toth TE, Meng XJ: **Use of a swine bioassay and a RT-PCR assay to assess the risk of transmission of swine hepatitis E virus in pigs.** *J Virol Methods* 2002, **101**:71–78.

49. Tian DY, Chen Y, Xia NS: **Significance of serum IgA in patients with acute hepatitis E virus infection.** *World J Gastroenterol* 2006, **12**:3919–3923.

50. Osterman A, Vizoso-Pinto MG, Jung J, Jaeger G, Eberle J, Nitschko H, Baiker A: **A novel indirect immunofluorescence test for the detection of IgG and IgA antibodies for diagnosis of Hepatitis E Virus infections.** *J Virol Methods* 2013, **191**:48–54.

51. Suneetha PV, Pischke S, Schlaphoff V, Grabowski J, Fytili P, Gronert A, Bremer B, Markova A, Jaroszewicz J, Bara C, Manns MP, Cornberg M, Wedemeyer H: **Hepatitis E virus (HEV)-specific T-cell responses are associated with control of HEV infection.** *Hepatology* 2012, **55**:695–708.

52. Tsarev SA, Tsareva TS, Emerson SU, Yarbough PO, Legters LJ, Moskal T, Purcell RH: **Infectivity titration of a prototype strain of hepatitis E virus in cynomolgus monkeys.** *J Med Virol* 1994, **43**:135–142.

53. Aggarwal R, Kamili S, Spelbring J, Krawczynski K: **Experimental studies on subclinical hepatitis E virus infection in cynomolgus macaques.** *J Infect Dis* 2001, **184**:1380–1385.

54. Kumar Acharya S, Kumar Sharma P, Singh R, Kumar Mohanty S, Madan K, Kumar Jha J, Kumar Panda S: **Hepatitis E virus (HEV) infection in patients with cirrhosis is associated with rapid decompensation and death.** *J Hepatol* 2007, **46**:387–394.

55. Wolf P: **Biochemical diagnosis of liver disease.** *Indian J Clin Biochem* 1999, **14**:59–90.

56. Pennington CR, Ross PE, Bouchier IAD: **Serum bile acids in patients with viral hepatitis.** *Scand J Gastroenterol* 1978, **13**:77–80.

57. Gupta P, Jagya N, Pabhu SB, Durgapal H, Acharya SK, Panda SK: **Immunohistochemistry for the diagnosis of hepatitis E virus infection.** *J Viral Hepat* 2012, **19**:e177–e183.

58. da Costa Lana MV, Gardinali NR, da Cruz RA, Lopes LL, Silva GS, Caramori Júnior JG, de Oliveira AC, de Almeida SM, Colodel EM, Alfieri AA, Pescador CA: **Evaluation of hepatitis E virus infection between different production systems of pigs in Brazil.** *Trop Anim Health Prod* 2014, **46**:399–404.

59. Lee YH, Ha Y, Ahn KK, Cho KD, Lee BH, Kim SH, Chae C: **Comparison of a new synthetic, peptide-derived, polyclonal antibody-based, immunohistochemical test with in situ hybridisation for the detection of swine hepatitis E virus in formalin-fixed, paraffin-embedded tissues.** *Vet J* 2009, **182**:131–135.

60. Ha SK, Chae C: **Immunohistochemistry for the detection of swine hepatitis E virus in the liver.** *J Viral Hepat* 2004, **11**:263–267.

61. Choi C, Chae C: **Localization of swine hepatitis E virus in liver and extrahepatic tissues from naturally infected pigs by in situ hybridization.** *J Hepatol* 2003, **38**:827–832.

62. Crispe IN: **Liver antigen-presenting cells.** *J Hepatol* 2011, **54**:357–365.

63. Li W, Sun Q, She R, Wang D, Duan X, Yin J, Ding Y: **Experimental infection of Mongolian gerbils by a genotype 4 strain of swine hepatitis E virus.** *J Med Virol* 2009, **81**:1591–1596.

64. Aggarwal R, Jameel S: **Hepatitis E.** *Hepatology* 2011, **54**:2218–2226.

65. Wedemeyer H, Rybczynska J, Pischke S, Krawczynski K: **Immunopathogenesis of hepatitis E virus infection.** *Semin Liver Dis* 2013, **33**:71–78.

66. Agrawal V, Goel A, Rawat A, Naik S, Aggarwal R: **Histological and immunohistochemical features in fatal acute fulminant hepatitis E.** *Indian J Pathol Microbiol* 2012, **55**:22–27.

12

Efficient strategy for constructing duck enteritis virus-based live attenuated vaccine against homologous and heterologous H5N1 avian influenza virus and duck enteritis virus infection

Zhong Zou[1,2†], Yong Hu[1,3†], Zhigang Liu[1,2,4], Wei Zhong[1,2], Hangzhou Cao[1,2], Huanchun Chen[1,2] and Meilin Jin[1,2*]

Abstract

Duck is susceptible to many pathogens, such as duck hepatitis virus, duck enteritis virus (DEV), duck tembusu virus, H5N1 highly pathogenic avian influenza virus (HPAIV) in particular. With the significant role of duck in the evolution of H5N1 HPAIV, control and eradication of H5N1 HPAIV in duck through vaccine immunization is considered an effective method in minimizing the threat of a pandemic outbreak. Consequently, a practical strategy to construct a vaccine against these pathogens should be determined. In this study, the DEV was examined as a candidate vaccine vector to deliver the hemagglutinin (HA) gene of H5N1, and its potential as a polyvalent vaccine was evaluated. A modified mini-F vector was inserted into the gB and UL26 gene junction of the attenuated DEV vaccine strain C-KCE genome to generate an infectious bacterial artificial chromosome (BAC) of C-KCE (vBAC-C-KCE). The HA gene of A/duck/Hubei/xn/2007 (H5N1) was inserted into the C-KCE genome via the mating-assisted genetically integrated cloning (MAGIC) to generate the recombinant vector pBAC-C-KCE-HA. A bivalent vaccine C-KCE-HA was developed by eliminating the BAC backbone. Ducks immunized with C-KCE-HA induced both the cross-reactive antibodies and T cell response against H5. Moreover, C-KCE-HA-immunized ducks provided rapid and long-lasting protection against homologous and heterologous HPAIV H5N1 and DEV clinical signs, death, and primary viral replication. In conclusion, our BAC-C-KCE is a promising platform for developing a polyvalent live attenuated vaccine.

Introduction

Ducks are considered one of the most important waterfowl for its various usages in different aspects. In China and southeast Asia, duck farming is not only a traditional agribusiness for nourishment, but also critical for habiliment. However, this traditional business is seriously threatened by numerous pathogens, such as avian influenza virus (AIV), duck hepatitis virus, duck enteritis virus (DEV), and duck tembusu virus [1,2].

Waterfowl is considered a larger and key natural reservoir of influenza A viruses. It is currently known that almost all the subtypes can be isolated from waterfowl with the exception of the H13 and H16 subtypes [3-5]. Notably, a novel reassorting avian-origin influenza A (H7N9) virus has been isolated from the ducks of live poultry markets [6]. As of October 25, 2013, the virus had caused 137 human cases and 45 human deaths during both epidemic waves in China [7]. The highly pathogenic avian influenza virus (HPAIV) H5N1 is a potential pandemic threat that has caused global concern in many Asian countries, and the duck is believed to be the primary source of infection [2]. Since 2003, a total of 694 human beings have been infected with HPAIV H5N1, with fatality rates approaching 60% [8]. Although many measures have been taken to control AIV infection and transmission, AIV is still a huge threat to public health and the duck industry.

Under these circumstances, vaccination, as an adjunct for improving bio-security and stamping-out policies, contributes to protecting ducks against AIV infection [9].

* Correspondence: jml8328@126.com
†Equal contributors
[1]State Key Laboratory of Agricultural Microbiology, Huazhong Agricultural University, Wuhan 430070, China
[2]College of Veterinary Medicine, Huazhong Agricultural University, Wuhan 430070, China
Full list of author information is available at the end of the article

Currently, conventional inactivated vaccines are largely used for routine preventative vaccination and target vaccination programs [10]. However, inactivated vaccine production is costly and time-consuming, and the oil emulsion adjuvant can cause severe adverse reactions [11]. Furthermore, the risk of contamination by avian pathogens in the egg supply or microbial contaminants during processing has previously jeopardized vaccine supplies [12]. Additionally, inactivated vaccines usually need several weeks to provide solid immune protection [13], which is a major limitation in emergency vaccination to establish a buffer zone. Considering the drawbacks aforementioned, alternative vaccine manufacturing strategies are needed.

Duck viral enteritis is caused by the DEV which belongs to *Anatid herpesvirus* 1; it is an acute, contagious, and lethal disease of ducks, geese, and swans [14]. The DEV genome consists of approximately 160 kilobase pairs (kbp), each pair is composed of two unique sequences, unique long (UL) and unique short (US). The latter is flanked by inverted repeated sequences (IRS and TRS) [15]. A live C-KCE vaccine strain attenuated in the embryonated chicken egg has been developed and utilized to control duck viral enteritis for many years. Furthermore, the ability to induce DEV immunity is not significantly interfered by pre-existing antibodies [16]. Additionally, DEV possesses a wide tropism and can establish latency in the trigeminal ganglia, lymphoid tissues, and peripheral blood lymphocytes [17], in which they efficiently induce both strong humoral immune and cellular immune responses. Thus, the potential of C-KCE as a DNA-based platform for developing polyvalent vaccine deserves in-depth study.

Efficient genetic modification of herpesviruses, such as DEV, has come to rely on bacterial artificial chromosome (BAC) for generating recombinant viruses [18]. In this technology, a BAC-containing clone of the complete viral genome has to be generated, enabling propagation of the viral genome in *Escherichia coli* (*E.coli*) and avoiding the need for cumbersome cloning techniques [19]. Mating-assisted genetically integrated cloning (MAGIC) [20] utilizes bacterial mating, in vivo site-specific endonuclease cleavage and homologous recombination to catalyze the transfer of a DNA fragment between a donor vector in one bacterial strain and recipient plasmid in another separate bacterial strain. The recombination between these plasmids can be forced by inducing *I-SceI* to site-specific cleavage and the *red-gam* recombinase to homologous recombination. Recombination events of MAGIC are genetically selected and result in placement of the gene of interest under the control of new regulatory elements with high efficiency [21].

In the present study, we established a BAC of the C-KCE strain. The hemagglutinin (HA) gene of HPAIV H5N1 was accurately inserted into the C-KCE genome based on MAGIC. A bivalent vaccine C-KCE-HA was generated by eliminating the BAC backbone via *Cre/Lox*p-mediated recombination [22]. Our data indicate that the HA gene inserted into that C-KCE genome was robustly expressed under the control of chicken β-actin promoter and cytomegalovirus immediate enhancer. We further demonstrated C-KCE-HA-immunized ducks induced both cross-reactive antibodies and T cell response against H5. Meanwhile this recombinant C-KCE-HA conferred 100% protection against two antigenically distinct strains of HPAIV H5N1 and virulent DEV challenge in the duck. Therefore, our BAC-C-KCE offers a suitable platform to generate polyvalent live attenuated vaccine against multiple pathogens.

Materials and methods
Virus strain and cells
The attenuated DEV C-KCE vaccine strain, obtained from the China Institute of Veterinary Drugs Control, was propagated and titrated in primary chicken embryo fibroblasts (CEF) propagated in Eagle's minimal essential medium (EMEM, Biochrom), which was supplemented with 100 μg/mL penicillin, 100 μg/mL streptomycin, and 10% fetal bovine serum (FBS) at 37 °C under a 5% CO_2 atmosphere. A virulent DEV strain (HB/10) isolated from Hubei Province in the central part of China was propagated and titrated in duck embryo fibroblasts (DEF). AIV H5N1 A/duck/Hubei/xn/2007 (H5N1) (XN/07) (clade 2.3.2) (GenBank accession number of HA: AHI43271.1) and A/duck/Hubei/HangMei01/2006 (HM/06) (clade 2.3.4) (GenBank accession number of HA: ACF16400.1) were propagated in the allantoic cavities of 10-day-old specific-pathogen-free (SPF) embryonated chicken eggs and stored at −80 °C.

Plasmids and bacterial strains
All the plasmids and *E.coli* strains were kindly donated by Dr Lixin Ma. The mini-F plasmid pBlue-lox was maintained in *E.coli* strain DH10B-IS2 (umuC:araC-ParaBAD-I-Sce-I-FRT) which was constructed in Lixin Ma's laboratory and expresses enzyme *I-SceI* stimulated by 0.2% w/v L-arabinose [21]. The plasmid pML300 contained in DH10B-IS2 carries the *red-gam* recombinase gene stimulated by rhamnose, and is unable to replicate when the bacteria are grown at 42 °C [23]. DH10b was used for generating the recombinant donor plasmid pRThGA. DH10b, but not DH10B-IS2, provided a trans-acting factor π, which could support the conditional origin of replication from R6K, *ori*γ, which contained the donor vector plasmid pRThGA1-HA [24]. The plasmid pCAGGS-NLS/cre expressing Cre recombinase has been previously described [25].

Generation of pBlue-lox-gB-UL26-Amp insertion plasmid and of donor plasmid pRThGA1-HA

The plasmid pBlue-lox-gB-UL26-Amp contains two copies of the *Pac*I restriction site, an enhanced red fluorescent protein (RFP) gene and its cassette, two copies of the direct orientation 34 bp *Lox*p, and two copies of the reverse complement 18 bp *I-sce*I. To insert the 8.28 kb spanning BAC mini-F plasmid into the C-KCE genome, a 454 bp inter-genic region [15] between the gB and UL26/UL26.5 genes was found to be suitable. The inter-genic region is flanked by two poly A sites (Figure 1B). The gB (UL27) is transcribed from left to right and its poly A site is located between nucleotides 65676 and 68678, whereas the UL26/UL26.5 genes are transcribed from right to left and their shared poly A site is located between nucleotides 69131 and 71254 on the complementary strand. Hence, for the insertion of the BAC plasmid sequence within the gB-UL26 junction region, a BAC insertion plasmid containing a *Pac*I insertion site within the gB-UL26 inter-genic region (nucleotides 68678 to 69131) and flanked by the upstream gB gene and the downstream UL26 gene was constructed. In brief, the gB upstream (partial) region and the inter-genic region were

amplified as a 1.1 kb fragment using primers gB-F/gB-R (Table 1). The inter-genic region and downstream UL26 (partial) region were then amplified as a 1.2 kb fragment using primers UL26-F/UL26-R (Table 1). Briefly, the RFP gene under the control of the immediate early promoter of human cytomegalovirus (PHCMV) was amplified from pRTRA as a 1.8 kb fragment using primers Red-F/Red-R (Table 1). The three PCR products described above were used as the templates for "a ligation PCR" using primers UL26-F/Red-R (Table 1). A 4.3 kb fragment was then cloned into the *Sal* I/*Not* I sites of pBlue-lox, resulting in pBlue-lox-gB-UL26. To increase the copy number of pBlue-lox, the ampicillin resistance gene replicon fragment was amplified from pcdna3.1 (+) with the primers Amp-F/Amp-R (Table 1), and inserted into *Pac*I-digested pBlue-lox-gB-UL26 to obtain the plasmid pBlue-lox-gB-UL26-amp. Fragments from the CMV.IE enhancer to rabbit β-globin poly A were amplified from pCAGGS using the primers pCA-I-SceI-H1-F/pCA-I-SceI-H2-R flanked by 50-bp homology arms and *I-sce*I restriction sites. The fragment cut by *I-sce*I was ligated into the pRThGA vector (also cut by the same enzymes), resulting in the recombinant plasmid pRThGA1. The H5

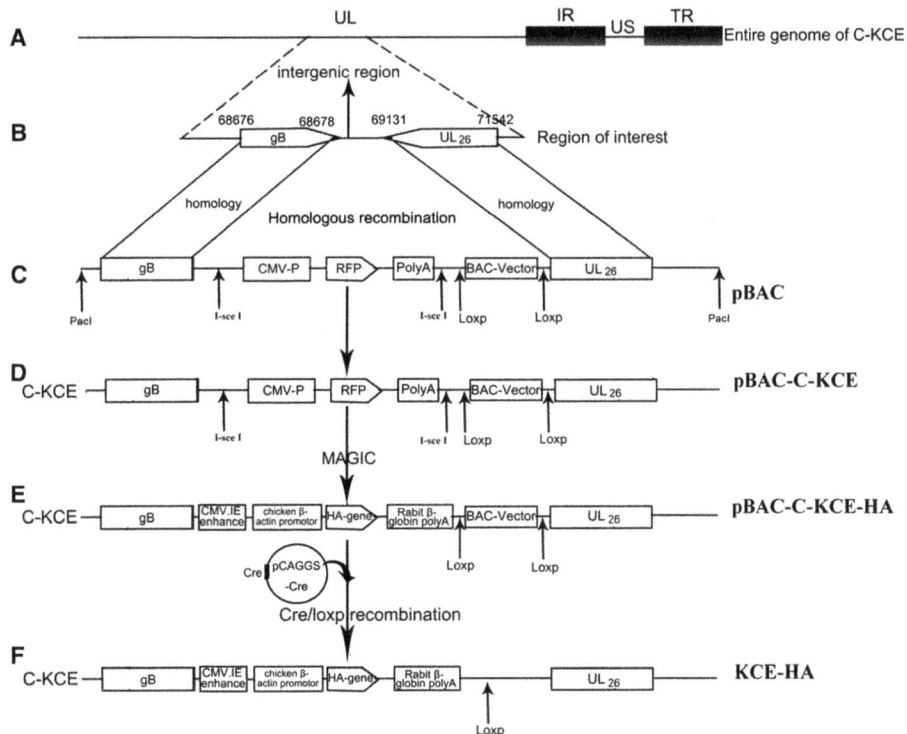

Figure 1 Generation and characterization of H5 HA gene recombinant C-KCE-HA. (A) The organization of the 158-kbp attenuated commercial DEV vaccine strain (C-KCE). **(B)** A portion of the genome C-KCE expanded to show the gB, UL26 gene and inter-genic region is depicted. **(C)** The organization of transfer vector pBlue-lox-gB-UL26-Amp digested by *Pac*I contains an enhanced red fluorescent protein gene and its expression cassette, two copies of the direct orientation 34-bp *Lox*p and two copies of the reverse complement 18-bp *I-sce*I. **(D)** After homologous recombination, pBlue-lox-gB-UL26 was inserted into the genome of C-KCE with the red fluorescent protein as a selection marker. **(E)** After MAGIC, the red fluorescent gene, CMV promoter, and ploy A were entirely replaced by the HA gene and its cassette. **(F)** After *Cre/Lox*p–mediate recombination, the BAC backbone was excised only 34-bp *Lox*p sequence positioned in C-KCE-HA genome.

Table 1 Primers used for generating pBAC-C-KCE, donor plasmid pRThGA and identification of the pBAC-C-KCE-HA

Purpose and primer	Sequence (5′ → 3′)	Sequence designation, restriction enzyme site and introduction sequence
BAC insertion[a]		
UL26-F	aaa**gtcgac**_ataacttcgtatagcatacattatacgaagttat_gccgtatgaatgcgctgac	*Sal* I site (bold), *Lox* p sequence (italic)
UL26-R	**ttaattaa**cgcggacaaaacgacgattac	*Pac* I site (bold)
gB-F	gtaatcgtcgttttgtccgcg**ttaattaa**tgaaaaagacggcggtacaat	*Pac* I site (bold)
gB-R	aagaatgcattcggcctgg	
Red-F	ccaggccgaatgcattcttcgtggggtgtggtgcttttggt	
Red-R	tcga**gcggccgc**_tagggataacagggtaat_ccccaccttatatattctttcccaccct	*Not* I site (bold), *I-isce* I sequence (italic)
Amp-F	aaa**ttaattaa**ggggataacgcaggaaagaac	*Pac* I site (bold)
Amp-R	aaa**ttaattaa**acgtcaggtggcacttttcg	*Pac* I site (bold)
Modification pRThGA[b]		
pCA-*I-Sce*I-H1-F	aaa**tagggataacagggtaat**_gttgagccttttttgtgggagtgggttaaattgtactagcg cgtttcgctttg_cagtacatctacgtattagtcatcgctatta	*I-isce* I sequence (bold), Homology arm H1 (italic)
pCA-*I-Sce*I-H2-R	aaa**tagggataacagggtaat**_tagcatgcataacttcgtataatgtatgctatacgaagt tatgcggccgc_cacacaggaaacagctatgaccatgattac	*I-isce* I sequence (bold), Homology arm H2 (italic)
Amp t-*I-Sce*I-F	aaa**attaccctgttatcccta**cacgttaagggattttggtcat	*I-isce* I sequence (bold)
OriT-R6K-*I-Sce*I-R	aaa**attaccctgttatcccta**	*I-isce* I sequence (bold)
Identification HA[c]		
BAC-F	gagaacagaaaagaaagcgcgt	
BAC-R	cgcagccacagaaaagaaacga	

[a]Primers used for the construction of the BAC insertion vector. The restriction are marked in italics. [b]Primers used for modification of donor plasmid pRThGA. [c]Primers used for verification HA gene insertion into pBAC-C-KCE base on MAGIC.

gene was represented as AI A/duck/Hubei/2911/2007 (H5N1) (GenBank ID: FJ784852.1) flanked by *Smal* I and *Xho* I restriction sites synthesized by Sangon Biotech Life Science Products & Services with several mutations at the cleavage site as previously described [26]. The fragment then was cloned into the *Smal* I and *Xho* I sites present in pRThGA1 to generate the donor vector plasmid pRThGA1-HA.

Construction of a C-KCE BAC clone

After C-KCE was incubated to CEF cells at a multiplicity of infection (MOI) of 50 for 2 h at 37 °C, pBlue-lox-gB-amp linearized with *Pac*I (Figure 2C) was transfected by calcium phosphate precipitation. When the complete cytopathic effect was observed, the total supernatant was harvested. The infected virus was diluted and then plated on the fresh CEF, and overlaid with DMEM-FBS containing 0.5% methylcellulose. When red fluorescent plaques were observed, plaque-purification was carried out as previously described [25] to obtain a fluorescent plaque population, termed vBAC-C-KCE. Circular viral DNA was extracted from CEF by the method of Hirt [27]. Approximately 5 µg of genomic DNA was used to electroporate *DH10B-IS2* with 0.1 cm cuvettes under the following conditions: 1.5 kV, resistance of 200 Ω,

and capacitance of 25 µF. The plasmid pBAC-C-KCE was isolated from chloramphenicol-resistant colonies using QIAprep miniprep kit (Qiagen), and transfected into CEF by the calcium phosphate precipitation method.

Generating the recombinant pBAC-C-KCE-HA vector by MAGIC and deleting the BAC vector

E. coli DH10b containing the donor vector pRThGA1-HA was grown in LB broth containing 100 µg/mL ampicillin. The recipient strain DH10B-IS2, containing the plasmid pML300 and recipient plasmid pBAC-C-KCE, was grown in LB broth containing 50 µg/mL spectinomycin, 34 µg/mL chloramphenicol, 100 µg/mL streptomycin, and 0.2% w/v glucose overnight. The recipient strain was washed twice with two units of LB the next day. The donor and recipient strains were separately diluted to 1:25, 1:50, 1:100, or 1:200 with LB containing 0.2% w/v rhamnose, and grown at 30 °C for 2 h to an A600 of 0.15–0.25. The donor and recipient strains were mixed to a ratio of 1:1 based on their A600 in the presence of 0.2% w/v L-arabinose. The mixture was incubated at 37 °C for 2 h without shaking, and then for a further 2 h with shaking. The recombinant culture was diluted at a ratio of 1:100, plated on selective plates containing 34 µg/mL chloramphenicol, 100 µg/mL streptomycin, and

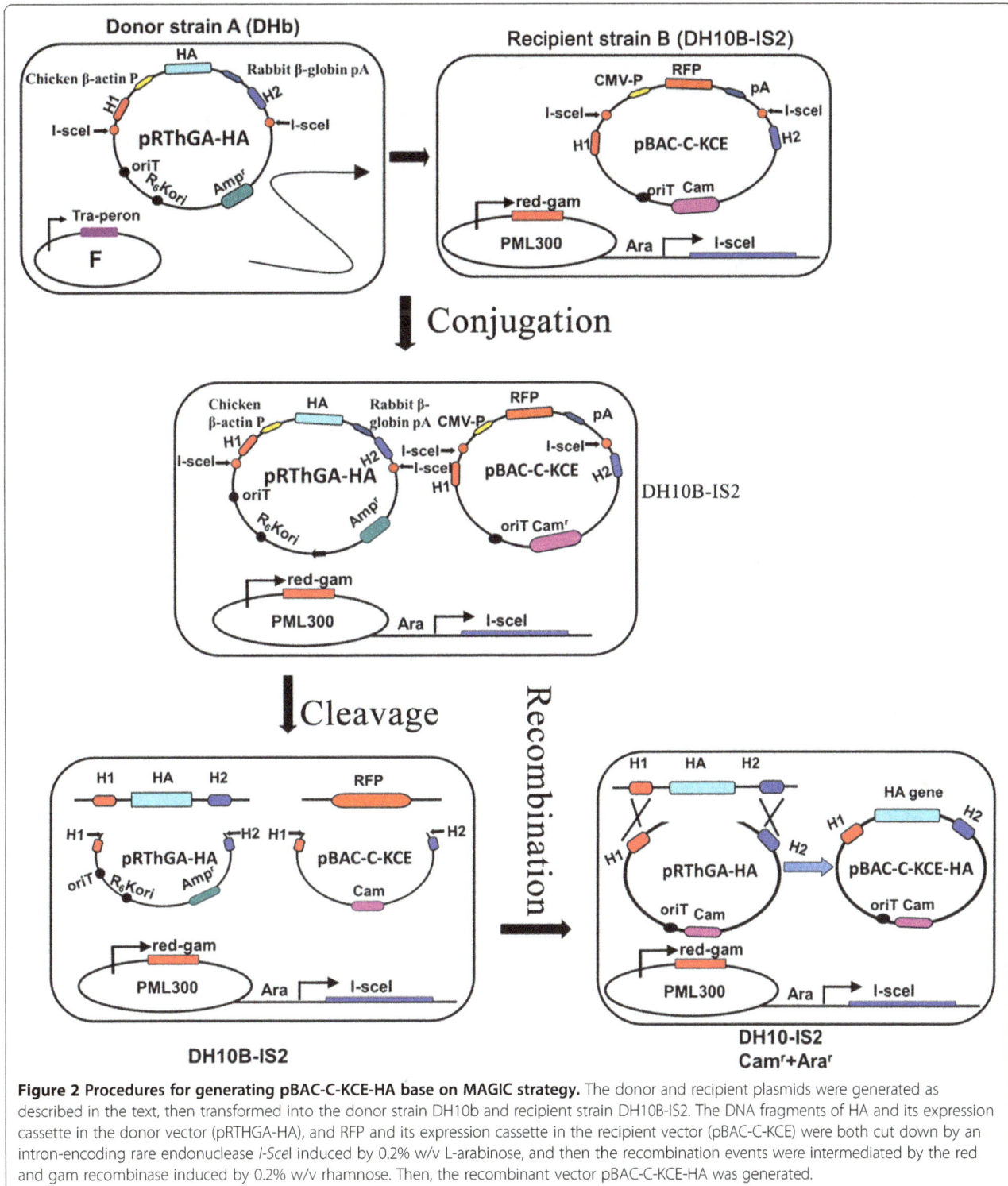

Figure 2 Procedures for generating pBAC-C-KCE-HA base on MAGIC strategy. The donor and recipient plasmids were generated as described in the text, then transformed into the donor strain DH10b and recipient strain DH10B-IS2. The DNA fragments of HA and its expression cassette in the donor vector (pRTHGA-HA), and RFP and its expression cassette in the recipient vector (pBAC-C-KCE) were both cut down by an intron-encoding rare endonuclease *I-Sce*I induced by 0.2% w/v L-arabinose, and then the recombination events were intermediated by the red and gam recombinase induced by 0.2% w/v rhamnose. Then, the recombinant vector pBAC-C-KCE-HA was generated.

0.2% w/v L-arabinose, and finally incubated at 42 °C overnight. The positive clone was named pBAC-C-KCE-HA. To excise the BAC vector sequence, pC-KCE-BAC–HA was co-transfected with pCAGGS-NLS/cre into CEF. The excised BAC vector named C-KCE-HA virus was purified by plaque.

Confirmation of the expression of the H5 HA gene in CEF infected with the C-KCE-HA

HA protein expression in the recombinant C-KCE-HA was evaluated by immunofluorescence (IFA) and Western blot. For IFA, the CEF grown on coverslips in six-well plates were infected at an MOI of 1 with C-KCE or

C-KCE-HA. The monoclonal antibody (mAb) against HA (previously prepared in our laboratory) or polyclonal antibody (pAb) against UL23 (previously prepared in our laboratory) were used as primary antibodies. The secondary antibodies were fluorescein isothiocyanate-conjugated goat anti-rabbit (for HA detection) or anti-mouse (for UL23 detection) IgG (Santa Cruz Biotechnology, CA, USA). The CEF nuclei were stained with 4'-6-diamidino-2-phenylindole (DAPI). The cells were observed using laser scanning confocal microscopy (Carl Zeiss, Zena, Germany). The results were analyzed using software Image J (NIH, USA). For western blot analysis, HA expression was analyzed in CEF in six-well plates infected with C-KCE-HA and C-KCE at an MOI of 1. mAb against HA, pAb against UL23, and mAb against GAPDH (Santa Cruz Biotechnology, CA, USA) for the control were used as primary antibodies. Goat HRP-conjugated anti-rabbit or anti-mouse IgG were used as secondary antibodies. The bands were visualized using Electro-Chemi-Luminescence kit (Thermo, USA) according to the manufacturer's instructions.

Stability and growth properties of the recovered virus C-KCE-HA

To analyze the genetic stability of the foreign gene in the recombinant virus, the virus was sequentially grown on primary CEF for 30 passages, and viral DNA was extracted and analyzed after each passage using HA-specific PCR (Table 1). To compare the growth of C-KCE and C-KCE-HA, a multi-step growth kinetic assay was performed and the plaque sizes were measured as previously described [28]. In order to observe the size of the plaques, the cells were stained with crystal violet, and the plaques were readily visible where the cells were destroyed by viral infection.

Animal experiments

SPF ducks were obtained from the Harbin Veterinary Research Institute, China. Total of 405 one-month-old SPF ducks were used for our studies. Six animal experiments were conducted to evaluate the safety, immunogenicity, and protective efficacy of the C-KCE-HA vaccine against challenge with both homologous and heterologous HPAIV H5N1 and DEV.

For safety experiments, three groups of ducks (five per group) were subcutaneously inoculated with 10^7 PFU of C-KCE-HA (a recommended dose for DEV vaccine is 10^5 PFU), C-KCE, or PBS as a control.

For immunogenicity experiments against DEV, we subcutaneously inoculated three groups of ducks (five per group) with 10^5 PFU of C-KCE-HA, C-KCE, or PBS as a control. At 0, 1, 2, 3, and 4 weeks post-vaccination (pv), serum samples were obtained weekly from all ducks to screen the neutralizing (NT) antibody against DEV.

For clinical protection of C-KCE-HA against virulent DEV challenge, three groups of ducks (twenty per group) were inoculated subcutaneously with 10^5 PFU of C-KCE or C-KCE-HA, whereas naive control ducks were inoculated with PBS. Then, each groups of ducks were randomly subdivided into four groups (five per group). The ducks were challenged with a 100-fold 50% duck lethal dose (DLD_{50}) of HB/10 by intramuscular injection either at 3 days, 1 week, 2 weeks, or 12 weeks pv.

To test the serological responses against HPAIV XN/07 and HM/06 stimulated by immunized C-KCE-HA in ducks, ducks randomly divided into three groups of ducks (five per group) received one immunization subcutaneously with 10^5 PFU of C-KCE-HA, C-KCE, or PBS as a negative control. Serum samples were obtained weekly for 12 weeks from all the groups to monitor the hemagglutination inhibition (HI) and neutralization antibodies.

To detect the cellular response primed by immunized C-KCE-HA in ducks, three groups of ducks (twenty per group) were subcutaneously inoculated with C-KCE-HA (10^5 PFU), C-KCE (10^5 PFU), or PBS (control). At 1, 4, 12, and 36 weeks pv, five ducks of each group were sacrificed humanely. Their spleens were collected to evaluate the cellular immune responses.

To evaluate the clinical protection of C-KCE-HA against HPAIV XN/07, 120 ducks were randomly divided into 12 groups (ten per group). Four groups of ducks were inoculated subcutaneously with 10^5 PFU of C-KCE-HA, and eight groups were inoculated with 10^5 PFU of C-KCE (four groups) or PBS (four groups) as a negative control. Each treatment ducks were then intramuscularly challenged with a 100-fold DLD_{50} of XN/07 at 3 days, 1 week, 2 weeks, or 12 weeks pv. Three ducks in each group were humanely euthanized on day 3 post-challenge (pc), and their organs, including lung, spleen, kidney, and brain, were collected to determine virus titration in 10-day-old SPF embryonated chicken eggs as previously described [29]. Oropharyngeal and cloacal swabs were collected on days 3, 5, and 7 pc for virus titration in eggs. Ducks were monitored daily for signs of disease and death pc for 2 weeks. The animal experimental design about evaluating the clinical protection of C-KCE-HA against HPAIV XM/06 is the same as the XN/07 mentioned above.

Serologic tests and virus titration

NT antibody against HB/10 was tested in DEF as previously described [12]. Serum samples were obtained to monitor HA-specific antibodies via HI assays using chicken red blood cells. The NT antibody against homologous XN/07 and heterologous HM/06 of AIV was determined in MDCK cells as described previously [30]. Each swab was washed in 1 mL of PBS with 200 µg/mL penicillin and 200 µg/mL streptomycin. One gram of each organ was collected and mixed into 1.0 mL of PBS, homogenized, and clarified by centrifugation. Virus titration was conducted in 10-day-old SPF embryonated chicken eggs, and calculated using the method of Reed and Muench [31].

Interferon-γ (IFN-γ) ELISpot assay

Duck spleens were homogenized and washed with Hank Balanced Salt Solution media. Gey solution was added to remove the red blood cells. Splenocytes in Complete Tumor Medium were added into a 96-well (1×10^5–2×10^5 cells per well) plate pretreated with 70% ethanol and coated with anti-duck IFN-γ mAb. Cells were re-stimulated with the HA 518 epitope conserved in both H5N1 viruses used in this study, including currently circulating avian and human H5N1 viruses, and some H9N2 viruses [32]. The cultures were incubated at 37 °C and 5% CO_2 for 48 h, and developed according to an ELISpot protocol (TSZ, USA). Spots were counted using an AID ViruSpot Reader (Cell Technology, Inc.).

Statistical analysis

All experiments were reproducible and performed in triplicate. Statistical analyses were conducted by a one-way ANOVA test to compare the data of the difference groups using GraphPad Prism version 5.0 (GraphPad Software, La Jolla, CA, USA). p-values of < 0.05 were considered statistically significant.

Laboratory facility

All experiments related to HPAIV were conducted in a bio-security level-3 facility.

Results

Establishing a full-length C-KCE clone harboring mini-F plasmid sequences

Establishing a full-length C-KCE clone in *E. coli* first requires the insertion of a BAC vector into the viral genome (Figure 1A). Thus, the BAC vector was inserted into a large junction of the gB and UL26 genes in the C-KCE genome (Figure 1B). The resulting virus, vBAC-C-KCE, was plaque-purified based on the expression of RFP (Figure 3A). The virus was passaged in CEF for 20 rounds to evaluate the genetic stability of the purified vBAC-C-KCE (Figure 3B). The circular viral DNA from the vBAC-C-KCE-infected CEF was extracted, and transformed into the *E. coli* strain DH10B-IS2. pBAC-C-KCE (Figure 1D) was isolated using a QIAprep miniprep kit and transfected into CEF. At 5 days after transfection, approximately 90% of the clones resulted in cytopathic effects. Two clones were selected randomly and sequenced in Shanghai Southgene Technology Co., Ltd. We found that one of the two clones covered the entire 158 kb C-KCE genome (GenBank ID: KF263690.1). Restriction fragment length polymorphisms (RFLP) of C-KCE and BAC-C-KCE were analyzed to confirm that a full-length C-KCE BAC clone

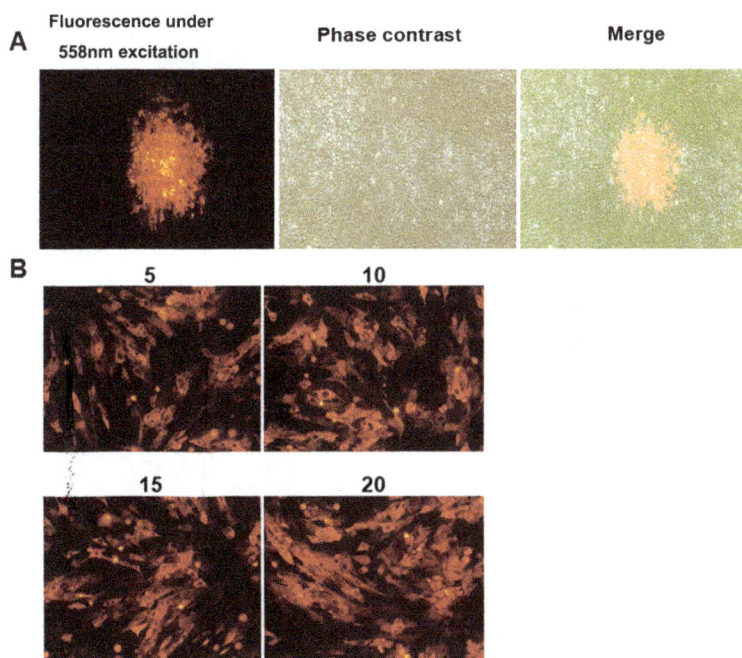

Figure 3 Characterization of the recombinant virus BAC-C-KCE. (A) Plaques of recombinant virus vBAC-C-KCE and parental virus C-KCE were shown under green light excitation, phase contrast, or merge (400×). **(B)** Investigation of the genetic stability of vBAC-C-KCE. The numbers represent the passages of the vBAC-C-KCE (400×). Red fluorescent protein as a selection marker was observed under fluorescence microscopy.

was indeed generated (Figure 4A). This clone was termed pBAC-C-KCE for subsequent studies. The findings confirm that BAC was stably inserted into the gB and UL26 junction region in a site-specific manner.

Rapid generation of the C-KCE-HA vaccine encoding H5N1 HA

The red fluorescent gene, CMV promoter, and poly A were entirely replaced by the HA gene and its cassette. Thus, the HA gene was expressed under the control of the chicken β-actin promoter. The colonies were randomly selected and screened by PCR. A 1.2 kb fragment was amplified from the positive recombinant plasmid pBAC-C-KCE-HA (Figure 1E), and the region around the recombination site was further confirmed by sequencing. Among the randomly selected 24 colonies, 22 contained the expected recombinant vector pBAC-C-KCE-HA (Figure 4B). The efficiency of the positive clone was as high as 90%. BAC vector sequences were flanked by two direct orientation Loxp sequences. pBAC-C-KCE-HA was co-transfected with pCAGGS-NLS/cre to remove the BAC vector sequence. After Cre-mediated removal of the BAC vector sequences, non-fluorescent plaques

appeared and were collected. The resulting C-KCE-HA virus (Figure 1F) without the BAC backbone was plaque-purified and then confirmed by PCR (data not shown). Based on our experimental results, we found that the HA gene could be inserted into pBAC-C-KCE via MAGIC. Moreover, the C-KCE-HA virus, whose BAC backbone was eliminated, was successfully generated by Cre/Loxp–mediate recombination, and only the 34 bp Loxp sequences were positioned in the C-KCE-HA genome.

Biological characterization and stability of the rescued C-KCE-HA recombinant viruses

To assess the genetic stability and growth kinetics of C-KCE-HA, the virus was grown on CEF sequentially for 30 passages. The viral DNA was extracted and analyzed after each passage using HA-specific PCR (data not shown).

To compare the growth of C-KCE and C-KCE-HA, the assays of multi-step growth kinetics and measurements of plaque size were performed. The growth kinetics of C-KCE-HA was similar to that of C-KCE (Additional file 1A). The plaque sizes were also similar (Additional file 1B). These results reveal that the HA gene was stably

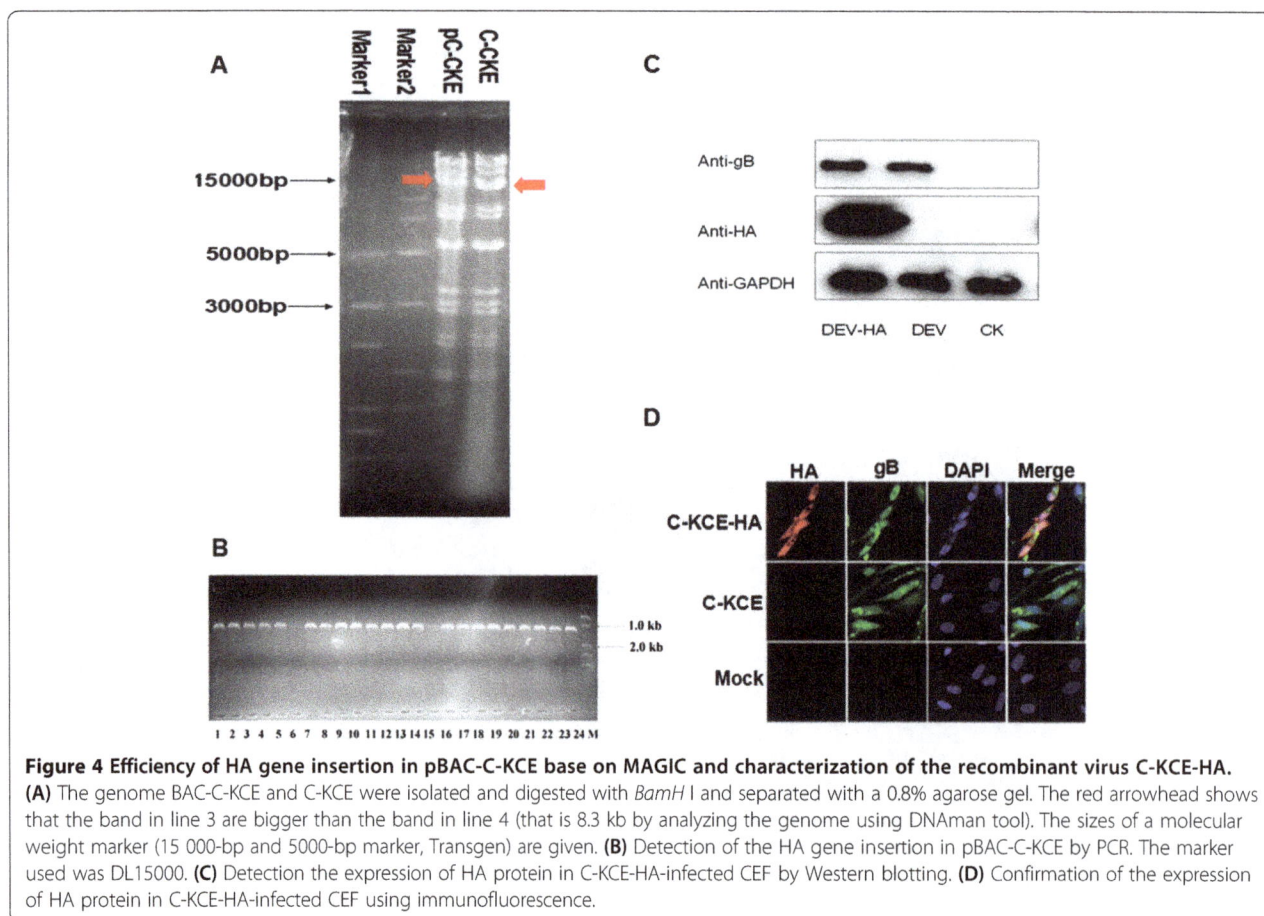

Figure 4 Efficiency of HA gene insertion in pBAC-C-KCE base on MAGIC and characterization of the recombinant virus C-KCE-HA. (A) The genome BAC-C-KCE and C-KCE were isolated and digested with *BamH* I and separated with a 0.8% agarose gel. The red arrowhead shows that the band in line 3 are bigger than the band in line 4 (that is 8.3 kb by analyzing the genome using DNAman tool). The sizes of a molecular weight marker (15 000-bp and 5000-bp marker, Transgen) are given. (B) Detection of the HA gene insertion in pBAC-C-KCE by PCR. The marker used was DL15000. (C) Detection the expression of HA protein in C-KCE-HA-infected CEF by Western blotting. (D) Confirmation of the expression of HA protein in C-KCE-HA-infected CEF using immunofluorescence.

inserted into the C-KCE genome, and exerted no adverse reaction on C-KCE replication in vitro. The expression of the HA protein was determined by western blot and IFA. As expected, the cells infected with C-KCE-HA reacted well. Strong signals were visualized using ECL detection reagents with mAb for HA or pAb for UL23. By contrast, the parental virus C-KCE reacted well with mAb for UL23, and the blank cells did not react with either of the antibodies (Figure 4C). The results of IFA matched those of western blot well. As shown in Figure 4D, diffused HA and UL23 expression were observed, indicating that the HA protein was expressed in the C-KCE-HA-infected CEF. These results also imply that the E protein was robustly expressed during C-KCE-HA replication.

Virulence and immunogenicity evaluation of C-KCE-HA

In our safety experiments, all the ducks remained healthy during the observation period, demonstrating that the insertion of the HA gene did not increase the virulence of the vector C-KCE virus.

To evaluate whether inserting a foreign gene influences the immunogenicity of the parental virus C-KCE, serum samples were obtained weekly for four weeks from all ducks vaccinated with C-KCE-HA, C-KCE, or PBS to screen the NT antibody, a marker of immunogenicity, against HB/10. The NT antibody titers of the PBS-inoculated groups were lower than 3 $\log_2$ and considered negative (Additional file 2). By contrast, the NT antibody titers of three ducks exceeded 2^3 in C-KCE and C-KCE-HA vaccinated groups at one week pv. The NT antibody titers of four ducks reached 2^4 at two weeks pv, but the titers of the two groups started to drop rapidly since then; however, they were still higher than those of the control group (Additional file 2).

Although the NT antibody titers primed by C-KCE or C-KCE-HA were low and short-lived, no significant difference was observed, indicating that the insertion of the HA gene did not change the immunogenicity of the parental virus C-KCE.

Clinical protection of C-KCE-HA against virulent DEV challenge

Animal experiments were conducted to examine the effect of the inserted exogenous gene on the protective efficacy of the parental virus C-KCE, and evaluate the efficacy of the C-KCE-HA vaccine against HB/10 challenge. The ducks immunized with C-KCE or C-KCE-HA survived the lethal challenge regardless of when they were challenged with HB/10 in our experiments. However, two ducks that received C-KCE-HA and were challenged on day 3 pv (Figure 5) showed slight and transient symptoms, including polydipsia and slight loss of appetite, at the beginning of the experimental period. Conversely, the PBS-inoculated ducks showed severe symptoms and

succumbed to infection within 8 days (Figure 5). The protective efficacy of C-KCE-HA and C-KCE against lethal DEV challenge showed no difference. These results demonstrate that the insertion of the HA gene did not alter the protective efficacy of C-KCE.

Induction of antibody response in C-KCE-HA-vaccinated ducks

Antigenic drift is associated more with HA compared with other genes [10]. The HA gene of XN/07 shares approximately 95% identity with HM/06 (Additional file 3). The HA gene of XN/07 shares approximately 95% identity with HM/06 (Additional file 3). To determine whether the serological responses induced by C-KCE-HA vaccine can cross-react with more recent H5N1 viruses isolated from ducks, XN/07 and HM/06 were analyzed by HI and NT. No detectable HI and NT were observed against XN/07 antigens tested in ducks that received mock vaccination (data not shown). Tests were carried out on the sera of C-KCE-HA-immunized ducks to detect the HI antibody against XN/07. The earliest detection of an immune response to XN/07 was at week 2. The antibody level started to increase at week 3 with titers of $2^4 \pm 2^2$, and it peaked at week 4 with titers of $2^6 \pm 2^1$. However, the antibody level began to decline at week 5. Ultimately, the HI antibody was not detected from any duck at 12 weeks pv until the end of our analysis (Figure 6A). The HI antibody responses against HM/06 were consistent with those observed in XN/07, but the HI level was approximately 2^2 titers lower (Figure 6B).

Sera from vaccinated ducks were also evaluated using the NT assay to detect functional antibodies with neutralization activity against the XN/07 (Figure 6C) and HM/06 (Figure 6D) viruses. The trends of NT and HI antibody responses in the C-KCE-HA-inoculated groups were similar, but the levels of the NT antibody were higher than those of the HI antibody at all time points tested (Figure 6). These results demonstrate that vaccination with C-KCE-HA induced cross-reactive antibody responses, and primarily induced antibody responses specific to the delivery of the HA strain.

Cellular response to C-KCE-HA virus vaccination

IFN-γ ELISpot assays were performed to evaluate whether C-KCE-HA can prime cellular immune responses. As expected, ducks that received the C-KCE-HA vaccine demonstrated significantly increased numbers of IFN-γ-secreting cells in spleen cells, regardless of the time the spleen cells were stimulated with the conserved HA 518 epitope (Figure 7). By contrast, numbers of IFN-γ-secreting cells in the groups of C-KCE and PBS were limited. These data demonstrate that C-KCE-HA vaccination robustly generated cellular immune responses to HA.

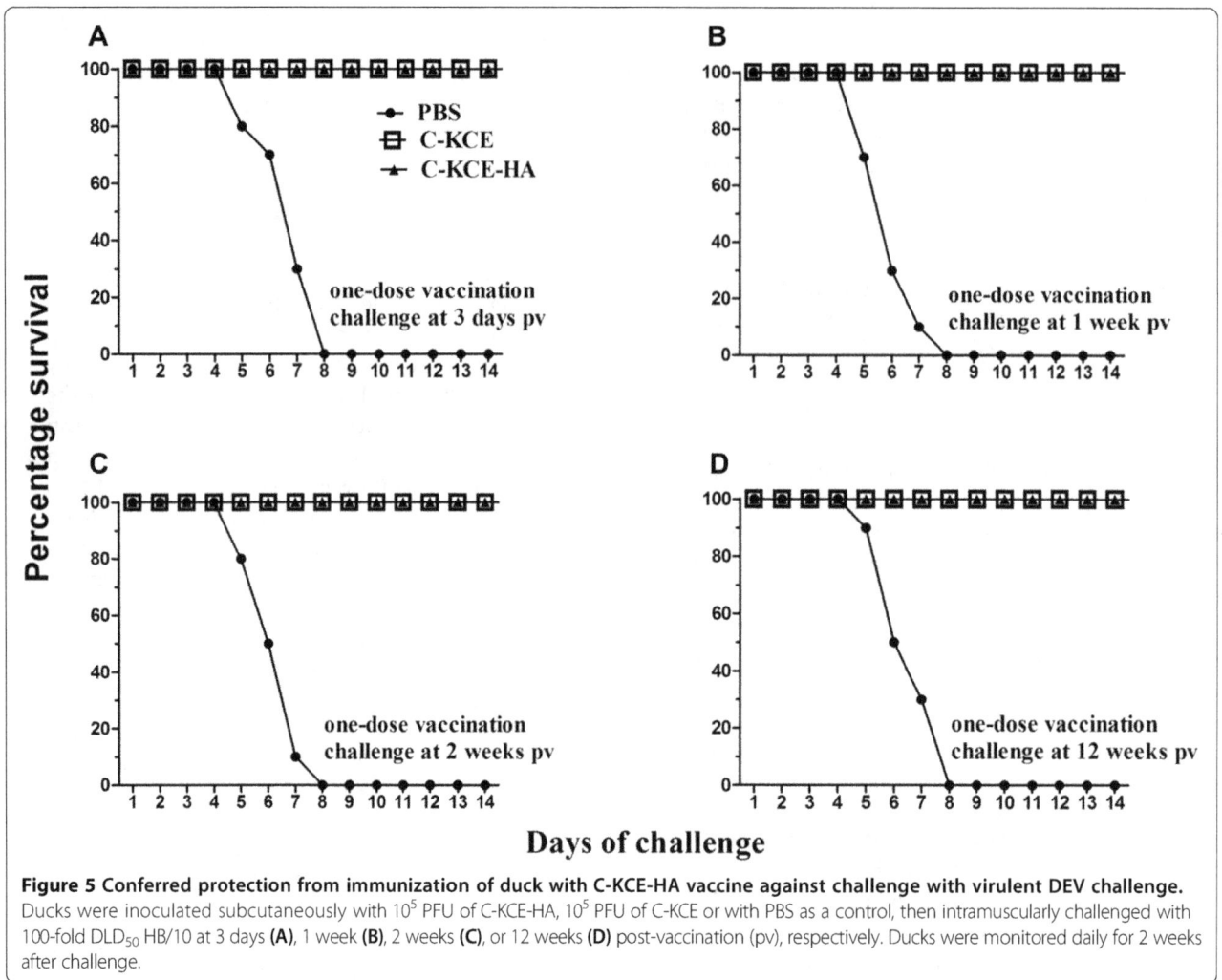

Figure 5 Conferred protection from immunization of duck with C-KCE-HA vaccine against challenge with virulent DEV challenge. Ducks were inoculated subcutaneously with 10^5 PFU of C-KCE-HA, 10^5 PFU of C-KCE or with PBS as a control, then intramuscularly challenged with 100-fold DLD_{50} HB/10 at 3 days **(A)**, 1 week **(B)**, 2 weeks **(C)**, or 12 weeks **(D)** post-vaccination (pv), respectively. Ducks were monitored daily for 2 weeks after challenge.

Vaccine efficacy against lethal H5N1 AIV challenge in ducks

To evaluate whether C-KCE-HA can induce cross-protection against H5 AIV, we challenged the vaccinated ducks with the homologous AIV XN/07 and heterologous AIV HM/06. When we challenged the ducks that received a dose of C-KCE-HA with a 100-fold DLD_{50} of AIV, they were fully protected from challenge with both homologous (Table 2) and heterologous (Table 3) AIV H5N1. The challenged virus was neither recovered from any organs tested nor detected in the oropharynx and cloacae (Tables 2 and 3). All the ducks remained healthy during the observation period. In the control groups of ducks challenged with XN/07 and HM/06 viruses, both viruses were detected in the lung, kidney, spleen, and brain, with titers ranging from 4.3 to 8.6 $\log_{10}$ 50% egg infectious doses ($lgEID_{50}/g$) (Additional file 4). All the ducks shed the virus through both the oropharynx and cloacae on day 3 and died after days 4 to 5 pc (Tables 2 and 3). These data indicate that a single dose of 10^5 PFU of C-KCE-HA could induce solid cross-protection against

homologous and heterologous H5N1 AIV challenge. Thus, it completely blocked replication and shedding of the challenged virus at early stages in ducks.

Discussion

Several infectious pathogens, particularly HPAIV H5N1, can seriously threaten the progression of the duck industry. Vaccines are the most effective method to control these pathogens, and several approaches are being taken worldwide to develop vaccines against these pathogens. However, all of them can pose both practical and immunological challenges [33]. Therefore, a novel vaccine must meet a number of criteria, including low production cost, ease of production, high production yield, and ease of administration. An appealing strategy for improving the immunology of the virus vaccine in a pratical manner involves the use of a live *Anatid herpesvirus* which can deliver foreign antigens of other viruses and can therefore serve as a dual vaccine. Thus, we established a BAC clone of DEV attenuated strain C-KCE. The HA gene of HPAIV H5N1 was inserted into the

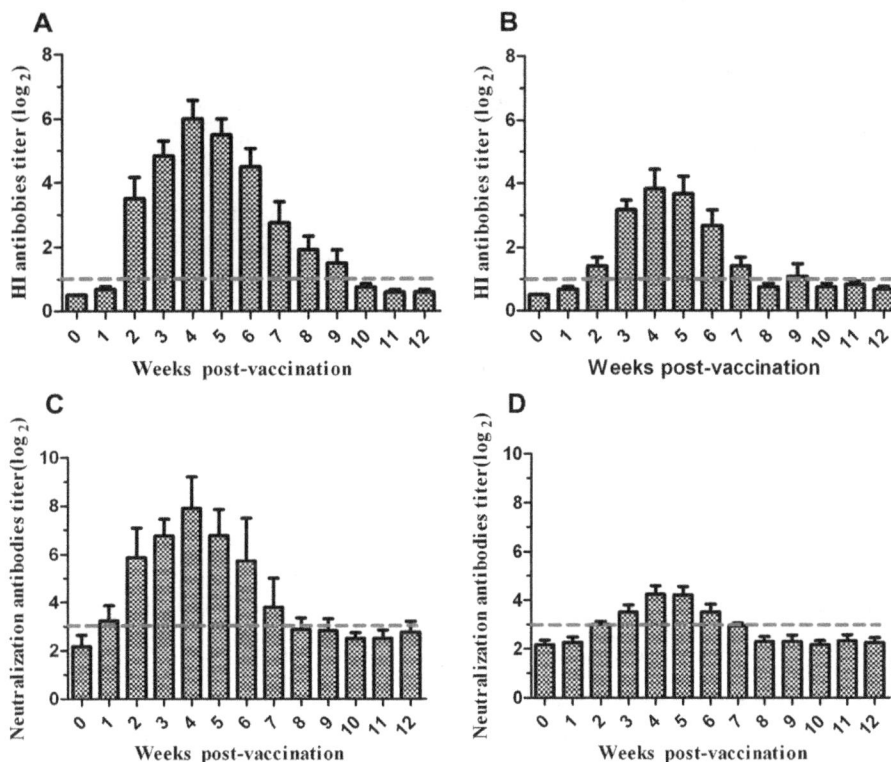

Figure 6 Serological response against homologous and heterologous avian influenza virus strains in duck immunized with C-KCE-HA. Ducks were inoculated subcutaneously with 10^5 PFU of C-KCE-HA. Sera were collected from ducks weekly for HI antibody and NT antibody detection. **(A)**. HI responses were assessed against the homologous XN/07 virus. **(B)**. HI responses were assessed against the heterologous HM/06 virus. **(C)**. NT responses were assessed against the homologous XN/07 virus. **(D)**. NT responses were assessed against the heterologous HM/06 virus. Dotted lines indicate the thresholds for a positive response.

C-KCE genome through MAGIC. Although C-KCE-HA contained an HA gene and its cassette, insertion exerted no adverse effect on C-KCE replication in vitro, and it did not alter the pathogenicity and immunogenicity of C-KCE in vivo. After a single immunization, C-KCE-HA induced humoral immune and cellular immune responses to HA.

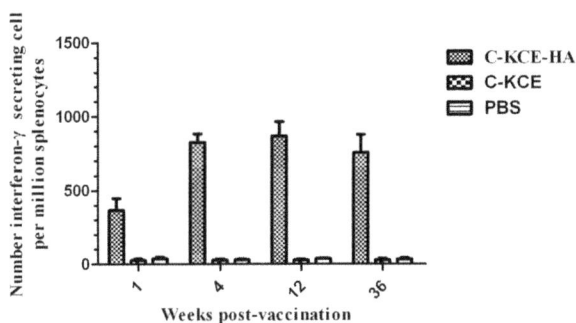

Figure 7 Induction of HA-518-epitope-specific and IFN-γ-secreting spleen cells in ducks immunized with C-KCE-HA vaccine. HA-specific responses of splenocytes taken 1, 4, 12, 36 weeks post-vaccination as determined by IFN-γ-ELISPOT assay inducing HA-518-epitope-specific. Data represent means standard errors of the mean of triplicate determinations for a minimum of three ducks per group.

As early as one week pv, ducks provided solid protection against challenge with homologous and heterologous H5N1 virus without viral shedding, clinical signs, and death. Therefore, the use of C-KCE-HA could simultaneously prevent two deadly infectious diseases, namely, AI and DEV, with a single live virus vaccine.

Viral vectors have been widely explored for developing vaccines. Fowlpox virus, varicella-zoster virus, pseudorabies virus, turkey herpesvirus, adenovirus, baculovirus, and Newcastle disease virus-based vectors [11,32,34-38] are the most extensively studied viral vectors. Some recombinant vaccines have even been granted licenses by some governments, and they are currently utilized for preventing the spread of pathogens. Attenuated DEV vaccine strains, including C-KCE and clone03, are ideal avian vaccine vector candidates because these viruses can induce long-lasting protection against DEV in ducks, and they have a natural host range limited to avian species [39].

Herpesvirus mutagenesis has come to rely on BAC and recombinant technology to generate recombinant viruses. Construction of the BAC of C-KCE can be used to develop a bivalent vaccine as well as facilitate the study of DEV pathogenesis. For example, the virulent

Table 2 Protective efficacy of C-KCE-HA against H5N1 lethal virus XN/07 challenge in ducks

Challenge virus	Challenge time pv	Vaccine	Virus isolation from the swabs (shedding/total log$_{10}$ EID$_{50}$/mL)						No. surviving/ total
			Day 3 pc		Day 5 pc		Day 7 pc		
			Oropharyngeal	Cloacal	Oropharyngeal	Cloacal	Oropharyngeal	Cloacal	
XN/07	1 week	C-KCE-HA	0/7	0/7	0/7	0/7	0/7	0/7	7/7
		C-KCE	7/7(3.1 ± 0.6)	5/7(2.4 ± 0.5)	—	—	—	—	0/7
		PBS	7/7(4.2 ± 0.5)	6/7(3.8 ± 0.4)	—	—	—	—	0/7
	3 weeks	C-KCE-HA	0/7	0/7	0/7	0/7	0/7	0/7	7/7
		C-KCE	7/7(2.7 ± 0.6)	6/7(2.4 ± 0.6)	—	—	—	—	0/7
		PBS	7/7(4.3 ± 0.7)	7/7(4.3 ± 0.7)	—	—	—	—	0/7
	12 weeks	C-KCE-HA	0/7	0/7	0/7	0/7	0/7	0/7	7/7
		C-KCE	7/7(2.7 ± 0.7)	7/7(2.6 ± 1.1)	—	—	—	—	0/7
		PBS	7/7(2.1 ± 0.9)	4/7(1.8 ± 1.2)	—	—	—	—	0/7
	36 weeks	C-KCE-HA	0/7	0/7	0/7	0/7	0/7	0/7	7/7
		C-KCE	7/7(3.1 ± 0.3)	6/7(2.1 ± 0.5)	—	—	—	—	0/7
		PBS	7/7(2.7 ± 0.7)	7/7(1.8 ± 0.6)	—	—	—	—	0/7

One-month-old SPF ducks were used in these studies. Groups of seven ducks were inoculated subcutaneously with 10^5 PFU of C-KCE-HA, 10^5 PFU of C-KCE or with PBS as a control. They then were challenged intramuscularly with 100-fold DLD$_{50}$ homologous (XN/07) AIVs at 1 week, 3 weeks, 12 weeks or 24 weeks post-vaccination (pv). Oropharyngeal and cloacal swabs were collected on days 3, 5, and 7 post-challenge (pc) and titrated in SPF eggs. All of the ducks in C-KCE and PBS groups died within 5 days. The horizontal line indicates that the animals had died by that time point.

strain 2085 is the first established infectious BAC used to evaluate the function of the gC gene [25]. Two general approaches to infectious clone design could be applied to establish a BAC clone of the C-KCE. In one approach, the BAC vector could be inserted into a viral gene dispensable for viral growth and pathogenesis. In another approach, the BAC vector was inserted into the gene junction of the C-KCE genome. The expression of the neighboring genes could not be interfered in this junction. Currently, the full genomes of the three strains

of DEV are available in GenBank [15,40,41]. Molecular characterization of the genome of DEV is similar to other herpesvirus type 1. Those areas have been proven to be suitable for foreign gene insertion, including the sites within gG, gB, US2, and gD [42-45]. The insertion site of the foreign gene could alter the immunogenicity and vaccine efficacy of recombinant DEV [39]. Hence, we inserted a mini-F vector into the gB and UL26 gene junction, which is the longest among all the junctions within the C-KCE genome (454 bp). The stability of

Table 3 Protective efficacy of C-KCE-HA against H5N1 lethal virus HM/06 challenge in ducks

Challenge virus	Challenge time pv	Vaccine	Virus isolation from the swabs (shedding/total log$_{10}$ EID$_{50}$/mL)						No. surviving/ total
			Day 3 pc		Day 5 pc		Day 7 pc		
			Oropharyngeal	Cloacal	Oropharyngeal	Cloacal	Oropharyngeal	Cloacal	
HM/06	1 week	C-KCE-HA	0/7	0/7	0/7	0/7	0/7	0/7	7/7
		C-KCE	7/7(2.1 ± 0.9)	6/7(2.5 ± 0.3)	—	—	—	—	0/7
		PBS	7/7(3.4 ± 1.2)	7/7(3.8 ± 0.4)	—	—	—	—	0/7
	3 weeks	C-KCE-HA	0/7	0/7	0/7	0/7	0/7	0/7	7/7
		C-KCE	7/7(4.1)	7/7(3.3 ± 0.5)	—	—	—	—	0/7
		PBS	7/7(3.6 ± 0.7)	7/7(2.5 ± 1.1)	—	—	—	—	0/7
	12 weeks	C-KCE-HA	0/7	0/7	0/7	0/7	0/7	0/7	7/7
		C-KCE	7/7(2.6 ± 0.8)	7/7(3.1 ± 0.6)	—	—	—	—	0/7
		PBS	7/7(2.9 ± 0.6)	6/7(2.3 ± 1.1)	—	—	—	—	0/7
	36 weeks	C-KCE-HA	0/7	0/7	0/7	0/7	0/7	0/7	7/7
		C-KCE	7/7(2.5 ± 0.6)	5/7(2.8 ± 0.3)	—	—	—	—	0/7
		PBS	7/7(2.7 ± 0.9)	6/7(2.4 ± 0.6)	—	—	—	—	0/7

One-month-old SPF ducks were used in these studies. Groups of seven ducks were inoculated subcutaneously with 10^5 PFU of C-KCE-HA, 10^5 PFU of C-KCE or with PBS as a control. They then were challenged intramuscularly with 100-fold DLD$_{50}$ heterologous (HM/06) AIVs at 1 week, 3 weeks, 12 weeks or 24 weeks post-vaccination (pv). Oropharyngeal and cloacal swabs were collected on days 3, 5, and 7 post-challenge (pc) and titrated in SPF eggs. All of the ducks in C-KCE and PBS groups died within 5 days. The horizontal line indicates that the animals had died by that time point.

vBAC-C-KCE was confirmed by assaying vBAC-C-KCE, which was serial passaged 20 times, in CEF. This finding indicates that the junction of C-KCE was an ideal location for foreign gene insertion.

We accurately and efficiently inserted the HA gene into pBAC-C-KCE via MAGIC. Notably, the efficiency of the positive clone was approximately 90%. MAGIC has been explored in many viruses, such as adenoviruses and baculovirus [21,46]. In contrast to other traditional systems, this novel strategy is highly efficient, time-efficient, and uses a low level of background nonrecombinants to construct a recombinant virus. The vaccine strains for AI control have been frequently updated; AIV have undergone rapid genetic evolution, and expanded their host range and virulent properties in mammals [12]. Thus, BAC-C-KCE based on MAGIC could be considered for the development of the AI vaccine against newly emerging AIV in ducks. Once the HA sequence of an emerging AIV is known, a bivalent vaccine can be rapidly generated. For example, the recent emergence of the AIV (H7N9) strain in poultry and its subsequent transmission to humans in China have raised great concerns about the potential pandemic spread of lethal diseases [47]. Utilizing MAGIC, we successfully constructed and obtained the recombinant vaccine expression of HA of H7N9 within two weeks of acquiring the HA gene (data not shown).

Generally, the expression level has two important determinants, including the inserted gene itself and its promoter. Previous studies have demonstrated that the expression of HA in the pCAGGS vector can display higher levels than that in other vectors [11,15]. We reasoned that the amount of HA expression was critical to the efficacy of C-KCE-HA for inducing protective neutralization antibodies against AIV. To this end, we also selected the chicken β-actin promoter driving a high-level of protein expression across a wide range of species and cell types. Indeed, our results show that HA protein was robustly expressed during C-KCE-E replication, and the protection efficiency of C-KCE-HA also improved [39].

The neutralization antibody against influenza virus is the hallmark of protective immunity [32]. Serological data revealed that the antibodies could be barely detected at 1 and 12 weeks pv. Of note, our challenge studies showed that the C-KCE-HA provided protection from a lethal challenge with homologous virus XN/07 and early isolate HM/06, which is antigenically different. Thus, in addition to neutralizing, antibodies play a role in this protection but T-cell responses, which have been shown to aid in virus clearance, also contribute to this protection [32]. Clearly, the HA protein is the major surface glycoprotein of the influenza virus; it not only induces HA-specific antibodies, but also stimulates cellular responses [36]. Our study builds upon these findings,

going one step further in trying to understand the role of the T-cell response to the C-KCE-HA influenza virus HA vaccine. The presence of heterotypic H5N1 protection without a sufficient humoral neutralizing response, further reinforced by the ability of the C-KCE-HA vaccine to fully protect the immunized duck, strongly suggests a complementary role for the cellular response to its humoral counterpart. Moreover, the provision of long-term immunity with a single dose of C-KCE-HA had obvious benefits to layers and breeder flocks [39]. Overall, the C-KCE-based vaccine could be utilized to offset traditional inactivated AIV vaccines.

Our findings highlight the potential of a BAC-C-KCE-vector-based delivery system, which offers stockpiling options for the development of a pandemic influenza vaccine. In addition to insertion of HA alone, due to the huge capacity of the BAC system, viral NP and M2 can be inserted to generate a universal influenza vaccine [48] against newly emerging antigenic drift and shift variants. Similarly, immunogenic genes of other pathogens, such as duck hepatitis virus, duck tembusu virus, and AIV H9N2, could also be inserted at the same time to generate a polyvalent vaccine. We expect that the application of this novel BAC-C-KCE platform to develop a series of vaccines in the near future will greatly decrease those pathogens in poultry.

Additional files

Additional file 1: Comparsion of the growth between C-KCE and C-KCE-HA. (A). Multi-step growth kinetics of C-KCE-HA and C-KCE in CEF cells. Data were shown for the indicated time points after infection with an MOI of 0.01. Titers are given as plaque forming units in 0.1 mL. Means of virus titers as determined by three independent experiments are shown; standard deviations are shown with the error bars. (B). Plaque phenotype of C-KCE-HA and C-KCE in CEF cells. After titration of viruses, cells were fixed in 4% paraformaldehyde and stained with crystal violet.

Additional file 2: Humoral immune response against virulent DEV in ducks vaccinated with C-KCE-HA or its parental strain C-KCE. Groups of 5 ducks were inoculated subcutaneously with 10^5 PFU of C-KCE-HA, C-KCE or with PBS as a control. Sera were collected range from 0 to 4 weeks to detect the NT antibody against virulent DEV in DEF cells. NT antibody titers for ducks are expressed as a $\log_2$. Dotted lines indicate the thresholds for a positive response.

Additional file 3: Phylogenetic relationships of the HA genes of H5N1 AIV. The tree includes AIV that were isolated from some provinces in China during 2004 to 2010. The phylogenetic tree was generated with the MEGA (version 5.0) by using the neighbor-joining algorithm and based on bootstrap values of 1000. The HA gene donor virus for the recombinant vaccine generation and the challenge viruses used in this study are marked in red.

Additional file 4: Replication of challenge virus in ducks. Homologous and heterologous H5N1 replication in the organs of ducks that were vaccinated with C-KCE-HA. Groups of three ducks were inoculated subcutaneously with 10^5 PFU of C-KCE-HA, C-KCE or with PBS as a control. They then were challenged with homologous (XN/07) or heterologous (HM/06) AIV intramuscularly at 1 week, 3 weeks, 12 weeks or 36 weeks pv. Day 3 after challenge, the ducks were euthanized and their organs were harvested for virus titration in eggs. Data represent means ± standard deviations of $\log_{10}$ EID$_{50}$s. The backslash indicates that the challenge virus was not detected by that time point.

Competing interests

The authors declare that they have no competing interests.

Authors' contributions

Conceived and designed the experiments: ZZ, HY. Performed the experiments: ZZ, ZGL, WZ, HZC. Analyzed the data: ZZ, HY, HCC, MLJ. Contributed reagents/materials/analysis tools: ZZ, HY. Wrote the paper: ZZ, MLJ. All authors read and approved the final manuscript.

Acknowledgments

This research was supported by the Research Fund for the Doctoral Program of Higher Education of China (20100480912). We should like to thank Dr Lixin Ma, (Science and Technology, HuBei University, Wuhan, 430070, China) for kindly donating plasmids and *E.coli* strains. Special acknowledgments go to Prof. Yanxiu Liu (College of Foreign Languages, Huazhong Agricultural University, Wuhan 430070, China) and Dr Kui Zhu (Department of Veterinary Sciences, Ludwig-Maximilians-Universität München, 85764 Oberschleissheim, Germany) for editing the manuscript.

Author details

[1]State Key Laboratory of Agricultural Microbiology, Huazhong Agricultural University, Wuhan 430070, China. [2]College of Veterinary Medicine, Huazhong Agricultural University, Wuhan 430070, China. [3]Hubei Collaborative Innovation Center for Industrial Fermentation, Hubei University of Technology, Wuhan 430068, China. [4]College of Life Sciences, AnQing Normal University, AnQing 246011, China.

References

1. Chen P, Liu J, Jiang Y, Zhao Y, Li Q, Wu L, He X, Chen H (2014) The vaccine efficacy of recombinant duck enteritis virus expressing secreted E with or without PrM proteins of duck tembusu virus. Vaccine 32:5271–5277

2. Liu X, Wei S, Liu Y, Fu P, Gao M, Mu X, Liu H, Xing M, Ma B, Wang J (2013) Recombinant duck enteritis virus expressing the HA gene from goose H5 subtype avian influenza virus. Vaccine 31:5953–5959

3. Wilcox BR, Knutsen GA, Berdeen J, Goekjian V, Poulson R, Goyal S, Sreevatsan S, Cardona C, Berghaus RD, Swayne DE, Yabsley MJ, Stallknecht DE (2011) Influenza-A viruses in ducks in northwestern Minnesota: fine scale spatial and temporal variation in prevalence and subtype diversity. PLoS One 6:e24010

4. Olsen B, Munster VJ, Wallensten A, Waldenstrom J, Osterhaus AD, Fouchier RA (2006) Global patterns of influenza a virus in wild birds. Science 312:384–388

5. Munster VJ, Baas C, Lexmond P, Waldenstrom J, Wallensten A, Fransson T, Rimmelzwaan GF, Beyer WE, Schutten M, Olsen B, Osterhaus AD, Fouchier RA (2007) Spatial, temporal, and species variation in prevalence of influenza A viruses in wild migratory birds. PLoS Pathog 3:e61

6. Cowling BJ, Freeman G, Wong JY, Wu P, Liao Q, Lau EH, Wu JT, Fielding R, Leung GM (2013) Preliminary inferences on the age-specific seriousness of human disease caused by avian influenza A(H7N9) infections in China, March to April 2013. Euro Surveill 18:20475

7. World Health Origination [http://www.who.int/influenza/human_animal_interface/influenza_h7n9/10u_ReportWebH7N9Number.pdf?ua=1]

8. World Health Origination [http://www.who.int/influenza/human_animal_interface/EN_GIP_20150106CumulativeNumberH5N1cases_corrected.pdf?ua=1]

9. Swayne DE, Pavade G, Hamilton K, Vallat B, Miyagishima K (2011) Assessment of national strategies for control of high-pathogenicity avian influenza and low-pathogenicity notifiable avian influenza in poultry, with emphasis on vaccines and vaccination. Rev Sci Tech 30:839–870

10. Li Y, Reddy K, Reid SM, Cox WJ, Brown IH, Britton P, Nair V, Iqbal M (2011) Recombinant herpesvirus of turkeys as a vector-based vaccine against highly pathogenic H7N1 avian influenza and Marek's disease. Vaccine 29:8257–8266

11. Sonoda K, Sakaguchi M, Okamura H, Yokogawa K, Tokunaga E, Tokiyoshi S, Kawaguchi Y, Hirai K (2000) Development of an effective polyvalent vaccine against both Marek's and Newcastle diseases based on recombinant Marek's disease virus type 1 in commercial chickens with maternal antibodies. J Virol 74:3217–3226

12. Wong SS, Webby RJ (2013) Traditional and new influenza vaccines. Clin Microbiol Rev 26:476–492

13. Kapczynski DR, Swayne DE (2009) Influenza vaccines for avian species. Curr Top Microbiol Immunol 333:133–152

14. Yu X, Jia R, Huang J, Shu B, Zhu D, Liu Q, Gao X. Lin M, Yin Z, Wang M, Chen S, Wang Y, Chen X, Cheng A (2012) Attenuated Salmonella typhimurium delivering DNA vaccine encoding duck enteritis virus UL24 induced systemic and mucosal immune responses and conferred good protection against challenge. Vet Res 43:56

15. Li Y, Huang B, Ma X, Wu J, Li F, Ai W, Song M, Yang H (2009) Molecular characterization of the genome of duck enteritis virus. Virology 391:151–161

16. Jiang Y, Yu K, Zhang H, Zhang P, Li C, Tian G, Li Y, Wang X, Ge J, Bu Z, Chen H (2007) Enhanced protective efficacy of H5 subtype avian influenza DNA vaccine with codon optimized HA gene in a pCAGGS plasmid vector. Antiviral Res 75:234–241

17. Shawky S, Schat KA (2002) Latency sites and reactivation of duck enteritis virus. Avian Dis 46:308–313

18. Warden C, Tang Q, Zhu H (1997) Herpesvirus BACs: past, present, and future. J Biomed Biotechnol 2011:124595

19. Messerle M, Crnkovic I, Hammerschmidt W, Ziegler H, Koszinowski UH (1997) Cloning and mutagenesis of a herpesvirus genome as an infectious bacterial artificial chromosome. Proc Natl Acad Sci U S A 94:14759–14763

20. Li MZ, Elledge SJ (2005) MAGIC, an in vivo genetic method for the rapid construction of recombinant DNA molecules. Nat Genet 37:311–319

21. Tan R, Li C, Jiang S, Ma L (2006) A novel and simple method for construction of recombinant adenoviruses. Nucleic Acids Res 34:e89

22. Seidler B, Schmidt A, Mayr U, Nakhai H, Schmid RM, Schneider G, Saur D (2008) A Cre-loxP-based mouse model for conditional somatic gene expression and knockdown in vivo by using avian retroviral vectors. Proc Natl Acad Sci U S A 105:10137–10142

23. Wang ZW, Sarmento L, Wang Y, Li XQ, Dhingra V, Tseggai T, Jiang B, Fu ZF (2005) Attenuated rabies virus activates, while pathogenic rabies virus evades, the host innate immune responses in the central nervous system. J Virol 79:12554–12565

24. Metcalf WW, Jiang W, Wanner BL (1994) Use of the rep technique for allele replacement to construct new Escherichia coli hosts for maintenance of R6K gamma origin plasmids at different copy numbers. Gene 138:1–7

25. Wang J, Osterrieder N (2011) Generation of an infectious clone of duck enteritis virus (DEV) and of a vectored DEV expressing hemagglutinin of H5N1 avian influenza virus. Virus Res 159:23–31

26. Chowdhury SI, Batterson W (1994) Transinhibition of herpes simplex virus replication by an inducible cell-resident gene encoding a dysfunctional VP19c capsid protein. Virus Res 33:67–87

27. Hirt B (1967) Selective extraction of polyoma DNA from infected mouse cell cultures. J Mol Biol 26:365–369

28. Adler H, Messerle M, Wagner M, Koszinowski UH (2000) Cloning and mutagenesis of the murine gammaherpesvirus 68 genome as an infectious bacterial artificial chromosome. J Virol 74:6964–6974

29. Zhou H, Zhu J, Tu J, Zou W, Hu Y, Yu Z, Yin W, Li Y, Zhang A, Wu Y, Yu Z, Chen H, Jin M (2010) Effect on virulence and pathogenicity of H5N1 influenza A virus through truncations of NS1 eIF4GI binding domain. J Infect Dis 202:1338–1346

30. Stephenson I, Wood JM, Nicholson KG, Charlett A, Zambon MC (2004) Detection of anti-H5 responses in human sera by HI using horse erythrocytes following MF59-adjuvanted influenza A/Duck/Singapore/97 vaccine. Virus Res 103:91–95

31. Reed LJ, Muench H (1938) A simple method of estimating fifty percent endpoints. Am J Hyg 27:493–497

32. Hoelscher MA, Garg S, Bangari DS, Belser JA, Lu X, Stephenson I, Bright RA, Katz JM, Mittal SK, Sambhara S (2006) Development of adenoviral-vector-based pandemic influenza vaccine against antigenically distinct human H5N1 strains in mice. Lancet 367:475–481

33. Subbarao K, Murphy BR, Fauci AS (2006) Development of effective vaccines against pandemic influenza. Immunity 24:5–9

34. Bublot M, Pritchard N, Swayne DE, Selleck P, Karaca K, Suarez DL, Audonnet JC, Mickle TR (2006) Development and use of fowlpox vectored vaccines for avian influenza. Ann N Y Acad Sci 1081:193–201

35. DiNapoli JM, Nayak B, Yang L, Finneyfrock BW, Cook A, Andersen H, Torres-Velez F, Murphy BR, Samal SK, Collins PL, Bukreyev A (2010) Newcastle disease

virus-vectored vaccines expressing the hemagglutinin or neuraminidase protein of H5N1 highly pathogenic avian influenza virus protect against virus challenge in monkeys. J Virol 84:1489–1503

36. Gao W, Soloff AC, Lu X, Montecalvo A, Nguyen DC, Matsuoka Y, Robbins PD, Swayne DE, Donis RO, Katz JM, Barratt-Boyes SM, Gambotto A (2006) Protection of mice and poultry from lethal H5N1 avian influenza virus through adenovirus-based immunization. J Virol 80:1959–1964

37. Ge J, Deng G, Wen Z, Tian G, Wang Y, Shi J, Wang X, Li Y, Hu S, Jiang Y, Yang C, Yu K, Bu Z, Chen H (2007) Newcastle disease virus-based live attenuated vaccine completely protects chickens and mice from lethal challenge of homologous and heterologous H5N1 avian influenza viruses. J Virol 81:150–158

38. Somboonthum P, Yoshii H, Okamoto S, Koike M, Gomi Y, Uchiyama Y, Takahashi M, Yamanishi K, Mori Y (2007) Generation of a recombinant Oka varicella vaccine expressing mumps virus hemagglutinin-neuraminidase protein as a polyvalent live vaccine. Vaccine 25:8741–8755

39. Liu J, Chen P, Jiang Y, Wu L, Zeng X, Tian G, Ge J, Kawaoka Y, Bu Z, Chen H (2012) A duck enteritis virus-vectored bivalent live vaccine provides fast and complete protection against H5N1 avian influenza virus infection in ducks. J Virol 85:10989–10998

40. Wu Y, Cheng A, Wang M, Yang Q, Zhu D, Jia R, Chen S, Zhou Y, Wang X, Chen X (2012) Complete genomic sequence of Chinese virulent duck enteritis virus. J Virol 86:5965

41. Wang J, Hoper D, Beer M, Osterrieder N (2012) Complete genome sequence of virulent duck enteritis virus (DEV) strain 2085 and comparison with genome sequences of virulent and attenuated DEV strains. Virus Res 160:316–325

42. Gabev E, Fraefel C, Ackermann M, Tobler K (2009) Cloning of Bovine herpesvirus type 1 and type 5 as infectious bacterial artifical chromosomes. BMC Res Notes 2:209

43. Liu ZF, Brum MC, Doster A, Jones C, Chowdhury SI (2008) A bovine herpesvirus type 1 mutant virus specifying a carboxyl-terminal truncation of glycoprotein E is defective in anterograde neuronal transport in rabbits and calves. J Virol 82:7432–7442

44. Smith GA, Enquist LW (2000) A self-recombining bacterial artificial chromosome and its application for analysis of herpesvirus pathogenesis. Proc Natl Acad Sci U S A 97:4873–4878

45. Wang K, Kappel JD, Canders C, Davila WF, Sayre D, Chavez M, Pesnicak L, Cohen JI (2012) A herpes simplex virus 2 glycoprotein D mutant generated by bacterial artificial chromosome mutagenesis is severely impaired for infecting neuronal cells and infects only Vero cells expressing exogenous HVEM. J Virol 86:12891–12902

46. Yao LG, Liu ZC, Zhang XM, Kan YC, Zhou JJ (2007) A highly efficient method for the generation of a recombinant Bombyx mori nuclear-polyhedrosis-virus Bacmid and large-scale expression of foreign proteins in silkworm (B. mori) larvae. Biotechnol Appl Biochem 48:45–53

47. Gao HN, Lu HZ, Cao B, Du B, Shang H, Gan JH, Lu SH, Yang YD, Fang Q, Shen YZ, Xi XM, Gu Q, Zhou XM, Qu HP, Yan Z, Li FM, Zhao W, Gao ZC, Wang GF, Ruan LX, Wang WH, Ye J, Cao HF, Li XW, Zhang WH, Fang XC, He J, Liang WF, Xie J, Zeng M, et al. (2013) Clinical findings in 111 cases of influenza A (H7N9) virus infection. N Engl J Med 368:2277–2285

48. Fiers W (2006) A universal vaccine against influenza. Bull Mem Acad R Med Belg 161:237–239

13

Role of γ-glutamyltranspeptidase in the pathogenesis of *Helicobacter suis* and *Helicobacter pylori* infections

Guangzhi Zhang, Richard Ducatelle, Ellen De Bruyne, Myrthe Joosten, Iris Bosschem, Annemieke Smet, Freddy Haesebrouck[*†] and Bram Flahou[*†]

Abstract

Helicobacter (*H.*) *suis* can colonize the stomach of pigs as well as humans, causing chronic gastritis and other gastric pathological changes including gastric ulceration and mucosa-associated lymphoid tissue (MALT) lymphoma. Recently, a virulence factor of *H. suis*, γ-glutamyl transpeptidase (GGT), has been demonstrated to play an important role in the induction of human gastric epithelial cell death and modulation of lymphocyte proliferation depending on glutamine and glutathione catabolism. In the present study, the relevance of GGT in the pathogenesis of *H. suis* infection was studied in mouse and Mongolian gerbil models. In addition, the relative importance of *H. suis* GGT was compared with that of the *H. pylori* GGT. A significant and different contribution of the GGT of *H. suis* and *H. pylori* was seen in terms of bacterial colonization, inflammation and the evoked immune response. In contrast to *H. pylori*Δ*ggt* strains, *H. suis*Δ*ggt* strains were capable of colonizing the stomach at levels comparable to WT strains, although they induced significantly less overall gastric inflammation in mice. This was characterized by lower numbers of T and B cells, and a lower level of epithelial cell proliferation. In general, compared to WT strain infection, *ggt* mutant strains of *H. suis* triggered lower levels of Th1 and Th17 signature cytokine expression. A pronounced upregulation of B-lymphocyte chemoattractant CXCL13 was observed, both in animals infected with WT and *ggt* mutant strains of *H. suis*. Interestingly, *H. suis* GGT was shown to affect the glutamine metabolism of gastric epithelium through downregulation of the glutamine transporter ASCT2.

Introduction

Helicobacter (*H.*) *pylori* is a Gram-negative bacterium that colonizes the stomach of more than half of the world's population. Infection with this bacterium can cause gastritis, peptic ulcer disease, gastric adenocarcinoma and mucosa-associated lymphoid tissue (MALT) lymphoma [1-3]. Besides *H. pylori*, non-*H. pylori* helicobacters (NHPH) have also been detected in the stomach of humans and these bacteria cause similar gastric diseases. The risk of developing gastric MALT lymphoma is higher during NHPH infection compared to infection with *H. pylori* [4-9]. *H. suis* is the most prevalent gastric NHPH in humans. Pigs are the natural host of this bacterium, with prevalences reaching 90% or more [10] and most likely, pigs and possibly also pork are the main sources of human *H. suis* infection [4,11-13].

H. suis infection seems to persist for life, at least in pigs and rodents used as models for human infections [14]. In pigs, infection causes development of gastritis and a decrease in body weight gain. Moreover, the bacterium seems to play a role in the development of ulceration of the non-glandular pars oesophagea [15]. In mice and Mongolian gerbil models of human gastric disease, experimental *H. suis* infection causes severe gastric pathology [4,16,17], including gastritis, parietal cell necrosis and the development of gastric MALT lymphoma-like lesions, resembling the lesions observed in *H. suis*-infected humans.

Previous studies have shown that this bacterium lacks a homologue for several virulence factors of *H. pylori*, such as the *cytotoxin associated genes* pathogenicity island (*cag*-PAI) and the vacuolating cytotoxin (VacA) [18]. We were,

---

* Correspondence: freddy.haesebrouck@ugent.be; bram.flahou@ugent.be
†Equal contributors
Department of Pathology, Bacteriology and Avian Diseases, Faculty of Veterinary Medicine, Ghent University, 9820 Merelbeke, Belgium

however, capable of identifying the γ-glutamyl transpepti-dase (GGT) as an important virulence factor of *H. suis*. This enzyme has been described to cause gastric epithelial cell damage [19] and modulation of lymphocyte proliferation [20] through the interaction of the enzyme with two of its substrates, L-glutamine and reduced glutathione, making it the first identified and investigated *H. suis* virulence determinant.

The role of GGT during *H. pylori* infection *in vivo* has been investigated in mice. Conflicting conclusions have been drawn regarding the importance of GGT for colonization. Some groups have concluded that *H. pylori* GGT is required for persistent infection in mice [21], while others have made contrary conclusions [22]. In addition, there is accumulating evidence that *Helicobacter* GGT is a crucial virulence factor involved in immune evasion and immune tolerance [23-25].

Currently, it is unknown if and how *H. suis* GGT influences the course of *H. suis* infection *in vivo*. The aim of the present study was to extend our previous *in vitro* findings with *H. suis* GGT, and to study the role of this virulence factor in the pathogenesis of *H. suis* infection *in vivo*. At the same time, we aimed at comparing its relative importance with that of the GGT of *H. pylori*. The current experiments were performed in BALB/c mice and outbred Mongolian gerbils, since these animal models have indeed been shown to be valuable tools to investigate the role of *Helicobacter* species in gastric pathology. Typically, in Mongolian gerbils, a more rapid and severe development of gastric lesions can be observed compared to mice [4,26,27].

Material and methods
Animal and bacterial strains
Sixty 4-week-old, female specific-pathogen-free (SPF) BALB/c mice were purchased from Harlan NL (Horst, The Netherlands). Twenty-five 4-week-old, female SPF outbred Mongolian gerbils (Crl:MON) were obtained from Charles River Laboratories (Lille, France).

For *H. suis* infection in mice and Mongolian gerbils, strain HS5cLP was used. This strain has been isolated in 2008 from the stomach of a slaughterhouse pig [28]. For experimental *H. pylori* infection in Mongolian gerbils, strain PMSS1 [29] was used, since this strain has no history of *in vivo* adaptation in mice, in contrast to the mouse-adapted strain SS1. In BALB/c mice, *H. pylori* strain SS1 [29] was used, since strain PMSS1 has previously been demonstrated not to be able to colonize the stomach of BALB/c mice [29].

Construction of isogenic *ggt* mutant strains of *H. suis* and *H. pylori*
An isogenic *H. suis ggt* mutant strain (HS5cLPΔ*ggt*) was prepared as described previously [20]. The isogenic *ggt* mutant strain of *H. pylori* was obtained using the same strategy as for creation of the *H. suis* isogenic *ggt* mutant, except that a kanamycin resistance cassette was used instead of a chloramphenicol resistance cassette [20]. Very briefly, deletion of *ggt* in *H. pylori* SS1 and PMSS1 was introduced by allelic exchange using pBluescript II SK (+) phagemid vector (Agilent Technologies, California, USA) in which ~440 bp of the 5′ –end and ~430 bp of the 3′ –end of the target gene and the kanamycin resistance cassette from plasmid pKD4 [30] were ligated through a PCR-mediated strategy with 2 cycles of inverse PCR and fusion PCR [20]. All primers used for PCR-mediated construction of the recombinant plasmids are shown in Table 1. The resultant plasmid was amplified in XL1-Blue MRF′ *E. coli* (Agilent Technologies) and used as a suicide plasmid in *H. pylori* SS1 and PMSS1 (a kind gift from Sara Lindén and Anne Muller, respectively). The *H. pylori* SS1 *ggt* mutant (SS1Δ*ggt*) and *H. pylori* PMSS1 *ggt* mutant (PMSS1Δ*ggt*)

Table 1 Primers used for construction of the *H. pylori ggt* isogenic mutant strains

Primer name	Sequence (5′- 3′)	Primer use
pBlue linear Fwd 1	GGGGATCCACTAGTTCTAGAGCG	Linearization of plasmid
pBlue linear Rev1	CGGGCTGCAGGAATTCGATATCAAG	Linearization of plasmid
HpGGT-flank_fusion1F	CTTGATATCGAATTCCTGCAGCCCGTAACCGGTAAAATCAACACGGACGC	Amplification *H. pylori ggt* and partial up- and downstream flanking genes
HpGGT-flank_fusion1R	CGCTCTAGAACTAGTGGATCCCCGCGCTCTTATAAAAAGAAGCCGC	Amplification *H. pylori ggt* and partial up- and downstream flanking genes
pBluelinear_Hpggtflank1F	CCAAGGAAAGAATTTTAATCCTATTTAG	Linearization of the recombinant plasmid
pBluelinear_Hpggtflank1R	CTGTTTTCCTTTCAATCAACAATAATC	Linearization of the recombinant plasmid
Hpkana_fusion_1F	ATTATTGTTGATTGAAAGGAAAACAGATGATTGAACAAGATGGATTGC	Amplification kanamycin resistance gene
Hpkana_fusion_1R	CTAAATAGGATTAAAATTCTTTCCTTGGTCAGAAGAACTCGTCAAGAAG	Amplification kanamycin resistance gene
T7 prom3	TAATACGACTCACTATAGGG	Sequencing
M13R	CAGGAAACAGCTATGAC	Sequencing

were obtained by electrotransformation [31] or natural transformation [32] as described previously. Finally, bacteria were selected on columbia agar plates (Oxoid, Basingstoke, UK) with Vitox supplement (Oxoid), 5% (v/v) defibrinated sheep blood (E&O Laboratories Ltd, Bonnybridge, UK), and kanamycin (25 μg/mL). The plates were incubated for 5–9 days. The isogenic *ggt* mutants were verified by a GGT activity assay [19], PCR and nucleotide sequencing.

Culture conditions of bacterial strains

Wild-type (WT) *H. suis* strain HS5cLP was grown for 48 h as described previously [29]. HS5cLPΔ*ggt* bacteria were grown under the same conditions as strain HS5cLP, except that the cultivation plates were supplemented with chloramphenicol (30 μg/mL) as described previously [20].

WT *H. pylori* strains SS1 and PMSS1 were grown on Columbia agar plates containing 5% (v/v) defibrinated sheep blood for 48–72 h at 37 °C under microaerobic conditions as described previously [29]. Subsequently, colonies were picked up and cultured in Brucella broth supplemented with Vitox (Oxoid) and 5% fetal calf serum (HyClone) on a rotational shaker under microaerobic conditions (16 h, 125 rpm). SS1Δ*ggt* and PMSS1Δ*ggt* strains were cultured under the same conditions as the corresponding WT strains on plates supplemented with kanamycin (25 μg/mL).

Experimental design

Upon arrival, sixty BALB/C mice and twenty-five Mongolian gerbils were divided into 5 groups, and the animals were allowed to acclimate to the new environment for 1 week. Animals were inoculated intragastrically 3 times at 48 h intervals. Animals from group 1 and 2 (both mice and Mongolian gerbils) were inoculated with Brucella broth containing 8×10^7 viable bacteria of strains HS5cLP and HS5cLPΔ*ggt*, respectively. Animals in group 3 and 4 were inoculated with Brucella broth containing 3×10^8 viable bacteria of strains SS1 and SS1Δ*ggt* (mice) or 1×10^9 viable bacteria of strains PMSS1 and PMSS1Δ*ggt* (gerbils). Animals in the fifth group were inoculated with Brucella broth and served as uninfected controls. For mice, at 4 weeks, 9 weeks and 6 months post infection (pi), 4 animals from each group were euthanized by cervical dislocation under isoflurane anaesthesia. For Mongolian gerbils, all animals were sacrificed at 9 weeks pi. The stomachs of the animals were resected for further processing as described previously [27,29].

Animal experiments were approved by the Ethical Committee of the Faculty of Veterinary Medicine, Ghent University, Belgium (EC2013/29).

Histopathological examination and immunohistochemistry (IHC)

Three longitudinal strips of gastric tissue from mice and Mongolian gerbils were cut from the oesophagus to the duodenum along the greater curvature. Tissue was fixed in 4% phosphate buffered formaldehyde, processed by standard methods and embedded in paraffin for light microscopy. Five serial sections of 5 μm were cut. The first section was stained with haematoxylin/eosin (H&E) to score the degree of gastritis according to the Updated Sydney System with some modifications [33]. After deparaffinization and rehydration for the remaining sections, heat-induced antigen retrieval was performed in citrate buffer (pH = 6.0). In order to block endogenous peroxidase activity and non-specific reactions, all the slides were incubated with 3% H_2O_2 in methanol (5 min) and 30% goat serum (30 min), respectively. For the differentiation between T and B lymphocytes, CD3 and CD20 antigens were stained on sections two and three, using a polyclonal rabbit anti-CD3 antibody (1/100; DakoCytomation, Glostrup, Denmark) and a polyclonal rabbit anti-CD20 antibody (1/25; Thermo Scientific, Fremont, USA), respectively. These sections were further processed with Envision + System-HPR (DAB) (DakoCytomation) for use with rabbit primary antibodies. On the fourth and fifth section, epithelial cell proliferation and the number of parietal cells were determined by IHC staining, using a mouse monoclonal anti-Ki67 antibody (1/25; Menarini Diagnostics, Zaventem, Belgium) and mouse monoclonal anti-hydrogen potassium ATPase β-subunit (H^+/K^+ ATPase) antibody (1/25 000; Abcam Ltd, Cambridge, UK), respectively. Subsequent visualization was done with Envision + System-HPR (DAB) (DakoCytomation) for use with mouse primary antibodies. Quantification of T cells, B cells and epithelial cells were performed as described previously [4]. Briefly, the numbers of cells belonging to defined cell populations (T cells, B cells, and epithelial cells) were determined by counting the positive cells in five randomly chosen High Power Fields (magnification: × 400), both in the antrum and corpus region.

In order to assess the possible development of pseudo-pyloric metaplasia induced by *Helicobacter* infection, alcian blue-periodic acid-schiff stain staining (AB/PAS) was performed.

Quantification of colonizing bacteria in the stomach of mice and Mongolian gerbils

Strips of gastric tissue containing all regions for mice and separate pieces (antrum and corpus) for Mongolian gerbils were stored in 0.5 mL RNA*later* solution (Ambion, Austin, TE, USA) at –70 °C until RNA and DNA extraction. Quantitative Real-Time PCR (qRT-PCR) was used to determine the number of colonizing bacteria in the gastric tissue as described previously [29,34].

RNA extraction and reverse transcription

qRT-PCR was used to determine gene expression in the gastric tissue from mice and Mongolian gerbils. Total RNA was extracted using the RNeasy Mini Kit (Qiagen, Hilden, Germany) according to the manufacturer's instructions. The concentration of RNA was measured using a NanoDrop spectrophotometer (Isogen Life Science, PW De Meern, Utrecht, The Netherlands). The purity of the RNA was evaluated with the Experion automated electrophoresis system using StdSens RNA chips (Bio-Rad, Hercules CA, USA). The RNA concentration from all samples was adjusted to 1 µg/µL and cDNA was synthesized immediately after RNA purification using the iScript™ cDNA Synthesis Kit (Bio-Rad).

Design and validation of primers and determination of gene expression

The housekeeping genes *H2afz*, *PPIA* and *HPRT* were included as reference genes for mice [29]. For Mongolian gerbils, a set of reference genes was tested based on the fact that they are extensively used in other animal species. Primers were designed based on the conserved regions of *ACTB*, *β-actin*, *RPS18*, *GAPDH*, *HPRT1*, *SDHA* and *UBC* complete or partial coding sequences available for humans, pigs, mice and rats.

The mRNA expression levels of various cytokines (IFN-γ, IL-4, IL-5, IL-17, IL-1β, IL-6, IL-10), previously shown to be differentially expressed during *H. suis* infection, as well as other genes (Foxp3, CXCL13, ASCT2, ATP4a, and ATP4b) were quantified using SYBR Green based RT-PCR with iQ™ SYBR Green Supermix. Reactions were performed using a CFX96 RT PCR System in a C1000 Thermal Cycler (Bio-Rad) as described previously [29]. All reactions were performed in 12 µL volumes containing 0.05 µL of each primer (1.25 pmol/µL), 6 µL iQ™ SYBR Green Supermix, 3.9 µL HPLC water and 2 µL cDNA. The experimental program consisted of 95 °C for 15 min, followed by 40 cycles of denaturation at 95 °C for 20 s, annealing at 60 °C for 30 s, and extension at 72 °C for 30 s. The threshold cycle values (Ct) were normalized to the geometric means of the reference genes and the normalized mRNA levels of all target genes were calculated using the method of $2^{-\Delta\Delta Ct}$ [35].

Due to the unavailability of gene information for Forkhead/winged helix transcription factor (Foxp3) and the chemokine CXC ligand 13 (CXCL13) from Mongolian gerbils, primers were designed based on the conserved regions of Foxp3 and CXCL13 complete or partial coding sequences available for humans, pigs, mice and rats with the same strategy as described above. The mRNA expression levels of Foxp3 and CXCL13 were

determined using the same method as described above. Sequence information of all the primers for mice and for Mongolian gerbils is shown in Tables 2 and 3.

Statistical analysis

Differences in colonization capacity were analyzed using a non-parametric Mann–Whitney *U* test. Differences in lymphocytic infiltration, cytokine expression and IHC analysis were assessed with one-way ANOVA followed by a Bonferroni post hoc test. Statistical analyses were performed using SPSS Statistics 20 software (IBM). Pairwise comparisons were done for each individual time-point and on pooled data using time as stratification factor. *P* values less than 0.05 were considered statistically significant. All data are expressed as mean ± SD. All the figures were created using GraphPad Prism5 software (GraphPad Software Inc., San Diego, CA, USA).

Table 2 List of genes and primers used for qRT-PCR in Mongolian gerbils

Gene	Primer	Sequence (5'- 3')	References
Foxp3	sense	GCCCCTMGTCATGGTGGCA	This study
	antisense	CCGGGCCTTGAGGGAGAAGA	
CXCL13	sense	GAATGGCTGCCCCAAAACTGAA	This study
	antisense	TCACTGGAGCTTGGGGAGTTGAA	
GAPDH	sense	AACGGGAAGCTCACTGGCATG	This study
	antisense	CTGCTTCACCACCTTCTTGATGTCA	
HPRT1	sense	GCCCCAAAATGGTTAAGGTTGCA	This study
	antisense	TCAAGGGCATATCCAACAACAAAC	
RPS18	sense	CGAGTACTCAACACCAACATCGATGG	This study
	antisense	ATGTCTGCTTTCCTCAACACCACATG	
IL-1β	sense	GGCAGGTGGTATCGCTCATC	[64]
	antisense	CACCTTGGATTTGACTTCTA	
IFN-γ	sense	CCATGAACGCTACACACTGCATC	[65]
	antisense	GAAGTAGAAAGAGACAATCTGG	
IL-5	sense	AGAGAAGTGTGGCGAGGAGAGACG	[27]
	antisense	ACAGGGCAATCCCTTCATCGG	
IL-6	sense	GAGGTGAAGGATCCAGGTCA	[66]
	antisense	GAGGAATGTCCTCAGCTTGG	
IL-10	sense	GGTTGCCAAGCCTTATCAGA	[27]
	antisense	GCTGCATTCTGAGGGTCTTC	
IL-17	sense	AGCTCCAGAGGCCCTCGGAC	[64]
	antisense	AGGACCAGGATCTCTTGCTG	
ATP4b	sense	GGGGGTAACCTTGAGACCTGATG	[27]
	antisense	AAGAAGTACCTTTCCGACGTGCAG	
β-actin	sense	TCCTCCCTGGAGAAGAGCTA	[66]
	antisense	CCAGACAGCACTGTGTTGGC	

Table 3 List of genes and primers used for qRT-PCR in mice

Gene	Primer	Sequence (5'- 3')	References
IL-1β	sense	GGGCCTCAA AGGAAAGAATC	[29]
	antisense	TACCAGTTGGGGAACTCTGC	
IFN-γ	sense	GCGTCATTGAATCACACCTG	[29]
	antisense	TGAGCTCATTGAATGCTTGG	
IL-4	sense	ACTCTTTCGGGCTTTTCGAT	[29]
	antisense	AAAAATTCATAAGTTAAAGCATGGTG	
IL-10	sense	ATCGATTTCTCCCCTGTGAA	[29]
	antisense	CACACTGCAGGTGTTTTAGCTT	
IL-17	sense	TTTAACTCCCTTGGCGCAAAA	[29]
	antisense	CTTTCCCTCCGCATTGACAC	
Foxp3	sense	GCCCCTMGTCATGGTGGCA	This study
	antisense	CCGGGCCTTGAGGGAGAAGA	
CXCL13	sense	CTCTCCAGGCCACGGTATT	[67]
	antisense	TAACCATTTGGCACGAGGAT	
ATP4a	sense	TGCTGCTATCTGCCTCATTG	[68]
	antisense	GTGCTCTTGAACTCCTGGTAG	
ATP4b	sense	AACAGAATTGTCAAGTTCCTC	[68]
	antisense	AGACTGAAGGTGCCATTG	
HPRT	sense	CAGGCCAGACTTTGTTGGAT	[29]
	antisense	TTGCGCTCATCTTAGGCTTT	
PPIA	sense	AGCATACAGGTCCTGGCATC	[29]
	antisense	TTCACCTTCCCAAAGACCAC	
H2afz	sense	CGTATCACCCCTCGTCACTT	[29]
	antisense	TCAGCGATTTGTGGATGTGT	

Results

Colonization density

All control animals were negative for *Helicobacter*. Results of infected animals showed that WT *H. suis* can persistently colonize the mouse stomach with colonization levels as high as 5.42×10^4 ($\pm 1.46 \times 10^4$) bacteria/mg gastric tissue even at 6 months pi (Figure 1C). *H. pylori* strain SS1 was shown to colonize the mouse stomach at a much lower bacterial density, being 1.68×10^3 ($\pm 1.73 \times 10^3$) bacteria/mg tissue at 6 months pi (Figure 1C, $p < 0.05$).

Interestingly, *H. suis* strain HS5cLPΔ*ggt* was able to colonize the corpus of the stomach of the mice to a similar extent as the WT strain, and this was observed for all timepoints (Figures 1A-1C). In contrast, *H. pylori* strain SS1Δ*ggt* was shown to have an impaired colonization capacity in mice at all three timepoints (Figures 1A-1C, $p < 0.05$). Similar colonization data were demonstrated in the antrum of *Helicobacter* infected-mice at all three timepoints (data not shown).

Both the HS5cLP and HS5cLPΔ*ggt* strain successfully colonized the antrum and corpus of the stomach of Mongolian gerbils, although colonization rates were much lower in the corpus compared to the antrum. No statistically significant differences were observed between both strains (Figure 1D, $p > 0.05$). *H. pylori* strain PMSS1Δ*ggt* was able to colonize the antrum and corpus of the stomach at similar levels compared to PMSS1 (Figure 1D, $p > 0.05$), although 2 out 5 Mongolian gerbils were negative for the presence of PMSS1Δ*ggt* in the corpus of the stomach (data not shown).

Infection-induced inflammation

All control mice and gerbils showed normal gastric histomorphology at all timepoints. The correlation between inflammation scores and bacterial colonization is displayed in Figure 1.

Compared to mice with WT strain infection, infection with *H. suis* strain HS5cLPΔ*ggt* generally induced significantly less overall inflammation both in the antrum ($p < 0.01$) and corpus ($p < 0.01$), whereas only in the corpus region ($p < 0.01$), infection with *H. pylori* strain SS1Δ*ggt* induced less inflammation, compared to that seen in WT strain infected mice. At 6 months pi, the corpus region in 2 out of 4 mice with HS5cLP infection contained large lymphoid aggregates or lymphoid follicles accompanied by destruction of the normal mucosal architecture (Figure 2A), which was not observed in animals from other groups.

For Mongolian gerbils, infection with HS5cLP or PMSS1 induced severe antrum-dominant gastritis with formation of lymphocytic aggregates in the lamina propria and/or sub-mucosa of the stomach (Figures 1D, 2E, and 2G). No significant differences were observed between the WT and mutant strain of *H. suis* with respect to the inflammatory response induced in gerbils (Figures 1D, 2E and 2F), although all animals infected with strain HS5cLP showed inflammation in the corpus region, whereas this was only the case for some animals infected with HS5cLPΔ*ggt* (data not shown). In one gerbil infected with *H. suis* strain HS5cLP, a pronounced inflammatory response was observed, in which more than 65% of the area in the lamina propria and submucosa of the antrum was densely infiltrated with inflammatory cells, fused lymphoid aggregates and lymphoid follicles (Additional file 1).

Inflammation induced by *H. pylori* strain PMSS1Δ*ggt* in the antrum of gerbils was less severe compared to that seen in WT infected animals ($p < 0.05$) (Figures 1D, 2G and 2H).

Inflammatory cell infiltration

In general, an increase of T cell numbers was observed in the corpus (Figure 3A, $p < 0.05$) of mice infected with *H. suis* strain HS5cLP and *H. pylori* strain SS1 at all three timepoints. Compared to the mice infected with WT *H. suis*, HS5cLPΔ*ggt* induced a lower T cell response in the

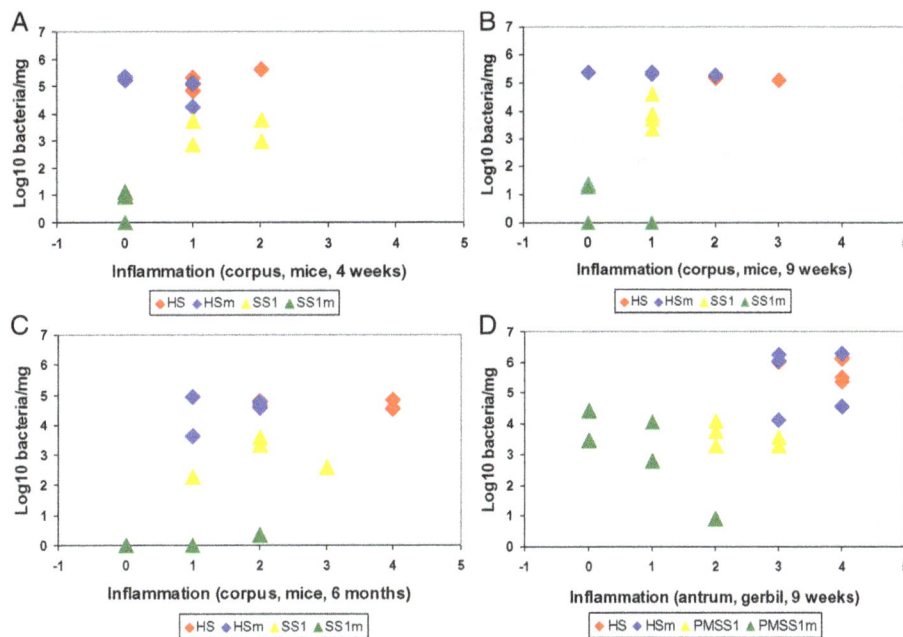

Figure 1 Correlation between bacterial colonization capacity and inflammation score in the stomach of mice and Mongolian gerbils. The colonization capacity is shown as log10 values of *H. suis* or *H. pylori* per mg tissue, determined with qRT-PCR in the corpus of mice **(A-C)** and antrum of Mongolian gerbils **(D)**. 0, no infiltration with mononuclear and/or polymorphonuclear cells; 1, very mild diffuse infiltration with mononuclear and/or polymorphonuclear cells or the presence of one small (20–50 cells) aggregate of inflammatory cells; 2, mild diffuse infiltration with mononuclear and/or polymorphonuclear cells or the presence of one small (50–200 cells) aggregate of inflammatory cells; 3, moderate diffuse infiltration with mononuclear and/or polymorphonuclear cells and/or the presence of 2–4 inflammatory aggregates; 4, marked diffuse infiltration with mononuclear and/or polymorphonuclear cells and/or the presence of at least five inflammatory aggregates. HS vs. HSm: Colonization: $p > 0.05$; Inflammation: $p < 0.05$. SS1 vs. SS1m: Colonization: $p < 0.05$; Inflammation: $p < 0.05$. PMSS1 vs. PMSS1m: Colonization: $p > 0.05$; Inflammation: $p < 0.05$. HS: animals infected with WT *H. suis* srain HS5cLP; HSm: animals infected with *H. suis* strain HS5cLPΔggt; SS1: animals infected with WT *H. pylori* SS1; SS1m: animals infected with *H. pylori* SS1Δggt; PMSS1: animals infected with WT *H. pylori* PMSS1; PMSS1m: animals infected with *H. pylori* PMSS1Δggt.

corpus at 6 months pi ($p < 0.01$). *H. pylori* strain SS1Δggt induced a reduced T cell response in the corpus region ($p < 0.01$) compared to WT infected animals, at both 9 weeks and 6 months pi (Figure 3A). Similar results were observed in the antrum of mice (data not shown).

An increase of B cell numbers was observed in the corpus mucosa of mice infected with strain HS5cLP ($p < 0.01$) and SS1 ($p < 0.01$) at 6 months pi (Figure 3B). Compared to the WT *H. suis* infected mice, HS5cLPΔggt induced a lower B cell response in the corpus region of mice at 6 months pi ($p < 0.05$) and a similar reduction was observed in SS1Δggt infected mice ($p < 0.01$) (Figure 3B).

For Mongolian gerbils, an exact quantification of T and B lymphocytes was not performed since the inflammation was characterized by a marked diffuse infiltration with large numbers of lymphocytes and large inflammatory aggregates. Histopathological analysis showed a pronounced increase of T cell numbers as well as lymphocytic aggregates and follicles in the lamina propria and tunica submucosa in all groups (Figures 4A-4D), although this was most pronounced in the antrum of both WT and mutant *H. suis* infected animals (Figures 4A-4B). T cell

infiltration levels induced by PMSS1Δggt infection were lower compared to that seen in WT *H. pylori* infected animals (Figures 4C and 4D).

WT and mutant strains of *H. suis* induced similar levels of B cell infiltration, mainly in the centre of lymphocytic aggregates/follicles in the antrum (Figures 4E and 4 F). WT *H. pylori* induced mild B cell infiltration in the antrum of gerbils, whereas animals with PMSS1Δggt infection did not show an obvious B cell infiltration (Figures 4G and 4H). A marked proliferation of B cells in germinal centers was observed in gerbils infected with *H. suis* strains HS5cLP (Additional file 2A) and HS5cLPΔggt (Additional file 2B) but not in *H. pylori* infected animals.

Epithelial cell-related changes

For mice, IHC staining did not reveal a clear decrease of the number of parietal cells in the stomach, except for mice infected with *H. suis* strain HS5cLP for 6 months ($p < 0.05$). For Mongolian gerbils, a clear loss of parietal cells was only observed in the transition zone between corpus and antrum in *H. suis* strain HS5cLP (Additional file 3B) and HS5cLPΔggt (Additional file 3C) infected

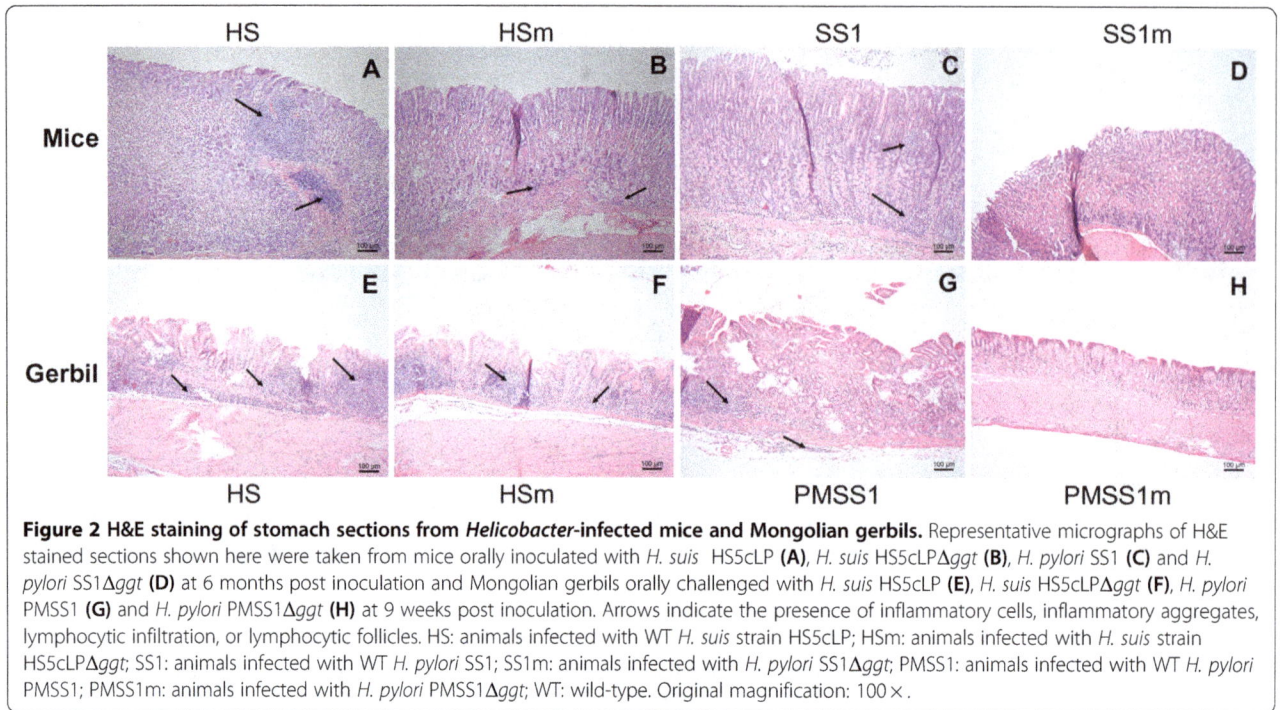

Figure 2 H&E staining of stomach sections from *Helicobacter*-infected mice and Mongolian gerbils. Representative micrographs of H&E stained sections shown here were taken from mice orally inoculated with *H. suis* HS5cLP **(A)**, *H. suis* HS5cLPΔ*ggt* **(B)**, *H. pylori* SS1 **(C)** and *H. pylori* SS1Δ*ggt* **(D)** at 6 months post inoculation and Mongolian gerbils orally challenged with *H. suis* HS5cLP **(E)**, *H. suis* HS5cLPΔ*ggt* **(F)**, *H. pylori* PMSS1 **(G)** and *H. pylori* PMSS1Δ*ggt* **(H)** at 9 weeks post inoculation. Arrows indicate the presence of inflammatory cells, inflammatory aggregates, lymphocytic infiltration, or lymphocytic follicles. HS: animals infected with WT *H. suis* strain HS5cLP; HSm: animals infected with *H. suis* strain HS5cLPΔ*ggt*; SS1: animals infected with WT *H. pylori* SS1; SS1m: animals infected with *H. pylori* SS1Δ*ggt*; PMSS1: animals infected with WT *H. pylori* PMSS1; PMSS1m: animals infected with *H. pylori* PMSS1Δ*ggt*; WT: wild-type. Original magnification: 100×.

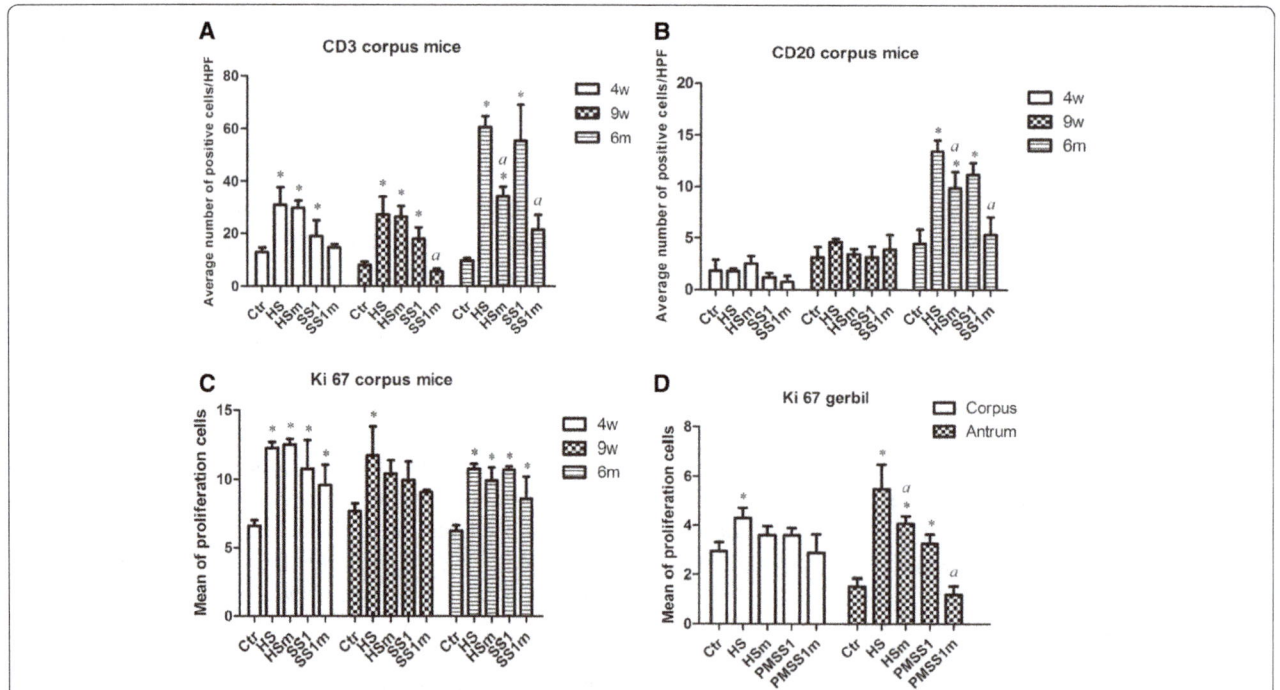

Figure 3 Quantitative analysis of defined cell populations with immunohistochemistry. (A-B) Shown are the average (± SD) numbers of cells/ High Power Field, including T cells (CD3-positive) and B cells (CD20-positive) in the corpus of the stomach of mice. **(C-D)** Shown are the average (± SD) numbers of epithelial cells in five randomly chosen microscopic fields at the level of the gastric pits in the stomach from mice and Mongolian gerbils. An * represents a statistically significant difference ($p < 0.05$) between infected and control groups. An *a* represents a statistically significant difference ($p < 0.05$) between WT *Helicobacter* infected groups and isogenic *ggt* mutant infected groups. Ctr: animals from control group; HS: animals infected with WT *H. suis* strain HS5cLP; HSm: animals infected with *H. suis* strain HS5cLPΔ*ggt*; SS1: animals infected with WT *H. pylori* SS1; SS1m: animals infected with *H. pylori* SS1Δ*ggt*; PMSS1: animals infected with WT *H. pylori* PMSS1; PMSS1m: animals infected with *H. pylori* PMSS1Δ*ggt*; WT: wild-type; 3w: 3 weeks post infection; 9w: 9 weeks post infection; 6 m: 6 months post infection.

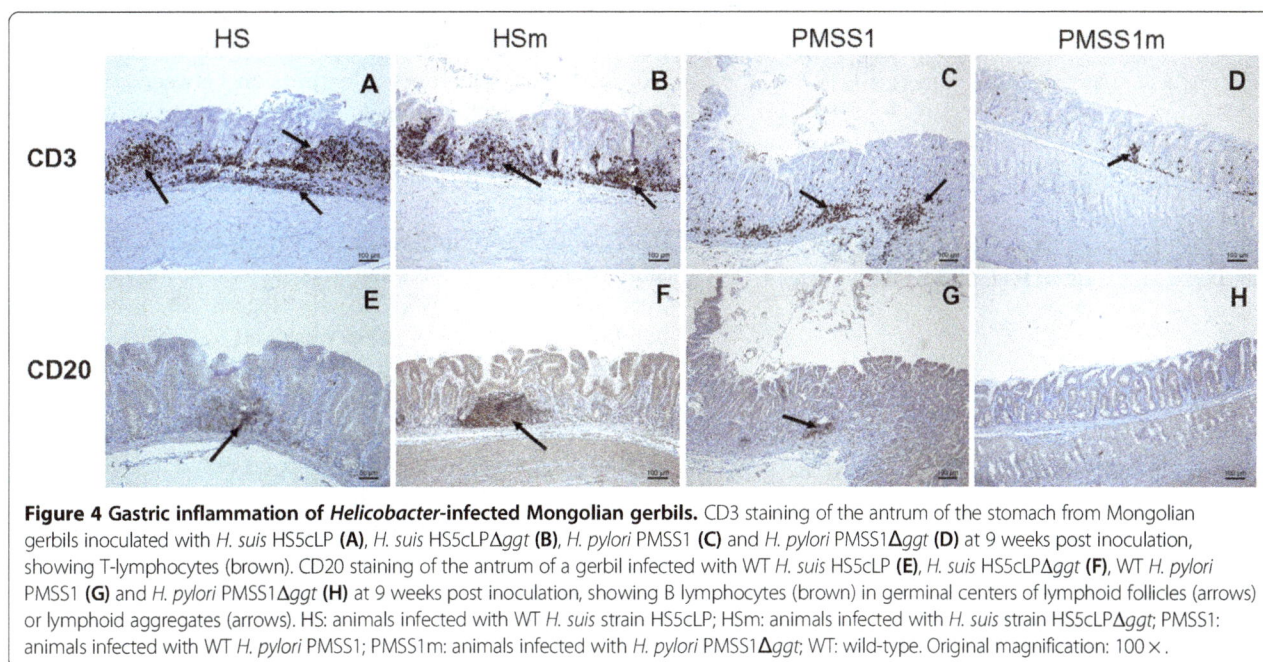

Figure 4 Gastric inflammation of *Helicobacter*-infected Mongolian gerbils. CD3 staining of the antrum of the stomach from Mongolian gerbils inoculated with *H. suis* HS5cLP **(A)**, *H. suis* HS5cLPΔ*ggt* **(B)**, *H. pylori* PMSS1 **(C)** and *H. pylori* PMSS1Δ*ggt* **(D)** at 9 weeks post inoculation, showing T-lymphocytes (brown). CD20 staining of the antrum of a gerbil infected with WT *H. suis* HS5cLP **(E)**, *H. suis* HS5cLPΔ*ggt* **(F)**, WT *H. pylori* PMSS1 **(G)** and *H. pylori* PMSS1Δ*ggt* **(H)** at 9 weeks post inoculation, showing B lymphocytes (brown) in germinal centers of lymphoid follicles (arrows) or lymphoid aggregates (arrows). HS: animals infected with WT *H. suis* strain HS5cLP; HSm: animals infected with *H. suis* strain HS5cLPΔ*ggt*; PMSS1: animals infected with WT *H. pylori* PMSS1; PMSS1m: animals infected with *H. pylori* PMSS1Δ*ggt*; WT: wild-type. Original magnification: 100×.

animals, but not in *H. pylori* PMSS1 or PMSS1Δ*ggt* infected animals (Additional files 3D and 3E).

Data on gastric epithelial cell proliferation in the corpus region are summarized in Figures 3C and 3D. Compared to control mice, an increased epithelial cell proliferation was seen in the corpus (Figure 3C, $p < 0.05$) of HS5cLP infected mice at all timepoints, and a similar increase was observed for SS1 infected mice (Figure 3C, $p < 0.05$). In general, mice infected with *H. suis* and *H. pylori* strains mutated for the GGT revealed somewhat lower epithelial cell proliferation rates compared to WT strain infected mice (Figure 3C), which was, however, not statistically significant. Compared to WT strain infected Mongolian gerbils, both HS5cLPΔ*ggt* ($p < 0.05$) and PMSS1Δ*ggt* ($p < 0.01$) infected animals revealed a significantly lower level of epithelial cell proliferation in the antrum (Figure 3D).

AB/PAS staining showed that *H. suis* infection triggered the development of pseudopyloric metaplasia to a varying degree in the corpus region of mice at 6 months pi (Additional files 4B and 4C). Compared to WT *H. suis* infection, infection with HS5cLPΔ*ggt* in general led to less obvious regions affected by pseudopyloric metaplasia. Infection with WT *H. pylori* also induced pseudopyloric metaplasia to a varying degree in the corpus region of mice at 6 months pi (Additional file 4D), whereas strain SS1Δ*ggt* did not (Additional file 4E).

Cytokine secretion in response to bacterial infection

Data on gene expression levels are presented in Figures 5 and 6.

Primers for housekeeping genes of Mongolian gerbils were chosen based on the specificity and amplification efficiency of the primers, and stable expression levels of the genes. *β-actin*, *RPS18*, *GAPDH* and *HPRT1* were included as the final reference genes for qRT-PCR performed in gerbils.

IFN-γ and IL-1β

In general, only *H. pylori* strain SS1 infection induced a significant up-regulation of the Th1 signature cytokine IFN-γ in mice (Figure 5A, $p < 0.05$). WT and mutant strains of *H. suis* ($p < 0.01$) and *H. pylori* ($p < 0.01$) induced a pronounced upregulation of IFN-γ expression in the antrum of infected Mongolian gerbils (Figure 5C), and no significant differences were observed between WT infected- and mutant infected animals.

No significant differences of IL-1β expression were observed between groups (data not shown). In Mongolian gerbils, similarly increased expression levels of IL-1β were seen in animals infected with WT and mutant strains of *H. suis* (data not shown).

IL-4, IL-5, IL-6, IL-10

In general, compared to control mice, the expression of anti-inflammatory IL-10 was upregulated in *H. suis* strain HS5cLP and HS5cLPΔ*ggt* infected mice (Figure 5A, $p < 0.01$). A very similar expression pattern was observed for Foxp3 (Figure 5B, $p < 0.01$), an important cell marker of CD4$^+$/CD25$^+$ regulatory T cells (Tregs), which are one of the most important cell types secreting IL-10 [36].

In Mongolian gerbils, a clear increase of IL-10 expression, compared to control animals, was demonstrated

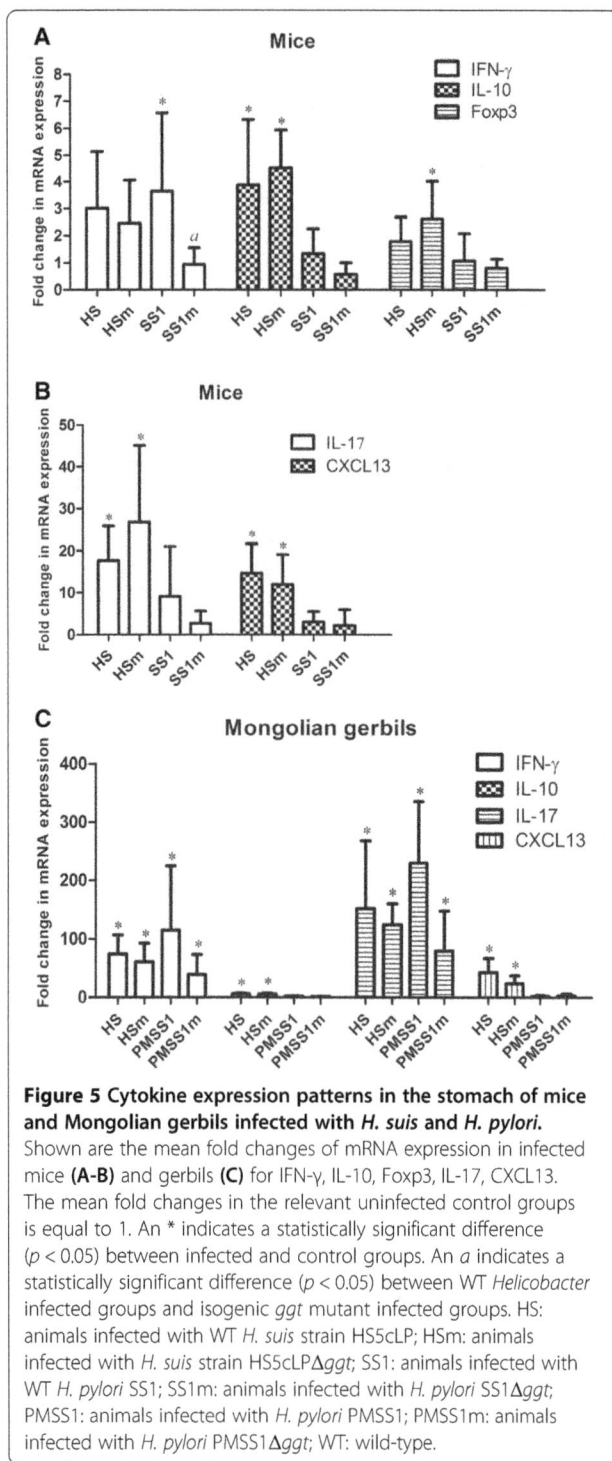

Figure 5 Cytokine expression patterns in the stomach of mice and Mongolian gerbils infected with *H. suis* and *H. pylori*.
Shown are the mean fold changes of mRNA expression in infected mice **(A-B)** and gerbils **(C)** for IFN-γ, IL-10, Foxp3, IL-17, CXCL13. The mean fold changes in the relevant uninfected control groups is equal to 1. An * indicates a statistically significant difference ($p < 0.05$) between infected and control groups. An *a* indicates a statistically significant difference ($p < 0.05$) between WT *Helicobacter* infected groups and isogenic *ggt* mutant infected groups. HS: animals infected with WT *H. suis* strain HS5cLP; HSm: animals infected with *H. suis* strain HS5cLPΔ*ggt*; SS1: animals infected with WT *H. pylori* SS1; SS1m: animals infected with *H. pylori* SS1Δ*ggt*; PMSS1: animals infected with *H. pylori* PMSS1; PMSS1m: animals infected with *H. pylori* PMSS1Δ*ggt*; WT: wild-type.

both in the antrum of gerbils infected with strain HS5cLP ($p < 0.01$) and strain HS5cLPΔ*ggt* (Figure 5C, $p < 0.01$). Compared to control animals, no significant changes of IL-10 and Foxp3 expression levels were observed in animals infected with *H. pylori* (Figures 5A and 5C).

Compared to control animals, an upregulation of IL-6 expression was only demonstrated in gerbils with

HS5cLP and HS5cLPΔ*ggt* infection, but no difference was observed between both groups (data not shown). No significant differences in expression between control animals and infected animals could be demonstrated for IL-4 and IL-5 (data not shown).

IL-17
IL-17 is a Th17 response signature cytokine. A notable increase of IL-17 expression was generally observed in mice infected with WT *H. suis* (Figure 5B, $p < 0.05$). Similar expression levels were observed for HS5cLPΔ*ggt* infected mice (Figure 5B, $p < 0.05$).

In Mongolian gerbils, both WT and mutant *H. suis* and *H. pylori* infection generally induced increased levels of IL-17 expression (Figure 5C, $p < 0.01$). These levels were lower in HS5cLPΔ*ggt* and PMSS1Δ*ggt* infected gerbils compared to WT infected animals, which was, however, not statistically significant (Figure 5C, $p > 0.05$), most likely due to the limited number of animals in each group.

CXCL13
CXCL13 plays an important role during the B-cell homing to follicles in lymph nodes and spleen and formation of gastric lymphoid follicles [37], and it is involved in the pathogenesis of *Helicobacter* infection [14,37]. In general, infection with both HS5cLP and HS5cLPΔ*ggt* induced a marked upregulation of CXCL13 in mice (Figure 5B, $p < 0.01$). Moreover, an even higher increase of CXCL13 expression levels was observed in the antrum of gerbils infected with *H. suis* strains HS5cLP and HS5cLPΔ*ggt* compared to control gerbils (Figure 5C, $p < 0.01$). No statistically significant differences of CXCL13 expression levels were observed between HS5cLP and HS5cLPΔ*ggt* infected animals (Figures 5B and 5C).

Changes of epithelial cell-related factors in the stomach
The H^+/K^+ ATPase is responsible for gastric acid secretion by parietal cells [38]. Compared to uninfected control mice, a clear decrease of *Atp4a* (Figure 6A, $p < 0.05$) and *Atp4b* ($p < 0.05$, data not shown) mRNA expression levels was detected in the stomach of HS5cLP and SS1 infected mice at 9 weeks pi. In addition, a statistically higher expression of *Atp4a* (Figure 6A, $p < 0.05$) and *Atp4b* ($p < 0.05$, data not shown) was observed in HS5cLPΔ*ggt* infected mice compared to WT infected animals.

ASCT2 is an important glutamine transporter for the growth of epithelial cells and other cell types [39]. Compared to control animals, infection with *H. suis* strain HS5cLP resulted in a downregulation of ASCT2 expression in mice at 9 weeks pi (Figure 6B, $p < 0.05$), and infection with *H. suis* strain HS5cLPΔ*ggt* revealed significantly higher ASCT2 expression levels compared to

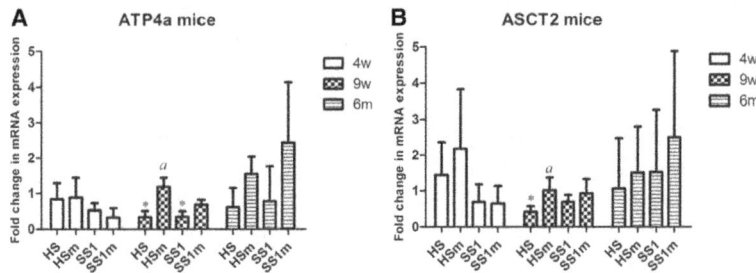

Figure 6 Expression of epithelial cell-associated factors. Shown are the mean fold changes of mRNA expression in infected mice for ATP4a **(A)** and ASCT2 **(B)**. The mean fold changes in the relevant uninfected control groups is equal to 1. An * indicates a statistically significant difference ($p < 0.05$) between infected and control groups. An *a* indicates a statistically significant difference ($p < 0.05$) between WT *Helicobacter* infected groups and isogenic *ggt* mutant infected groups. HS: animals infected with WT *H. suis* strain HS5cLP; HSm: animals infected with *H. suis* strain HS5cLPΔ*ggt*; SS1: animals infected with WT *H. pylori* SS1; SS1m: animals infected with *H. pylori* SS1Δ*ggt*; PMSS1: animals infected with *H. pylori* PMSS1; PMSS1m: animals infected with *H. pylori* PMSS1Δ*ggt*; WT: wild-type; 3w: 3 weeks post infection; 9w: 9 weeks post infection; 6 m: 6 months post infection.

WT *H. suis* infection (Figure 6B, $p < 0.05$). Similar results were observed in *H. pylori* infected mice, without being statistically significant (Figure 6, $p > 0.05$).

Discussion

Although, in the present study, *H. suis* strain HS5cLPΔ*ggt* was shown to be able to colonize the stomach of mice at similar levels compared to WT *H. suis*, it induced significantly less overall inflammation in both corpus and antrum. This suggests that the *H. suis* GGT is involved in the induction and regulation of the inflammatory response, without being an essential factor for colonization. However, in Mongolian gerbils, *H. suis* strain HS5cLPΔ*ggt* was shown to induce only a slightly milder inflammatory response compared to the WT *H. suis* strain. This implies that, besides GGT, *H. suis* harbours other virulence factors or bacterial components, involved in the generation and modulation of the host immune response. In a previous study performed *in vitro*, lysate from HS5cLPΔ*ggt* indeed was shown to still have an effect on the proliferation and function of T lymphocytes, further suggesting the presence of hitherto unidentified factors in *H. suis* that can modulate the host immune and inflammatory response [20]. These factors remain to be investigated in the future.

Interestingly and in contrast to what we observed for *H. suis* lacking GGT, *H. pylori* strains SS1Δ*ggt* and PMSS1Δ*ggt* failed to persistently colonize the stomach of mice and gerbils, highlighting the different relative contributions of *H. pylori* GGT and *H. suis* GGT to the colonization ability in these rodent models. In any case, data from the current study as well as previous studies on the *H. pylori* GGT show that the *H. pylori* GGT confers a benefit to *H. pylori* in terms of its colonization capacity, at least in mice and gerbils, whereas the *H. suis* GGT mainly affects the inflammatory response evoked during *H. suis* infection without having a notable impact on the levels of bacterial colonization. Since *H. suis* lacks

several other virulence determinants of *H. pylori*, such as VacA, the role of *H. suis* GGT in inducing or shaping the host immune response appears to be relatively important.

Our study reveals that *H. suis* infection induces a Th17 response in mice, without a significant upregulation of Th1 cytokines such as IFN-γ. This confirms the results of a previous study in which both Th1- and Th2-prone mouse strains were used [29]. However, the use of Mongolian gerbils in the present study demonstrated that *H. suis* infection can induce a marked upregulation of IFN-γ expression in this animal model, which is accompanied by a more pronounced gastritis compared to that seen in mice. For *H. pylori*, it has been demonstrated that infection induces the expression of IFN-γ in both mice and gerbils, which plays a pivotal role in promoting mucosal inflammation. This in turn contributes to more pronounced gastric mucosal damage [40]. Thus, the higher levels of IFN-γ expression in gerbils infected with *H. suis* most likely contribute to the more pronounced inflammation observed in this animal model compared to that in mice.

IL-10 is considered an important anti-inflammatory cytokine, which is mainly produced by regulatory T cells and dendritic cells [41], and this cytokine has been described to be upregulated in WT *H. suis* infected mice [29]. In the present study, we observed a similar expression pattern for IL-10 and Foxp3 in mice. This may indicate that the secretion of IL-10 mainly occurs through Tregs in the stomach, which needs to be confirmed in future studies. It may be postulated that the higher levels of IL-10 expression in HS5cLPΔ*ggt* infected mice are partially responsible for the attenuated inflammatory response, when compared to WT-infected animals. Previously published data from *in vitro* experiments have shown that *H. pylori* GGT suppresses IL-10 secretion by activated human CD4+ T cells [42], which is supported by our findings. The enzyme has, however, also been described to reprogram DC towards a tolerogenic phenotype, which was shown to depend upon increased secretion of IL-10 [43].

A pronounced upregulation of CXCL13 expression levels was observed in *H. suis*-infected animals, which was shown to be independent of the presence of *H. suis* GGT. Interestingly, a similar upregulation was completely absent in *H. pylori*-infected animals. Possibly, however, a longer experimental period (e.g. 12–18 months) may induce upregulation of CXCL13 expression in the stomach of these animals as well. CXCL13, also named B-cell-attracting chemokine-1 or B-lymphocyte chemoattractant, is a CXC subtype member of the chemokine superfamily [44], and it may play a pivotal role in various immune and inflammatory conditions as well as *H. pylori*-associated gastritis in humans [45,46]. It has been shown that the expression of CXCL13 is significantly upregulated in gastric MALT lymphoma in both humans [47] and mice [48]. The pronounced upregulation of CXCL13 as well as the presence of a clear proliferation of B-cells in germinal centers in the present study seem to be in line with the higher risk to develop gastric MALT lymphoma in humans infected with NHPH compared to *H. pylori* infected patients [5,49-51]. A recent report showed that the formation of gastric lymphoid follicles after challenge with gastric mucosal homogenate from a monkey harbouring *H. suis* was efficiently suppressed by the administration of anti-CXCL13 antibodies [14]. Taken together, this shows that CXCL13 might be one of the key cytokines involved in the development of gastric MALT lymphoma associated with *H. suis* infection.

In previous experiments we have shown that *H. suis* GGT inhibits the proliferation of lymphocytes *in vitro* through the interaction with glutamine [20]. This seems contradictory to the results of the present *in vivo* study showing that animals infected with *H. suis* strain HS5cLPΔ*ggt* exhibited a lower lymphocytic infiltration rate in the gastric mucosa. Besides lymphocytes, however, *H. suis* and its GGT also target gastric mucosal epithelial cells [19]. The uncontrolled loss of epithelial cells by cell death, e.g. necrosis, also triggers the influx of inflammatory cells, in turn promoting the further development of inflammation. In line with some of our previous studies [4], *H. suis* infection indeed affected the function of gastric acid secreting parietal cells, as shown by the decreased expression levels of *Atp4a* and *Atp4b*, and the mutant work demonstrated that *H. suis* GGT indeed plays a role. In addition, the present study indicates that the epithelial (hyper)proliferation observed in WT *H. suis* infected mice is more pronounced than in HS5cLPΔ*ggt* infected mice. This suggests that *H. suis* lacking GGT causes less damage to the epithelium compared to WT bacteria. Probably, this also has an implication on the subsequent development of inflammation in the presence of a more or less damaged epithelium. However, it remains to be determined whether the impact of the *H. suis* GGT on the health of gastric epithelial cells is stronger compared to its direct effects on lymphocytes residing in the deeper tissue layers, including the inhibitory effect on their proliferation.

As mentioned above, infection with *H. suis* strain HS5cLP in mice induced a clear downregulation of *Atp4a* and *Atp4b* expression levels in the stomach at 9 weeks and 6 months pi, and such an effect was not observed in the HS5cLPΔ*ggt* infected animals, showing that *H. suis* GGT contributes to alterations in gastric acid secretion by parietal cells. Previous reports have shown that *H. suis* is often observed near or inside the canaliculi of parietal cells in the stomach of mice, and colonization of *H. suis* is also closely linked with necrosis of parietal cells in mice and Mongolian gerbils [4]. Besides the direct effect of *H. suis* GGT on the acid secretion by parietal cells, altered expression levels of IL-1β may also affect the acid production through multiple pathways [52,53], including a decreased histamine release from enterochromaffin-like cells [54]. The impaired gastric acid secretion and subsequent development of mucous metaplasia observed in the present study, may lead to the development of gastric atrophy, hypochlorhydria and gastric cancer [55,56].

For the first time, we were able to show an effect of *H. suis* GGT on the glutamine metabolism of gastric epithelial cells. This amino acid, targeted by the enzymatic activity of *H. suis* GGT [20], is a major fuel for rapidly dividing cells, including enterocytes, macrophages and lymphocytes [57,58]. It is supportive in improving digestion, absorption, and retention of nutrients through affecting tissue anabolism, stress, and immunity, and it also plays an important role in animal nutrition and health. WT *H. suis* infection was shown to cause a significant downregulation of ASCT2 mRNA in mice, while HS5cLPΔ*ggt* did not show this effect. This suggests that glutamine depletion catalysed by GGT activity at the level of the gastric mucosa resulted in the downregulation of glutamine transporter ASCT2. ASCT2 is a Na^+-dependent, broad-scope neutral amino acid transporter [59,60], which is essential for glutamine uptake by fast growing epithelial cells and tumor cells [39,61,62], and ASCT2 expression levels depend on glutamine availability [63].

In summary, our data show that *H. suis* GGT is not an essential factor for colonization in mice and gerbils, whereas it is involved in the induction of an inflammatory response. This differs to what has been described for the *H. pylori* GGT. In addition, we demonstrated that *H. suis* infection causes a considerable increase of IFN-γ expression levels in Mongolian gerbils, which differs from the situation in mice, where *H. suis* infection is not accompanied by increased expression of this Th1 signature cytokine. This Th1 response was shown to be attenuated in the absence of *H. suis* GGT. CXCL13 expression levels were shown to be upregulated during *H. suis* infection, in contrast to what we observed for *H. pylori* infection, and this was shown not to depend on the presence of *H. suis* GGT. WT *H. suis* infection was shown to suppress expression levels of *Atp4a* and *Atp4b*, involved in gastric acid secretion, and to suppress expression levels of the glutamine transporter ASCT2. These effects on the gastric epithelium were clearly related to the presence of *H. suis* GGT.

Additional files

Additional file 1: H&E staining of the stomach section from a *Helicobacter suis* infected Mongolian gerbil. The vast majority of the antrum of the stomach from this WT *H. suis*-infected animal was densely infiltrated with inflammatory cells, fused lymphoid aggregates and lymphoid follicles. Original magnification: 25 ×.

Additional file 2: Proliferation of B cells in germinal centers. Representative micrographs of a Ki67 staining of the stomach from a WT *H. suis* infected (A) and *H. suis*Δ*ggt* infected gerbil (B) are shown. Proliferating germinal centers were observed in animals from both groups, but mainly in WT *H. suis* infected animals. WT: wild-type. Original magnification: 50× and 200 ×.

Additional file 3: Immunohistochemical staining of the hydrogen potassium ATPase of parietal cells in the stomach mucosa of Mongolian gerbils. Moderate numbers of parietal cells (brown) are present at the transition zone between the corpus and antrum of the stomach of control Mongolian gerbils (A). A clear loss of parietal cells is observed in the transition zone between the corpus and antrum of the stomach from Mongolian gerbils infected with WT *H. suis* strain HS5cLP (B) or *H. suis* strain HS5cLPΔ*ggt* (C) at 9 weeks post inoculation. No clear change of parietal cell numbers is seen in the transition zone between the corpus and antrum of the stomach from Mongolian gerbils infected with WT *H. pylori* PMSS1 (D) or *H. pylori* PMSS1Δ*ggt* (E) at 9 weeks post inoculation. WT: wild-type. Original magnification: 100 ×.

Additional file 4: Determination of mucous metaplasia in the stomach from *Helicobacter*-infected mice. An AB/PAS staining was applied to determine the presence of pseudopyloric metaplasia (arrows) in the stomachs of control mice (A), WT *H. suis* infected mice (B), *H. suis*Δ*ggt* infected mice (C), WT *H. pylori* infected mice (D), and *H. pylori*Δ*ggt* infected mice (E) at 6 months post infection. WT: wild-type; AB/PAS: alcial blue-periodic acid-Schiff stain. Original magnification: 100 ×.

Competing interests

The authors declare that they have no competing interests.

Authors' contributions

GZZ and BF coordinated the study, designed the study, carried out the experiments, analysed the data and drafted the manuscript. FH coordinated the study, designed the study and drafted the manuscript. EDB, MJ, IB and AS contributed to the experiments, and RD participated in the design of this study and drafting of the manuscript. All authors read and approved the final manuscript.

Authors' information

Freddy Haesebrouck and Bram Flahou share senior authorship.

Acknowledgements

This work was supported by grants from China Scholarship Council (CSC) (Grant No. 2010676001) and from the Research Fund of Ghent University, Ghent, Belgium (Grant No. GOA01G00408 and 01SC2411). The authors are grateful to Sofie De Bruyckere and Nathalie Van Rysselberghe for their excellent technical support with qRT-PCR, and we thank Christian Puttevils, Delphine Ameye and Sarah Loomans for their excellent technical help with animal tissue staining, Shaoji Li for the help with animal experiments, and Anja Roevens for the assistance with the experiment.

References

1. Parsonnet J, Friedman GD, Vandersteen DP, Chang Y, Vogelman JH, Orentreich N, Sibley RK (1991) *Helicobacter pylori* infection and the risk of gastric carcinoma. N Engl J Med 325:1127–1131
2. Huang JQ, Sridhar S, Chen Y, Hunt RH (1998) Meta-analysis of the relationship between *Helicobacter pylori* seropositivity and gastric cancer. Gastroenterology 114:1169–1179
3. Ernst PB, Gold BD (2000) The disease spectrum of *Helicobacter pylori*: the immunopathogenesis of gastroduodenal ulcer and gastric cancer. Annu Rev Microbiol 54:615–640
4. Flahou B, Haesebrouck F, Pasmans F, D'Herde K, Driessen A, Van Deun K, Smet A, Duchateau L, Chiers K, Ducatelle R (2010) *Helicobacter suis* causes severe gastric pathology in mouse and mongolian gerbil models of human gastric disease. PLoS One 5:e14083
5. Haesebrouck F, Pasmans F, Flahou B, Chiers K, Baele M, Meyns T, Decostere A, Ducatelle R (2009) Gastric helicobacters in domestic animals and nonhuman primates and their significance for human health. Clin Microbiol Rev 22:202–223
6. Joosten M, Flahou B, Meyns T, Smet A, Arts J, De Cooman L, Pasmans F, Ducatelle R, Haesebrouck F (2013) Case report: *Helicobacter suis* infection in a pig veterinarian. Helicobacter 18:392–396
7. Trebesius K, Adler K, Vieth M, Stolte M, Haas R (2001) Specific detection and prevalence of *Helicobacter heilmannii*-like organisms in the human gastric mucosa by fluorescent in situ hybridization and partial 16S ribosomal DNA sequencing. J Clin Microbiol 39:1510–1516
8. O'Rourke JL, Dixon MF, Jack A, Enno A, Lee A (2004) Gastric B-cell mucosa-associated lymphoid tissue (MALT) lymphoma in an animal model of '*Helicobacter heilmannii*' infection. J Pathol 203:896–903
9. Lee A, Eckstein RP, Fevre DI, Dick E, Kellow JE (1989) Non *Campylobacter pylori* spiral organisms in the gastric antrum. Aust N Z J Med 19:156–158
10. Hellemans A, Chiers K, De Bock M, Decostere A, Haesebrouck F, Ducatelle R, Maes D (2007) Prevalence of '*Candidatus* Helicobacter suis' in pigs of different ages. Vet Rec 161:189–192
11. De Cooman L, Houf K, Smet A, Flahou B, Ducatelle R, De Bruyne E, Pasmans F, Haesebrouck F (2014) Presence of *Helicobacter suis* on pork carcasses. Int J Food Microbiol 187:73–76
12. De Cooman L, Flahou B, Houf K, Smet A, Ducatelle R, Pasmans F, Haesebrouck F (2013) Survival of *Helicobacter suis* bacteria in retail pig meat. Int J Food Microbiol 166:164–167
13. Van den Bulck K, Decostere A, Baele M, Driessen A, Debongnie JC, Burette A, Stolte M, Ducatelle R, Haesebrouck F (2005) Identification of non-*Helicobacter pylori* spiral organisms in gastric samples from humans, dogs, and cats. J Clin Microbiol 43:2256–2260
14. Yamamoto K, Nishiumi S, Yang L, Klimatcheva E, Pandina T, Takahashi S, Matsui H, Nakamura M, Zauderer M, Yoshida M, Azuma T (2014) Anti-CXCL13 antibody can inhibit the formation of gastric lymphoid follicles induced by *Helicobacter* infection. Mucosal Immunol 7:1244–1254
15. De Bruyne E, Flahou B, Chiers K, Meyns T, Kumar S, Vermoote M, Pasmans F, Millet S, Dewulf J, Haesebrouck F, Ducatelle R (2012) An experimental *Helicobacter suis* infection causes gastritis and reduced daily weight gain in pigs. Vet Microbiol 160:449–454
16. O'Rourke JL, Lee A (2003) Animal models of *Helicobacter pylori* infection and disease. Microbes Infect 5:741–748
17. Rogers AB, Fox JG (2004) Inflammation and cancer. I. Rodent models of infectious gastrointestinal and liver cancer. Am J Physiol Gastrointest Liver Physiol 286:G361–G366
18. Vermoote M, Vandekerckhove TT, Flahou B, Pasmans F, Smet A, De Groote D, Van Criekinge W, Ducatelle R, Haesebrouck F (2011) Genome sequence of *Helicobacter suis* supports its role in gastric pathology. Vet Res 42:51
19. Flahou B, Haesebrouck F, Chiers K, Van Deun K, De Smet L, Devreese B, Vandenberghe I, Favoreel H, Smet A, Pasmans F, D'Herde K, Ducatelle R (2011) Gastric epithelial cell death caused by *Helicobacter suis* and

Helicobacter pylori gamma-glutamyl transpeptidase is mainly glutathione degradation-dependent. Cell Microbiol 13:1933–1955

20. Zhang G, Ducatelle R, Pasmans F, D'Herde K, Huang L, Smet A, Haesebrouck F, Flahou B (2013) Effects of *Helicobacter suis* gamma-glutamyl transpeptidase on lymphocytes: modulation by glutamine and glutathione supplementation and outer membrane vesicles as a putative delivery route of the enzyme. PLoS One 8:e77966

21. Chevalier C, Thiberge JM, Ferrero RL, Labigne A (1999) Essential role of *Helicobacter pylori* gamma-glutamyltranspeptidase for the colonization of the gastric mucosa of mice. Mol Microbiol 31:1359–1372

22. McGovern KJ, Blanchard TG, Gutierrez JA, Czinn SJ, Krakowka S, Youngman P (2001) Gamma-Glutamyltransferase is a *Helicobacter pylori* virulence factor but is not essential for colonization. Infect Immun 69:4168–4173

23. Oertli M, Noben M, Engler DB, Semper RP, Reuter S, Maxeiner J, Gerhard M, Taube C, Muller A (2013) *Helicobacter pylori* gamma-glutamyl transpeptidase and vacuolating cytotoxin promote gastric persistence and immune tolerance. Proc Natl Acad Sci U S A 110:3047–3052

24. Salama NR, Hartung ML, Muller A (2013) Life in the human stomach: persistence strategies of the bacterial pathogen *Helicobacter pylori*. Nat Rev Microbiol 11:385–399

25. Schmees C, Prinz C, Treptau T, Rad R, Hengst L, Voland P, Bauer S, Brenner L, Schmid RM, Gerhard M (2007) Inhibition of T-cell proliferation by *Helicobacter pylori* gamma-glutamyl transpeptidase. Gastroenterology 132:1820–1833

26. Wiedemann T, Loell E, Mueller S, Stoeckelhuber M, Stolte M, Haas R, Rieder G (2009) *Helicobacter pylori* cag-Pathogenicity island-dependent early immunological response triggers later precancerous gastric changes in Mongolian gerbils. PLoS One 4:e4754

27. Joosten M, Blaecher C, Flahou B, Ducatelle R, Haesebrouck F, Smet A (2013) Diversity in bacterium-host interactions within the species *Helicobacter heilmannii* sensu stricto. Vet Res 44:65

28. Baele M, Decostere A, Vandamme P, Ceelen L, Hellemans A, Mast J, Chiers K, Ducatelle R, Haesebrouck F (2008) Isolation and characterization of *Helicobacter suis* sp. nov. from pig stomachs. Int J Syst Evol Microbiol 58:1350–1358

29. Flahou B, Deun KV, Pasmans F, Smet A, Volf J, Rychlik I, Ducatelle R, Haesebrouck F (2012) The local immune response of mice after *Helicobacter suis* infection: strain differences and distinction with *Helicobacter pylori*. Vet Res 43:75

30. Van Parys A, Boyen F, Verbrugghe E, Leyman B, Bram F, Haesebrouck F, Pasmans F (2012) *Salmonella* Typhimurium induces SPI-1 and SPI-2 regulated and strain dependent downregulation of MHC II expression on porcine alveolar macrophages. Vet Res 43:52

31. Ferrero RL, Cussac V, Courcoux P, Labigne A (1992) Construction of isogenic urease-negative mutants of *Helicobacter pylori* by allelic exchange. J Bacteriol 174:4212–4217

32. Wang Y, Roos KP, Taylor DE (1993) Transformation of *Helicobacter pylori* by chromosomal metronidazole resistance and by a plasmid with a selectable chloramphenicol resistance marker. J Gen Microbiol 139:2485–2493

33. Stolte M, Meining A (2001) The updated Sydney system: classification and grading of gastritis as the basis of diagnosis and treatment. Can J Gastroenterol 15:591–598

34. Blaecher C, Smet A, Flahou B, Pasmans F, Ducatelle R, Taylor D, Weller C, Bjarnason I, Charlett A, Lawson AJ, Dobbs RJ, Dobbs SM, Haesebrouck F (2013) Significantly higher frequency of *Helicobacter suis* in patients with idiopathic parkinsonism than in control patients. Aliment Pharmacol Ther 38:1347–1353

35. Livak KJ, Schmittgen TD (2001) Analysis of relative gene expression data using real-time quantitative PCR and the 2(−Delta Delta C(T)) method. Methods 25:402–408

36. Josefowicz SZ, Lu LF, Rudensky AY (2012) Regulatory T cells: mechanisms of differentiation and function. Annu Rev Immunol 30:531–564

37. Ansel KM, Ngo VN, Hyman PL, Luther SA, Forster R, Sedgwick JD, Browning JL, Lipp M, Cyster JG (2000) A chemokine-driven positive feedback loop organizes lymphoid follicles. Nature 406:309–314

38. Chow DC, Forte JG (1995) Functional significance of the beta-subunit for heterodimeric P-type ATPases. J Exp Biol 198:1–17

39. McGivan JD, Bungard CI (2007) The transport of glutamine into mammalian cells. Front Biosci 12:874–882

40. Smythies LE, Waites KB, Lindsey JR, Harris PR, Ghiara P, Smith PD (2000) *Helicobacter pylori*-induced mucosal inflammation is Th1 mediated and exacerbated in IL-4, but not IFN-gamma, gene-deficient mice. J Immunol 165:1022–1029

41. Eaton KA, Mefford M, Thevenot T (2001) The role of T cell subsets and cytokines in the pathogenesis of *Helicobacter pylori* gastritis in mice. J Immunol 166:7456–7461

42. Beigier-Bompadre M, Moos V, Belogolova E, Allers K, Schneider T, Churin Y, Ignatius R, Meyer TF, Aebischer T (2011) Modulation of the CD4⁺ T-cell response by *Helicobacter pylori* depends on known virulence factors and bacterial cholesterol and cholesterol alpha-glucoside content. J Infect Dis 204:1339–1348

43. Engler DB, Reuter S, van Wijck Y, Urban S, Kyburz A, Maxeiner J, Martin H, Yogev N, Waisman A, Gerhard M, Cover TL, Taube C, Muller A (2014) Effective treatment of allergic airway inflammation with *Helicobacter pylori* immunomodulators requires BATF3-dependent dendritic cells and IL-10. Proc Natl Acad Sci U S A 111:11810–11815

44. Gunn MD, Ngo VN, Ansel KM, Ekland EH, Cyster JG, Williams LT (1998) A B-cell-homing chemokine made in lymphoid follicles activates Burkitt's lymphoma receptor-1. Nature 391:799–803

45. Galamb O, Gyorffy B, Sipos F, Dinya E, Krenacs T, Berczi L, Szoke D, Spisak S, Solymosi N, Nemeth AM, Juhasz M, Molnar B, Tulassay Z (2008) *Helicobacter pylori* and antrum erosion-specific gene expression patterns: the discriminative role of CXCL13 and VCAM1 transcripts. Helicobacter 13:112–126

46. Nakashima Y, Isomoto H, Matsushima K, Yoshida A, Nakayama T, Nakayama M, Hisatsune J, Ichikawa T, Takeshima F, Hayashi T, Nakao K, Hirayama T, Kohno S (2011) Enhanced expression of CXCL13 in human *Helicobacter pylori*-associated gastritis. Dig Dis Sci 56:2887–2894

47. Mazzucchelli L, Blaser A, Kappeler A, Scharli P, Laissue JA, Baggiolini M, Uguccioni M (1999) BCA-1 is highly expressed in *Helicobacter pylori*-induced mucosa-associated lymphoid tissue and gastric lymphoma. J Clin Invest 104: R49–R54

48. Nobutani K, Yoshida M, Nishiumi S, Nishitani Y, Takagawa T, Tanaka H, Yamamoto K, Mimura T, Bensuleiman Y, Ota H, Takahashi S, Matsui H, Nakamura M, Azuma T (2010) *Helicobacter heilmannii* can induce gastric lymphoid follicles in mice via a Peyer's patch-independent pathway. FEMS Immunol Med Microbiol 60:156–164

49. Stolte M, Kroher G, Meining A, Morgner A, Bayerdorffer E, Bethke B (1997) A comparison of *Helicobacter pylori* and *H. heilmannii* gastritis. A matched control study involving 404 patients. Scand J Gastroenterol 32:28–33

50. Morgner A, Lehn N, Andersen LP, Thiede C, Bennedsen M, Trebesius K, Neubauer B, Neubauer A, Stolte M, Bayerdorffer E (2000) *Helicobacter heilmannii*-associated primary gastric low-grade MALT lymphoma: complete remission after curing the infection. Gastroenterology 118:821–828

51. Joo M, Kwak JE, Chang SH, Kim H, Chi JG, Kim KA, Yang JH, Lee JS, Moon YS, Kim KM (2007) *Helicobacter heilmannii*-associated gastritis: clinicopathologic findings and comparison with *Helicobacter pylori*-associated gastritis. J Korean Med Sci 22:63–69

52. Beales IL, Calam J (1998) Interleukin 1 beta and tumour necrosis factor alpha Inhibit acid secretion in cultured rabbit parietal cells by multiple pathways. Gut 42:227–234

53. Wallace JL, Cucala M, Mugridge K, Parente L (1991) Secretagogue-specific effects of interleukin-1 on gastric-acid secretion. Am J Physiol 261:G559–G564

54. Prinz C, Neumayer N, Mahr S, Classen M, Schepp W (1997) Functional impairment of rat enterochromaffin-like cells by interleukin 1 beta. Gastroenterology 112:364–375

55. Kapadia CR (2003) Gastric atrophy, metaplasia, and dysplasia: a clinical perspective. J Clin Gastroenterol 36:S29–S36

56. Correa P (1992) Human gastric carcinogenesis: a multistep and multifactorial process–first american cancer society award lecture on cancer epidemiology and prevention. Cancer Res 52:6735–6740

57. Rhoads JM, Argenzio RA, Chen W, Rippe RA, Westwick JK, Cox AD, Berschneider HM, Brenner DA (1997) L-glutamine stimulates intestinal cell proliferation and activates mitogen-activated protein kinases. Am J Physiol 272:G943–G953

58. Wu G (2009) Amino acids: metabolism, functions, and nutrition. Amino Acids 37:1–17

59. Utsunomiya-Tate N, Endou H, Kanai Y (1996) Cloning and functional characterization of a system ASC-like Na + −dependent neutral amino acid transporter. J Biol Chem 271:14883–14890

60. Kekuda R, Prasad PD, Fei YJ, Torres-Zamorano V, Sinha S, Yang-Feng TL, Leibach FH, Ganapathy V (1996) Cloning of the sodium-dependent,

broad-scope, neutral amino acid transporter Bo from a human placental choriocarcinoma cell line. J Biol Chem 271:18657–18661

61. Wang Q, Beaumont KA, Otte NJ, Font J, Bailey CG, van Geldermalsen M, Sharp DM, Tiffen JC, Ryan RM, Jormakka M, Haass NK, Rasko JE, Holst J (2014) Targeting glutamine transport to suppress melanoma cell growth. International journal of cancer. Int J Cancer 135:1060–1071

62. Bode BP, Fuchs BC, Hurley BP, Conroy JL, Suetterlin JE, Tanabe KK, Rhoads DB, Abcouwer SF, Souba WW (2002) Molecular and functional analysis of glutamine uptake in human hepatoma and liver-derived cells. Am J Physiol Gastrointest Liver Physiol 283:G1062–G1073

63. Bungard CI, McGivan JD (2004) Glutamine availability up-regulates expression of the amino acid transporter protein ASCT2 in HepG2 cells and stimulates the ASCT2 promoter. Biochem J 382:27–32

64. Sugimoto M, Ohno T, Graham DY, Yamaoka Y (2009) Gastric mucosal interleukin-17 and −18 mRNA expression in Helicobacter pylori-induced Mongolian gerbils. Cancer Sci 100:2152–2159

65. Crabtree JE, Court M, Aboshkiwa MA, Jeremy AH, Dixon MF, Robinson PA (2004) Gastric mucosal cytokine and epithelial cell responses to Helicobacter pylori infection in Mongolian gerbils. J Pathol 202:197–207

66. Sugimoto M, Ohno T, Graham DY, Yamaoka Y (2011) Helicobacter pylori outer membrane proteins on gastric mucosal interleukin 6 and 11 expression in Mongolian gerbils. J Gastroenterol Hepatol 26:1677–1684

67. Lee HS, Park JH, Kang JH, Kawada T, Yu R, Han IS (2009) Chemokine and chemokine receptor gene expression in the mesenteric adipose tissue of KKAy mice. Cytokine 46:160–165

68. Jain RN, Brunkan CS, Chew CS, Samuelson LC (2006) Gene expression profiling of gastrin target genes in parietal cells. Physiol Genomics 24:124–132

14

Monoclonal antibody specific to HA2 glycopeptide protects mice from H3N2 influenza virus infection

Xing Xie, Yan Lin, Maoda Pang, Yanbing Zhao, Dildar Hussain Kalhoro, Chengping Lu and Yongjie Liu*

Abstract

Canine influenza virus (CIV) subtype H3N2 is a newly identified, highly contagious respiratory pathogen that causes cough, pneumonia and other respiratory symptoms in dogs. Data indicate that the virus is responsible for recent clinical cases of dog disease in China. However, therapeutic options for this disease are very limited. In this study, seven monoclonal antibodies (mAbs) against CIV JS/10 (an H3N2 subtype virus) were produced and characterized. Among them, mAb D7, which is specific for the HA2 glycopeptide (gp), induced the highest neutralization titers. The protection provided by mAb D7 was evaluated in BALB/c mice challenged with homologous or heterologous strains of H3N2 influenza virus, including two strains of CIV and one strain of swine influenza virus (SIV). The data show that mAb D7 protected the mice from infection with the three viral strains, especially the homologous strain, which was indicated by the recovery of body weight, reduction of viral load, and reduction of tissue damage. Moreover, the levels of IFN-γ and TNF-α in the lungs, as detected by ELISA, were reduced in the infected mice treated with the mAb D7 compared with those without mAb D7 treatment. Thus, our findings demonstrate, for the first time, that a mAb could reduce the release of IFN-γ and TNF-α associated with tissue damage by CIV infection and that the mAb might be of great therapeutic value for CIV infection.

Introduction

Influenza A virus, a highly contagious pathogen, can infect both birds and mammals. It has undergone significant genetic variation to adapt to different hosts [1]. Its interspecific transmission is achieved by the recombination or direct transfer of genetic material [2]. The first case of dog infection with H3N8 canine influenza virus (CIV) was reported in the USA in 2004 [3,4], followed by a report of CIV in South Korea, which subsequently demonstrated that CIV was able to transmit directly from dog to dog [5,6]. Recently, the first case of H3N2 CIV infection was reported in Guangdong Province in 2010 [7]. Over recent years, infection with H3N2 CIV in dogs has developed from scattered cases to wide distribution across the country [8-10]. Dogs have no natural immunity to this virus, thus a number of preventive and therapeutic measures against CIV have been attempted to control the prevalence of this virus. Among them, vaccination is an important method to prevent and control influenza virus infection [11-13]. Current vaccine research against CIV has made some progress. In 2009, the U.S. Department of Agriculture (USDA) approved a list of vaccines against H3N8 CIV, which could effectively reduce viral shedding [14]. In 2012, the patent for an H3N2 CIV vaccine in South Korea was also approved [15]. Preventive vaccination is historically the primary measure to control influenza virus infection, but it has some limitations [16]. For example, influenza vaccines may not be effective enough to prevent against divergent viral strains, or may be less immunogenic and effective in certain groups, such as the very young, the old, and the immunocompromised [17]. Therefore, it is crucial to develop other measures to protect animals from infection/disease [18]. For example, passive immunity by transferring a specific antibody to a recipient could protect animals from infection [19]. Monoclonal antibodies (mAbs) can neutralize viruses, thus preventing virus attachment to, or fusion with, the host cell [20]. Many studies have demonstrated that mAbs are an effective and preventive treatment against human-origin [21-23] or avian-origin influenza virus infection [11,24,25]. However, to date, there are no neutralizing mAbs available to prevent and control H3N2 CIV infection.

* Correspondence: liuyongjie@njau.edu.cn
College of Veterinary Medicine, Nanjing Agricultural University, Nanjing, China

In this study, we identified seven mAbs against H3N2 CIV, and tested one of them, the D7 mAb, against three different H3N2 subtype virus strains in animal experiments. This is the first description of a neutralizing mAb against H3N2 CIV.

Materials and methods

Virus strains, cells and medium

Three viral strains of the H3N2 subtype, including A/Canine/Jiangsu/06/2010 (JS/10), A/Canine/Guangdong/12/2012 (GD/12) and A/swine/Shandong/3/2005 (SD/05) were used in this study. The GenBank accession numbers of JS/10, GD/12 and SD/05 are JN247616 to JN247623, KF826944 to KF826951 and EU116037 to EU116044, respectively. The three viral strains were adapted to mice by passaging 3 times. They were propagated in 10-day-old specific-pathogen free (SPF) embryonated chicken eggs and stored at −70 °C before use.

Madin-Darby canine kidney (MDCK) cells were cultured in Dulbecco's modified essential medium (DMEM) containing 10% (v/v) fetal bovine serum (Hyclone, tah, USA) and maintained at 37 °C and in a 5% (v/v) CO_2 atmosphere.

Experimental animals

BALB/c mice (6 weeks old, female) were purchased from the Animal Experiment Center, Yangzhou University. All animal experiments complied with the guidelines of the Animal Welfare Council of China, and the Animal Ethics Committee of Nanjing Agricultural University approved the study.

Fifty-percent tissue culture infective dose ($TCID_{50}$) assays

One day before infection, a 96-well dish containing a monolayer of MDCK cells was prepared. The next day, serial dilutions of the three influenza virus strains were made, and the cell monolayers were laterally inoculated; each dilution had three replicates. The cytopathic effect (CPE) was observed daily and the numbers of wells for a virus dilution that showed more than and less than 50% pathological changes were recorded. $TCID_{50}$ titers were calculated in accordance with the Reed-Muench method [26].

Generation of H3N2 mAbs

Canine influenza virus JS/10 was grown in 10-day-old SPF embryonated chicken eggs at 37 °C for 72 h. Allantoic fluids were harvested and the hemagglutination (HA) activity of the allantoic fluids was tested at room temperature using 1% chicken red blood cells (RBC). HA titers more than or equal to 1:64 were selected, and the virus was purified using differential centrifugation and sucrose density gradient centrifugation. Preparation of anti-H3 mAbs followed standard hybridoma technology,

as previously described [27]. Six-week-old female BALB/c mice were injected intracutaneously with 100 μg of purified virus JS/10 using complete Freund's adjuvant (Sigma, Beijing, China) as the primary adjuvant, followed by incomplete Freund's adjuvant. Three days before harvesting the splenocytes, 100 μg of JS/10 were inoculated intravenously. Isolation and screening of the hybridomas was performed as described previously [28]. MAbs were prepared by injecting hybridoma cells into the peritoneal cavities of pristane-primed BALB/c mice. The ascetic fluid was collected after 9–12 days and inactivated at 56 °C for 30 min.

Hemagglutination inhibition (HI) and microneutralization tests

The HI test was performed to assess antibody reactivity against three H3N2 strains, JS/10, GD/12 and SD/05, as previously described [29]. Briefly, 25 μL of serial two-fold dilutions of the purified 5-fold diluted ascetic fluid of the mAb were mixed with 4 HA units of virus in disposable hemagglutination plates and incubated at 37 °C for 30 min. Then, 25 μL of 1% chicken RBC were added to each well and incubated at room temperature for 30 min. To rule out non-specific inhibition, in the HI assay, we used the ascetic fluid produced with the injection of SP2/0 myeloma cells as a negative control. The HI titer was expressed as the reciprocal of the highest serum dilution that completely inhibited hemagglutination of 4 HA units of the virus [30].

Cell-based neutralization assays were performed as previously described [31]. A dose of 100 $TCID_{50}$ of viruses was used in the assays. Supernatants of ascites were tested at a starting dilution of 1:25. Briefly, two-fold dilutions of hybridoma supernatants were mixed with virus suspension containing 100 $TCID_{50}$ of purified H3N2 virus and incubated at 37 °C in a 5% CO_2 incubator for 1 h before their addition to a monolayer of MDCK cells in 96-well plates. One hundred microliters of serum-free DMEM was added to each well and incubation at 37 °C continued for 1 h. The cytopathic effect was observed every 24 h for 48 to 72 h.

Antigen identification of MAbs

To determine the recognized HA domain of the MAbs, we recombinantly expressed the HA, HA1 and HA2 proteins of virus JS/10. The recombinant proteins were subjected to SDS-PAGE under reducing conditions. The proteins were then electro-transferred and immobilized on a nitrocellulose membrane. The membrane was blocked with 5% nonfat milk in phosphate buffered saline (PBS) containing 0.1% Tween 20 (PBST) at 37 °C for 1 h. The membrane was subsequently incubated with the mAb prepared in this study, rinsed in PBST, and incubated with horseradish peroxidase (HRP)-conjugated rabbit anti-mouse immunoglobulin (Bio-Rad, Shanghai,

China), followed by incubation with chromogenic reagents (Tiangen, Beijing, China) [32].

Cross-protection by H3-specific mAb

BALB/c mice were used to determine the protective efficacy of mAb D7. Intranasal inoculations with 10^7 $TCID_{50}$ of virus strains JS/10, GD/12 and SD/05 were given to experimental groups I (n = 45), II (n = 45) and III (n = 45), respectively; the control group received PBS (n = 15). Each experimental group was divided into three subgroups (n = 15 for each subgroup), which were the virus-infected, mAb D7 and irrelevant mAb IgG subgroups, respectively. Mice injected with PBS or irrelevant mAb IgG were considered as blank and negative controls, respectively. For the mAb D7 and irrelevant mAb IgG subgroups, mice were pretreated intraperitoneally with mAb D7 (36 µg/mL) or irrelevant mAb IgG (32 µg/mL) against IgM from Chinese breams developed in our laboratory, at a dose of 20 mg per kg of body weight in 100 µL of PBS before the viral challenge [24,33,34]. After 24 h, mice were challenged with three different H3N2 strains. Mice were observed daily to monitor body weight and clinical symptoms for up to 14 days.

Three mice from each subgroup were euthanized humanely according to a pre-designated schedule. At 2, 4, 6, 10 and 14 days post-infection (dpi), blood samples and tissues including heart, spleen, lung, brain and intestine, as well as feces were collected. Virus shedding was detected by screening fecal samples. Detection of viral RNA was used to determine tissue distribution and virus shedding. Tissues and feces were homogenized in lysates at a ratio of 1:1 (g/mL), respectively, centrifuged at 10 000 × g for 30 min, and the supernatants were collected for the extraction of viral RNA using the Virus Nucleic Acid Extraction Kit II (Geneaid, Taiwan). All tissues collected above, including blood, were used for virus titration; the lung, brain and heart were also used for histological and immunohistochemical analysis at 6 dpi.

Real-time PCR for quantitation of viral loads

Quantitative assays were carried out to measure viral loads in the blood and main organs [33]. Total RNA from tissues and blood samples was reverse transcribed using the PrimeScript™ RT reagent Kit with gDNA Eraser (Perfect Real Time) (Takara, Dalian, China) and then run on an ABI 7500 Real Time PCR System using the SYBR1 Premix Ex TaqTM (Perfect Real Time) kit (Takara). Reverse transcription and cDNA amplification were carried out as described previously [8]. The primers used were designed against a region of the matrix gene: 5′- TCTATCGTCCCATCAGGC/GGTCTTGTCTTTAG CCATTC-3′. A reference standard was prepared using pMD19-T Simple Vector (50 ng/µL; Takara) that contained

the corresponding target virus sequences. A series of eight 10-fold dilutions equivalent to 1×10^3–1×10^{10} copies per reaction were prepared to generate calibration curves and were run in parallel with the test samples [35]. RNA of the amount of the two avian-origin CIV and human-origin influenza viruses was calculated from the standard curve by real-time RT-PCR. The detection limit of this assay was 1120 copies of RNA per mL.

Histopathology and immunohistochemical analysis

After euthanasia at 6 dpi, the heart, brain and lung from the mice inoculated with JS/10, GD/12, SD/05 or PBS were collected and placed into 10% neutral buffered formalin. After fixation the tissues were embedded in paraffin, sectioned at 4 µm and stained with hematoxylin and eosin for histological evaluation. Sequential slides were stained using an immunoperoxidase method [8]. Expression of hemagglutinin in tissues was examined by immunohistochemical staining of histological sections. In brief, sections were blocked with 1% bovine serum albumin/PBS, stained with mAb D7 at a dilution of 1:5000 for one hour at 37 °C, followed by biotin conjugated goat anti-mouse immunoglobulin (Bio-Rad) at a dilution of 1:200 for 30 min at 37 °C. The sections were subsequently incubated with HRP conjugated streptavidin (Bio-Rad) at 37 °C for 30 min. Sections were then developed with HRP-DAB chromogenic substrate kit (Tiangen) for 10 min and counterstained with hematoxylin. The lungs were assigned a grade of 0 to 3 based on the histological character of the lesions. Score criteria of different grades were in accordance with a previous study [36].

Measurement of cytokines

We further investigated if there was a correlation between severe disease and inflammatory cytokine production in virus-challenged mice, and ascertained whether passive immunization with antibodies affected the levels of cytokines involved in defense against three different influenza virus infections. Sections of the lungs (alternating right and left lungs) from all the mice were homogenized in 1 mL of PBS per 1 g of lung tissue. The homogenates were centrifuged, and the supernatants were frozen at −70 °C until tested. The supernatants were assayed for gamma interferon (IFN-γ) and tumor necrosis factor (TNF-α) using ELISA kits (Sigma-Aldrich, Beijing). The minimum detection limits of such assays were as follows: 25 pg/mL for TNF-α and 10 pg/mL for IFN-γ, as previously determined by the manufacturer.

Statistical analysis

Data were collected and analyzed using MS Excel 2010 and SPSS Statics v20.0 software. Weight loss, viral titers, cytokine levels and histological score were analyzed by analysis of variance (ANOVA), followed by Turkey's multiple comparison test with $P < 0.05$ considered to be a significant difference, while $P < 0.01$ was considered to be statistically extremely significant.

Results

Virus titers

CIV was propagated in MDCK cells and the titers of three viral strains, JS/10, GD/12 and SD/05 were determined to be $10^{7.13}$ TCID$_{50}$/mL, $10^{7.25}$ TCID$_{50}$/mL and 10^8 TCID$_{50}$/mL, respectively.

Characterization of mAbs

After fusion between spleen cells from H3N2 virus-immunized mice and sp2/0 myeloma cells, we obtained seven mAbs against the JS/10 virus. Isotyping tests showed that all of these mAbs were IgG2b isotypes, except for one that was IgG2a. Of the seven mAbs identified, four mAbs reacted with HA. Among these four mAbs, mAb D7 reacted with HA2 and three other mAbs reacted with HA1 (Figure 1), as demonstrated by western blotting. HI and neutralization titers of the seven mAbs showed that mAb D7 had the highest neutralization activity, but had no HI activity (Table 1). Further analysis indicated that mAb D7 could react with virus strains JS/10, GD/12 and SD/05, and produce high

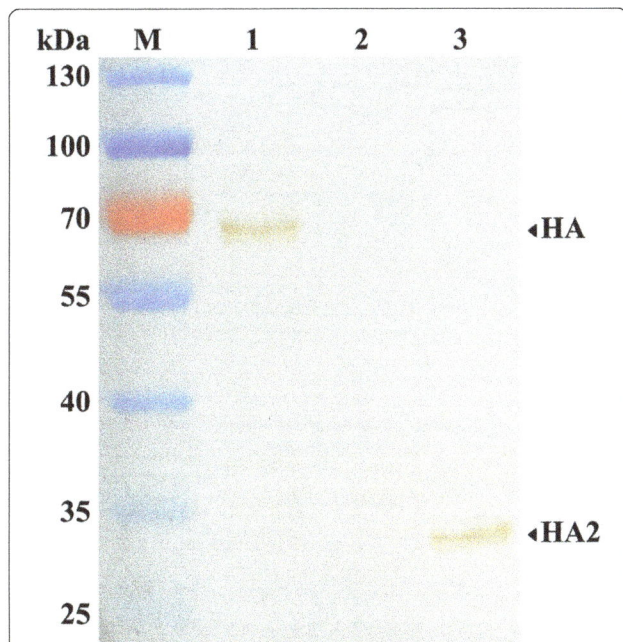

Figure 1 Antigen identification of mAb D7 by western blotting using recombinant proteins HA, HA1 and HA2. Lane M, protein pre-stained mass markers; Lane 1, mAb D7 reacted with expressed viral protein HA; Lane 2, mAb D7 reacted with recombinant protein HA1 (not visualized here); Lane 3, mAb D7 reacted with expressed protein HA2. Viral proteins were identified by DAB staining with HRP-labeled goat anti-mouse secondary antibody.

Table 1 Characteristics of seven monoclonal antibodies (mAbs) direct against JS/10

mAb	Isotype	Neutralization titer	HI titer
B6	IgG2a	1600	320
B7	IgG2b	1600	80
B8	IgG2b	800	40
D7	IgG2b	12800	0
D8	IgG2b	6400	160
G6	IgG2b	400	20
H9	IgG2b	100	20

neutralization activities against the three viral strains, especially against the homologous strain JS/10 (Table 2).

MAb D7 in the treatment of influenza in mice

To access the protective efficacy of mAb D7, we inoculated mice with three different H3N2 strains one day after treatment with mAb D7. Three days after the inoculation, all mice challenged with the three virus strains exhibited clinical signs of infection, including depression, decreased activity and huddling. Similar clinical signs were observed in irrelevant mAb IgG pretreated groups. However, similar to the PBS control group, mice in mAb D7 pretreated groups seemed to be energetic and had a good appetite during the infection.

In terms of body weight, mice challenged with JS/10 after treatment with D7 showed a similar increase in body weight compared with the PBS control group and there was no significant difference between the two groups (Figures 2A, B and C). At 14 dpi, mice treated with mAb D7 showed a body weight increase of nearly 30%. Although the body weights in the virus-infected group and irrelevant mAb IgG group both demonstrated an upward trend, the growth rate was slower than that in the mAb D7 group. The extent of the increase in body weight was significantly slower compared with that of the mAb D7 group at 10, 12 and 14 dpi ($P < 0.05$) (Figure 2A). In the group of mice infected with GD/12, the body weights of the mice in the three experimental groups all showed an upward trend, but the growth rate of the mice treated with mAb D7 was much higher than in the other two groups. In addition, the body weight changes of mice in the mAb D7 group at 10, 12 and 14

Table 2 Characteristics of monoclonal antibody (mAb) D7 direct against virus strains JS/10, GD/12 and SD/05

Virus strains	mAb D7		mAb IgG	
	Neutralization titer	HI titer	Neutralization titer	HI titer
JS/10	12800	0	0	0
GD/12	6400	0	0	0
SD/05	3200	0	0	0

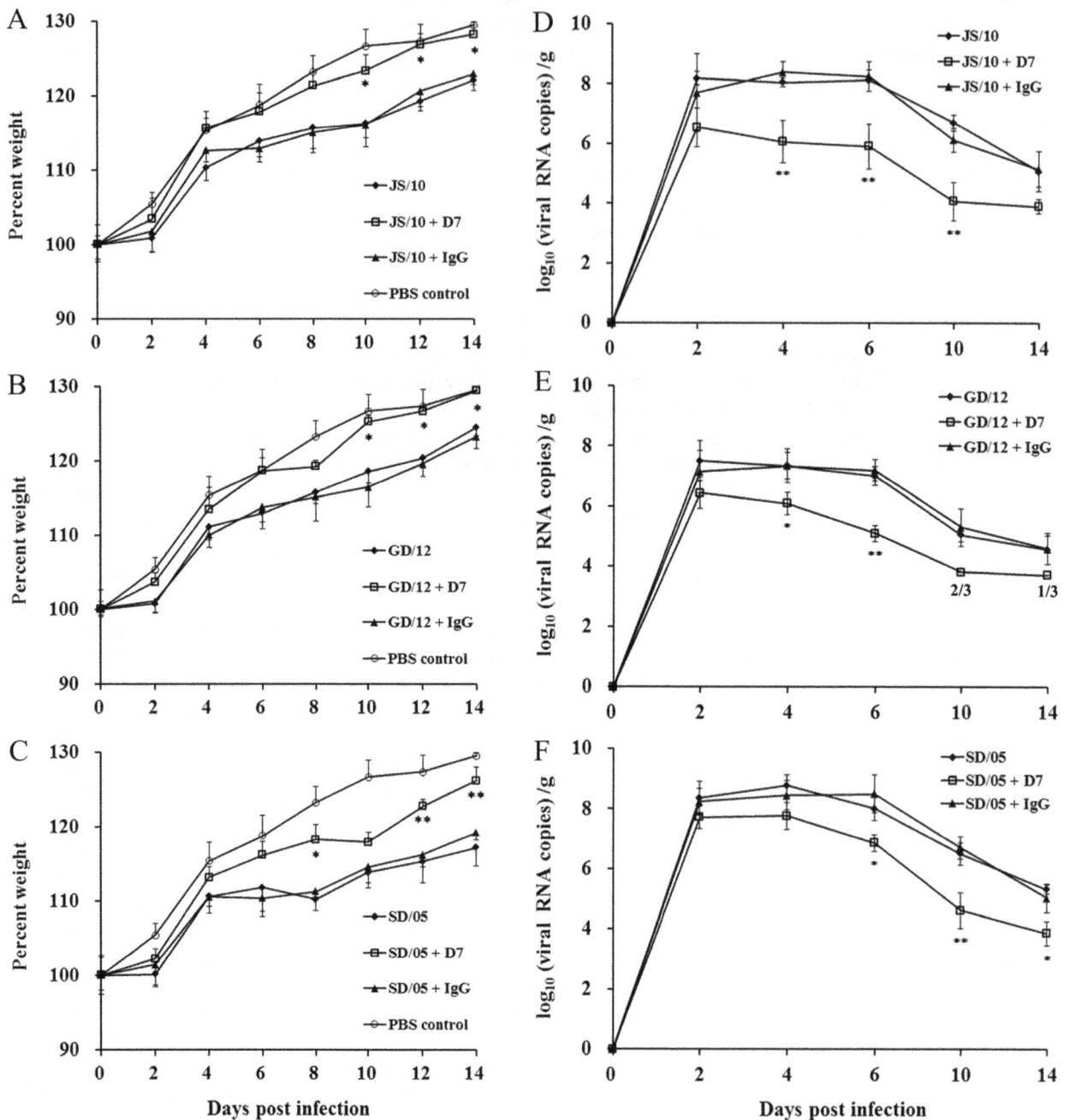

Figure 2 Body weight changes and viral loads in the lungs of mice treated with mAb D7. Three groups of 6-week-old BALB/c mice were challenged with approximately 10^7 $TCID_{50}$ of strains JS/10 **(A, D)**, GD/12 **(B, E)** and SD/05 **(C, F)**, respectively. In each virus group, mice were pretreated with 20 mg/kg of mAb D7, mAb IgG or PBS 1 day before viral challenge. Mice were monitored for body weight loss throughout the 14-day observation period. For body weight change **(A, B, C)**, the results are expressed in terms of percent body weight. *$P < 0.05$, or **$P < 0.01$, indicates a significant difference in weight data for the mAb D7 treated groups compared with the virus-infected groups and irrelevant mAb IgG groups. # $P < 0.05$, indicates a significant difference in weight data for the PBS group compared with the mAb D7 treated group. For viral loads in the lungs **(D, E, F)**, the results are expressed in terms of mean log10 number of copies/g of RNA standard deviation. *$P < 0.05$, or **$P < 0.01$, indicates a significantly different virus titer for the mAb D7 group compared with the other two groups. 2/3, and 1/3, indicate the proportion of the lungs in which virus could be detected.

dpi were significantly different from those of the other two experimental groups ($P < 0.05$). The mice in the mAb D7 group showed weight gains of nearly 30%, which was not significantly different from the PBS control group (Figure 2B). However, after infection with SD/05, mice in the virus-infected group showed a slight decrease in body weight at 6 dpi and mice in the mAb IgG group displayed a slight decline at 8 dpi. By contrast, mice in the mAb D7 group continued to grow at 8 ($P < 0.05$), 12 ($P < 0.01$) and 14 dpi ($P < 0.01$). The growth rate in the mAb D7 group was significantly higher than that in the virus-infected group and mAb IgG group, but slightly lower than in the PBS control group at 14 dpi; mice body weight gain in the mAb group reached approximately 25% (Figure 2C).

Quantitation of viral RNA loads

Real-time PCR was used to evaluate the kinetics of viral RNA loads in the lung, heart, brain, spleen, intestine, feces and blood of the infected mice. The viral titers were expressed as the number of copies of viral RNA. The dynamic changes of viral titers in the lungs of mice in the virus-infected group, mAb D7 group and irrelevant mAb IgG group were similar: peak viral titers were observed at 2, 4 and 6 days after infection, after which the viral titer declined at 10 and 14 dpi (Figures 2D, E and F). However, viral titers in the lungs of mice treated with mAb D7 were significantly lower than in the mice in the other two groups at specific time points. After challenge with JS/10, viral loads in lungs of mice treated with mAb D7 were significantly lower than those in the other two groups at 4, 6 and 10 dpi ($P < 0.01$) (Figure 2D). For strain GD/12, viral titers of the lungs in the mAb D7 group were significantly lower compared with the other two experimental groups at 4 ($P < 0.05$) and 6 dpi ($P < 0.01$). In addition, at 10 and 14 dpi, viral RNA could not be detected in some lung samples (1/3 and 2/3, respectively) in the mAb D7 group (Figure 2E). For virus SD/05, the viral titer of mice in the mAb D7 group was significantly lower than in the other two groups at 6 ($P < 0.05$), 10 ($P < 0.01$) and 14 dpi ($P < 0.05$) (Figure 2F). For mice in the virus-infected group, peak viral titers of three virus strains JS/10, GD/12 and SD/05 were $10^{8.4}$, $10^{7.3}$, $10^{8.5}$ copies/g, respectively, while for mice in the mAb D7 group, peak values were $10^{6.5}$, $10^{6.4}$ and $10^{7.8}$ copies/g, respectively.

Considering that mAb D7 resulted in a significant reduction in viral titers in the lungs of mice infected with three different virus strains at 6 dpi, we chose that time point to determine the viral RNA loads in different tissues and fecal samples. We found that viral loads in collected feces, blood and other tissues at 6 dpi in the mAb D7 group were also lower than those in the other two groups (Figure 3). After mice were challenged with virus JS/10, viral titers of the lung, heart, intestine, feces and blood in the mAb D7 group decreased by 192 ($P < 0.01$), 145 ($P < 0.05$), 20 ($P < 0.05$), 82 ($P < 0.01$) and 26 ($P < 0.01$) fold, respectively, compared to the other two groups (Figure 3A). For mice challenged with virus GD/12, viral titers of the lung, heart, spleen, feces and

blood of mice treated with mAb D7 were found to be reduced by 103 ($P < 0.01$), 30 ($P < 0.01$), 25 ($P < 0.05$), 13 ($P < 0.05$) and 31 ($P < 0.05$) fold in comparison with the other two groups (Figure 3B). For virus SD/05, mAb D7 resulted in a reduction in viral titers of the lung, spleen, intestine, feces and blood by 13 ($P < 0.05$), 21 ($P < 0.05$), 57 ($P < 0.05$), 33 ($P < 0.05$) and 10 ($P < 0.05$) fold, respectively (Figure 3C).

Generally, mAb D7 could reduce viral loads of the three virus strains in the infected mice. Notably, in the virus-infected group and irrelevant mAb IgG group, after infection with virus JS/10, even till 14 dpi, virus RNA was detected in most tissues, while for the mice treated with mAb D7, virus RNA could not be detected in the brain and almost all the other tissues, except for the lung and blood, at 14 dpi (Additional file 1). For virus GD/12, at 10 dpi, viral titers in all the detected tissues were much lower compared with the other two viruses, in all three groups. Viral titers in some tissues were undetectable. Mice in the mAb D7 group showed a much faster virus clearance rate than the other two groups. At 10 dpi, no virus was detected in the intestines and feces of three mice in the mAb D7 group and at 14 dpi, virus was undetectable in all the other tissues in mice treated with mAb D7, except for the lungs in one mouse (Additional file 2). However, in mice infected with SD/05, the virus showed the longest retention time. At 14 dpi, nearly all tissues from mice in virus-infected and irrelevant mAb IgG groups showed detectable virus RNA. Even in the mAb D7 group, all mice showed positive virus RNA in the detected tissues, except for the intestines and feces (Additional file 3).

Histopathological and immunohistochemical findings

To compare the above results with pathological findings in mice infected with three different virus strains, and treated with mAb D7 and irrelevant mAb IgG, we chose the heart, brain and lung from different treatment groups at 6 dpi to perform histopathological and immunohistochemical analysis. All the sampled tissues from mice in the virus-infected group showed significant lesions and viral antigen staining, while those from the control group did not show any lesions. Mice treated with mAb D7 had markedly fewer lesions compared with the virus-infected group (Figure 4). Histological lesions in the mAb IgG group showed similar results with those in the virus-infected group (data not shown).

Regardless of virus strain, the lung interstitial space was obviously widened, and the bronchial lumen became narrow, with the alveolar septum thickened by the infiltration of a number of inflammatory cells (Figures 4A and C). Large areas of the lung appeared consolidated, with symptoms of pulmonary congestion (Figure 4E). Interstitial pneumonia was also obvious, with the alveolar

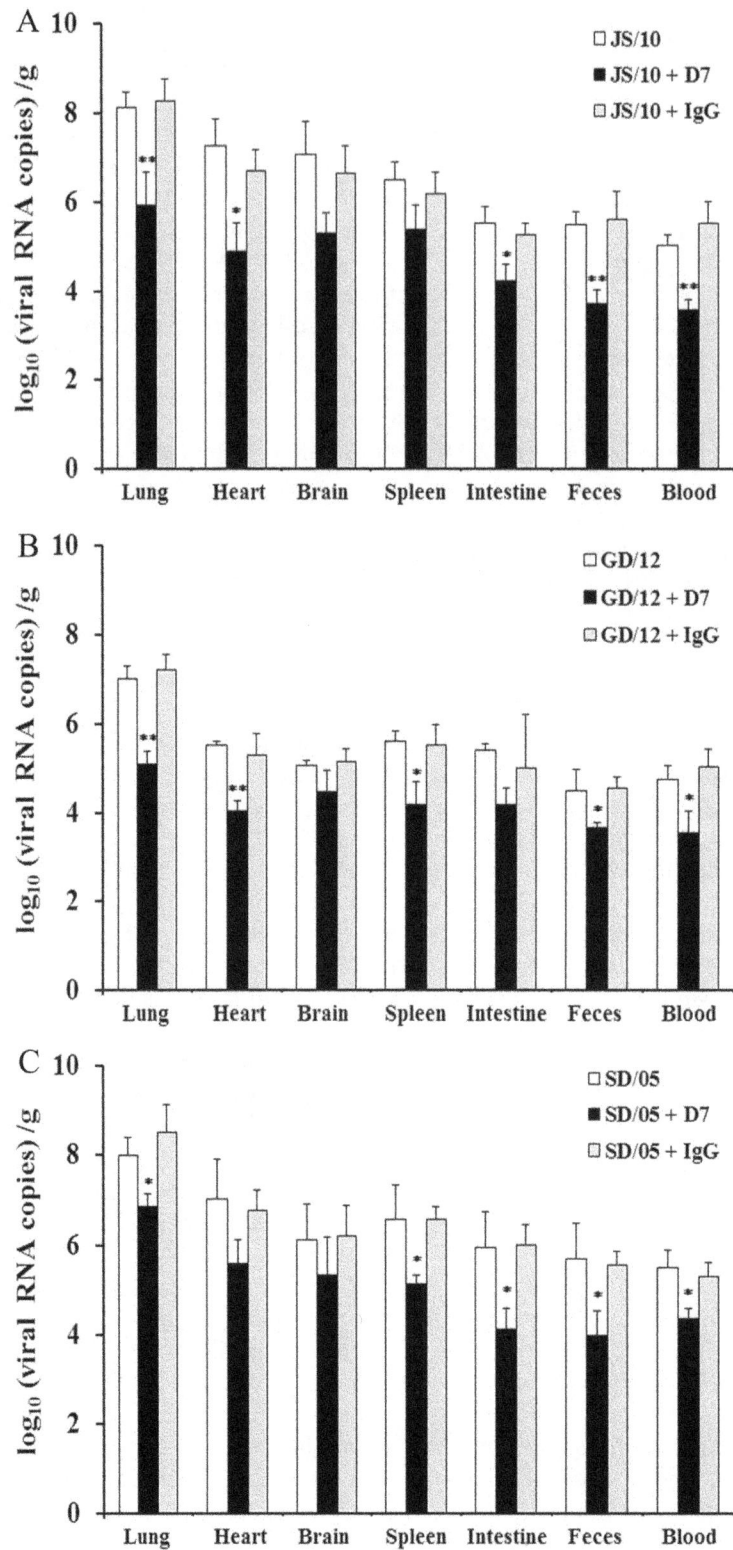

Figure 3 Viral loads in collected tissues and fecal samples of mice at 6 dpi. Mice were pretreated with 20 mg/kg of mAb D7, mAb IgG or PBS 1 day before viral challenge with virus JS/10 **(A)**, GD/12 **(B)** or SD/05 **(C)**, respectively. In each virus group, the lung, heart, brain, spleen, intestine, feces and blood of mice were collected for determination of viral loads using real-time PCR at 6 days post-challenge. *$P < 0.05$, or **$P < 0.01$, indicates significantly different virus titers compared with the other two groups.

septum and proliferation of connective tissue infiltrated with numerous macrophages around the bronchioli and blood vessels (Figures 4C and E). In brief, histological lesions were characterized by multifocal to coalescing reddish consolidation in mice infected with the virus JS/10, GD/12 or SD/05 in both the virus-infected and irrelevant mAb IgG groups. However, the degree of histological lesions observed for SD/05 was the most severe, and GD/12 showed the least severe lesions among these three viruses. Mice treated with mAb D7 showed only mild necrotizing bronchiolitis and ciliated tracheal epithelium with mild hyperplasia (Figure 4F). In addition, very small gaps were observed between the alveoli and there were no excessive amounts of alveolar macrophages in the lung (Figures 4B and D). For virus strain GD/12, mAb D7 demonstrated the best protective efficacy compared with the other two viruses. Mice in the PBS group showed bronchia with a simple ciliated columnar epithelium and the alveolar cavity as a vacuolated thin-walled structure (Figure 4G). Viral antigen staining was present in almost all bronchiolar epithelial cells and some alveolar cells at 6 dpi after virus challenge (Figures 5A, C and E), while mice in mAb D7 showed only a little virus antigen staining surrounding vessels near the alveoli (Figures 5B, D and F). The PBS control group had no viral staining (Figure 5G). Lung grades for degree of injury at 6 dpi are shown in Figure 6. There was significantly less injury to the lungs in the mAb D7 group than in the virus-infected group and mAb IgG group for all virus strains.

Similar to the lung, all mice in the virus-infected groups showed histological lesions in the brain. The extent of histological lesions infected was the most severe with SD/05 and was the least severe for GD/12. The severity of the infection may depend on the differences in virus titer. In the cerebrum, congestion and hemorrhage were evident. Nerve fibers were dissolved and neurons had necrolysis-like vacuoles; glial nodules and neuronophagia were also observed (Figures 4O and Q). Dilation and hyperemia were found in the capillaries (Figure 4S). Moreover, microglial cells and nerve cells showed a satellite phenomenon. The cytoplasm of the neurons was basophilic because of contraction (Figures 4O and Q). Viral antigens could be detected in glial nodules and microglial-gathered areas (Figures 5O, Q, and S). The brains of mice treated with mAb D7 had only mild lesions surrounding microglial cells and nerve cells (Figures 4P and T), and almost no antigen staining was found (Figures 5R and T). The PBS control group showed no histological findings (Figure 4U) and no viral staining (Figure 5U).

In the heart, for all mice in virus-infected groups, the cardiac striated muscle was disordered and full of vacuoles, characterized by myocarditis, and lymphocyte infiltration was observed (Figure 4H). Lymphoproliferation was also found among the muscle fibers (Figure 4J). The nuclei showed pyknosis, with some myocardial cells showing coagulative necrosis (Figures 4J and L), which was consistent with heavy antigen staining (Figures 5H, J and L). No significant differences in microscopic lesions (Figures 4I, K, M and N) and viral antigen staining (Figures 5I, K, M and N) were found between the mAb D7 and PBS groups.

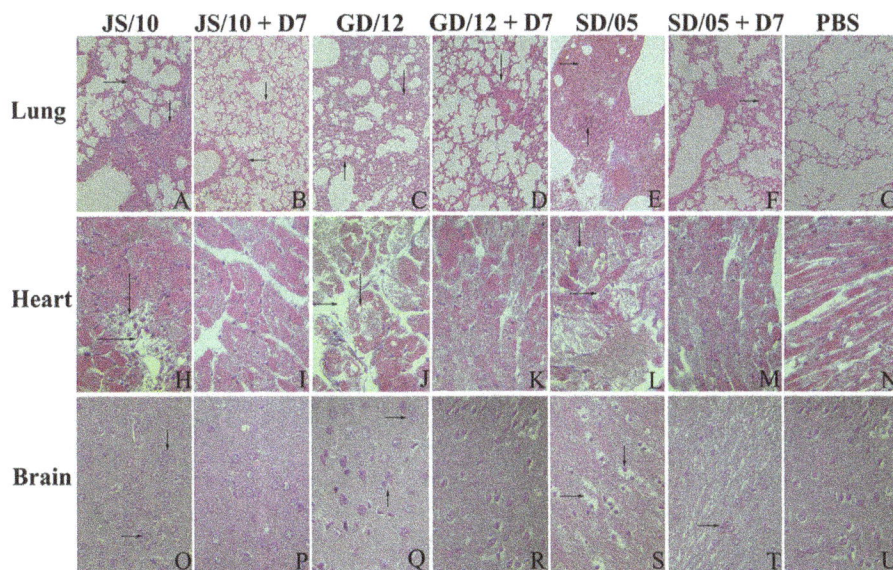

Figure 4 Histopathological changes shown by H&E staining in the lung, heart and brain at 6 dpi. For each virus, selected tissues from mice in the virus-infected group (**A, C, E, H, J, L, O, Q, S**), the mAb D7 treated group (**B, D, F, I, K, M, P, R, T**) and the PBS group (**G, N, U**) are shown, respectively. Short arrows indicate the lesions. All the images are shown at 100 × magnification.

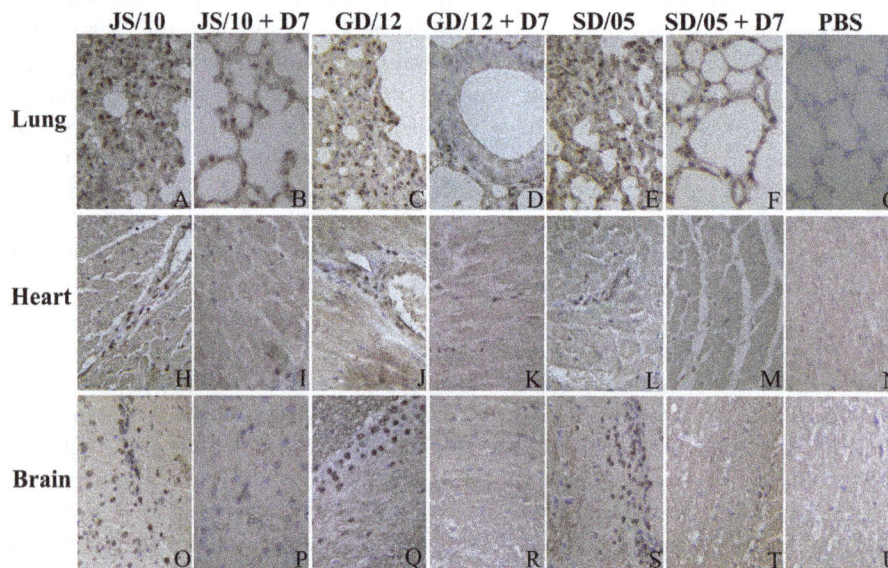

Figure 5 Immunohistochemical detection of influenza viral antigen in the lung, heart and brain at 6 dpi. For each virus, selected tissues from mice in the virus-infected group (**A, C, E, H, J, L, O, Q, S**), the mAb D7 treated group (**B, D, F, I, K, M, P, R, T**) and the PBS group (**G, N, U**) are shown, respectively. All the images are shown at 400 × magnification.

Cytokine response in lung tissue

To gain a better understanding of the effect of CIV on the innate immune response and to ascertain whether passive immunization with monoclonal antibody affected the levels of cytokines, we examined the levels of IFN-γ and TNF-α in the lungs of mice in the virus-infected and mAb D7 groups.

As shown in Figure 7, the level of IFN-γ in response to all three virus strains showed an identical trend, higher at

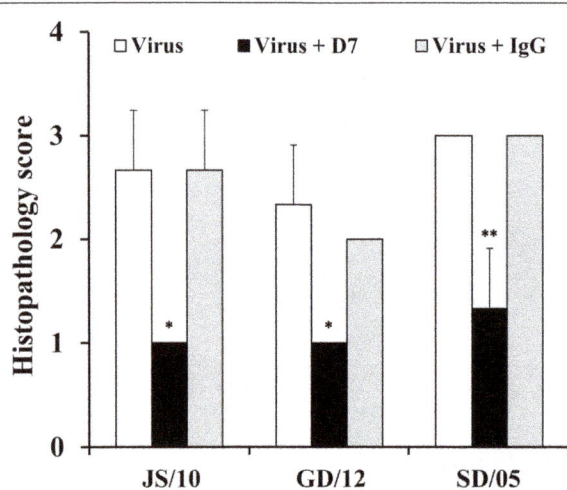

Figure 6 The degree of lung injury after infection with virus JS/10, GD/12 and SD/05 at 6 dpi. The lungs were assigned a grade 0 to 3 based on the histological character of the lesions. *$P < 0.05$, or **$P < 0.01$, indicates a significantly different score for the mAb D7 group compared with the other two groups.

2, 4 and 6 dpi than at 10 and 14 dpi. The IFN-γ levels in mAb D7 group in all three virus strains were significantly lower than the virus-infected group or mAb IgG group, especially at 6, 10 and 14 dpi. However, the cytokine levels differed with the various virus strains.

For virus strain JS/10, the IFN-γ level of all groups reached its peak at 2 dpi, and then exhibited an overall downward trend. The cytokine levels in the mAb D7 group at 6 ($P < 0.01$) and 10 dpi ($P < 0.05$) were significantly lower than that in the virus-infected or mAb IgG group; however, the IFN-γ level did not show any significant difference among the three groups at other time points (Figure 7A). The IFN-γ level in the mAb D7 group returned to normal after 10 dpi, while the other two groups returned to the normal level at 14 dpi.

For virus strain GD/12, the IFN-γ levels of the three experimental groups were significantly higher than in the mice in the PBS group at 2 ($P < 0.01$), 4 ($P < 0.01$) and 6 dpi ($P < 0.01$), sustaining a relatively high level until 10 dpi, after which it decreased. The peak level of IFN-γ in the mAb IgG group was lower compared with the other two virus strains at 2 dpi (Figure 7B). Although the IFN-γ levels in the three experimental groups challenged with GD/12 did not show much difference compared with each other, the IFN-γ level in the mAb D7 group at 10 dpi returned to a normal level, which was significantly lower ($P < 0.05$) compared with the other two groups; all the three groups showed normal levels at 14 dpi.

For virus strain SD/05, this virus induced the largest rise in IFN-γ levels. The level in the SD/05-infected

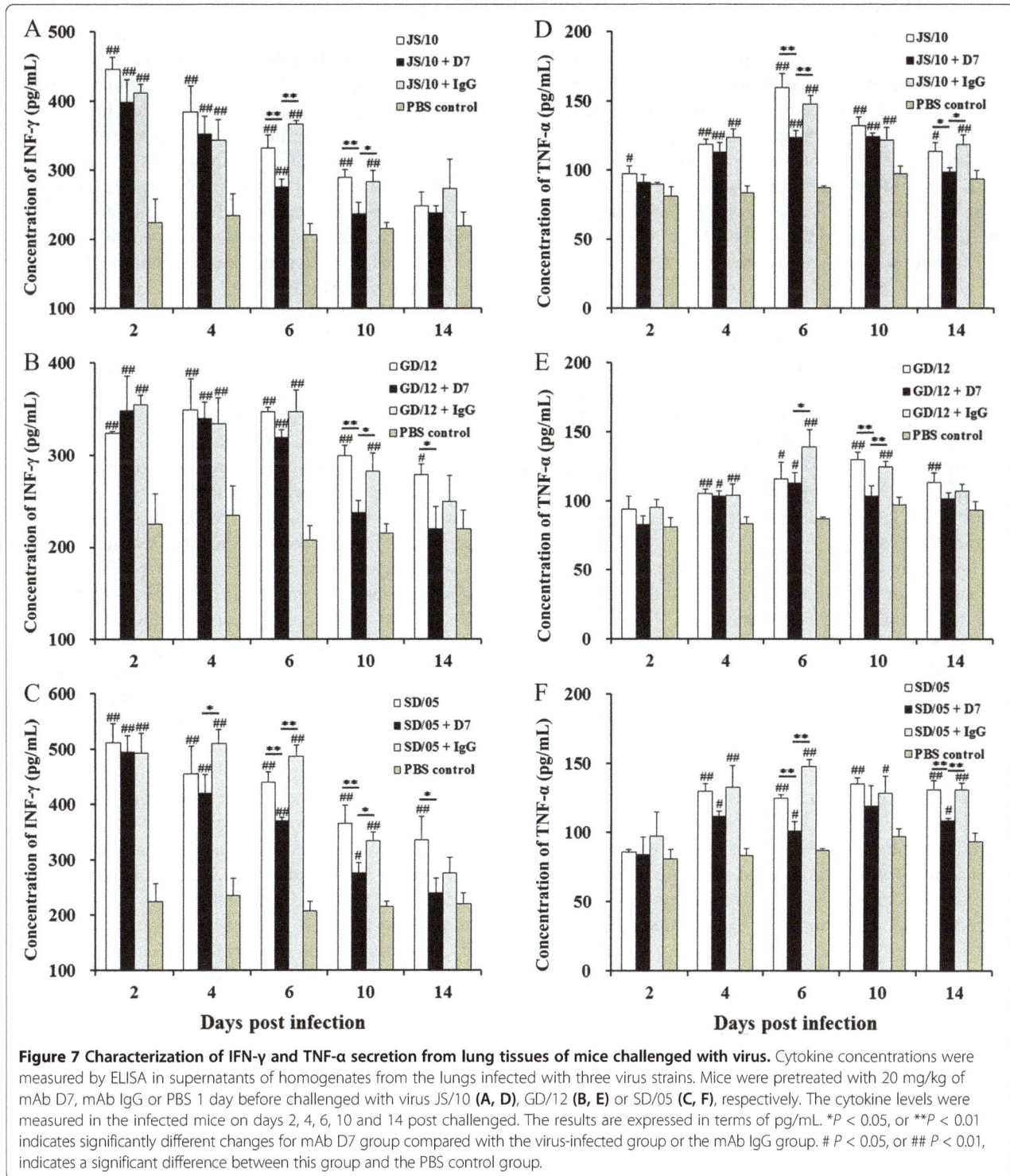

Figure 7 Characterization of IFN-γ and TNF-α secretion from lung tissues of mice challenged with virus. Cytokine concentrations were measured by ELISA in supernatants of homogenates from the lungs infected with three virus strains. Mice were pretreated with 20 mg/kg of mAb D7, mAb IgG or PBS 1 day before challenged with virus JS/10 **(A, D)**, GD/12 **(B, E)** or SD/05 **(C, F)**, respectively. The cytokine levels were measured in the infected mice on days 2, 4, 6, 10 and 14 post challenged. The results are expressed in terms of pg/mL. *$P < 0.05$, or **$P < 0.01$ indicates significantly different changes for mAb D7 group compared with the virus-infected group or the mAb IgG group. # $P < 0.05$, or ## $P < 0.01$, indicates a significant difference between this group and the PBS control group.

group was significantly higher than that of the other two viruses at 2 dpi. In addition, mice in virus-infected and mAb IgG groups both demonstrated the same trend in the period of 2 to 10 dpi ($P < 0.01$), i.e., significant elevation followed by a downward trend (Figure 7C).

Although the IFN-γ level in the mAb D7 group at 2 to 10 dpi was relatively high compared with the PBS group, the IFN-γ levels were significantly lower than those of the other two groups at 6 ($P < 0.01$) and 10 dpi ($P < 0.05$), and then declined to the normal level at 14 dpi.

Changes in TNF-α level were not the same as those for IFN-γ. After infection with the three virus strains, TNF-α levels of mice in all groups were only slightly higher than those of the PBS group at 2 dpi and increased at 4 and 6 dpi. Levels reached their maximum at 10 dpi and decreased at 14 dpi, however, the cytokine level was still higher than that of the control group at 14 dpi which was quite different compared with the IFN-γ level. The increase in TNF-α level was lower compared with the IFN-γ level. In addition, the TNF-α level in the mAb D7 group was apparently lower than the virus-infected group or mAb IgG group, especially at 10 and 14 dpi.

For virus strain JS/10, TNF-α levels in the virus-infected group and mAb IgG group showed a small rise at 2 dpi, reaching its peak at 6 dpi, and then declined; however, the cytokine level was still significantly higher ($P < 0.05$) than that of the PBS group (Figure 7D). The TNF-α level in the mAb D7 group at 14 dpi ($P < 0.05$) was remarkably lower than that in the virus-infected group and mAb IgG group, and decreased to a similar level as the PBS group.

For virus strain GD/12, the TNF-α level of all three experimental groups increased from 2 to 6 dpi, and then returned to normal at 14 dpi (Figure 7E). The TNF-α level of the mAb D7 group at 10 dpi was significantly lower ($P < 0.05$) than in the other two groups, while the cytokine level did not show much difference in these three groups at the other time points.

For virus strain SD/05, the TNF-α levels in the virus-infected group and mAb D7 group were markedly higher than those of the PBS group from 4 to 14 dpi (Figure 7F). Although the TNF-α level in the mAb D7 group was also significantly higher ($P < 0.05$) than the PBS group, except at 2 and 10 dpi, the level in the mAb D7 group was significantly lower ($P < 0.01$) compared with the virus-infected and irrelevant mAb IgG groups at 6 and 14 dpi.

Discussion

H3N2 CIV is a newly identified avian influenza virus (AIV) subtype that can infect dogs and transmit directly from dog to dog [5,8]. CIV infection has been reported in several countries, including South Korea and China [9,10,37]. It is important to develop a set of measures to prevent and control CIV infection in dogs.

Antibody-mediated passive immunity can provide protection against invading pathogens [38,39]. In this study, we developed seven mAbs against JS/10, whose pathogenicity has been characterized both in mice [8] and dogs [40]. Among them, four mAbs reacted with HA. The HA glycoprotein is the primary target of antibodies that confer protective immunity to influenza viruses [41]. Therefore, the generation of neutralizing antibodies

against antigenic sites on the HA glycoprotein is regarded as a criterion for evaluating immunity to influenza viruses and is believed to constitute the main correlate of protection [42,43]. Anti-HA globular head mAbs have potent neutralizing activity against homologous strains, but have very limited breadth of reactivity because of the high variability of amino-acid changes in the HA1 globular head [44]. HA2, which is the HA stalk, however, is a conserved region of HA among all influenza A virus subtypes [33,45] and is responsible for the fusion of the virus and the endosomal membrane during the entry of the virus into the cell [20]. Here, western blotting showed that MAb D7 recognized the HA2 domain of H3, and had highest neutralization activities. Although MAb D7 lacked HI activity, some previous studies reported that a lack of in vitro HI activity of anti-HA2 MAbs does not rule out protective activity in vivo [33,45]. Therefore, we selected the anti-HA2 MAb D7 for further evaluation in regards to protection against different influenza virus strains.

To investigate the protection of mAb D7 against homologous and heterologous strains of H3N2 influenza viruses, we selected three virus strains to perform the challenge experiment in mice, including two strains of CIV (JS/10 and GD/12) and one strain of swine influenza virus (SIV) (SD/05). Considering that almost all H3N2 CIV isolates reported were not lethal to mice or dogs in challenge experiment [5,8,10,15,40], we evaluated the protection efficacy by body weights, viral loads and histological lesions. Body weight loss is the parameter most commonly used to evaluate influenza viral pathogenicity in mice [46]. Our study shows that all three virus strains could remarkably reduce the growth rate of the mice after infection, while pretreatment with mAb D7 helped to control the declination to some extent. From the pathological point of view, the lung, heart and brain in mAb D7 treated groups showed markedly fewer lesions compared with the virus-infected group and mAb IgG group, with all virus strains. The pathological scores of the lungs in mAb D7 group were lower than those in the virus-infected group and mAb IgG group, suggesting that mAb D7 could mitigate the damage caused by influenza virus. These results suggest that mAb D7 could offer a protective effect against the three virus strains.

To further evaluate the effects of the anti-influenza virus mAb, we monitored viral loads by real-time PCR. The mAb D7 decreased the viral loads in the lungs to significantly lower levels, relative to those in the virus-infected group and mAb IgG group. Similar results were also found in other tissues. For JS/10, the virus in the brain and other organs of all three mice treated with mAb D7 had been cleared by 10 dpi, except for the lungs. For virus GD/12, the application of mAb D7 caused virus clearance from the intestine and feces 4 days earlier than that in the other two groups; moreover, there was no detectable virus RNA at 14 dpi. For virus SD/05, a slower rate of clearance of viral load was observed. This virus could persist and be detected in most tissues in the mAb D7 group until 14 dpi, but virus in the intestine and feces had been cleared by 14 dpi. These results indicate that protection against the virus strains provided by mAb D7 might be caused by earlier clearance of the virus from the tissues or shortening the time of virus shedding. A previous study has reported that mAbs could reduce the period of virus clearance [23].

Our study indicates that mAb D7 could provide good protection against challenge with homologous, as well as heterologous, virus strains of H3N2 influenza virus. This finding was in accordance with a previous report [47] that HA2 mAbs are highly cross-reactive among strains of the same subtype, and even within different subtypes. In spite of this, we found that this mAb was relatively less effective against the swine-lineage than canine-lineage H3 virus strains. Sequence analysis of amino acids showed that JS/10 had higher sequence identity to canine-lineage GD/12 (98.6%) than to swine-lineage SD/05 (84.8%), with 3 and 16 different amino acids, respectively, in HA2 (data not shown). The difference in amino acid sequence may affect antigen-antibody recognition. This may explain why the mAb induced by canine-lineage influenza virus strain JS/10 is not strong enough to react against more distantly related strains within the same subtype.

Cytokines are important in establishing an innate immune response, as well as in determining the magnitude of the inflammatory response to influenza virus infection. The most important feature of the mechanism of immune suppression with influenza virus H5N1 is the cytokine storm [11,48]. Here, to gain a better understanding of how virus infection and mAb treatment affected host immune response, we analyzed the levels of IFN-γ and TNF-α in the lung.

An important finding in this study is that the TNF-α levels peaked two days later than IFN-γ levels in all groups. A previous study showed similar results: IFN-γ and TNF-α in the lungs of pigs infected with human H1N1 influenza virus peaked at 3 dpi, and 6 dpi respectively [49]. IFN-γ has important immune-regulatory functions and antiviral activity, and is primarily produced by natural killer (NK) and T cells. NK cells are a major player in innate immune responses. We speculated that early production of IFN-γ during infection probably arises from NK cells, whereas TNF-α functions relatively late in the inflammatory cycle induced by infection, at a time when virus is already being contained and the response is centered on resolution of the inflammation [50,51]. TNF-α in mice challenged by JS/10 and

SD/05 maintained higher levels until 14 dpi. A previous study demonstrated that the depletion of TNF-α in influenza or respiratory syncytial virus-infected animals significantly reduced pulmonary inflammation and cytokine production, without compromising viral clearance [52]. We speculated that the elevated level of TNF-α at 14 dpi might be correlated with the uncleared virus loads in the lungs.

In the present study, three strains of H3N2 CIV were shown to induce elevated levels of cytokines in the lungs. This was in agreement with previous reports on H3N2 CIV [37,53]. During H5N1 influenza virus infection, the elevated pro-inflammatory cytokine response has been proposed as the main cause of the increased severity of the disease [54]. The study of Lee et al. [55] reported that the levels of IFN-γ and TNF-α in the lungs of dogs infected with H3N2 influenza virus increased quickly, while the infected dogs developed severe bronchointerstitial pneumonia accompanied with massive infiltration of immune cells. This result suggests that the dysregulation of chemokines during H3N2 CIV infection might contribute to viral pneumonia characterized by extensive immune cell infiltration. In support of this hypothesis, we observed that elevated levels of cytokines accompanied the clinical manifestations in the CIV infected dogs.

We found that IFN-γ and TNF-α levels in the mAb D7 group were significantly lower than in the virus-infected group or mAb IgG group, while the histopathological findings showed more significant lesions in lungs of mice from the latter two groups than in the mAb D7 group. These observations indicate that mAb D7 treatment may reduce the virus-induced cytokine production and pathological lesions caused by virus infection. The effect is likely to be mediated by inhibition of CIV replication by the mAb. Fritz et al. [50] reported that active influenza virus replication is required for the induction of potent pro-inflammatory, regulatory and chemotactic factors.

Our study and a previous report [55] demonstrate that active replication of CIV in the canine respiratory system results in intense inflammatory responses. Considering that it is important for the host to maintain a balance of the cytokine levels, we speculated that inhibition of the inflammatory cytokine response might offer a therapy for CIV infection. However, Salomon et al. [56] demonstrated that inhibition of the cytokine response during H5N1 influenza virus infection is not sufficient to protect against death, and proposed that therapies targeting the virus would be preferable.

In conclusion, our results suggest that the HA2-specific mAb D7 could contribute to early recovery from influenza infection with different H3N2 virus strains. This mAb will further our understanding of the antigenic properties of H3N2 virus and might contribute to the prevention and control of H3N2 virus epidemic in dogs.

Additional files

Additional file 1: Viral RNA detection in collected samples of mice inoculated with virus strain JS/10. Numbers 1, 2 and 3 represent the three mice euthanized from each group at different dpi. + represents viral loads in terms of mean log10 number of copies/g of RNA. Numbers of +'s represent the magnitude of RNA copies.

Additional file 2: Viral RNA detection in collected samples of mice inoculated with virus strain GD/12. Numbers 1, 2 and 3 represent the three mice euthanized from each group at different dpi. + represents viral loads in terms of mean log10 number of copies/g of RNA. Numbers of +'s represent the magnitude of RNA copies.

Additional file 3: Viral RNA detection in collected samples of mice inoculated with virus strain SD/05. Numbers 1, 2 and 3 represent the three mice euthanized from each group at different dpi. + represents viral loads in terms of mean log10 number of copies/g of RNA. Numbers of +'s represent the magnitude of RNA copies.

Competing interests

The authors declare that they have no competing interests.

Authors' contributions

XX carried out most of the experiments described in the manuscript and wrote the article; YL, MDP participated in the design of the study and performed the statistical analysis; YBZ, DHK, CPL helped with the animal experiments. YJL conceived the study and contributed in its design and coordination. All authors read and approved the final manuscript.

Acknowledgements

This work was supported by the International S&T Cooperation Program of China (ISTCP 2014DFG32770) and the Priority Academic Program Development of Jiangsu Higher Education Institutions (PAPD).

References

1. Ali A, Daniels JB, Zhang Y, Rodriguez-Palacios A, Hayes-Ozello K, Mathes L (2011) Pandemic and seasonal human influenza virus infections in domestic cats: prevalence, association with respiratory disease, and seasonality patterns. J Clin Microbiol 49:4101–4105
2. Neumann G, Kawaoka Y (2006) Host range restriction and pathogenicity in the context of influenza pandemic. Emerg Infect Dis 12:881–886
3. Crawford PC, Dubovi EJ, Castleman WL, Stephenson I, Gibbs EP, Chen L, Smith C, Hill RC, Ferro P, Pompey J, Bright RA, Medina MJ, Johnson CM, Olsen CW, Cox NJ, Klimov AI, Katz JM, Donis RO (2005) Transmission of equine influenza virus to dogs. Science 310:482–485
4. Payungporn S, Crawford PC, Kouo TS, Chen LM, Pompey J, Castleman WL, Dubovi EJ, Katz JM, Donis RO (2008) Influenza A virus (H3N8) in dogs with respiratory disease, Florida. Emerg Infect Dis 14:902–908
5. Song D, Kang B, Lee C, Jung K, Ha G, Kang D, Park S, Park B, Oh J (2008) Transmission of avian influenza virus (H3N2) to dogs. Emerg Infect Dis 14:741–746
6. Song D, Lee C, Kang B, Jung K, Oh T, Kim H, Park B, Oh J (2009) Experimental infection of dogs with avian-origin canine influenza A virus (H3N2). Emerg Infect Dis 15:56–58
7. Li S, Shi Z, Jiao P, Zhang G, Zhong Z, Tian W, Long LP, Cai Z, Zhu X, Liao M, Wan XF (2010) Avian-origin H3N2 canine influenza A viruses in Southern China. Infect Genet Evol 10:1286–1288
8. Lin Y, Zhao Y, Zeng X, Lu C, Liu Y (2012) Genetic and pathobiologic characterization of H3N2 canine influenza viruses isolated in the Jiangsu Province of China in 2009–2010. Vet Microbiol 158:247–258
9. Sun Y, Sun S, Ma J, Tan Y, Du L, Shen Y, Mu Q, Pu J, Lin D, Liu J (2013) Identification and characterization of avian-origin H3N2 canine influenza viruses in northern China during 2009–2010. Virology 435:301–307
10. Teng Q, Zhang X, Xu D, Zhou J, Dai X, Chen Z, Li Z (2013) Characterization of an H3N2 canine influenza virus isolated from Tibetan mastiffs in China. Vet Microbiol 162:345–352
11. Rockman S, Brown LE, Barr IG, Gilbertson B, Lowther S, Kachurin A, Kachurina O, Klippel J, Bodle J, Pearse M, Middleton D (2013) Neuraminidase-inhibiting antibody is a correlate of cross-protection against lethal H5N1 influenza virus in ferrets immunized with seasonal influenza vaccine. J Virol 87:3053–3061
12. Cada DJ (2013) Influenza vaccine progress. Hosp Pharm 48:266
13. Yamazaki T, Ichinohe T (2014) Inflammasomes in antiviral immunity: clues for influenza vaccine development. Clin Exp Vaccine Res 3:5–11
14. Deshpande MS, Jirjis FF, Tubbs AL, Jayappa H, Sweeney D, Spencer SJ, Lakshmanan N, Wasmoen TL (2009) Evaluation of the efficacy of a canine influenza virus (H3N8) vaccine in dogs following experimental challenge. Vet Ther 10:103–112
15. Cho YS, Ha GW, Oh JS, Kang DS, Song D, Kang B, Lee CS. Canine influenza virus and vaccine therefore. United States Patent 2012. Patent N0: US 8,246,962 B2.
16. Friesen RH, Koudstaal W, Koldijk MH, Weverling GJ, Brakenhoff JP, Lenting PJ, Stittelaar KJ, Osterhaus AD, Kompier R, Goudsmit J (2010) New class of monoclonal antibodies against severe influenza: prophylactic and therapeutic efficacy in ferrets. PLoS One 5:e9106
17. Smith NM, Bresee JS, Shay DK, Uyeki TM, Cox NJ, Strikas RA (2006) Prevention and control of influenza: recommendations of the advisory committee on immunization practices (ACIP). MMWR Recomm Rep 55:1–42
18. Greenough TC, Babcock GJ, Roberts A, Hernandez HJ, Thomas WD, Jr, Coccia JA, Graziano RF, Srinivasan M, Lowy I, Finberg RW, Subbarao K, Vogel L, Somasundaran M, Luzuriaga K, Sullivan JL, Ambrosino DM (2005) Development and characterization of a severe acute respiratory syndrome-associated coronavirus-neutralizing human monoclonal antibody that provides effective immunoprophylaxis in mice. J Infect Dis 191:507–514
19. Keller MA, Stiehm ER (2000) Passive immunity in prevention and treatment of infectious diseases. Clin Microbiol Rev 13:602–614
20. Skehel JJ, Wiley DC (2000) Receptor binding and membrane fusion in virus entry: the influenza hemagglutinin. Annu Rev Biochem 69:531–569
21. Rahim MN, Selman M, Sauder PJ, Forbes NE, Stecho W, Xu W, Lebar M, Brown EG, Coombs KM (2013) Generation and characterization of a new panel of broadly reactive anti-NS1 mAbs for detection of influenza A virus. J Gen Virol 94:593–605
22. Gocnik M, Fislova T, Sladkova T, Mucha V, Kostolansky F, Vareckova E (2007) Antibodies specific to the HA2 glycopolypeptide of influenza A virus haemagglutinin with fusion-inhibition activity contribute to the protection of mice against lethal infection. J Gen Virol 88:951–955
23. Tumpey TM, Renshaw M, Clements JD, Katz JM (2001) Mucosal delivery of inactivated influenza vaccine induces B-cell-dependent heterosubtypic cross-protection against lethal influenza A H5N1 virus infection. J Virol 75:5141–5150
24. Chen Y, Qin K, Wu WL, Li G, Zhang J, Du H, Ng MH, Shih JW, Peiris JS, Guan Y, Chen H, Xia N (2009) Broad cross-protection against H5N1 avian influenza virus infection by means of monoclonal antibodies that map to conserved viral epitopes. J Infect Dis 199:49–58
25. Du L, Jin L, Zhao G, Sun S, Li J, Yu H, Li Y, Zheng BJ, Liddington RC, Zhou Y, Jiang S (2013) Identification and structural characterization of a broadly neutralizing antibody targeting a novel conserved epitope on the influenza virus H5N1 hemagglutinin. J Virol 87:2215–2225
26. Reed LJ, Muench H (1938) A simple method for estimating fifty percent endpoints. Am J Hyg 27:493–497
27. Vareckova E, Betakova T, Mucha V, Solarikova L, Kostolansky F, Waris M, Russ G (1995) Preparation of monoclonal antibodies for the diagnosis of influenza A infection using different immunization protocols. J Immunol Methods 180:107–116
28. Peterson EM, Cheng X, Pal S, de la Maza LM (1993) Effects of antibody isotype and host cell type on in vitro neutralization of Chlamydia trachomatis. Infect Immun 61:498–503
29. Wu WL, Chen Y, Wang P, Song W, Lau SY, Rayner JM, Smith GJ, Webster RG, Peiris JS, Lin T, Xia N, Guan Y, Chen H (2008) Antigenic profile of avian H5N1 viruses in Asia from 2002 to 2007. J Virol 82:1798–1807
30. Lee C, Jung K, Oh J, Oh T, Han S, Hwang J, Yeom M, Son D, Kim J, Park B, Moon H, Song D, Kang B (2010) Protective efficacy and immunogenicity of an inactivated avian-origin H3N2 canine influenza vaccine in dogs challenged with the virulent virus. Vet Microbiol 143:184–188
31. Kaverin NV, Rudneva IA, Ilyushina NA, Varich NL, Lipatov AS, Smirnov YA, Govorkova EA, Gitelman AK, Lvov DK, Webster RG (2002) Structure of antigenic sites on the haemagglutinin molecule of H5 avian influenza virus and phenotypic variation of escape mutants. J Gen Virol 83:2497–2505

32. Narasaraju T, Sim MK, Ng HH, Phoon MC, Shanker N, Lal SK, Chow VT (2009) Adaptation of human influenza H3N2 virus in a mouse pneumonitis model: insights into viral virulence, tissue tropism and host pathogenesis. Microbes Infect 11:2–11

33. Prabhu N, Prabakaran M, Ho HT, Velumani S, Qiang J, Goutama M, Kwang J (2009) Monoclonal antibodies against the fusion peptide of hemagglutinin protect mice from lethal influenza A virus H5N1 infection. J Virol 83:2553–2562

34. Wallach MG, Webby RJ, Islam F, Walkden-Brown S, Emmoth E, Feinstein R, Gronvik KO (2011) Cross-protection of chicken immunoglobulin Y antibodies against H5N1 and H1N1 viruses passively administered in mice. Clin Vaccine Immunol 18:1083–1090

35. To KK, Chan KH, Li IW, Tsang TY, Tse H, Chan JF, Hung IF, Lai ST, Leung CW, Kwan YW, Lau YL, Ng TK, Cheng VC, Peiris JS, Yuen KY (2010) Viral load in patients infected with pandemic H1N1 2009 influenza A virus. J Med Virol 82:1–7

36. Alymova IV, Green AM, van de Velde N, McAuley JL, Boyd KL, Ghoneim HE, McCullers JA (2011) Immunopathogenic and antibacterial effects of H3N2 influenza A virus PB1-F2 map to amino acid residues 62, 75, 79, and 82. J Virol 85:12324–12333

37. Jeoung HY, Lim SI, Shin BH, Lim JA, Song JY, Song DS, Kang BK, Moon HJ, An DJ (2013) A novel canine influenza H3N2 virus isolated from cats in an animal shelter. Vet Microbiol 165:281–286

38. Casadevall A, Pirofski LA (2004) New concepts in antibody-mediated immunity. Infect Immun 72:6191–6196

39. Parren PW, Geisbert TW, Maruyama T, Jahrling PB, Burton DR (2002) Pre- and postexposure prophylaxis of Ebola virus infection in an animal model by passive transfer of a neutralizing human antibody. J Virol 76:6408–6412

40. Zeng XJ, Lin Y, Zhao YB, Lu CP, Liu YJ (2013) Experimental infection of dogs with H3N2 canine influenza virus from China. Epidemiol Infect 141:2595–2603

41. Wang TT, Tan GS, Hai R, Pica N, Petersen E, Moran TM, Palese P (2010) Broadly protective monoclonal antibodies against H3 influenza viruses following sequential immunization with different hemagglutinins. PLoS Pathog 6:e1000796

42. Waddington CS, Walker WT, Oeser C, Reiner A, John T, Wilkins S, Casey M, Eccleston PE, Allen RJ, Okike I, Ladhani S, Sheasby E, Hoschler K, Andrews N, Waight P, Collinson AC, Heath PT, Finn A, Faust SN, Snape MD, Miller E, Pollard AJ (2010) Safety and immunogenicity of AS03B adjuvanted split virion versus non-adjuvanted whole virion H1N1 influenza vaccine in UK children aged 6 months-12 years: open label, randomised, parallel group, multicentre study. BMJ 340:c2649

43. Martinez O, Tsibane T, Basler CF (2009) Neutralizing anti-influenza virus monoclonal antibodies: therapeutics and tools for discovery. Int Rev Immunol 28:69–92

44. de Jong JC, Palache AM, Beyer WE, Rimmelzwaan GF, Boon AC, Osterhaus AD (2003) Haemagglutination-inhibiting antibody to influenza virus. Dev Biol 115:63–73

45. Gerhard W, Mozdzanowska K, Zharikova D (2006) Prospects for universal influenza virus vaccine. Emerg Infect Dis 12:569–574

46. Bouvier NM, Lowen AC (2010) Animal models for influenza virus pathogenesis and transmission. Viruses 2:1530–1563

47. Vareckova E, Cox N, Klimov A (2002) Evaluation of the subtype specificity of monoclonal antibodies raised against H1 and H3 subtypes of human influenza A virus hemagglutinins. J Clin Microbiol 40:2220–2223

48. Matthaei M, Budt M, Wolff T (2013) Highly pathogenic H5N1 influenza A virus strains provoke heterogeneous IFN-alpha/beta responses that distinctively affect viral propagation in human cells. PLoS One 8:e56659

49. Kim HM, Lee YW, Lee KJ, Kim HS, Cho SW, van Rooijen N, Guan Y, Seo SH (2008) Alveolar macrophages are indispensable for controlling influenza viruses in lungs of pigs. J Virol 82:4265–4274

50. Fritz RS, Hayden FG, Calfee DP, Cass LM, Peng AW, Alvord WG, Strober W, Straus SE (1999) Nasal cytokine and chemokine responses in experimental influenza A virus infection: results of a placebo-controlled trial of intravenous zanamivir treatment. J Infect Dis 180:586–593

51. Hayden FG, Fritz R, Lobo MC, Alvord W, Strober W, Straus SE (1998) Local and systemic cytokine responses during experimental human influenza A virus infection. Relation to symptom formation and host defense. J Clin Invest 101:643–649

52. Hussell T, Pennycook A, Openshaw PJ (2001) Inhibition of tumor necrosis factor reduces the severity of virus-specific lung immunopathology. Eur J Immunol 31:2566–2573

53. Jung K, Lee CS, Kang BK, Park BK, Oh JS, Song DS (2010) Pathology in dogs with experimental canine H3N2 influenza virus infection. Res Vet Sci 88:523–527

54. Szretter KJ, Gangappa S, Lu X, Smith C, Shieh WJ, Zaki SR, Sambhara S, Tumpey TM, Katz JM (2007) Role of host cytokine responses in the pathogenesis of avian H5N1 influenza viruses in mice. J Virol 81:2736–2744

55. Lee YN, Lee HJ, Lee DH, Kim JH, Park HM, Nahm SS, Lee JB, Park SY, Choi IS, Song CS (2011) Severe canine influenza in dogs correlates with hyperchemokinemia and high viral load. Virology 417:57–63

56. Salomon R, Hoffmann E, Webster RG (2007) Inhibition of the cytokine response does not protect against lethal H5N1 influenza infection. Proc Natl Acad Sci U S A 104:12479–12481

15

Interactions of highly and low virulent *Flavobacterium columnare* isolates with gill tissue in carp and rainbow trout

Annelies Maria Declercq[1*], Koen Chiers[2], Wim Van den Broeck[1], Jeroen Dewulf[3], Venessa Eeckhaut[2], Maria Cornelissen[4], Peter Bossier[5], Freddy Haesebrouck[2] and Annemie Decostere[1]

Abstract

The interactions of *Flavobacterium columnare* isolates of different virulence with the gills of carp (*Cyprinus carpio* L.) and rainbow trout (*Oncorhynchus mykiss* Walbaum) were investigated. Both fish species were exposed to different high (HV) or low virulence (LV) isolates and sacrificed at seven predetermined times post-challenge. Histopathological and ultrastructural examination of carp and rainbow trout inoculated with the HV-isolate disclosed bacterial invasion and concomitant destruction of the gill tissue, gradually spreading from the filament tips towards the base, with outer membrane vesicles surrounding most bacterial cells. In carp, 5-10% of the fish inoculated with the LV-isolate became moribund and their gill tissue displayed the same features as described for the HV-isolate, albeit to a lesser degree. The bacterial numbers retrieved from the gill tissue were significantly higher for HV- compared to LV-isolate challenged carp and rainbow trout. TUNEL-stained and caspase-3-immunostained gill sections demonstrated significantly higher apoptotic cell counts in carp and rainbow trout challenged with the HV-isolate compared to control animals. Periodic acid-*Schiff*/alcian blue staining demonstrated a significantly higher total gill goblet cell count for HV- and LV-isolate challenged compared to control carp. Moreover, bacterial clusters were embedded in a neutral matrix while being encased by acid mucins, resembling biofilm formation. Eosinophilic granular cell counts were significantly higher in the HV-isolate compared to LV-isolate inoculated and control carp. The present data indicate a high colonization capacity, and the destructive and apoptotic-promoting features of the HV-isolate, and point towards important dynamic host mucin–*F. columnare* interactions warranting further research.

Introduction

Columnaris disease, caused by the Gram-negative bacterium *Flavobacterium columnare*, is notorious in freshwater aquaculture, amongst others of carp (*Cyprinus carpio* L.) and rainbow trout (*Oncorhynchus mykiss* Walbaum), in which it induces severe economic losses due to gill, skin and fin lesions often resulting in high mortality [1-10]. Recently, the bacterium-host interactions of columnaris disease were reviewed, whereby the various prevailing knowledge gaps were highlighted [11]. The mechanisms adopted by the pathogen to establish itself and to maintain a grip on the skin and the gill tissue, and consequently to elicit disease and mortality, are far from fully elucidated. Especially the interplay of *F. columnare* with the gill tissue still puzzles the research community. Hitherto, only a few studies explored the interaction between *F. columnare* and the gill tissue [12-15] focussing on host mucosal responses. Sun et al. studied the transcriptomic profiling of host responses in the gill tissue to columnaris disease following experimental challenge in catfish and found a rhamnose-binding lectin with putative roles in bacterial attachment and aggregation, and several immune suppressive pathways being stimulated after infection with *F. columnare* [15]. Accordingly, Peatman et al. found resistant catfish to have a higher expression of immune stimulating genes in the gills following challenge with *F. columnare* as compared to susceptible fish which showed high expression levels of a rhamnose-binding lectin and several

* Correspondence: andclerc.declercq@ugent.be
[1]Department Morphology, Ghent University, Faculty of Veterinary Medicine, Salisburylaan 133, 9820 Merelbeke, Belgium
Full list of author information is available at the end of the article

mucosal immune suppression factors, possibly predisposing them to *F. columnare* infection [14].

In a recent study, variation in virulence between different *F. columnare* strains isolated from carp and rainbow trout was shown and the highly virulent isolates induced severe gill lesions in experimentally infected carp and rainbow trout [16]. The carp showed a diffuse lesion pattern, affecting all gill arches bilaterally and the animals died within 12 h after inoculation. In rainbow trout, the distribution pattern of the gill lesions was more focal and only present in the first gill arches. Mortality started 15 to 18 h after inoculation, also reaching 100% within 72 h.

To obtain better insights in the interaction of *F. columnare* isolates of differential virulence with the gills of carp and rainbow trout, the sequence of events taking place at the level of the gill tissue following challenge with a highly and a low virulent isolate was mapped. Gill health status, pathogen localisation and spread, degree of apoptosis, changes in chloride cell number, quantitative and qualitative mucus changes and bacterial cell counts were investigated at seven predetermined sampling points post-challenge. By merging the retrieved data, we sought to further elucidate the *F. columnare*-gill interplay.

Materials and methods
Fish
Two-day old carp fry were obtained from a Belgian hatchery and grown to a mean length of six centimetres before inclusion in the experiment. Rainbow trout with an average length of five centimetres were purchased from a Belgian hatchery (Villers-le-Gambon, Belgium) and acclimatized for one month in our facilities. The fish were maintained in one cubic metre stocking tanks filled with 800 L of recirculating and aerated tapwater. The water temperature was $22 \pm 1\,°C$ for the carp and $19 \pm 1\,°C$ for the rainbow trout. Starting from two weeks before the experimental challenge, the water temperature of the stocking tanks was gradually increased by $1\,°C$ every two days until a temperature of $25 \pm 1\,°C$ and $22 \pm 1\,°C$ was reached for the carp and rainbow trout, respectively. This water temperature was then kept constant until the onset of the challenge. Free and ionized ammonia and nitrite concentrations were determined daily and were below detectable levels at all times. A photoperiod of 12 h light/ 12 h darkness was provided and the fish were fed a commercial diet (rainbow trout: Trouw Nutrition, carp: Fin Perfect Feed, Sonubaits) to satiation twice daily. Fish were deprived from food 24 h prior to the experimental challenge. Twenty-five carp and twenty-five rainbow trout were sacrificed with an overdose of benzocaine (ethylaminobenzoate; Sigma, Belgium; 10 g/100 mL acetone). Parasites were not observed during microscopic

examination of wet mount preparations, made from scrapings of the gill and skin tissue. Gill and skin were also screened for the presence of *F. columnare* by means of Polymerase Chain Reaction (PCR) and bacteriological examination using cultivation onto modified Shieh agar [17,18] containing 1 µg/mL tobramycin [19]. For the PCR, DNA from the tissue samples was extracted using a DNeasy blood and tissue kit (Qiagen, Venlo, the Netherlands), according to the guidelines of the manufacturer. PCR mixtures, primer sequences and cycle conditions were as described before [20,21]. *F. columnare* or its DNA were not detected in these samples.

Bacterial propagation
For each fish species, a highly virulent (HV) and a low virulent (LV) isolate with a known virulence profile, as described by Declercq et al., were used [16]. Isolates that were able to elicit 80% mortality or more within 72 h were assigned as HV, whereas isolates causing 20% mortality or less within the time-course of the 7 days experiment were designated LV [16]. Carp were experimentally inoculated with isolates 0901393 (HV) and CDI-A (LV), obtained from diseased carp. Rainbow trout were challenged by isolates P11/91 (HV) and JIP 44/87 (LV), sampled from diseased trout [20]. All four isolates belonged to genomovar I, as determined at the Aquatic Microbiology Laboratory of Auburn University (USA) using 16S-Restriction Fragment Length Polymorphism according to the protocol described by Olivares-Fuster et al. [22]. For more information concerning origin of the isolates, the reader is referred to Declercq et al. [20].

The isolates were grown for 36 h at 28 °C on modified Shieh agar plates [17,18]. For each isolate, five colonies per plate were sampled and transferred to 15 mL Falcon tubes filled with 4 mL of modified Shieh broth, which were placed overnight on a shaker at 28 °C at 100 rpm. The content of two Falcon tubes of these initial broth cultures was added to an additional 392 mL of modified Shieh broth in 500 mL glass bottles and again incubated for 24 h at 28 °C on a shaker at 100 rpm. The content of these bottles was used in the immersion challenge studies and the bacterial titres were determined by making tenfold dilution series in triplicate on modified Shieh agar plates.

Experimental challenge
A group of 27 randomly chosen carp or rainbow trout was removed from the stocking tanks and placed in a 10 L inoculation tank filled with 4.6 L of aerated water at $27 \pm 1\,°C$ (carp) or $23 \pm 1\,°C$ (rainbow trout). Per fish species, three predetermined groups were included in duplicate; fish to be inoculated with either the HV- or LV-isolate and a control group. Then, 400 mL of

cultivated modified Shieh broth containing the *F. columnare* isolates was added to the proper water tank. For the carp, the bacterial titres of the HV-isolate were 3.2 or 6.4×10^7, for the LV-isolate 1.6 or 4.0×10^7 CFU/mL. For the trout, the bacterial titres of the HV-isolate were 6.4×10^7 or 1.6×10^8 CFU/mL, and for the LV-isolate 3.2 or 6.4×10^7 CFU/mL. A control group was included, constituting fish immersed in a tank with water supplemented with 400 mL modified Shieh broth not containing *F. columnare*. After a 90 min inoculation period, each group of 27 fish was transferred to a 60 L tank with trickling filter filled with 48 L of recirculated, aerated tapwater of $25 \pm 1\,^{\circ}C$ for the carp or $22 \pm 1\,^{\circ}C$ for the rainbow trout. The fish were clinically monitored every 30 min and three fish per tank were sacrificed with an overdose of benzocaine (10 g/100 mL acetone) at nine predetermined time-points i.e., 1, 2.5, 4, 6, 8, 9.5, 15.5, 24 and 36 h post inoculation (pi). As soon as the humane endpoints (isolation in a corner, swimming at the water surface, loss of balance) were reached, the fish were sacrificed with an overdose of benzocaine. In case dead fish were encountered, these were immediately removed from the aquaria and sampled only for bacteriological analysis, and not for histological nor ultrastructural examination. Of all sacrificed fish, the gill arches were inspected and the first two left gill arches were removed and sampled for histological, (immuno) histochemical, scanning (SEM) and transmission (TEM) electron microscopic examination. In all animals, the counterpart right gill arches served for bacteriological examination for *F. columnare* by means of bacterial titration by making tenfold dilution series of the gill tissue in triplicate on modified Shieh agar plates; additionally in the control animals PCR was performed as described before [16]. All experiments were approved by the Ethical Committee of the Faculty of Veterinary Medicine, Ghent University under the project number EC2012/60.

Histological and (immuno)histochemical examination

Histological sections were used to enable a step-by-step tracking of microscopically discernible gill lesions in the course of time. Particular attention was paid to the localisation and arrangement of long slender bacterial cells with the typical *F. columnare* morphology, possible shifts in amount and type of mucins, and the type and spread of gill lesions (top, middle or base of the filaments and lamellae).

The gill tissue sections were fixed for 24 h in 4% phosphate-buffered formaldehyde, dehydrated in graded alcohol-xylene series and embedded in paraffin wax using the STP 420 Microm Tissue Processor and the embedding station EC 350–1 and 2 (Microm, Prosan, Merelbeke, Belgium), respectively. All tissues were sectioned (8 μm) (Microm microtome HM 360, Prosan) and stained with haematoxylin and eosin (H&E). A combined periodic acid Schiff/alcian blue (PAS/AB) stain at pH 2.5 was additionally applied, allowing mucous cells/mucin to stain blue (AB-positive, acid mucins), purple (PAS/AB-positive, neutral combined with acid mucins) or magenta (PAS-positive, neutral mucins).

In addition, (immuno)histochemistry was adopted to visualize apoptotic cells and ATP-ase activity of chloride cells. Therefore, 5 μm thin paraffin embedded tissue sections were mounted on 3-aminopropyl-triethoxysilane-coated slides (APES, Sigma, St. Louis, MO, USA), dried for 1 h at $60\,^{\circ}C$ on a hot plate and further dried overnight at $37\,^{\circ}C$. To discern apoptosis, the terminal deoxynucleotidyl transferase (TdT)-mediated deoxyuridine triphosphate (dUTP) nick end-labelling (TUNEL) methodology was used for discerning DNA fragmentation. The TACS™ TdT in situ apoptosis detection kit (R&D Systems Europe Ltd, Abingdon, UK) was adopted following the protocol as described by Van Cruchten et al. [23]. In addition, caspase-3 activity was determined using a polyclonal rabbit IgG human/mouse active caspase-3 antibody (1/400, R&D Systems Europe Ltd, Abingdon, UK) and the Anti-Rabbit HRP-AEC Cell & Tissue Staining Kit (R&D Systems Europe Ltd, Abingdon, UK). The protocol employed was modified from Van Cruchten et al. [23] with the difference that 50 μL of a labelled polymer of the Dako EnVision + System/HRP, Rabbit (DAB+) kit was used according to the instructions of the manufacturer. To detect the ATPase activity of the chloride cells, a monoclonal mouse antibody Na, K- ATPase (1/200, University of Iowa, Department of Biological Sciences) and the Dako EnVision + System/HRP, Mouse (DAB+) (DakoCytomation, Glostrüp, Denmark) staining kit (Ref.K4007) were applied according to the instructions of the manufacturer.

The (immuno)reactive cells on the (immuno)histochemically stained sections and the PAS-positive, PAS/AB-positive, AB-positive goblet cells and eosinophilic granular cells (EGC) on PAS/AB-stained sections were quantified on three randomly selected gill filaments. Counting was done at the tip, middle and base of these filaments. For all goblet, EGC- and chloride cell counts, results are expressed as the number of cells per 100 μm gill filament. For the TUNEL- and caspase-3-techniques, the results are presented as the number of positive cells per 1000 μm lamellar surface. Apoptosis and chloride cell activity were only determined at the first four sampling points.

Electron microscopy

For SEM, the gill samples were preserved in a HEPES-glutaraldehyde solution. Tissue samples were postfixed in 1% buffered osmium tetroxide for 2 h and dehydrated in an increasing alcohol series followed by increasing ethanol–acetone series up to 100% acetone. The samples were then dried to the critical point with a Balzers CPD 030 critical point drier (Sercolab bvba, Merksem, Belgium) and further mounted on metal bases and sputtered with platinum using the JEOL JFC 1300 Auto Fine Coater (Jeol Ltd, Zaventem, Belgium). The samples were examined with a JEOL JSM 5600 LV scanning electron microscope (Jeol Ltd). For TEM processing, a protocol as described by De Spiegelaere et al. [24] was used. For examination of the TEM-samples, a JEM-1400 plus Jeol electron microscope (Jeol Ltd) operating at 80 kV was used. Micrographs were taken digitally.

Statistical analysis

The effect of three independent variables (degree of virulence of bacterial strain, time point after inoculation and localization on the gill filament) on nine dependent variables (number of recovered bacteria, presence of chloride cells, EGC (only in carp), PAS-positive, PAS/AB-positive, AB-positive, total goblet, TUNEL- and caspase-3 positive cell counts), was assessed. Since a clearly distinct result was noted in some carps inoculated with the LV-isolate in terms of mortality and macroscopically discernible gill lesions, this group was further subdivided into a group of fish displaying no macroscopic abnormalities (further denoted as the carp inoculated with the LV-isolate) and a group of fish that died with grossly visible gill lesions comparable to the macroscopic lesions as seen in fish exposed to the HV-isolate (further denoted as the LV-isolate affected fish).

As the bacterial titration counts for carp and rainbow trout were not normally distributed, the data were log transformed for further statistical analysis.

Depending on the distribution of the dependent variables, two different statistical assays were performed. Firstly, the effect of the independent variables on the outcome of bacterial titrations, PAS/AB-positive goblet cells, total goblet cells, chloride cells, TUNEL and caspase-3 positive cells in carp, and chloride cells, TUNEL, and caspase-3 positive cells in rainbow trout were assessed using a multivariate linear mixed model. When a significant effect on one of the independent variables was observed in the multivariate model, post hoc comparisons were performed using Scheffe or least significant difference (LSD) tests.

Secondly, the data of PAS-positive goblet cells, AB-positive goblet cells and EGC in carp, and PAS-positive goblet cells, PAS/AB-positive goblet cells, AB-positive goblet cells and total gill goblet cells in rainbow trout, were transformed into a binary dataset with values "absence of cells (=0)" and "presence of cells (=1)" and analysed by means of a multivariate logistic regression model.

Statistical results were considered to be significant when p-values were below 0.05. All analyses were performed using SPSS version 21.0.

Results

At the last two sampling points (SPs) i.e. 24 h and 36 h pi, no fish in the groups challenged with the HV-isolates were remaining. Therefore, these SPs were omitted. As the disease progressed markedly faster in trout challenged with the HV-isolate from SP5 onwards, the remaining trout of all groups were sacrificed 3.5 h earlier compared to the carp hence advancing the last SP to 12 h instead of 15.5 h pi.

The control animals of both carp and rainbow trout remained clinically healthy throughout the experiment and no mortality occurred. No lesions nor *F. columnare* bacterial cells were observed upon macroscopic, light microscopic and ultrastructural examination of the gill tissue. Additional light microscopic images display the normal gill histology of a carp (Additional files 1 and 2). Additional scanning electron microscopic images demonstrate the intact gill filaments and gill lamellae in the control animals (Additional files 3 and 4). Skin lesions were not observed in any of the animals during the trials.

Carp

Chronological changes in type and extent of gill lesions
Following challenge with the HV-isolate
SP 1 and 2 (1 and 2.5 h pi, respectively) No macroscopic lesions were noted and none of the 12 fish sampled or any of the fish present in the tank displayed any clinical signs of discomfort or disease. No dead fish were encountered.

Histological imaging revealed bacteria clustered focally in an eosinophilic matrix encompassing the tips of one to three (first SP) and two to six (second SP) out of the six discernible filaments. The lamellae that were in the vicinity of these bacterial clusters were oedematous at the first SP. The lamellae visualized on the sections of the second SP revealed fusion and necrosis. In these necrotic areas, the bacteria were closely associated with the denuded lamellar epithelium with only pillar cells still showing an intact structure. In addition, the bacterial cells had further migrated to the middle of the filaments (Figure 1). Filamental architecture was safeguarded in all fish examined.

PAS-staining showed a PAS-positive matrix immediately surrounding the bacteria that in turn was enclosed by AB-positive mucins (Figure 2). Both layers exhibited the same thickness of 3-30 μm, with the thickness of the surrounding layer increasing with the size of the bacterial cluster.

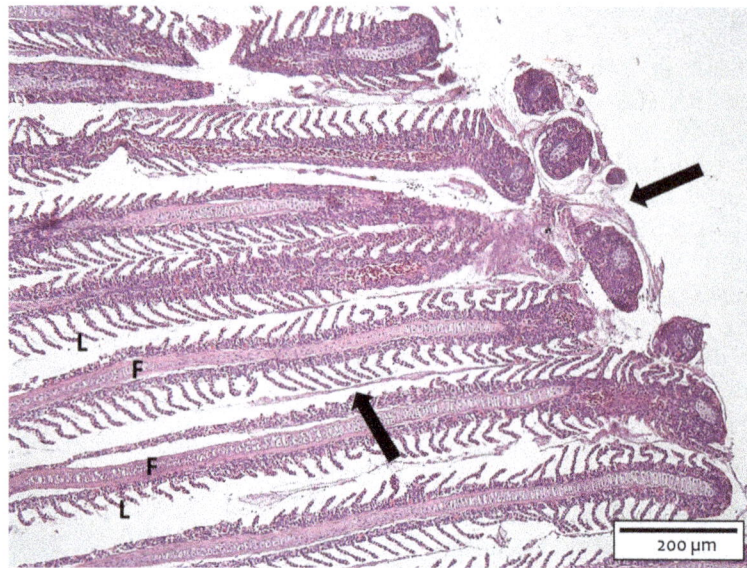

Figure 1 Gill section of a carp challenged with the HV-isolate at SP 2. The bacterial cells (arrows) are clustered focally in an eosinophilic matrix encompassing the tips of the gill filaments (F) and extending to the middle of the gill filaments. L = gill lamella (H&E, bar = 200 µm).

SEM (Figure 3) and TEM revealed aggregates of long, slender bacterial cells, with large clumps of these bacterial cells encompassing the filament tips at the second SP.

SP 3 and 4 (4 h and 6 h pi, respectively) At 6 h pi, the first moribund fish appeared. These two fish were hanging at the surface or in a corner of the tanks, displayed loss of balance and were gasping for air. These two (out of the six) sampled fish displayed macroscopic lesions.

The latter consisted of foci of whitish discolouration of the first gill arch on both sides. One dead fish was encountered.

Upon inspection of the histological sections from the six fish sacrificed at 4 h pi, assembled bacterial cells were noted in close proximity to the lamellar epithelium of the filament tips with focal loss of filamental architecture. In addition, bacterial cells had pursued their way to the filament base. The gill tissue of the fish sampled at

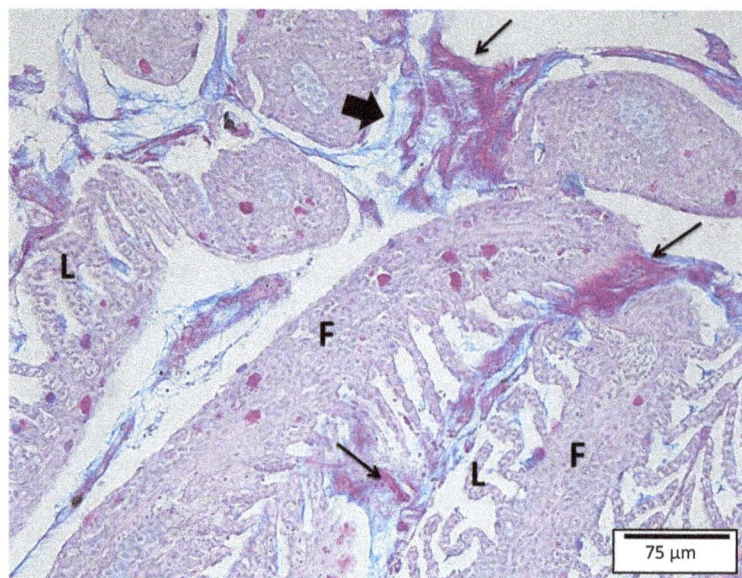

Figure 2 Gill section of a carp challenged with the HV-isolate at SP 2. The bacterial cells are surrounded by a PAS-positive matrix (thin arrows, magenta) enveloped by AB-positive mucins (thick arrow, blue). F = gill filament; L = gill lamella (PAS/AB, bar = 75 µm).

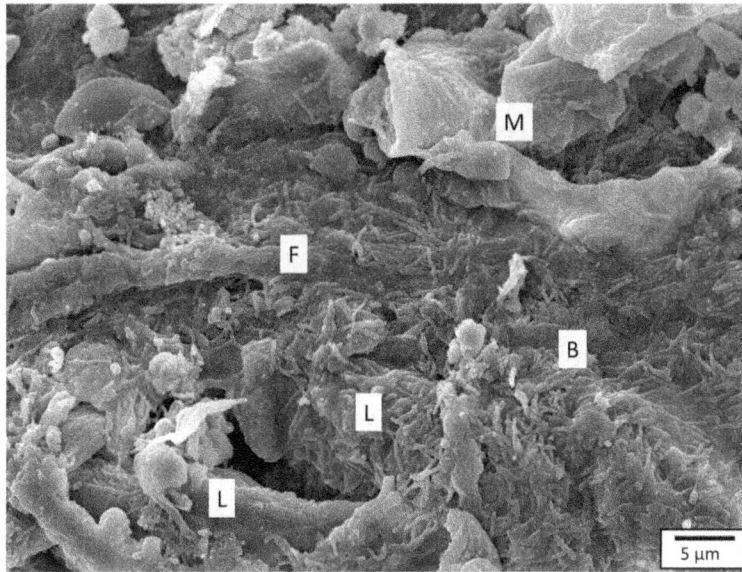

Figure 3 Carp gill after inoculation with HV-isolate at SP 2. The gill filament (F) and gill lamellae (L) are covered by long, slender bacterial cells (B), clustering in between mucus (M) and cell debris (SEM, bar = 5 μm).

6 h pi displayed multiple bacterial micro-colonies smothering half to all filament tips coinciding with lamellar fusion and filament destruction.

SEM confirmed the presence of huge clusters of densely packed bacterial cells wrapped in cellular debris and covering the gill tissue (Additional file 5). TEM-examination revealed bacterial cells directed parallel to and in intimate contact with the gill epithelia. In conjunction with bacterial presence, severe gill damage with oedema and cell necrosis was noted. The outer membrane of the bacteria was remarkably knurled and regularly surrounded by outer membrane vesicles (OMV) (Figure 4).

SP 5, 6 and 7 (8, 9.5 and 15.5 h pi, respectively) The vast majority of fish displayed overt signs of disease as exhibited by loss of equilibrium, isolation and respiratory distress, with an increase in severity at later SPs. All these fish showed macroscopic lesions, as manifested by multifocal discolouration of the first gill arches bilaterally. Thirteen dead fish were encountered. Two out of 18 sampled fish remained clinically healthy with no

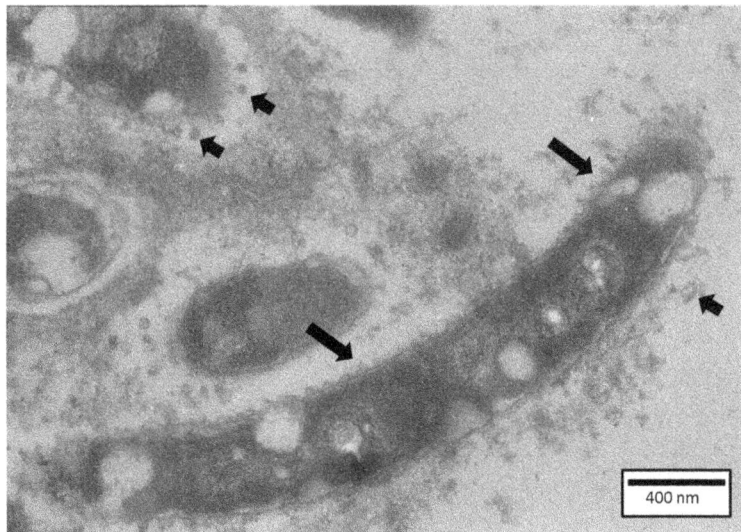

Figure 4 Carp gill after inoculation with the HV-isolate at SP 3. Bacterial cells present a knurled outer membrane (long arrows), and are regularly surrounded by outer membrane vesicles (short arrows) (TEM, bar = 400 nm).

apparent lesions. At the last SP, only four fish (two out of each aquarium) were remaining and sampled for (immuno)histochemical, ultrastructural and bacteriologic analysis.

The histological image changed into severe pathological lesions in all fish sampled, except for the two clinically healthy animals. Large clumps of bacterial micro-colonies, embedded in an eosinophilic matrix, covered all filament tips. Multifocally spread bacterial cells were seen in close contact with the lamellar epithelium over the full length of the gill filaments. Focal lamellar fusion and tissue necrosis were associated with the bacterial cells with significantly more fusion of the lamellae at the filament tips compared to the control animals. Areas of complete architectural loss in close proximity of bacterial clumps were additionally noted. At SP 7, overall oedema and total lamellar and filamental fusion were apparent (Figure 5).

TEM revealed all bacterial outer membranes consistently surrounded by OMV. SEM confirmed the histological findings and was demonstrated by large clumps of bacterial micro-colonies (Additional file 6), embedded in a matrix, covering all filament tips.

Following challenge with the LV-isolate

SP 1 and 2 (1 and 2.5 h pi, respectively) No clinical signs of discomfort nor macroscopic lesions were seen. No mortality was discerned.

Histological examination revealed the presence of clusters of bacterial cells in close contact with one to three (SP 1) and two to three (SP 2) out of six filament tips in all 12 fish sampled. These bacterial aggregates were also found in the middle of the filaments. The gill filament and lamellae did not exhibit any abnormalities, except for focal lamellar oedema in the filament tips in the presence of bacterial cells.

PAS-staining showed a PAS-positive matrix immediately surrounding the bacteria that in turn was enclosed by AB-positive mucins with the larger the bacterial cluster, the thicker the surrounding layers.

TEM examination revealed bacterial cells that appeared to be separated from the epithelium by a translucent layer (Figure 6). In one fish sampled at 2.5 h pi, close contact between the bacterial cell and the gill epithelium was noted, with a parallel orientation of the bacterium towards the lamellar epithelial cells and apparent bacterial cell division. The bacterium showed a cell wall with an apparently less knurled outer membrane compared to the bacterial cells of the HV-isolate. OMV were observed only in a minority of the bacterial cells. Bacteria could not be visualized using SEM examination. Indeed, only huge mucus clots and packed cells were evident mostly at the gill filaments tips, covering the gill tissue. In sites not covered by mucus, the normal fish gill fingerprinting pattern was visible.

SP 3 and 4 (4 and 6 h pi, respectively) Two fish out of twelve sampled exhibited severe signs of discomfort and were swimming at the surface, gasping for air. However, no macroscopic lesions were encountered in any of the fish sampled. No other clinical abnormalities nor dead fish were observed.

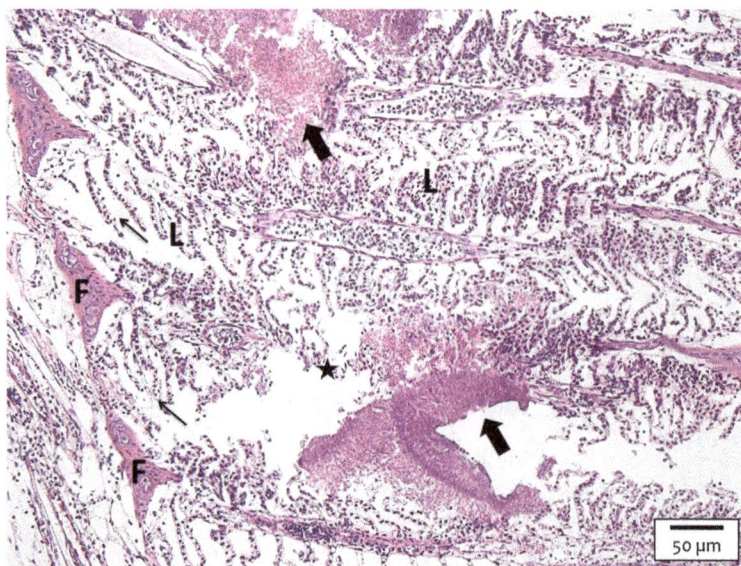

Figure 5 Gill section of a carp challenged with the HV-isolate at SP 7. Large clumps of bacterial micro-colonies (thick arrows) embedded in an eosinophilic matrix are discerned. Areas of complete architectural loss (asterisk) are noted in close proximity of bacterial clumps. Overall oedema (thin arrows) and total lamellar (L) and filament (F) fusion are apparent (H&E, bar = 50 μm).

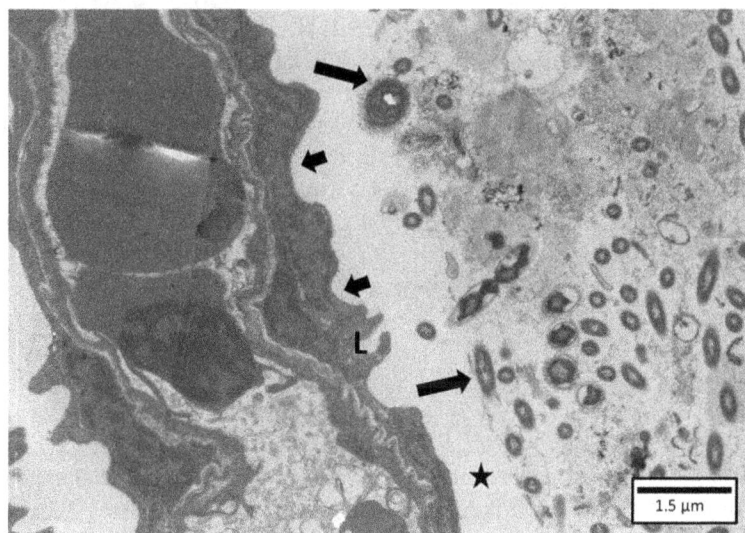

Figure 6 Gill of a carp inoculated with the LV-isolate at SP 2. A cluster of bacterial cells (long arrows) is separated from the lamellar epithelium (L) (short arrows) by a translucent layer (asterisk) (TEM, bar = 1.5 μm).

Histological examination revealed the presence of bacterial cells in nine out of the twelve fish sampled. Bacteria forming small micro-colonies surrounded by an eosinophilic matrix and necrotic cells were observed in close contact with the gill epithelium at the tips and middle of the filaments. The two clinically affected fish showed multifocal histological filament destruction as seen in the fish inoculated with the HV-isolate. No abnormalities were discerned in the outnumbering clinically healthy fish that were sacrificed.

SEM and TEM endorsed the histological results with bacterial cells being noted enclosed in mucus clots and in close contact with the gill epithelium, respectively. As in the HV-isolate, the outer membrane of the bacterial cell wall was surrounded by OMV, but only a minority of the bacterial cells revealed this phenomenon. Again, a less knurled outer membrane was noted.

SP 5, 6 and 7 (8, 9.5 and 15.5 h pi, respectively) Three fish were moribund at SP 6 and 7 and revealed macroscopic lesions consisting of multifocal whitish discolouration of the first gill arches. One dead fish was encountered.

The gills of the clinically healthy fish did not reveal any macroscopic or microscopic abnormalities and no bacterial cells were noted. The histological findings of the gills of the three moribund fish were comparable to those as described in the fish inoculated with the HV-isolate in terms of the elicited lesions and spread of the bacterial cells throughout the gill tissue. Indeed, huge clusters of bacteria embedded in an eosinophilic matrix with necrotic debris were sited at the filament tips, with offshoots of these in close contact with the gill epithelium over the entire length of the gill filaments. In these sites, severe oedema, lamellar fusion and

lamellar gill necrosis were present. Significantly more fusion of the lamellae was observed in the gills, especially at the filament tips, of fish inoculated with LV-isolate as compared to the control animals. At no time, the cartilaginous tissue was lysed nor were the gill filaments fused.

SEM and TEM of the gills of the moribund fish showed bacterial cells wrapped in a matrix of cells and mucus and contact with epithelial cells, respectively. No abnormalities in the clinically healthy fish were encountered.

Chronological changes in apoptotic, eosinophilic granular, goblet and chloride cells

With regard to the first four SPs, a borderline non-significant main effect of group for TUNEL-positive cells was observed ($p = 0.07$), but the post hoc tests (LSD) showed that the mean difference between the TUNEL-positive cell count per 1000 μm gill filament contour in the gills of carp challenged with the HV-isolate compared to the control animals was 1.65 ± 0.64 ($p < 0.05$). No other significant differences were noted for the TUNEL-positive cell counts. The main effect of group for caspase-3 immunoreactive cell counts per 1000 μm gill filament contour was highly significant ($p < 0.001$). The post hoc tests (LSD) revealed that the mean difference between the caspase-3 immunoreactive cell counts per 1000 μm gill filament contour in the gills of carp inoculated with the HV-isolate and the control animals was 2.3 ± 0.5 ($p < 0.001$); a comparable difference was noted between gill tissue of carp challenged with the LV-isolate and the control animals ($p < 0.001$). Most caspase-3-immunoreactive cells were noted at the second SP, followed by a decreasing trend. The vast majority of cells staining positive with either TUNEL or caspase-3 were epithelial cells, with only occasionally a positive goblet cell discerned. At no time, significant differences between the various groups were noted for the number of chloride cells per 100 µm gill filament length. Lysis of these cells was found, especially when oedema was present. The gills of fish exposed to the HV-or LV-isolate displayed lysis of chloride cells, although to a higher degree in the HV-isolate inoculated fish which showed more oedema.

The main effect of group for the total gill goblet cell counts was significant ($p < 0.01$). In the post hoc test (Scheffe), the mean difference between the total gill goblet cell count per 100 µm gill filament length of fish inoculated with the HV-isolate and the control animals was 0.83 ± 0.27 ($p < 0.05$), while the mean difference between fish inoculated with the LV-isolate and the control animals was 1.06 ± 0.31 per 100 µm gill filament length ($p < 0.01$), with no other significantly different results occurring in total goblet cell counts. For the PAS/AB-positive cell counts, no significant differences occurred between any of the groups. The main effect of group for PAS- and AB-positive cell counts was significant ($p < 0.01$). Upon comparing the cell counts in the gill tissue after HV-isolate inoculation with the control group, data revealed that the former had a 2.86 and 4.76 times higher odd ($p < 0.01$) for PAS-positive and AB-positive cell counts per 100 µm gill filament length, respectively. Higher counts were noted in the vicinity of bacterial cells, mostly at the tips of the gill filaments. Moreover, 3.85 times higher odds ($p < 0.01$) for the AB-positive cells per 100 µm gill filament length were encountered in the gills after challenge with the LV-isolate compared to the control animals and even 5.22 times higher odds ($p < 0.01$) were found for the AB-positive cells in the gills of LV-isolate affected fish compared to the control fish. The main effect of group for EGC positive cell counts was significant ($p < 0.05$). Upon comparing the cell counts in the gill tissue after inoculation with the HV-isolate with the control group, data revealed that the former had a 4.44 times higher odd per 100 µm gill filament length ($p < 0.01$). Data revealed that the EGC counts of control fish, fish inoculated with the LV-isolate and LV-isolate affected fish had a 0.23, 0.32 and 0.24 times lower odd ($p < 0.05$), respectively, upon comparing the cell counts in the gill tissue after HV-isolate inoculation. No other significant differences were found in the EGC count. In gill sections of fish exposed to the HV-isolate, upon inspection of sites of tissue damage, degranulation of EGC was noted along with their migration onto the gill lamellae. A dynamic overview of PAS-positive goblet cells, AB-positive goblet cells and eosinophilic granular cells in carp is presented in Figure 7.

Temporal changes in bacterial cell counts

The bacterial titres retrieved from the gill tissue at the first SP were the highest during the course of the experiment (7.8×10^8 CFU/g gill tissue and 5.6×10^7 CFU/g gill tissue for the fish inoculated with the HV- and LV-

isolate, respectively). A tenfold decrease was noted towards the third SP, after which titres increased again approaching the values of the first SP. Subsequently, the bacterial titres either stagnated or decreased gradually. An overview of the average bacterial titres retrieved from the gill tissue after exposure with the HV- and LV-isolates can be found in Figure 8. Overall, the mean bacterial logarithmic titres retrieved from gill tissue in the HV- and LV-challenged fish were ^{10}log 7.92 ± 0.15 CFU/g and ^{10}log 6.70 ± 0.18 CFU/g, respectively. The LV-isolate affected fish had a mean bacterial logarithmic titre of ^{10}log 7.15 ± 0.39 CFU/g. There was a clear significant main effect of group in the bacterial titres ($p < 0.001$). In the post hoc tests (Scheffe), the mean difference for the bacterial cell counts between the HV- and the LV-isolate challenged fish and the LV-isolate affected fish was ^{10}log 1.15 ± 0.21 ($p < 0.001$) and ^{10}log 1.10 ± 0.38 ($p < 0.05$) CFU/g, respectively. No *F. columnare* cells were detected in the gill tissue of the control animals.

Rainbow trout
Chronological changes in type and extensiveness of gill lesions
Following challenge with the HV-isolate
SP 1 and 2 (1 and 2.5 h pi, respectively) No clinical signs of discomfort nor macroscopic lesions were noted in any of the 12 sampled fish or any of the other fish present in the tanks. Three dead fish were encountered revealing no macroscopic abnormalities.

Histologically, the first lesions were noted as mild oedema and hyperplasia in six out of twelve sampled fish. The other half of the fish showed focal to generalized severe oedema with detachment of the epithelium from the underlying intact pillar cells. Bacterial cells were spotted focally, mostly encompassing the filament tips and middle of the gill filaments. Their presence was associated with localized lamellar necrosis, while the neighbouring lamellae remained intact, apart from slight oedema of the epithelium on the colonized side.

TEM confirmed the latter finding (Figure 9). Furthermore, TEM revealed the chromatin of the nucleus to be marginalized and clumped while the other cell organelles remained intact, as seen in apoptotic cells. SEM did not reveal abnormalities.

SP 3 and 4 (4 and 6 h pi, respectively) Clinical signs of discomfort and macroscopic lesions were absent in all fish. One dead fish occurred, showing no macroscopic lesions.

Histologically, bacterial cells were noted in six fish out of twelve fish sampled. Small clumps of bacterial cells were found very focally over the entire length of the filaments and in close contact with the epithelium. Their

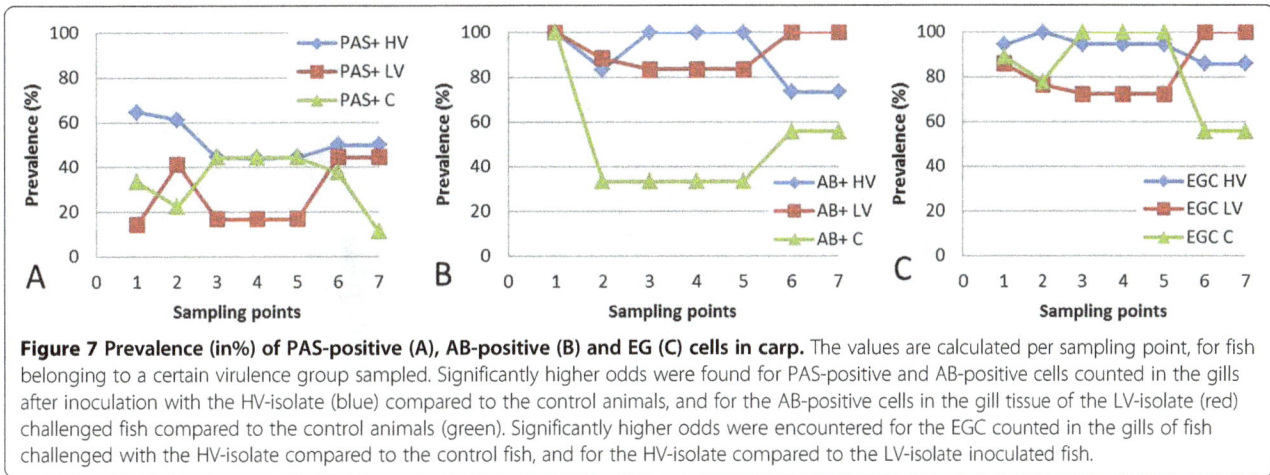

Figure 7 Prevalence (in%) of PAS-positive (A), AB-positive (B) and EG (C) cells in carp. The values are calculated per sampling point, for fish belonging to a certain virulence group sampled. Significantly higher odds were found for PAS-positive and AB-positive cells counted in the gills after inoculation with the HV-isolate (blue) compared to the control animals, and for the AB-positive cells in the gill tissue of the LV-isolate (red) challenged fish compared to the control animals (green). Significantly higher odds were encountered for the EGC counted in the gills of fish challenged with the HV-isolate compared to the control fish, and for the HV-isolate compared to the LV-isolate inoculated fish.

presence coincided with severe oedema, lamellar necrosis and sloughing of epithelial cells.

PAS-staining revealed the bacterial clusters to be wrapped in a PAS-positive matrix while being encased in AB-positive mucus.

The histological findings were confirmed by SEM- and TEM-pictures revealing bacterial clumps present at the gill filament tips and in close contact with the epithelium, respectively.

SP 5, 6 and 7 (8, 9.5 and 12 h pi, respectively) From SP 5 onwards, most remaining rainbow trout exhibited severe discomfort including an altered swimming pattern and gasping for air, and macroscopic focal whitish discolouration of the gill tissue. Eight dead fish were discerned. Only three fish out of the remaining 18 did not exhibit clinical nor macroscopic abnormalities the last three SPs.

Apart from the latter three fish mentioned, histological analysis showed small bacterial clumps in intimate contact with the gill epithelium over the entire length of the filaments, and affecting almost all lamellae. Consistent with the bacterial presence, severe, generalized oedema and lamellar necrosis occurred with shedding of the epithelial cells causing the underlying pillar cells to be denuded. The cartilaginous core of the filaments remained intact.

Likewise, SEM revealed bacterial clusters covering the gill epithelium as blankets and wrapped in between necrotic

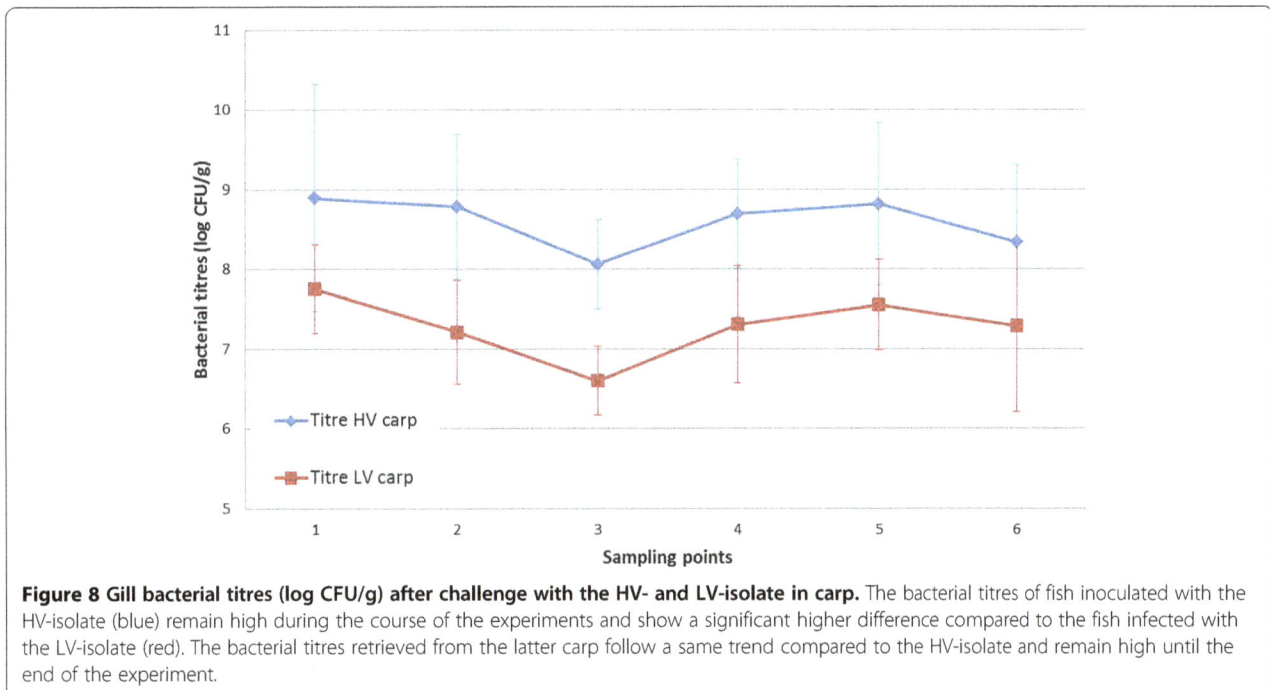

Figure 8 Gill bacterial titres (log CFU/g) after challenge with the HV- and LV-isolate in carp. The bacterial titres of fish inoculated with the HV-isolate (blue) remain high during the course of the experiments and show a significant higher difference compared to the fish infected with the LV-isolate (red). The bacterial titres retrieved from the latter carp follow a same trend compared to the HV-isolate and remain high until the end of the experiment.

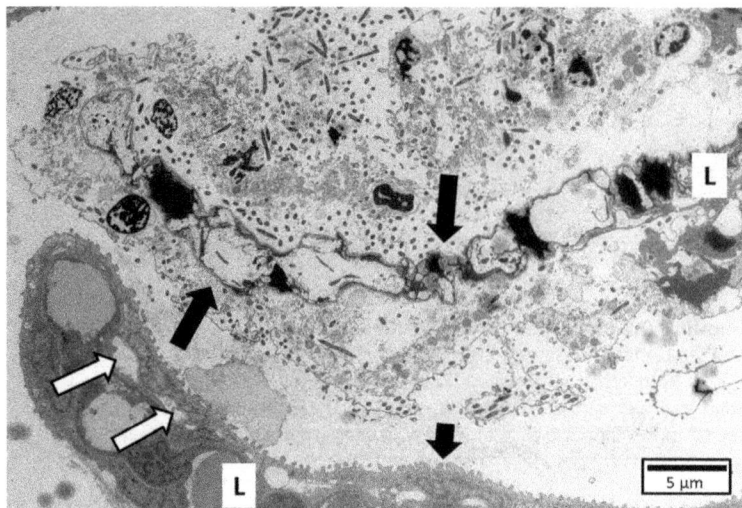

Figure 9 Gill tissue of a trout following exposure to HV-isolate at SP 1. Localized necrosis (long arrows) is observed in a gill lamella (L) while the neighbouring lamella remains intact (short arrow), apart from slight oedema (white arrows) of the epithelium on the sides where bacteria are present (TEM, bar = 10 µm).

cells and cellular debris. TEM revealed a knurled outer membrane in the majority of bacterial cells with the consistent occurrence of OMV.

Following challenge with the LV-isolate

Neither clinical signs nor macroscopic lesions were seen in rainbow trout challenged with the LV-isolate during the entire experiment. No dead fish were encountered.

At the first three SPs, 14 out of the 18 sampled fish showed mild gill oedema, either focal or generalized, associated with hypertrophia of the epithelial cells situated at the basis of the lamellae. At the last four SPs, two out of 24 fish showed mild oedema with no further abnormalities. Bacterial cells were never discerned in any sample. SEM and TEM showed normal gill tissue with no bacteria present.

Chronological changes in apoptotic, eosinophilic granular, goblet and chloride cells

With regard to the first four SPs, the main effect of group for TUNEL-positive cell counts was significant ($p < 0.05$). The post hoc tests (Scheffe) revealed that the mean difference between the TUNEL cell count per 1000 µm gill filament contour in the gills of fish challenged with the HV-isolate compared to the control animals was 2.67 ± 1.08 ($p < 0.05$). No other significant differences were noted for the TUNEL-positive cell counts. The main effect of place for TUNEL-positive cells was significant ($p < 0.01$). Post hoc results (Scheffe) showed that most TUNEL-positive cells per 1000 µm gill filament contour occurred at the filament tips with a mean difference of 3.30 ± 0.98 ($p < 0.01$) TUNEL-positive cells compared to the middle parts of the gill filaments. The main effect of group in caspase-3 immunoreactive

cell counts per 1000 µm gill filament contour was significant ($p < 0.01$). The post hoc tests (Scheffe) revealed that the mean difference between the caspase-3 immunoreactive cell counts per 1000 µm gill filament contour of the gills of rainbow trout challenged with the HV-isolate and the LV-isolate inoculated fish was 2.02 ± 0.54 ($p < 0.01$) while between the HV-isolate inoculated fish and the control animals, this difference was 1.91 ± 0.68 ($p < 0.05$) per 1000 µm gill filament contour. No other significant differences occurred. Cells staining positive with either TUNEL or caspase-3 were predominantly epithelial cells, including occasional goblet cells. No significant differences occurred for the number of chloride cells per 100 µm filament length in between the various groups. As described for the carp, fish exposed to the HV- or LV-isolate displayed lysis of chloride cells but, as more oedema was noted following challenge with the HV-isolate, markedly more lysis of chloride cells was perceived in the fish exposed to the latter isolate.

As for the goblet cell count, no significant differences were noted in between any of the goblet cell counts in between the various groups. An increase in AB-positive cell count was noted in the HV-group from the second to the third SP though.

EGC were not observed in the gill sections of rainbow trout.

Temporal changes in bacterial cell counts

Bacterial titres from the gill tissue inoculated with the HV- and LV-isolate were [10]log 8.03 ± 0.27 CFU and [10]log 2.76 ± 0.42 CFU per g gill tissue, respectively. There was a clear significant main effect of group in the bacterial titres ($p < 0.001$). In the post hoc tests (Scheffe), the mean difference for the bacterial cell counts in between the HV-isolate challenged fish and the LV-isolate inoculated fish was [10]log 5.26 ± 0.39 ($p < 0.001$) CFU/g. An overview of the bacterial titres retrieved from the gill tissue at the various SPs after challenge with the HV- and LV-isolate can be found in Figure 10. No *F. columnare* bacteria were retrieved from the control animals.

Discussion

The purpose of this study was to track the evolution and discern conspicuous features of the gill lesions in experimentally induced columnaris disease. This is the first description of the sequence of events taking place at the level of the gill tissue before the fish succumb to columnaris disease.

In carp, as soon as 1 h post challenge, bacterial cells of the HV-isolate were found in close contact with the epithelium of the filament tips. Only 1 h later, attachment was seen and the bacteria had pursued their way towards the middle of the filaments. The filament tips eventually were disintegrated and bacterial infiltrates were found in between necrotic tissue. Bacteria further invaded the base of the filaments, to ultimately colonize and break down the complete gill filament. Chondrolysis was a dominating feature in the last stages of disease coincided by infiltration of massive clusters of bacterial cells. When necrosis became generalized and severe oedema was evident, the lesions became visible macroscopically as bilaterally whitish discolouration of the gill tissue.

In 75% of the carp inoculated with the LV-isolate, bacterial cells were also able to attach to the epithelium of the filament tips from the first SP onwards and subsequently moved downwards to the middle of the filaments at the third and fourth SP. In contrast, at the fifth and following SPs, the gill sections of only 25% of the fish displayed bacterial cells. Nevertheless, the bacterial titres retrieved from the gill tissue remained high for all carp inoculated with the LV-isolate up until the last SP which seems inconsistent with the histological findings. This may signify that the bacterial cells were no longer as firmly attached to the gill tissue as they were during the first four SPs. Indeed, as described before [12,16], the bacteria might be part of the aqueous biofilm covering the gill tissue and hence be noted by bacteriological examination when plating out the gill sample. However, during processing for histological examination, they might have been washed away as this technique involves several washing steps hence visualizing only firmly attached bacteria. The fifth SP seems to be the turning point for the majority of carp to head for surmounting the LV-isolate *F. columnare* infection with colonization halted at the filament middle section, and bacterial cells allegedly being less firmly attached to the gills. In contrast, the gill tissue of the few carp succumbing to the disease at that time-point (and later) exhibited bacterial colonization over the entire filament length with necrosis of the gill lamellae as a result. Lysis of the cartilaginous tissue was never encountered following exposure to the LV-isolate, which stands in shrill contrast to what was observed in the gill sections of fish challenged with the HV-isolate.

The findings for the LV-isolate challenge both in carp and rainbow trout are intriguing as the bacterial cells seem to be able to colonize the gill tissue, albeit to a significantly lesser extent than those of the HV-isolate.

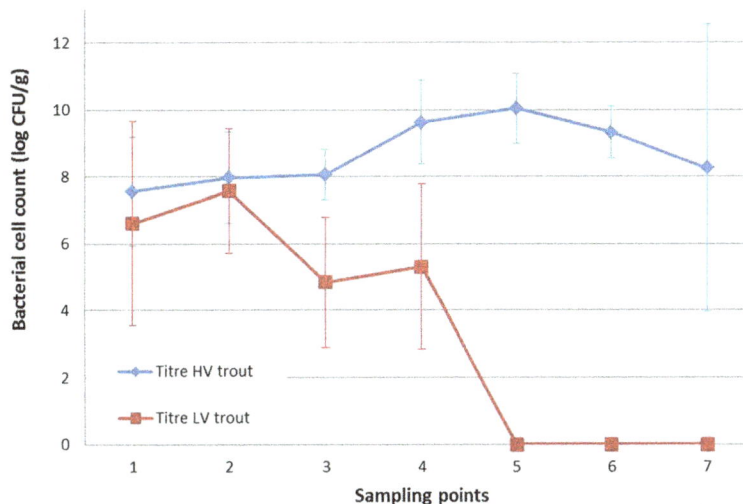

Figure 10 Gill bacterial titres (log CFU/g) after challenge with the HV- and LV-isolate in trout. The bacterial titres of fish inoculated with the HV-isolate (blue) remain high during the course of the experiments. The bacterial titres retrieved from fish infected with the LV-isolate (red) show progressively a substantially decreasing trend.

However, it appears that they cannot maintain a firm grip on this vital organ. The latter needs to be slightly toned down for the LV-isolate in carp where the gills of a few fish were colonized by *F. columnare* over the entire filament length. Why these few fish ultimately succumbed to the challenge with the LV-isolate and the majority of fish survived, warrants further research, as this might provide most relevant information concerning the susceptibility to this increasingly important disease.

In natural outbreaks of edible and ornamental fish, the same clinical and pathologic features have been perceived. Fish were described to firstly lose appetite, swim at the water surface with rapid opercular movements to finally lose balance and succumb to the disease. Acute to chronic massive mortality with [6,25,26] or without [25] macroscopic visible skin or gill lesions have been described. Histological examination of the affected gill tissue could reveal oedema, distortion of lamellae and clusters of bacterial cells situated at the filament tips [26] and bases [25]. In some cases, a total loss of gill architecture was observed [26].

Although skin lesions have been described in natural outbreaks of columnaris disease in salmonids [6], no skin lesions were observed in this study. Most probably, the disease pattern evolved too fast for skin lesions to be discernible, as the latter usually appear in more chronic cases of columnaris disease [1]. In the present studies, we aimed to mimic the natural situation as much as possible. Therefore, carp were inoculated with *F. columnare* strains isolated from carp, and rainbow trout with strains from trout. Our results therefore do not allow concluding whether the temporal differences in infection observed between rainbow trout and carp are fish species related or rather *F. columnare* strain dependent.

Virulence is determined by more than the process of colonization. Upon TEM examination of the carp and rainbow trout gill sections of fish inoculated with the HV-isolates, OMV were discerned surrounding the majority of bacterial cells. These OMV were markedly less frequent in the vicinity of the bacterial cells upon inspection of gill sections of fish exposed to the LV- carp isolate. The production and composition of OMV seem to be influenced by ambient factors that microbes sense inside the host during normal cell growth [27] and not during cell lysis [28]. OMV have been described to contain biologically active proteins important for nutrient acquisition, co-aggregation of bacteria and biofilm development, tissue lysis and virulence [29-31]. These bacterial "bombs" have been detected in *F. columnare* after in vitro research [32,33], but, as far as we know, they have never before been described in vivo.

The findings in the present study strongly point towards biofilm development as has been demonstrated

for *F. columnare* in in vitro experiments [34]. These in vivo findings comply with the demonstration of genes in *F. columnare* encoding biofilm formation by the research group of Tekedar et al. [35]. The recurring features stressing biofilm formation potentially being an important stage in the pathogenicity of *F. columnare*, warrant further investigation.

Another important parameter to investigate in the theme of virulence, is the myriad of ways adopted by the pathogen to escape the host's immune defence. A remarkable and hitherto unexplained lack of inflammatory response is typical of *F. columnare* infections, especially in the early stages, allowing progression of the infection. Apoptosis constitutes a cell death programme with a notably non-inflammatory outcome, which may provide an explanation for the impaired inflammatory response and the acuteness with which columnaris disease can strike. In the present study, TUNEL and caspase-3 staining showed that significantly higher apoptotic cell counts in the gill tissue of fish challenged with the HV- or LV-isolate compared to the control animals and in some cases even between fish gills challenged with either one of the bacterial isolates were perceived. Apoptosis mostly affected epithelial cells and only occasionally goblet cells. Sun et al. demonstrated an up-regulation of apoptosis pathways in the early stages after a challenge with *F. columnare*, which corresponds to our findings [15]. The initiation of an increase in apoptotic cells following exposure to *F. columnare* – as now also demonstrated morphologically – remains enigmatic [15]. Although different techniques for apoptosis detection are available, none of these are entirely specific or all-inclusive. Therefore, it was chosen to combine different techniques in our apoptosis research. The TUNEL assay was used, because it detects DNA fragmentation. However, DNA fragmentation has also been described to occur in oncosis (cell death with swelling) [36]. Therefore, the immunohistochemical detection of caspase-3 was also applied. It is generally accepted that the latter technique is entirely specific for apoptosis, although apoptosis can be independent of caspase-3 [37].

The presence of EGC or mast cells in teleosts may be demonstrated by using H&E and Giemsa stainings [38,39]. These EGC were described to stain negative using PAS [38]. However, precise and fully documented data on the staining characteristics of EGC remain scarce, while information on the impact of the organ and/or fish species and the effect of histological processing is almost fully lacking. In the current experiment, the granules of the EGC clearly stained PAS-positive in the gill tissue of carp. These cells were negative on alcian blue and toluidine blue stained sections (data not shown), with the well-delineated granules and staining features clearly differing from what was observed for the goblet cells. EGC have been associated with host defence actions towards bacteria [39] and parasites [39,40], although their exact role and the events they elicit are far from fully known. A significantly higher amount of these cells was noted in the carp gill tissue following exposure to the HV- as compared to the LV-isolate and control groups. EGC may be mobilized towards regions attacked by insults with acute tissue damage causing mast cell/eosinophilic granular cell degranulation and release of mediators of inflammation [39]. Degranulation of EGC was also noted in the carp in sites where tissue damage was visible. Whether this was favourable or disadvantageous for the host at this stage, is unclear. As this is the first time that a marked mobilization of EGC at the level of the gill tissue following *F. columnare* challenge is described, this phenomenon justifies further research into the function and significance of these cells in the pathogenesis of columnaris disease.

In this study, both fish species showed an increase in the total amount of producing goblet cells following challenge with either one of the *F. columnare* isolates compared to the control group, but only the carp showed significantly more producing goblet cells. A similar increase in goblet cells was seen after exposure to various parasites and bacteria [41,42].

Interestingly, gill mucus cell histochemistry demonstrated an increase of neutral mucin production in carp and a significant increase of PAS-positive cell numbers following challenge with the HV-isolate as compared to the control animals. A similar mucus shift has been described in Atlantic salmon after challenge with the causative agent of amoebic gill disease [41]. After exposure to the HV- or LV-isolate in carp, a significant increase in AB-positive productive goblet cells was also observed compared to the control animals. An increased number of goblet cells containing acid glycoconjugates has been noted in skin mucus of carp after exposure to water containing a high load of non-pathogenic bacteria [42]. Although not significant, an upward trend in acid mucus production was also noted in rainbow trout following challenge with the HV-isolate. Rainbow trout in general have been described to produce less acid mucins compared to other fish species such as Atlantic salmon [40], which might explain why the observed differences were not statistically significant.

The question arises how the mucus changes observed in this study are elicited and how these may impact both the pathogen and the host. A distinct possibility is that the bacterium itself can alter the composition of the mucins. This has been described for *Helicobacter pylori* infections in the acid environment of the stomach where *H. pylori* uses urea hydrolysis to elevate the pH of its environment. The elevation of pH to neutral transforms the viscoelastic mucin gel to a viscous liquid [43], enabling the helical cell-shaped bacterium to swim faster in the viscous solution [44]. It is unknown whether *F. columnare* can steer the pH of mucus as, to our knowledge, this is unknown for any gill-disease eliciting organism. A consistent finding throughout this study is the fact that *F. columnare* bacteria were immediately surrounded by a PAS-positive matrix whilst being encased by AB-positive mucins. As an acid environment has been described to be adverse for *F. columnare* bacteria [45], it is most tempting to speculate that the more neutral mucins in the immediate vicinity of the bacterial cells presumably are self-produced whilst the acid AB-positive mucus would be secreted by the host as a self-defence mechanism. Indeed, acid AB-positive mucins at pH 2.5 contain negative charges which reduce bacterial binding and are missing in PAS-positive mucins. In view of the importance of mucus in the fish's arsenal to combat disease, again, this finding should be further investigated.

In conclusion, the present study has revealed that, following immersion challenge, adhesion and aggregation of HV- *F. columnare* isolates adhere first at the tips of the gill filaments before the bacterial cells pursue their way to the middle and base of the filament, and eventually colonize the complete filament. Rainbow trout showed more focal tissue destruction compared to complete gill filament disintegration being most conspicuous in carp. Moreover, lysis of the cartilaginous tissue was perceived in carp. The production of OMV merits further attention, as these structures have been described to play a role in virulence and tissue lysis and have, as far as we know, never before been described in *F. columnare* in vivo. Furthermore, biofilm formation was discerned with bacterial cells wrapped in a PAS-positive matrix while being encased by AB-positive mucus. The observed shifts in goblet cells both quantitatively and qualitatively point towards the complex yet intriguing interplay of *F. columnare* with the gill mucus again warranting further research. The perceived increase in apoptotic cells and the higher EGC counts conclude the list of conspicuous features that provide pointers for future research on the pathogenesis of columnaris disease.

Additional files

Additional file 1: Gill section of a control carp at SP 7. The normal gill tissue structure is shown with parallel gill filaments (F) and sprouting from the filaments, intact gill lamellae (L) displayed (H&E, bar = 50 μm).

Additional file 2: Gill section of a control carp at SP 7. The normal gill tissue structure is shown with parallel gill filaments (F) and sprouting from the filaments, intact gill lamellae (L) displayed (PAS/AB, bar = 50 μm).

Additional file 3: Gill tissue of a control carp. One gill filament (upper structure) and the parallel orientated gill lamellae sprouting from this gill filament are visible (SEM, bar = 10 μm).

Additional file 4: Gill tissue of a control trout. The tops and middle parts of gill filaments are shown and sprouting from the latter, parallel ranked gill lamellae can be distinguished (SEM, bar = 100 μm).

Additional file 5: Carp gill after inoculation with HV-isolate at SP 3. Detail of densely packed bacterial cells wrapped between mucus and necrotic debris (SEM, bar = 2 μm).

Additional file 6: Carp gill after inoculation with HV-isolate at SP 7. A detail of densely packed bacterial cells wrapped between mucus and necrotic debris is shown, causing the gill lamellae to be covered (SEM, bar = 5 μm).

Competing interests

The authors declare that they have no competing interests.

Authors' contributions

AMD: executing the experimental trials, writing the outlines, writing the paper; KC: histopathological interpretation, reviewing and editing the paper; WVdB: histological interpretations, critically reviewing the manuscript; JD: statistical analysis; VE: genetic research and critically reviewing the manuscript; MC: aid in TEM-processing and critically reviewing the manuscript; PB: critically reviewing the manuscript; FH: aid in the set-up and execution of the in vivo experiments, critically reviewing the manuscript; AD: proposing the subject, aid in the set-up and execution of all experiments, reviewing and editing the paper. All authors agreed on outlines and the final version of the paper. All authors read and approved the final manuscript.

Acknowledgements

The isolates were kindly provided by Dr Jean-François Bernardet (Unité de Virologie & Immunologie Moléculaires, INRA Centre de Recherches de Jouy-en-Josas, France) and Dr. ir. Olga L.M. Haenen (Fish and Shellfish Diseases Laboratory, Central Veterinary Research Institute (CVI), Wageningen, the Netherlands). Prof. dr. Cova Arias and Drs. Haitham Mohammed of the Auburn University, USA, Alabama are thanked for the genomovar determination of the F. columnare isolates used in this study. We gratefully acknowledge Prof. dr. Simoens for his valuable comments on the manuscript. Furthermore, Jurgen De Craene, Lobke De Bels, Bart De Pauw, Marleen Foubert, Sarah Loomans, Leen Pieters, Christian Puttevils, Toke Thiron and Patrick Vervaet are thanked for their support during the trials. The Special Research Grant (Bijzonder Onderzoeksfonds, BOF, grant number 01Z06210) of Ghent University, Belgium and the Hercules foundation (grant number AUGE/11/009) are gratefully acknowledged for financial support.

Author details

[1]Department Morphology, Ghent University, Faculty of Veterinary Medicine, Salisburylaan 133, 9820 Merelbeke, Belgium. [2]Department of Pathology, Bacteriology and Poultry diseases, Ghent University, Faculty of Veterinary Medicine, Salisburylaan 133, 9820 Merelbeke, Belgium. [3]Department of Reproduction, Obstetrics and Herd Health, Ghent University, Faculty of Veterinary Medicine, Salisburylaan 133, 9820 Merelbeke, Belgium. [4]Department of Basic Medical Sciences, Faculty of Medicine and Health Sciences, Ghent University, De Pintelaan 185, 9000 Ghent, Belgium. [5]Ghent University, Laboratory of Aquaculture and Artemia Reference Center, Rozier 44, 9000 Ghent, Belgium.

References

1. Bernardet JF, Bowman JP (2006) The genus Flavobacterium. In: Dworkin M, Falkow S (ed) The Prokaryotes: A Handbook on the Biology of Bacteria. Proteobacteria: Delta and Epsilon Subclasses, vol 7. Deeply Rooting Bacteria. Springer Science + Business Media, LLC, New York, pp 481–531
2. Decostere A, Haesebrouck F, Devriese LA (1998) Characterization of four Flavobacterium columnare (Flexibacter columnaris) strains isolated from tropical fish. Vet Microbiol 44:35–45
3. Figueiredo HCP, Klesius PH, Arias CR, Evans J, Shoemaker CA, Pereira DJ, Jr, Peixoto MTD (2005) Isolation and characterization of strains of Flavobacterium columnare from Brazil. J Fish Dis 44:199–204
4. Lafrentz BR, LaPatra SE, Shoemaker CA, Klesius PH (2012) Reproducible challenge model to investigate the virulence of Flavobacterium columnare genomovars in rainbow trout Oncorhynchus mykiss. Dis Aquat Organ 101:115–122
5. Morley NJ, Lewis JW (2010) Consequences of an outbreak of columnaris disease (Flavobacterium columnare) to the helminth fauna of perch (Perca fluviatilis) in the Queen Mary reservoir, south-east England. J Helminthol 44:186–192
6. Řehulka J, Minařík B (2007) Blood parameters in brook trout Salvelinus fontinalis (Mitchill, 1815), affected by columnaris disease. Aquacult Res 44:1182–1197
7. Shoemaker CA, Klesius PH, Drennan JD, Evans J (2011) Efficacy of a modified live Flavobacterium columnare vaccine in fish. Fish Shellfish Immun 44:304–308
8. Soto E, Mauel MJ, Karsi A, Lawrence ML (2008) Genetic and virulence characterization of Flavobacterium columnare from channel catfish (Ictalurus punctatus). J Appl Microbiol 44:1302–1310
9. Suomalainen L-R, Bandilla M, Valtonen ET (2009) Immunostimulants in prevention of columnaris disease of rainbow trout, Oncorhynchus mykiss (Walbaum). J Fish Dis 44:723–726
10. Tripathi NK, Latimer KS, Gregory CR, Ritchie BW, Wooley RE, Walker RL (2005) Development and evaluation of an experimental model of cutaneous columnaris disease in koi Cyprinus carpio. J Vet Diagn Invest 44:45–54
11. Declercq AM, Haesebrouck F, Van den Broeck W, Bossier P, Decostere A (2013) Columnaris disease in fish: a review with emphasis on bacterium-host interactions. Vet Res 44:27
12. Decostere A, Haesebrouck F, Charlier G, Ducatelle R (1999) The association of Flavobacterium columnare strains of high and low virulence with gill tissue of black mollies (Poecilia sphenops). Vet Microbiol 67:287–298
13. Decostere A, Haesebrouck F, Van Driessche E, Charlier G, Ducatelle R (1999) Characterization of the adhesion of Flavobacterium columnare (Flexibacter columnaris) to gill tissue. J Fish Dis 22:465–474
14. Peatman E, Li C, Peterson BC, Straus DL, Farmer BD, Beck BH (2013) Basal polarization of the mucosal compartment in Flavobacterium columnare susceptible and resistant channel catfish (Ictalurus punctatus). Mol Immunol 56:317–327
15. Sun F, Peatman E, Li C, Liu S, Jiang Y, Zhou Z, Liu Z (2012) Transcriptomic signatures of attachment, NF-kB suppression and IFN stimulation in the catfish gill following columnaris bacterial infection. Dev Comp Immunol 38:169–180
16. Declercq AM, Chiers K, Haesebrouck F, Van Den Broeck W, Dewulf J, Cornelissen M, Decostere A (2015) Gill infection model for columnaris disease in common carp and rainbow trout. JAAH 27(Suppl 1):1–11
17. Shieh HS (1980) Studies on the nutrition of a fish pathogen, Flexibacter columnaris. Microbios Lett 13:129–133
18. Song Y-L, Fryer JL, Rohovec JS (1988) Comparison of six media for the cultivation of Flexibacter columnaris. Fish Pathol 23:91–94
19. Decostere A, Haesebrouck F, Devriese L (1997) Development of a medium for the selective isolation of Flavobacterium columnare from diseased fish. J Clin Microbiol 35:322–324
20. Declercq AM, Boyen F, Van den Broeck W, Bossier P, Karsi A, Haesebrouck F, Decostere A (2013) Antimicrobial susceptibility pattern of Flavobacterium columnare isolates collected worldwide from 17 fish species. J Fish Dis 36:45–55
21. Panangala VS, Shoemaker CA, Klesius PH (2007) TaqMan real-time polymerase chain reaction assay for rapid detection of Flavobacterium columnare. Aquacult Res 38:508–517
22. Olivares-Fuster O, Shoemaker CA, Klesius PH, Arias CR (2007) Molecular typing of isolates of the fish pathogen, Flavobacterium columnare, by single-strand conformation polymorphism analysis. FEMS Microbiol Lett 269:63–69
23. Van Cruchten S, Van den Broeck W, Duchateau L, Simoens P (2003) Apoptosis in the canine endometrium during estrous cycle. Theriogenology 60:1595–1608
24. De Spiegelaere W, Casteleyn C, Van den Broeck W, Simoens P (2008) Electron microscopic study of the porcine choroid plexus epithelium. Anat Histol Embryol 37:458–463
25. Amin NE, Abdallah IS, Faisal M, Easa M, El-S AT, Alyan SA (1988) Columnaris infection among cultured Nile tilapia Oreochromis niloticus. Antonie Van Leeuwenhoek 54:509–520
26. Decostere A, Ducatelle R, Haesebrouck F (2002) Flavobacterium columnare (Flexibacter columnaris) associated with severe gill necrosis in koi carp (Cyprinus carpio L). Vet Rec 150:694–695
27. Kuehn MJ, Kesty NC (2005) Bacterial outer membrane vesicles and the host-pathogen interaction. Genes Dev 19:2645–2655

28. Whitchurch CB, Tolker-Nielsen T, Ragas PC, Mattick JS (2002) Extracellular DNA required for bacterial biofilm formation. Science 295:1487

29. Berleman J, Auer M (2013) The role of bacterial outer membrane vesicles for intra- and interspecies delivery. Environ Microbiol 15:347–354

30. MacDonald IA, Kuehn MJ (2012) Offense and defense: microbial membrane vesicles play both ways. Res Microbiol 163:607–618

31. McMahon KJ, Castelli ME, Vescovi EG, Feldman MF (2012) Biogenesis of outer membrane vesicles in *Serratia marcescens* is thermoregulated and can be induced by activation of the Rcs phosphorelay system. J Bacteriol 194:3241–3249

32. Arias CR, LaFrentz S, Cai W, Olivares-Fuster O (2012) Adaptive response to starvation in the fish pathogen *Flavobacterium columnare*: cell viability and ultrastructural changes. BMC Microbiol 12:266

33. Laanto E, Penttinen RK, Bamford JKH, Sundberg L-R (2014) Comparing the different morphotypes of a fish pathogen - implications for key virulence factors in *Flavobacterium columnare*. BMC Microbiol 14:170

34. Cai W, De La Fuente L, Arias CR (2013) Biofilm formation by the fish pathogen *Flavobacterium columnare*: development and parameters affecting surface attachment. Appl Environ Microbiol 79:5633–5642

35. Tekedar HC, Karsi A, Gillaspy AF, Dyer DW, Benton NR, Zaitshik J, Vamenta S, Banes MM, Gülsoy N, Aboko-Cole M, Waldbieser GC, Lawrence ML (2012) Genome sequence of the fish pathogen *Flavobacterium columnare* ATCC 49512. J Bacteriol 194:2763–2764

36. Saikumar P, Dong Z, Mikhailov V, Denton M, Weinberg JM, Venkatachalam MA (1999) Apoptosis: definition, mechanisms, and relevance to disease. Am J Med 107:489–506

37. Hamatake M, Iguchi K, Hirano K, Ishida R (2000) Zinc induces mixed types of cell death, necrosis, and apoptosis in molt-4 cells. J Biochem 128:933–939

38. Holland JW, Rowley AF (1998) Studies on the eosinophilic granule cells in the gills of the rainbow trout, *Oncorhynchus mykiss*. Comp Biochem Physiol C Pharmacol Toxicol Endocrinol 120:321–328

39. Reite OB, Evensen Ø (2006) Inflammatory cells of teleostean fish: a review focusing on mast cells/eosinophilic granule cells and rodlet cells. Fish Shellfish Immun 20:192–208

40. Reite OB (2005) The rodlet cells of teleostean fish: their potential role in host defence in relation to the role of mast cells/eosinophilic granule cells. Fish Shellfish Immun 19:253–267

41. Roberts SD, Powell MD (2005) The viscosity and glycoprotein biochemistry of salmonid mucus varies with species, salinity and the presence of amoebic gill disease. J Comp Physiol B 175:1–11

42. van der Marel M, Caspari N, Neuhaus H, Meyer W, Enss ML, Steinhagen D (2010) Changes in skin mucus of common carp, *Cyprinus carpio* L., after exposure to water with a high bacterial load. J Fish Dis 33:431–439

43. Celli JP, Turner BS, Afdhal NH, Keates S, Ghiran I, Kelly CP, Ewoldt RH, McKinley GH, So P, Erramilli S, Bansil R (2009) *Helicobacter pylori* moves through mucus by reducing mucin viscoelasticity. Proc Natl Acad Sci U S A 106:14321–14326

44. Spagnolie SE, Liu B, Powers TR (2013) Locomotion of helical bodies in viscoelastic fluids: enhanced swimming at large helical amplitudes. Phys Rev Lett 111:068101

45. Fijan FJ (1968) Antibiotic additives for isolation of *Chondrococcus columnaris* from fish. Appl Microbiol 17:333–334

16

Multilocus sequence analysis of *Anaplasma phagocytophilum* reveals three distinct lineages with different host ranges in clinically ill French cattle

Amélie Chastagner[1*], Thibaud Dugat[2], Gwenaël Vourc'h[1], Hélène Verheyden[3], Loïc Legrand[4], Véronique Bachy[5], Luc Chabanne[6], Guy Joncour[7], Renaud Maillard[8], Henri-Jean Boulouis[2], Nadia Haddad[2], Xavier Bailly[1] and Agnès Leblond[1,9]

Abstract

Molecular epidemiology represents a powerful approach to elucidate the complex epidemiological cycles of multi-host pathogens, such as *Anaplasma phagocytophilum. A. phagocytophilum* is a tick-borne bacterium that affects a wide range of wild and domesticated animals. Here, we characterized its genetic diversity in populations of French cattle; we then compared the observed genotypes with those found in horses, dogs, and roe deer to determine whether genotypes of *A. phagocytophilum* are shared among different hosts. We sampled 120 domesticated animals (104 cattle, 13 horses, and 3 dogs) and 40 wild animals (roe deer) and used multilocus sequence analysis on nine loci (*ankA, msp4, groESL, typA, pled, gyrA, recG, polA*, and an intergenic region) to characterize the genotypes of *A. phagocytophilum* present. Phylogenic analysis revealed three genetic clusters of bacterial variants in domesticated animals. The two principal clusters included 98% of the bacterial genotypes found in cattle, which were only distantly related to those in roe deer. One cluster comprised only cattle genotypes, while the second contained genotypes from cattle, horses, and dogs. The third contained all roe deer genotypes and three cattle genotypes. Geographical factors could not explain this clustering pattern. These results suggest that roe deer do not contribute to the spread of *A. phagocytophilum* in cattle in France. Further studies should explore if these different clusters are associated with differing disease severity in domesticated hosts. Additionally, it remains to be seen if the three clusters of *A. phagocytophilum* genotypes in cattle correspond to distinct epidemiological cycles, potentially involving different reservoir hosts.

Introduction

Molecular characterization of the genetic diversity present within pathogen species provides valuable information that can be used to develop appropriate monitoring or control measures [1]. Understanding a pathogen's intraspecific genotypic diversity can aid in diagnosis, specifically by allowing the detection of different variants. Moreover, studies examining the host specificity of individual pathogen genotypes can aid in planning control measures for pathogens that circulate among multiple host species. Such measures could involve managing host diversity in order to reduce disease risk [2]. For example, in the UK, research on the genetics of the host-pathogen interaction between badgers and the tuberculosis-causing bacterium *Mycobacterium bovis* has helped to improve strategies for limiting tuberculosis in cattle [3]. Studies of genetic diversity can also clarify the epidemiology of vector-borne pathogens that, as a result of the low host specificity of their vector(s), circulate among multiple vertebrate hosts. This is the case for ticks, which may have different hosts during different developmental stages [4]. Transmission patterns of tick-borne pathogens can thus be quite complex and depend on a pathogen's ability to infect different host species. Initially, the *Ixodes*-borne pathogen *Borrelia burgdorferi* was thought to be a single bacterial species [5]. However, subsequent molecular

* Correspondence: chastagner.amelie@gmail.com
[1]INRA, UR346 Epidémiologie Animale, F-63122 Saint Genès Champanelle, France
Full list of author information is available at the end of the article

characterization revealed the presence of multiple variants, each with a specific host range, a result that has highlighted the complexity of the epidemiological cycles of this tick-pathogen association [6].

Anaplasma phagocytophilum is a pathogen that raises similar questions. This tick-borne bacterium is the etiologic agent of granulocytic anaplasmosis, an emerging disease that affects a wide range of mammals [7,8]. In cattle, it causes reduced milk yield, abortion, and immunosuppression, which facilitates secondary infections [9,10]. At present, disease control is limited to treating symptomatic cases with antibiotics; little preventive action is taken, since both the source(s) of the pathogen and the environmental conditions that favor the infection of cattle remain poorly documented.

In wild fauna, *A. phagocytophilum* is highly prevalent and persistent in cervids, which are consequently considered to be a reservoir for this bacterium. In areas where *A. phagocytophilum* is endemic, its prevalence is commonly higher than 70% in both roe deer *(Capreolus capreolus)* and red deer *(Cervus elaphus)* populations [11,12]. However, the strains carried by roe deer appear to be different from those carried by domesticated animals [13,14]. Indeed, molecular studies have shown that different variants of *A. phagocytophilum* circulate among different hosts, which suggests that each bacterial strain could be associated with a different epidemiological cycle [15-17]. A thorough genetic characterization of *A. phagocytophilum* could help determine which hosts contribute to each cycle and, more importantly, which hosts promote the spread of the bacterium in cattle.

Various molecular techniques have been used to characterize the genetic diversity of *A. phagocytophilum*. These include restriction fragment length polymorphism [18], pulsed-field gel electrophoresis [19], and multiple-locus variable number tandem repeat analysis [20]. Such techniques have yielded limited information due to either a lack of resolution (the two former techniques) or an excess of variability (the latter technique). The direct detection of polymorphism in DNA sequences has proven to be a more versatile method. Thus far, the characterization of *A. phagocytophilum* has been based on the sequencing of one or a few loci. The most frequently used markers are *groESL*, *ankA*, *msp4*, and 16S rRNA. All these markers except 16S rRNA have revealed high levels of diversity, but phylogenies based on single genes have yielded inconsistent results [13,21,22]. The use of seven or more markers can help resolve such phylogenetic incongruence. Different markers provide information that can be used to identify different genotypic groups, also called clonal complexes, that belong to a common lineage and that are closely related to each other [23]. Two recent studies have used this multilocus sequence typing approach to explore the intraspecific diversity of *A. phagocytophilum* in different host species. One examined dogs, sheep, roe deer, and humans in Europe [24], while the other investigated roe deer and red deer in Poland [25]. Using analyses of seven housekeeping genes and four loci, respectively, these studies have provided robust support for well-defined groups of strains.

In this study, we used multilocus sequence analysis to describe the genetic diversity of the *A. phagocytophilum* strains that infect domestic mammals in France. We employed nine loci, including three commonly studied genes (*groESL*, *ankA*, and *msp4*), and six new markers. Using this approach, we investigated the genetic diversity of *A. phagocytophilum* strains that were responsible for clinical cases of bovine granulocytic anaplasmosis throughout the country. Our goal was to identify the bacterial variants circulating within the cattle population. We then attempted to determine additional host species that could be involved in the circulation of bovine strains. To do this, we compared the genotypes associated with the bovine clinical cases to the genotypes circulating in horses, dogs, and roe deer in France. We discuss our results in the context of other studies that have investigated *A. phagocytophilum*'s genetic diversity in different reservoirs.

Materials and methods
Samples
All animal samples were collected in France between 2011 and 2013. We obtained samples from clinically ill domesticated animals via the network of veterinary clinics belonging to the French national association SNGTV (Société Nationale des Groupements Techniques Vétérinaires) and governmental veterinary laboratories (GVL). More precisely, blood or DNA extracts that had been prepared from different tissues (Additional file 1) were obtained from 104 cattle, 13 horses, and 3 dogs. All these animals had tested positive for granulocytic anaplasmosis after they expressed clinical symptoms compatible with the disease. During the same period, blood samples were taken from wild and captive-bred roe deer sampled as a result of deer management efforts and a population monitoring study. In total, 40 roe deer representing 3 regions were included in our study (Additional file 1).

To prepare the DNA extracts, whole blood samples were stabilized with EDTA, and 200 µL of each sample was used in the DNA extraction procedure. DNA extraction took place in a silica column, and we employed a Nucleospin Blood QuickPure Kit (Macherey-Nagel, Düren, Germany) in accordance with the manufacturer's instructions. Some DNA extracts arrived directly from the GVLs; all had been prepared in the same way, although the brand of column-based DNA extraction kits varied among laboratories and according to biological material.

The presence of *A. phagocytophilum* was assessed in each DNA sample with real-time PCR. For this, we used a protocol adapted from Courtney et al. [26] that targeted the *msp2* and *p44* genes. The reaction mix included 5 μL of DNA extract, 10 μL SsoFast Supermix (Biorad, Hercules, California), 2 μL of each primer (10 μM ApMSPf and ApMSP2r), and 0.5 μL of the Taqman probe ApMSP2p-HEX (10 μM), in a total volume of 20 μL.

Selection of loci

To characterize the genetic diversity of the bacteria causing the infections, we chose nine loci that are evenly distributed across the genome of *A. phagocytophilum*. Among these were *ankA*, *msp4*, and *groESL*, which have frequently been used to characterize the diversity of *A. phagocytophilum*. In addition, six other loci were specifically selected for this analysis. The biological function of the selected genes was not the principal criterion in locus selection, as had been initially proposed for MLST schemes by Maiden et al. [27]. Indeed, Konstantinidis et al. suggested that this strategy was rather conservative [28]. They showed that randomly chosen sets of orthologous genes always contain phylogenetic information that correlates with phylogenetic information at the whole genome scale. Furthermore, this pattern holds despite the fact that the strength of the correlation varies greatly among sets of genes, probably because of the species-specific recombination rate.

A single *A. phagocytophilum* genome was available at the beginning of this study (*A. phagocytophilum* strain HZ GenBank: NC_007797.1). Consequently, the choice of the six new loci could not be based on either the phylogenetic information they contained or the conservation of genes among *A. phagocytophilum* genomes. We thus selected markers by comparing the HZ genome with the genomes of *Anaplasma marginale* (strains St. Maries GenBank: NC_004842.2 & Florida GenBank: NC_012026.1) and the genome of the *Anaplasma centrale* Israel strain (GenBank: NC_013532.1). In particular, we looked for markers that were shared among *Anaplasma* strains and identified six targets: three house-keeping genes (*gyrA*, *polA*, and *recG*), a gene coding for a GTP-binding protein (*typA*), a gene encoding a response regulator linked to intracellular infection (pleD, [29]), and an intergenic spacer located in a region of high synteny (*APH_1099-APH_1100*).

Locus-specific amplification of DNA

Because of the low bacterial load within the blood samples, we first increased the amount of DNA so that more would be available for the amplification of the molecular markers. Multiple displacement amplification (MDA) was performed on positive samples using the

Illustra GenomiPhi V2 DNA Amplification Kit (GE Healthcare Life Sciences, Buckinghamshire, UK) in accordance with the manufacturer's recommendations. The DNA solution obtained was diluted in 80 μL of purified water.

Each locus was then amplified using nested PCR. In the first PCR, each reaction used 5 μL of pre-amplified DNA in a total reaction volume of 50 μL. The reaction mix included 2 units of Taq polymerase (Qiagen, Venlo, Netherlands), 4 μL of each primer (at a concentration of 10 μM), 4 μL of dNTPs (at a concentration of 25 mM), 10 μL of Q solution (Qiagen), and 2 μL of 25-mM MgCl$_2$. Prior to sample amplification, tests were performed to optimize the annealing temperatures. The PCR program began with an initial denaturation step of 3 min at 95 °C. This was followed by three cycles that consisted of a denaturation step of 1 min at 95 °C, an annealing step of 2 min at the temperature described for the published primers for *groEL* [30] and other primer pairs (Additional file 2), and an extension step of 90 s at 72 °C. The program continued with 40 cycles that differed from the first three by having a denaturation step of 1 min at 88 °C and ended with an extension step of 10 min at 72 °C. The nested PCR was performed using 5 μL of the product of the first PCR in a total volume of 50 μL, with the same mix and cycling conditions as in the primary amplification.

DNA sequencing and alignment

Nucleotide sequences were obtained from PCR products using Sanger sequencing (Beckman Coulter Genomic, Essex, UK). When PCR amplification with the external primers was successful in recovering an amount of PCR product that was sufficient for sequencing, we sequenced this longer fragment. However, when it was unsuccessful, the shorter fragment obtained from the nested PCR was used. For DNA fragments longer than 1000 bp, sequencing was performed on both strands. Base calls were checked manually in ChromasLite version 2.1, and IUPAC codes were used to indicate ambiguous states. DNA sequences were aligned using the "*Clustal Omega*" algorithm in SeaView version 4. The sequences analyzed in this study are available in Genbank under the accession numbers KJ832158-KJ833031.

Single-locus polymorphism analyses

Loci were amplified with differing degrees of success because bacterial DNA concentrations varied across samples. Additionally, the primers showed differing sensitivity to individual sequences. For this reason, each locus was initially examined independently in the polymorphism analyses. All samples were retained even if they had not yielded sequences for all target loci. We wanted to ensure that a similar amount of phylogenetic information could be obtained from the different sequences at each locus.

We therefore excluded from further analyses any sequences that were shorter than 70% of the expected length. We also excluded sequences containing ambiguous base-calls.

To estimate polymorphism at each locus, DnaSP 5.10 software was used to calculate haplotype diversity (Hd, the number of variable nucleotide sites) and nucleotide diversity (π, the average number of nucleotide differences per site between two sequences). We also investigated the potential impact of recombination on our alignments by calculating minimum recombination values (Rm).

Phylogenic tree building

Unless otherwise indicated, the following analyses were carried out with the packages "ape", "ade4", and "fpc" in R v2.15.1 [31].

For each locus, we first used the alignment constructed for the polymorphism analyses to build a DNA distance matrix. We then used a bio++ algorithm to integrate the parameters of the best model of evolution for that alignment (selected with the Akaike Criterion (AIC) value calculated using the *phymltest* function in "ape"). Using this DNA distance matrix, a phylogenic tree was built with the *bionj* function in "ape". When possible, similar analyses were performed using homologous data obtained from GenBank (data not shown).

Then, we restricted the alignment of each locus (except that of *ankA*) to samples for which at least five out of our eight loci had been successfully sequenced. The goal was to create a supertree. As before, the AIC of each locus was calculated from the restricted dataset in order to select the best model of sequence evolution. Then, the alignments of the eight loci were concatenated into a single alignment. As samples included in the supertree analysis could lack up to three loci, missing locus sequences were represented by gaps in the concatenated alignment. A supertree was built from the concatenated alignment with MrBayes 3.2 software, using a Bayesian method of construction that has been developed to highlight the information provided by the different markers while optimizing tree structure [32].

This method has been shown to be robust even when more than 50% of the data are missing [33].

The data were partitioned in MrBayes, and the respective best model of evolution was applied to each partition. Three runs of 500 000 generations were performed using a Metropolis-coupled Markov chain Monte Carlo (MCMCMC) approach based on six chains. Trees were sampled from the main chain every 500 generations. Assuming that convergence had not been reached, the first 25% of sampled trees were removed. Then, using the remaining trees, a supertree was generated from the 25% of trees with the highest posterior probabilities among the three runs. The robustness of the phylogenetic relationships among genotypes was evaluated using the Bayesian posterior probability of the branches.

Phylogenetic analyses

The presence of clusters in the phylogenic supertree was evaluated using the Ward's classification approach [34] based on the supertree distances; this was calculated using the *hclust* function in R. The number of clusters was determined using the minimum sum of squared errors and confirmed with the functions *pamk* and *kmeans* in the "fpc" package. Each sample present in the supertree was assigned to one cluster. The clusters from the supertree were mapped onto the *ankA* phylogenic tree in order to compare the two phylogenic structures.

We then wanted to explore if DNA polymorphism at each locus was linked with either host origin or the clusters identified in the supertree. To do this, a discriminant analysis was performed on the principal coordinate analysis of the DNA distance matrices using the *dudi. pco* function in the "ade4" package.

Results

Polymorphism analyses

All the results of the polymorphism analyses are summarized in Table 1.

Table 1 Genetic diversity measured for all loci with DnaSP

	APH 1099-1100	*Msp4*	*RecG*	*PolA*	*GyrA*	*TypA*	*GroESL*	*PleD*	*AnkA*	*AnkAI*	*AnkAII*	*AnkAIII*	*AnkAIV*	Mean
Nb indiv	98	136	88	79	54	114	100	63	101	34	6	16	45	
Length bp	435	390	351	333	837	462	630	597	654	661	753	710	702	
Nb site poly	19	38	12	21	20	27	35	27	352	47	22	36	74	
% site poly	3.37	9.74	3.41	6.30	2.39	5.84	5.55	4.52	53.82	7.11	2.92	5.07	10,54	6.575
Nb haplo	9	30	17	22	24	33	36	10	64	22	4	9	31	
Haplo Div (Hd)	0.565	0.875	0.807	0.838	0.93	0.86	0.923	0.661	0.983	0.961	0.8	0.908	0.958	0.827
Nucleo div (π)	0.0084	0.0237	0.0047	0.0106	0.0043	0.0087	0.01156	0.0168	0.2083	0.0176	0.0123	0.0076	0.0185	0.0178
Rm	1	7	1	5	6	7	7	2	NA	8	0	1	12	

Nb indiv: number of samples analyzed by loci; Length bp: length of the alignment in bp; Nb site poly and % site poly: number and proportion of polymorphic sites in the alignment; Nb haplo: number of haplotypes; Hd: haplotype diversity; π: nucleotide diversity; and Rm: number of estimated recombination events.

The sequence lengths of the alignments obtained for the different loci ranged from 333 to 837 bp, excluding gapped and missing sites (837 bp for *gyrA*, 630 bp for *groESL*, 654 bp for *ankA*, 597 bp for *pleD*, 462 bp for *typA*, 390 bp for *msp4*, 351 bp for *recG*, and 333 bp for *polA*). Haplotype diversity ranged from 0.565 to 0.983, with an average diversity of 0.827. The loci *msp4*, *gyrA*, *groESL*, and *ankA* demonstrated above-average haplotype diversity, while the haplotype diversity of *APH_1099-1100*, *recG*, and *pleD* was below average.

We treated *ankA* separately from the other loci because it is composed of four very divergent regions. Its overall average nucleotide diversity was 0.2. However, closer examination of this locus revealed that, while the start and the end regions of its sequences were obviously homologous, more than 50% of sites were polymorphic. As a result, it was difficult to estimate nucleotide diversity and the number of recombination events for the locus as a whole. Consequently, we chose to examine the sequences of the four clusters (named I to IV) separately.

When all loci were taken into account (including *ankA* I-IV), intralocus nucleotide diversity ranged from 4.7×10^{-3} to 2.3×10^{-2}, with an average of 1.8×10^{-2} nucleotides per site. The values for *msp4*, *groESL*, *pleD*, and *ankA* I-IV were higher than the mean, while *recG* and *gyrA* had the lowest diversity, with 4.7×10^{-3} and 4.3×10^{-3} nucleotide differences, respectively, per site between pairs of sequences.

Phylogenic trees and analyses

The different phylogenic trees built from single gene alignments were not directly comparable to each other because of both conflicting phylogenetic signals and missing data. Indeed, we were able to sequence all nine loci for only 11 samples. However, in each phylogenic tree, the genotypes obtained from roe deer clustered in one or two branches that were only distantly related to most other genotypes (Additional file 3). This clustering of roe deer genotypes was also supported by the discriminant analysis of all the loci (Additional file 4).

For each locus (with the exception of *ankA*), we generally found that measurements of diversity were relatively homogenous, while most branching patterns were heterogeneous. With this in mind, we decided to build a supertree, based on all loci except *ankA*, to obtain more insight into the phylogenetic relationships among *A. phagocytophilum* genotypes. The supertree was thus based on a sub-sample of 93 bacterial genotypes for which at least five loci had been characterized. This dataset included individual genotypes obtained from 72 cattle, 9 horses, 4 roe deer, and 3 dogs (Figure 1). Within the tree, the cluster analysis revealed the presence of three genetic groups. Cluster A included all the roe deer and two cattle genotypes (BR-BO-46 and BR-BO-08); cluster B was composed exclusively of cattle genotypes;

and cluster C was composed of the horse, dog, and remaining cattle genotypes. In general, the clusters identified in the supertree were not observed in the single-locus phylogenies, with the exception of the *pleD* phylogeny. No obvious geographical patterns were observed in the clustering of the different genotypes (Figure 2). However, we could not test the correlation between geographical and phylogenetic distance because of the low number of individual samples per host species, as well as the lack of precise information about sample location.

The *ankA* phylogeny generated here was structured in four clusters (designated I, II, III, and IV), as has been previously described [13]. For 95% of the genotypes, the pattern of clustering in the *ankA* phylogeny was highly similar to that of the supertree. In general, the genotypes of supertree cluster A grouped in *ankA* cluster II, the genotypes of supertree cluster B grouped in *ankA* cluster IV, and the genotypes of supertree cluster C grouped in *ankA* cluster I. Only four genotypes, all isolated from cattle, were found in a different cluster in the supertree than in the *ankA* phylogeny (BR-BO-09, RA-BO-03, BR-BO-14, and NO-BO-26). However, although the phylogenic relationships were topologically similar between the supertree and the *ankA* tree, the phylogenic distances between the clusters were very different. For example, we observed fewer than 0.05 substitutions per site between clusters B and C in the supertree; in contrast, the inferred divergence between clusters I and IV in the *ankA* tree (which contained the same genotypes) was nearly one substitution per site.

In the past, *ankA* cluster II had been reported to contain *A. phagocytophilum* genotypes isolated exclusively from ticks, roe deer, and red deer. However, our study found three cattle genotypes (BR-BO-46, BR-BO-08 and BR-BO-63) in this cluster. To our knowledge, this is a novel finding. Our results agree with previously published studies in showing that *ankA* cluster III only includes variants found in roe deer: six genotypes from roe deer grouped in this cluster [13]. Unfortunately, these samples could not be included in the supertree because the minimum criterion of having at least five sequenced loci was not met. The discriminant analysis of *ankA* revealed an association between host species and phylogenetic distance between genotypes, which was not found in the phylogenies of any of our other markers.

Discussion

High-resolution genetic data are important to decipher potentially genotype-dependent components of epidemiological cycles—such as sources and chains of transmission—and the spatial distributions of diseases. In this study, we characterized the diversity of *A. phagocytophilum* genotypes found in cattle using a combination of three commonly used markers and six new

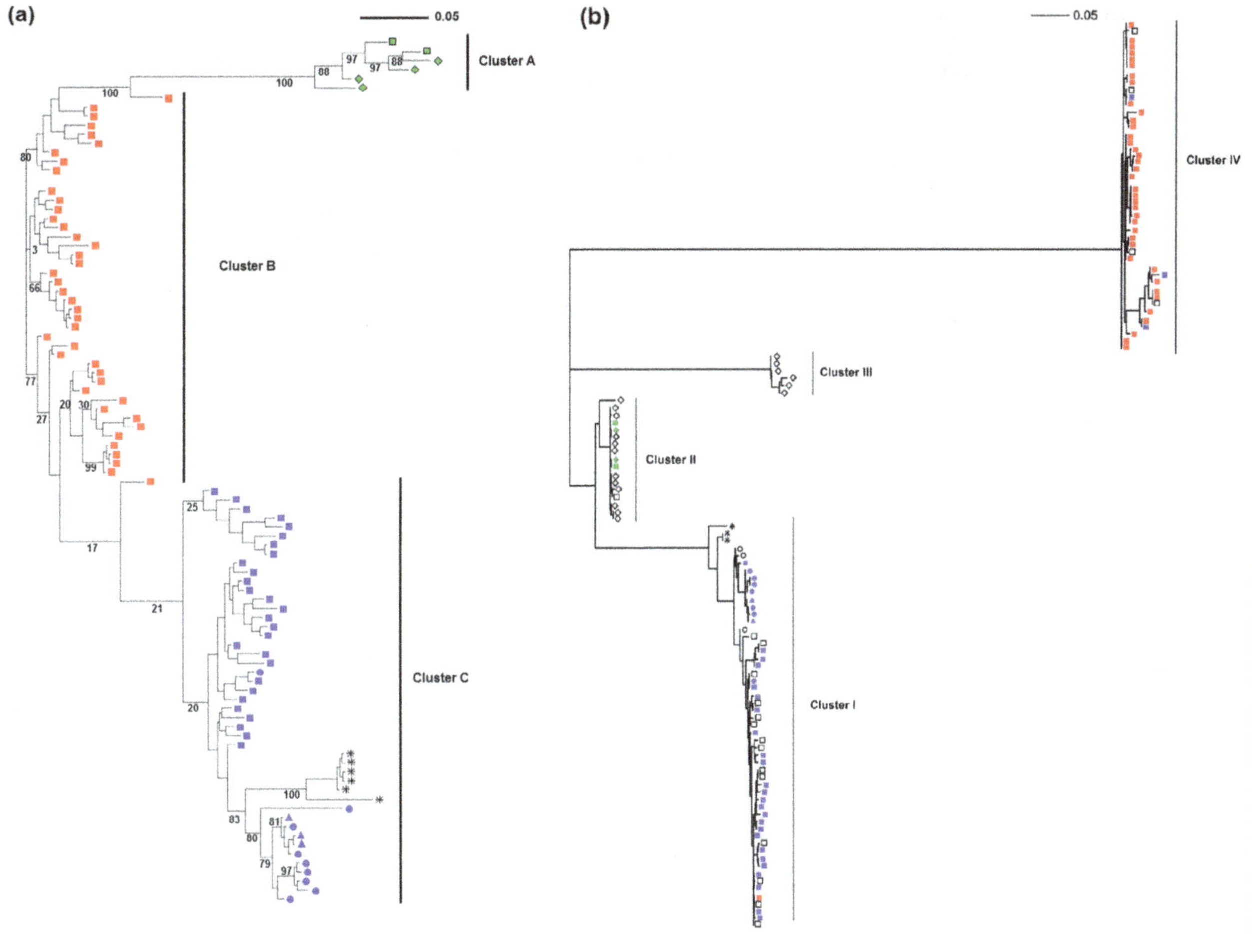

Figure 1 Unrooted supertree (a) & unrooted *ankA*tree (b). Each tree was built using a maximum likelihood approach. The supertree was built from parameters optimized by MCMCMC with MrBayes, and the *ankA* phylogeny was built using parameters optimized with *phymltest* in R. Each sample is identified by a symbol representing its host animal: □ for cattle, o for horses, ◊ for roe deer, and Δ for dogs; the different colors indicate the supertree cluster to which the sample was assigned.

ones. The new markers were included in order to improve the degree of resolution of our genotyping efforts. We constructed a supertree based on eight of those markers and compared its structure with that of a tree based on the *ankA* gene, which is linked to infection. In both trees, bovine *A. phagocytophilum* genotypes grouped into three major clusters. This finding strongly supports the existence of major genetic lineages in populations of *A. phagocytophilum*, a pattern that is probably due to host adaptation.

Our results support the value of these markers in studying the genetic diversity of *A. phagocytophilum*. Indeed, the degree of polymorphism found in our study allowed us to characterize multilocus genotypes that corresponded to most of the *ankA* groups described in the literature. The average pairwise divergence among genotypes (i.e., π) in our samples was lower for the new loci (*typA*, *gyrA*, *pleD*, *recG*, *polA*, and the intergenic spacer *APH_1099-APH_1100*) than it was for *groESL* and *msp4*.

It was also much lower than the *ankA* values, suggesting that the new genes we chose contain relevant phylogenic information. Haplotype diversity, which represents the probability of finding different alleles in a pair of samples, was similar across most loci; it had an average value of 0.8. This result also suggests that the added loci contributed to our ability to discriminate among genotypes of *A. phagocytophilum*.

Because of the unusual pattern of genetic diversity at the *ankA* locus, it was used to construct a separate tree, an approach that has been applied in other studies. The *ankA* locus is a widely used marker that enables large-scale genetic delineation among genotypes of *A. phagocytophilum*. Previous studies of *ankA* diversity have found that four highly divergent groups—designated groups I, II, III, and IV—exist within *A. phagocytophilum* [13]. The topology of our *ankA* phylogeny reflected this same grouping. However, the specific evolutionary constraints of *ankA* have resulted in a degree of genetic

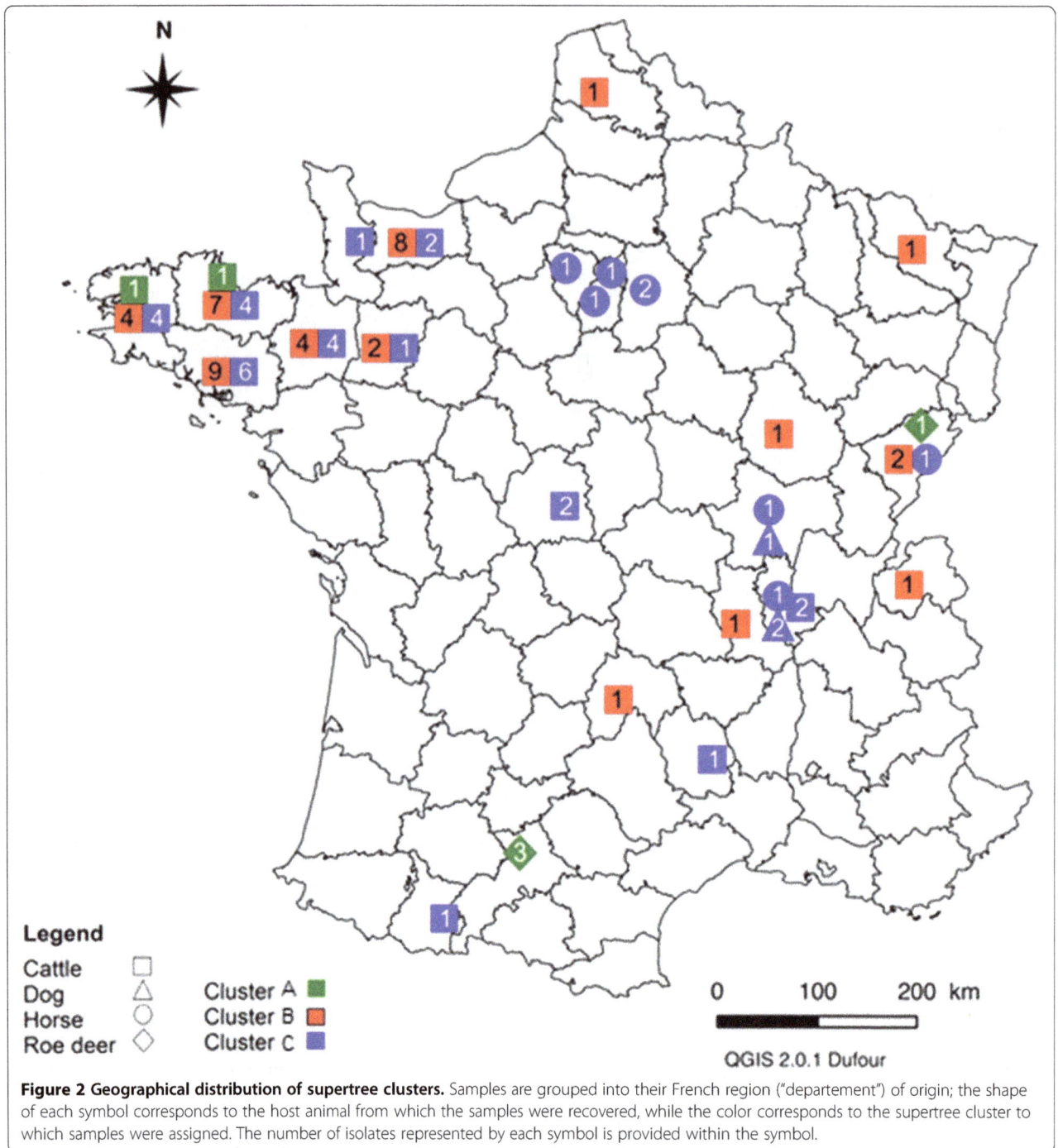

Figure 2 Geographical distribution of supertree clusters. Samples are grouped into their French region ("departement") of origin; the shape of each symbol corresponds to the host animal from which the samples were recovered, while the color corresponds to the supertree cluster to which samples were assigned. The number of isolates represented by each symbol is provided within the symbol.

divergence among groups that is too high to allow detailed inference about phylogenic relationships among *A. phagocytophilum* lineages (e.g., up to one substitution per site has been inferred between clusters I and IV). Likewise, within-group *ankA* diversity is too low to provide an informative degree of resolution.

As expected from previous studies [35], the other single-gene phylogenetic analyses generated different topologies. However, regardless of the gene under consideration, alleles

isolated from roe deer always grouped in one or two clusters that were distantly related to all other genotypes. There are several potential explanations for the phylogenetic incongruencies we observed among the single-tree phylogenies. First, they may reflect a lack of resolution resulting from the small number of informative sites per locus [23]. This could explain, for example, the presence of polytomies in the phylogenetic tree based on *typA*. Another potential explanation is the presence of recombination events.

Indeed, when we calculated the minimum recombination values, we found evidence of recombination events. Such events have the potential to bias the inference of phylogenetic relationships. This problem has already been reported in a phylogenetic study based on *msp4* and *ankA* markers [36,37]. Finally, the incongruencies we observed could also be the result of some individuals being co-infected by multiple strains [38]. In such cases, the phylogenetic locations of loci obtained from the same host individual would be expected to vary across the single-locus trees because the sequences would have come from different, co-infecting strains. In our data, the presence of ambiguous sites in some chromatograms suggests that multiple strains may have been present in some samples. This problem appeared to rarely affect the cattle samples but may have had an influence on around 30% of the roe deer samples. We thus excluded all samples with ambiguous sites at least one locus to avoid the risk of incongruence between loci.

These three factors may have increased inconsistency in the single-gene phylogenies. Because of this, we employed another approach that uses several markers—and thus the phylogenetic information they contain—to generate robust genotype clusters [23]. Indeed, the supertree approach, here based on a Bayesian method of construction, was designed to highlight the common information revealed by markers while optimizing tree structure [32]. Moreover, supertree construction is commonly used to deal with the problem of missing data [39]. This is another recurring problem in *A. phagocytophilum* studies, since the rate of successful amplification in naturally infected samples can be lower than 30% [17]. However, the dataset used to build our supertree contained less missing data and thus allowed us to obtain an informative clustering pattern [33,40].

In our supertree, we identified three divergence-based clusters that almost perfectly matched the topologies of *ankA* groups I, II, and IV [13]. Unfortunately, we were not able to include the roe deer genotypes assigned to *ankA* cluster III in our supertree. Their inclusion would have allowed us to further investigate the distribution of *ankA* alleles among *A. phagocytophilum* lineages and represents an interesting future research goal. From a phylogenetic point of view, the relationships among strains were more clearly resolved in the supertree than in the *ankA* phylogeny. This was the case even though most of the inner branches of the supertree were not as robustly supported, which was to be expected given the issues discussed above [33]. However, the various divergence-based clusters do not represent monophyletic groups in the supertree. The discovery of a related outgroup or the acquisition of more phylogenetic information could give further insight into the evolution of lineages within *A. phagocytophilum*. Indeed, a recent genomic study suggested that up to 50 markers may be required to achieve the resolution that is necessary to investigate the phylogenetic relationships among conspecific bacterial genotypes [23].

The similar genetic clusters formed in both the supertree and the *ankA* tree further support the idea that major genetic lineages exist within populations of *A. phagocytophilum*. The three clusters in our supertree appear to each be linked to a different host species community: cluster B was composed exclusively of cattle genotypes; cluster C was composed of genotypes found in cattle, horses, and dogs; and cluster A was composed of the all roe deer genotypes and two genotypes found in cattle. The strain divergence we observed may be explained by three factors. First, there may be epidemiological differences (e.g., different host reservoirs or vector species) leading to different epidemiological cycles [17,41,42]. Second, hosts may differ in their susceptibility, which could lead to the emergence of bacterial genotypes with different levels of virulence [43]. Third, different lineages may have emerged or evolved in different geographical areas [44]. Among these three possibilities, the first—that strain epidemiology may differ—seems to be the best supported by our results.

The hypothesis that different strains have different epidemiological cycles is supported by the observation that the topologies of the single-gene trees based on *pleD* and *ankA* showed the same clustering patterns as the supertree. These two genes are known to be involved in the infection process. The former is one of three response regulators of *pleC*, a gene predicted to encode a sensor kinase. Both *pleC* and *pleD* are synchronously upregulated during the exponential growth stage of *A. phagocytophilum* and downregulated prior to extracellular release in human patients [29]. The latter encodes an effector protein secreted by the type IV secretion system that has been implicated in several infection processes. In particular, AnkA facilitates intracellular infection by activating the Abl-1 signaling pathway [45] and by manipulating host cell processes in its interactions with the *Anaplasma* translocated substrate 1 (Ats-1) protein [46]. Furthermore, *ankA* interacts with other gene regulatory regions of host chromatin to downregulate expression of key host defense genes like CYBB (gp91^{phox}) [47]. From a phylogenetic point of view, genes involved in the infection process are highly relevant because selective pressures applied to those genes could promote host specialization. Indeed, phylogenetic analyses of *ankA* have identified clusters that are strongly linked to specific host communities. For example, clusters II and III are composed predominantly of strains isolated from roe and red deer [13], while the recently described cluster V includes only rodent strains [37]. However, it may also be that the evolution of *A. phagocytophilum* as a species is driven by two opposing selective pressures, one towards specialization in a given host species and the other favoring a broader host range [48,49]. The close association between the *ankA*-based genetic clusters and the host communities indicates that there may be a barrier to cross-species transmission, which could arise from the host-specific nature of infection pathways. This relationship also suggests that the optimized fitness of a strain in one host species comes at the cost of lower fitness when the strain infects other species. An alternative evolutionary strategy could involve infecting a large number of susceptible species in order to persist longer in host communities. This strategy could prove especially useful if the species composition of the community varies over time. Assuming that different bacterial variants have the opportunity to come in contact with different host species, the ability of a given *A. phagocytophilum* genotype to infect different host species would be key to its persistence in the local community. Selection may also favor an intermediate strategy—the maintenance of diverse variants with overlapping host ranges. This is what we found here, with three clusters of genotypes that each contained cattle-infecting strains. Other studies have shown that it is possible for populations of *A. phagocytophilum* to have co-existing epidemiological cycles, with different genotypes infecting different sets of hosts [12,17,41]. In this case, the divergence among strains would be linked to adaptation to different sets of hosts rather than to a single species [49].

The second hypothesis is that differences in host susceptibility have led to the emergence of divergent *A. phagocytophilum* genotypes that demonstrate different degrees of virulence. If genetic variation underlies the virulence of *A. phagocytophilum* genotypes, this fact may explain the variety of symptoms that have been described in cattle, including edema, fever, abortion, as well as acute or chronic symptoms [10]. Mathematical models support the idea that pathogen strains that differ in their degree of virulence can emerge within a single host species [43]. However, this outcome requires that a large degree of variation exist in individual susceptibility within that species (as a result of vaccination, for example). In contrast, the emergence of variable virulence is easier to observe in multihost systems [50]. In this case, a shift in the pathogen's host range would likely involve a concomitant evolutionary shift in virulence. It can be hypothesized that limited transmission between the respective reservoirs of different genotypes might eventually lead to variation in virulence. Consistent with this hypothesis is the observation that different *A. phagocytophilum* genotypes isolated from different host species showed different degrees of virulence when they were used to experimentally infect lambs [51] and mice [52]. In the present study, we found that the phylogenetic clustering of genotype groups in the supertree

mirrored the clustering observed in the single-gene trees that were based on infection-related genes. This pattern strongly suggests that the evolution of *A. phagocytophilum* genotypes is influenced by selective pressures on genes that regulate infection. The genetic variation that we observed in these genes may well be linked to variation in virulence, and it is possible that strains from different genotype clusters provoked different symptoms in infected animals. However, since we lacked sufficiently detailed information about the individual symptoms of each host animal, we were not able to test this hypothesis.

The third hypothesis states that genetically divergent strains of *A. phagocytophilum* may have evolved in different geographic regions. However, this hypothesis is not supported by our data, as we did not observe clear, broad-scale heterogeneity in the spatial distribution of the genotypes (Figure 2). It is nonetheless important to note that spatial (environmental or geographical) factors could structure pathogen populations. This could occur through drift or through changes in the host community involved in the transmission cycle. For example, there exists an European *A. phagocytophilum* genotype only observed in the Camargue and in Sardinia. This suggests that the environmental conditions of the Mediterranean region favor the dispersion of this genotype [36,53]. Similarly, it has been hypothesized that host distribution and other environmental constraints influence the local distribution of *A. phagocytophilum* lineages in Sicily [54]. In this study, however, we did not observe any clear clustering of genotype groups that could be attributed to geographical boundaries. Divergence among clusters is thus more likely explained by a difference in host communities rather than by geographical factors.

Consequently, of the three hypotheses discussed above, this study found support only for the first: that the genotype clustering we observed stems from strains having different epidemiological cycles. Therefore, we will further discuss the three clusters of *A. phagocytophilum* genotypes found in cattle, working from the assumption that they are the result of three independent epidemiological cycles.

In the supertree, clusters A, B, and C all included genotypes isolated from cattle. Within the latter, a subgroup of genotypes corresponded to those found in *ankA* cluster I. This subgroup contained genotypes associated with cattle as well as genotypes associated with dogs and horses. Although we had relatively few equine and canine samples, these results are consistent with those previously reported for *ankA* [13]. Furthermore, a recent study also showed that this cluster of *ankA* genotypes includes not only strains that infect horses and dogs, but also those that infect other hosts, such as humans, wild boar (*Sus scrofa*), hedgehogs *(Erinaceus europaeus)*, and red deer [24]. Since *A. phagocytophilum* has high levels of prevalence in red deer and hedgehogs (approximately 60% and 80% of individuals are infected, respectively [14,55-57]), further quantitative surveys are needed to assess whether these hosts play a role in the spread of this *A. phagocytophilum* strain in cattle.

In our analysis, supertree genotype cluster B, corresponding to *ankA* cluster IV, contained only strains isolated from cattle, although previous studies have reported related genotypes in sheep and, rarely, in roe and red deer [13,37]. The seemingly low level of prevalence of this bacterial lineage in wild mammals raises questions about the role of these animals in the spread of this genotype. Livestock are not generally thought of as reservoir species for *A. phagocytophilum* because they only sporadically exhibit clinical symptoms of anaplasmosis. However, a serological survey in cattle herds indicated that pathogen prevalence may be high—it varied from 31 to 77% at different times of the year [58]. Furthermore, longitudinal surveys in cattle herds have suggested that the immunity acquired following exposure to *A. phagocytophilum* does not suffice to prevent subsequent infection but is sufficient to prevent clinical signs of disease. This could result in a high proportion of asymptomatic carriers [59]. Interestingly, experimental studies have shown that *A. phagocytophilum* can persist in "reservoir tissues" in sheep; while they may be persistent carriers, PCR analyses of their blood will fail to detect infection [60]. It is possible that the bacteria present in "reservoir tissues" periodically circulate in the blood and infect feeding ticks. This possibility underscores the need for further experimental studies on *A. phagocytophilum* infection in cattle: if the same process occurs in cattle, the bovine population could act as a reservoir.

Finally, a few bovine genotypes were found in cluster A of the supertree, which corresponds to *ankA* cluster II. In the multigene phylogeny, this group was relatively distantly related to the others and was dominated by genotypes from roe deer. From an epidemiological point of view, it is likely that roe deer contribute to the spread of *A. phagocytophilum*, if only because the pathogen is highly prevalent in roe deer populations (up to 70% of infection detected by PCR, 11, 12). From a genetic point of view, a phylogenetic analysis of *ankA* indicated that the genotypes carried by roe deer and a few red deer were distantly related to the genotypes carried by other host species [13]. Similarly, previous studies using *groESL* have indicated that the strains carried by roe deer are different from the strains found in other hosts [14]. Finally, a recent study showed that both MLST genotypes and *ankA* sequences supported the existence of a roe deer-associated group of *A. phagocytophilum* genotypes [24]. After the publication of more than 800 *ankA* sequences and 380 MLST-characterized sequences in the literature, we report here, for the first time, that strains isolated from cattle are present within this cluster. Our results suggest that, however rare it may be, transmission can occur between cattle and roe deer and may be due to a spillover effect.

In conclusion, we used multilocus sequencing to describe the genetic diversity of *A. phagocytophilum* strains causing clinical illness in domesticated animals in France. In doing so, we discovered the presence of three groups of genotypes. These groups show a cross-country distribution and are probably associated with different host communities, an observation that suggests that *A. phagocytophilum* is propagated through different epidemiological cycles that involve different reservoir and host species. In order to gain further insights into the population dynamics of this bacterial pathogen, future epidemiological studies are needed. These studies should be organized on a subregional scale and focus on different potential reservoirs, domesticated hosts, and lineages of *A. phagocytophilum*. Such a sampling scheme would be challenging to carry out, so epidemiological modeling is also required to determine the number of infected individuals that should be sampled within a potential reservoir species to adequately describe pathogen flow. In addition, the detection and characterization of asymptomatic cases in cattle—whether these cases are due to variation in pathogen virulence or to differences in symptom manifestation in different hosts—represents an important research path to explore. In particular, the existence of healthy carriers that contribute to the maintenance and spread of virulent strains could have serious implications for efforts aimed at limiting bovine granulocytic anaplasmosis.

Additional files

Additional file 1: Description of the host and geographical origin of the samples and the classification of the *ankA* and supertree clusters to which the samples were assigned. The table contains information on the samples used in the study. a: "-" indicates ambiguous or too short sequences; "NA" indicates unsuccessful amplification. b: "-" indicates individuals not included in the supertree because less than five loci were characterized.

Additional file 2: Primers used in and information about the nested PCRs. The table contains information on the primers used in the study. * developed by Lotrič-Furlan [30].

Additional file 3: Unrooted trees based on the sequences of the following loci: a) *groEL*; b) *msp4*; c) *gyrA*; d) *pleD*; e) *polA*; f) *recG*; g) *typA*; and h) the intergenic region CtrA-APH_1100. Each tree was built using a maximum likelihood approach; parameter optimization was performed with *phymltest* in R. The colors indicate the supertree cluster to which the samples were assigned: green for the cluster A, red for the cluster B, and blue for the cluster C.

Additional file 4: Discriminant analysis by host based on the principal coordinates analyses of the following loci: a) *msp4*; b) *polA*; c) *typA*; d) *groEL*; e) *recG*; f) CtrA- APH_1100; g) *gyrA*; and h) *pleD*. The graphs show the results of the discriminant analysis conducted on the principal coordinates analysis of each locus.

Competing interests
The authors declare that they have no competing interests.

Authors' contributions

AL, XB, and GV participated in the design and coordination of the study and the drafting of the manuscript. TD, HV, LL, VB, LC, GJ, RM, H-JB, and NH contributed to data collection and help draft the manuscript. AC carried out all the experiments and analyses, contributed to data collection, and helped draft the manuscript. All authors read and approved the final manuscript.

Acknowledgements

We thank the teams of the LABÉO – Frank Duncombe, LDA 22, and LVD 69 for generously providing DNA extracts and blood samples from domesticated animals; the members of SNGTV for actively helping us to obtain samples from domesticated animals; Magalie René-Martellet and Jeanne Chêne for providing the dog samples; the members of the SAGIR network, which collected the roe deer samples; Lindsay Higgins and Jessica Pearce-Duvet for proofreading the manuscript; Nelly Dorr for creating the databases used in this study; and Angélique Pion and Valérie Poux, who were involved in laboratory work. Finally, we thank the French National Research Agency, which funded this work through the OSCAR project.

Author details

[1]INRA, UR346 Epidémiologie Animale, F-63122 Saint Genès Champanelle, France. [2]Université Paris-Est, Ecole Nationale Vétérinaire d'Alfort, UMR BIPAR, 23 avenue du Général de Gaulle, 94706 Maisons-Alfort, France. [3]INRA, CEFS, UR035, 24 chemin de Borde Rouge - Auzeville, CS 52627, F-31326 Castanet Tolosan, France. [4]LABÉO - Frank Duncombe, Unite Risques Microbiens (U2RM), Normandie Universite, EA 4655 Caen, Normandy, France. [5]Laboratoire Vétérinaire Départemental du Rhône, Campus vétérinaire VetAgro Sup, 1 avenue Bourgelat, 69280 Marcy l'Etoile, France. [6]Université de Lyon, VetAgro Sup, Jeune Equipe Hémopathogènes Vectorisés, F-69280 Marcy l'Etoile, France. [7]Groupe Vétérinaire de Callac, 26 rue du Cleumeur, 22160 Callac, France. [8]Ecole Nationale Vétérinaire de Toulouse, Unité pathologie des ruminants, 23 Chemin des Capelles, 31076 Toulouse, France. [9]Département Hippique, VetAgroSup, F-69280 Marcy L'Etoile, France.

References

1. Van Belkum A, Struelens M, de Visser A, Verbrugh H, Tibayrenc M (2001) Role of genomic typing in taxonomy, evolutionary genetics, and microbial epidemiology. Clin Microbiol Rev 14:547–560
2. Keesing F, Holt RD, Ostfeld RS (2006) Effects of species diversity on disease risk. Ecol Lett 9:485–498
3. Biek R, O'Hare A, Wright D, Mallon T, McCormick C, Orton RJ, et al. (2012) Whole genome sequencing reveals local transmission patterns of Mycobacterium bovis in sympatric cattle and badger populations. PLoS Pathog 8:e1003008
4. Anderson JF (1989) Epizootiology of Borrelia in Ixodes tick vectors and reservoir hosts. Rev Infect Dis 11(Suppl 6):S1451–S1459
5. Stanek G, Fingerle V, Hunfeld KP, Jaulhac B, Kaiser R, Krause A, et al. (2011) Lyme borreliosis: clinical case definitions for diagnosis and management in Europe. Clin Microb Infect 17:69–79
6. Kurtenbach K, De Michelis S, Etti S, Schäfer SM, Sewell H-S, Brade V, et al. (2002) Host association of Borrelia burgdorferi sensu lato–the key role of host complement. Trends Microbiol 10:74–79
7. Woldehiwet Z (2010) The natural history of Anaplasma phagocytophilum. Vet Parasitol 167:108–122
8. Stuen S, Granquist EG, Silaghi C (2013) Anaplasma phagocytophilum - a widespread multi-host pathogen with highly adaptive strategies. Front Cell Infect Microbiol 3:31
9. Macleod J, Gordon WS (1933) Studies in tick-borne fever of sheep, I: transmission by the tick, Ixodes ricinus, with a description of the disease produced. Parasitology 25:273–283
10. Joncour G, Pouliquen G, Kaufmann P, Mayaux P (2006) Anaplasma phagocytophilum, agent de l'ehrlichiose granulocytaire bovine (EGB) et avortements chez les bovins. Bull GTV 35:95–104 (in French)
11. Petrovec M, Bidovec A, Sumner JW, Nicholson WL, Childs JE, Avsic-Zupanc T (2002) Infection with Anaplasma phagocytophila in cervids from Slovenia: evidence of two genotypic lineages. Wien Klin Wochenschr 114:641–647
12. Silaghi C, Hamel D, Thiel C, Pfister K, Passos LMF, Rehbein S (2011) Genetic variants of Anaplasma phagocytophilum in wild caprine and cervid ungulates from the Alps in Tyrol, Austria. Vector Borne Zoonotic Dis 11:355–362
13. Scharf W, Schauer S, Freyburger F, Petrovec M, Schaarschmidt-Kiener D, Liebisch G, et al. (2011) Distinct host species correlate with Anaplasma phagocytophilum ankA gene clusters. J Clin Microbiol 49:790–796
14. Rymaszewska A (2008) Divergence within the marker region of the groESL operon in Anaplasma phagocytophilum. Eur J Clin Microbiol Infect Dis 27:1025–1036
15. Foley J, Nieto NC, Madigan J, Sykes J (2008) Possible differential host tropism in Anaplasma phagocytophilum strains in the Western United States. Ann N Y Acad Sci 1149:94–97
16. Rikihisa Y (2011) Mechanisms of obligatory intracellular infection with Anaplasma phagocytophilum. Clin Microbiol Rev 24:469–489
17. Rejmanek D, Bradburd G, Foley J (2012) Molecular characterization reveals distinct genospecies of Anaplasma phagocytophilum from diverse North American hosts. J Med Microbiol 61:204–212
18. Alberti A, Sparagano OA (2006) Molecular diagnosis of granulocytic anaplasmosis and infectious cyclic thrombocytopenia by PCR-RFLP. Ann N Y Acad Sci 1081:371–378
19. Dumler J, Asanovich K, Bakken J (2003) Analysis of genetic identity of North American Anaplasma phagocytophilum strains by pulsed-field gel electrophoresis. J Clin Microbiol 41:3392–3394
20. Bown K, Lambin X, Ogden N, Petrovec M, Shaw S, Woldehiwet Z, et al (2007) High-resolution genetic fingerprinting of European strains of Anaplasma phagocytophilum by use of multilocus variable-number tandem-repeat analysis. J Clin Microbiol 45:1771–1776
21. Liz J, Anderes L, Sumner J, Massung R, Gern L, Rutti B, et al. (2000) PCR detection of granulocytic ehrlichiae in Ixodes ricinus ticks and wild small mammals in western Switzerland. J Clin Microbiol 38:1002–1007
22. De La Fuente J, Massung RF, Wong SJ, Chu FK, Lutz H, Meli M, et al. (2005) Sequence analysis of the msp4 gene of Anaplasma phagocytophilum strains. J Clin Microbiol 43:1309–1317
23. Maiden MCJ, van Rensburg MJJ, Bray JE, Earle SG, Ford SA, Jolley KA, et al. (2013) MLST revisited: the gene-by-gene approach to bacterial genomics. Nat Rev Microbiol 11:728–736
24. Huhn C, Winter C, Wolfsperger T, Wüppenhorst N, Smrdel KS, Skuballa J, et al. (2014) Analysis of the population structure of Anaplasma phagocytophilum using multilocus sequence typing. PLoS One 3:e93725
25. Rymaszewska A (2014) Genotyping of Anaplasma phagocytophilum strains from Poland for selected genes. Folia Biol 62:35–46
26. Courtney JW, Kostelnik LM, Zeidner NS, Massung RF (2004) Multiplex real-time PCR for detection of Anaplasma phagocytophilum and Borrelia burgdorferi. J Clin Microbiol 42:3164–3168
27. Maiden MCJ, Bygraves JA, Feil E, Morelli G, Russell JE, Urwin R, et al. (1998) Multilocus sequence typing: a portable approach to the identification of clones within populations of pathogenic microorganisms. Proc Natl Acad Sci U S A 95:3140–3145
28. Konstantinidis KT, Ramette A, Tiedje JM (2006) Toward a more robust assessment of intraspecies diversity, using fewer genetic markers. Appl Environ Microbiol 72:7286–7293
29. Lai T-H, Kumagai Y, Hyodo M, Hayakawa Y, Rikihisa Y (2009) The Anaplasma phagocytophilum PleC histidine kinase and PleD diguanylate cyclase two-component system and role of cyclic Di-GMP in host cell infection. J Bacteriol 191:693–700
30. Lotrič-Furlan S, Petrovec M, Zupanc TA, Nicholson WL, Sumner JW, Childs JE, et al. (1998) Human granulocytic ehrlichiosis in Europe: clinical and laboratory findings for four patients from Slovenia. Clin Infect Dis 27:424–428
31. R Development Core Team (2008) R: a language and environment for statistical computing. In: Book R: A Language and Environment for Statistical Computing. R Foundation for Statistical Computing, City
32. Criscuolo A, Berry V, Douzery EJP, Gascuel O (2006) SDM: a fast distance-based approach for (super)tree building in phylogenomics. Syst Biol 55:740–755
33. Philippe H, Snell EA, Bapteste E, Lopez P, Holland PWH, Casane D (2004) Phylogenomics of eukaryotes: impact of missing data on large alignments. Mol Biol Evol 21:1740–1752
34. Ward JH, Jr (1963) Hierarchical grouping to optimize an objective function. J Am Stat Assoc 58:236–244
35. Silaghi C, Liebisch G, Pfister K (2011) Genetic variants of Anaplasma phagocytophilum from 14 equine granulocytic anaplasmosis cases. Parasit Vectors 4:161

36. Chastagner A, Bailly X, Leblond A, Pradier S, Vourc'h G (2013) Single genotype of *Anaplasma phagocytophilum* identified from ticks, Camargue. France Emerg Infect Dis 19:825–827

37. Majazki J, Wuppenhorst N, Hartelt K, Birtles R, von Loewenich FD (2013) *Anaplasma phagocytophilum* strains from voles and shrews exhibit specific *ankA* gene sequences. BMC Vet Res 9:235

38. Ladbury GAF, Stuen S, Thomas R, Bown KJ, Woldehiwet Z, Granquist EG, et al. (2008) Dynamic transmission of numerous *Anaplasma phagocytophilum* genotypes among lambs in an infected sheep flock in an area of anaplasmosis endemicity. J Clin Microbiol 46:1686–1691

39. Bininda-Emonds OR (2004) The evolution of supertrees. Trends Ecol Evol 19:315–322

40. Wiens JJ (1998) Combining data sets with different phylogenetic histories. Syst Biol 47:568–581

41. Bown KJ, Lambin X, Ogden NH, Begon M, Telford G, Woldehiwet Z, et al. (2009) Delineating *Anaplasma phagocytophilum* ecotypes in coexisting, discrete enzootic cycles. Emerg Infect Dis 15:1948–1954

42. Rejmanek D, Freycon P, Bradburd G, Dinstell J, Foley J (2013) Unique strains of Anaplasma phagocytophilum segregate among diverse questing and non-questing Ixodes tick species in the western United States. Ticks Tick Borne Dis 4:482–487

43. André JB, Gandon S (2006) Vaccination, within-host dynamics, and virulence evolution. Evolution 60:13–23

44. Zhaoqing Y, Miao J, Huang Y, Li X, Putaporntip C, Jongwutiwes S, et al. (2006) Genetic structures of geographically distinct Plasmodium vivax populations assessed by PCR/RFLP analysis of the merozoite surface protein 3β gene. Acta Trop 100:205–212

45. Lin M, den Dulk-Ras A, Hooykaas PJJ, Rikihisa Y (2007) Anaplasma phagocytophilum AnkA secreted by type IV secretion system is tyrosine phosphorylated by Abl-1 to facilitate infection. Cell Microbiol 9:2644–2657

46. Rikihisa Y, Lin M, Niu H (2010) Type IV secretion in the obligatory intracellular bacterium Anaplasma phagocytophilum. Cell Microbiol 12:1213–1221

47. Garcia-Garcia JC, Rennoll-Bankert KE, Pelly S, Milstone AM, Dumler JS (2009) Silencing of host cell CYBB gene expression by the nuclear effector AnkA of the intracellular pathogen Anaplasma phagocytophilum. Infect Immun 77:2385–2391

48. Keesing F, Belden LK, Daszak P, Dobson A, Harvell CD, Holt RD, et al. (2010) Impacts of biodiversity on the emergence and transmission of infectious diseases. Nature 468:647–652

49. Viana M, Mancy R, Biek R, Cleaveland S, Cross PC, Lloyd-Smith JO, et al. (2014) Assembling evidence for identifying reservoirs of infection. Trends Ecol Evol 29:270–279

50. Gandon S (2004) Evolution of multihost parasites. Evolution 58:455–469

51. Stuen S, Scharf W, Schauer S, Freyburger F, Bergström K, von Loewenich FD (2010) Experimental infection in lambs with a red deer (*Cervus elaphus*) isolate of *Anaplasma phagocytophilum*. J Wild Dis 46:803–809

52. Massung RF, Priestley RA, Miller NJ, Mather TN, Levin ML (2003) Inability of a variant strain of *Anaplasma phagocytophilum* to infect mice. J Infect Dis 188:1757–1763

53. Alberti A, Zobba R, Chessa B, Addis MF, Sparagano O, Parpaglia MLP, et al. (2005) Equine and canine *Anaplasma phagocytophilum* strains isolated on the island of Sardinia (Italy) are phylogenetically related to pathogenic strains from the United States. Appl Environ Microbiol 71:6418–6422

54. Torina A, Alongi A, Naranjo V, Estrada-Pena A, Vicente J, Scimeca S, et al. (2008) Prevalence and genotypes of Anaplasma species and habitat suitability for ticks in a Mediterranean ecosystem. Appl Environ Microbiol 74:7578–7584

55. Zeman P, Pecha M (2008) Segregation of genetic variants of *Anaplasma phagocytophilum* circulating among wild ruminants within a Bohemian forest (Czech Republic). Int J Med Microbiol 298:203–210

56. Silaghi C, Skuballa J, Thiel C, Pfister K, Petney T, Pfaffle M, et al. (2012) The European hedgehog (Erinaceus europaeus) - a suitable reservoir for variants of *Anaplasma phagocytophilum*? Ticks Tick Borne Dis 3:49–54

57. Stuen S, Pettersen KS, Granquist EG, Bergström K, Bown KJ, Birtles RJ (2013) *Anaplasma phagocytophilum* variants in sympatric red deer (Cervus elaphus) and sheep in southern Norway. Ticks Tick Borne Dis 4:197–201

58. Lempereur L, Lebrun M, Cuvelier P, Sépult G, Caron Y, Saegerman C, et al. (2012) Longitudinal field study on bovine *Babesia spp.* and *Anaplasma phagocytophilum* infections during a grazing season in Belgium. Parasitol Res 110:1525–1530

59. Pusterla N, Pusterla JB, Braun U, Lutz H (1998) Serological, hematologic, and PCR studies of cattle in an area of Switzerland in which tick-borne fever (caused by *Ehrlichia phagocytophila*) is endemic. Clin Diagn Lab Immunol 5:325–327

60. Stuen S, Casey AN, Woldehiwet Z, French NP, Ogden NH (2006) Detection by the polymerase chain reaction of *Anaplasma phagocytophilum* in tissues of persistently infected sheep. J Comp Pathol 134:101–104

17

Trend analysis of *Trichinella* in a red fox population from a low endemic area using a validated artificial digestion and sequential sieving technique

Frits Franssen[1][*], Gunita Deksne[2], Zanda Esíte[2], Arie Havelaar[1,3], Arno Swart[1] and Joke van der Giessen[1]

Abstract

Freezing of fox carcasses to minimize professional hazard of infection with *Echinococcus multilocularis* is recommended in endemic areas, but this could influence the detection of *Trichinella* larvae in the same host species. A method based on artificial digestion of frozen fox muscle, combined with larva isolation by a sequential sieving method (SSM), was validated using naturally infected foxes from Latvia. The validated SSM was used to detect dead *Trichinella* muscle larvae (ML) in frozen muscle samples of 369 red foxes from the Netherlands, of which one fox was positive (0.067 larvae per gram). This result was compared with historical *Trichinella* findings in Dutch red foxes. Molecular analysis using 5S PCR showed that both *T. britovi* and *T. nativa* were present in the Latvian foxes, without mixed infections. Of 96 non-frozen *T. britovi* ML, 94% was successfully sequenced, whereas this was the case for only 8.3% of 72 frozen *T. britovi* ML. The single *Trichinella* sp. larva that was recovered from the positive Dutch fox did not yield PCR product, probably due to severe freeze-damage. In conclusion, the SSM presented in this study is a fast and effective method to detect dead *Trichinella* larvae in frozen meat. We showed that the *Trichinella* prevalence in Dutch red fox was 0.27% (95% CI 0.065-1.5%), in contrast to 3.9% in the same study area fifteen years ago. Moreover, this study demonstrated that the efficacy of 5S PCR for identification of *Trichinella britovi* single larvae from frozen meat is not more than 8.3%.

Introduction

Trichinella species infect a wide range of mammals, including humans [1,2]. In the European Union, the magnetic stirrer method (EU reference method, EU-RM) according to European regulation EC 2075/2005 [3] is used for individual carcass control of *Trichinella* susceptible animals intended for human consumption and for surveillance of *Trichinella* infections in wildlife. This method includes two consecutive sedimentation steps to isolate *Trichinella* muscle larvae (ML) and has been validated for the detection of live larvae, for which critical control points are well described [4]. To analyse *Trichinella* in wildlife, some adjustments to the magnetic stirrer method are necessary to improve efficiency, like

prolongation of digestion time, since meat of wildlife is more difficult to digest. In Europe, the red fox is considered an indicator species for *Trichinella* infections in wildlife and many studies are being carried out to determine the prevalence and infection rate of *Trichinella* in red fox populations [5-13]. Since in Europe the red fox is also a final host for *Echinococcus multilocularis*, a zoonotic parasite and causative agent of alveolar echinococcosis in humans, fox carcasses are deep frozen at −80 °C for minimally one week, to inactivate the infective stage of this fox tapeworm prior to post mortem examination, according to WHO biosafety instructions [14]. Already between −18 and −30 °C, freezing kills *Trichinella* ML within one week [15-18], thereby altering their sedimentation characteristics [4], which is a key factor in the analysis with EU-RM. Gamble [19] showed that live larvae settled with a sedimentation speed of about 2 cm/min in meat digest at 40 °C. This is enough to pass

* Correspondence: frits.franssen@rivm.nl
[1]National Institute for Public Health and the Environment, Centre for Zoonoses and Environmental Microbiology, Bilthoven, The Netherlands
Full list of author information is available at the end of the article

through 2 litres of meat digest in a separatory funnel within 16 min. At 4 °C the sedimentation speed was less, which would prolong the sedimentation time to 24 – 28 min. In contrast, Dyer and Evje [20] recovered only 80% of spiked dead *Trichinella* ML in 2 litres *Trichinella*-free meat digest after one hour of sedimentation (twice the time routinely used in EU-RM).

Well before the EU-RM was established, Henriksen [21] successfully used a filtration method to isolate dead *Trichinella* ML from experimentally infected rabbits. Enemark et al. [9] used 22 µm disposable filters to retain ML after artificial digestion of fox fore legs that had been kept at –20 °C for three to ten months prior to analysis. Retained ML were visualized by subsequent iodine/hypochlorite staining, which renders these larvae unsuitable for molecular species identification.

Van der Giessen et al. [8] used the Trichomatic[35] method, an automated system by which naked *Trichinella* larvae were isolated on a 14 µm mesh size nylon filter for subsequent microscopical examination. Isolated individual larvae were identified as *Trichinella britovi*, using a single larva PCR and reversed line blot analysis as described by Rombout et al. [22].

In this study, we describe validation of an artificial digestion method using the magnetic stirrer method, followed by a sequential sieving step to isolate dead *Trichinella* larvae from naturally infected fox muscle samples. We show that the recovery rate of spiked dead *Trichinella* larvae in meat digest is 60% using EU-RM, while the recovery rate using SSM is 92%, making SSM the technique of choice to detect dead *Trichinella* larvae in frozen meat. Consequently, the most sensitive technique was used to analyse the recovery rate of *Trichinella* larvae before (EU-RM, live larvae) and after (SSM, dead larvae) freezing of naturally infected fox samples. Moreover, the efficacy of molecular identification was studied on isolated ML originating from foxes from an endemic area, before and after freezing. The validated sequential sieving method was used to study *Trichinella* prevalence in the red fox population in the eastern border region of the Netherlands. Obtained *Trichinella* prevalence was compared to historical data to analyse trends in time.

Materials and methods
Animals and *Trichinella* larvae
The left Foreleg of 35 *Trichinella* positive (EU-RM) [3] non-frozen red foxes from Latvia were collected during routine inspection at the Institute of Food Safety, Animal Health and Environment BIOR (Riga, Latvia). These animals originated from all four Latvian regions (Vidzeme 6, Zemgale 7, Latgale 9 and Kurzeme 11 individuals, 2 not specified). After primary analysis of the muscle samples by EU-RM without freezing, the forelegs were frozen and kept

at –80 °C for one to two weeks, after which a second muscle sample from the same foreleg was tested with SSM at BIOR. A digestion time of 30-40 min was used for artificial digestion as described [3,4]. After detection of ML, isolated *Trichinella* larvae were kept in 96% ethanol at room temperature until further use. For analysis with multiplex PCR [23], pools of five *Trichinella* ML were isolated from 30 foxes from all four regions of Latvia (Vidzeme 6, Zemgale 7, Latgale 8 and Kurzeme 9 individuals). For single larva PCR, individual *Trichinella* ML from the same 30 foxes that were found positive both before and after freezing, were transferred to 5 µL of DNAse free water and stored at –20 °C until further use.

Live *Trichinella britovi* larvae for the validation of detection by sequential sieving were obtained from a farmed wild boar, which tested positive during regular meat inspection in Latvia (Zemgale region, Latvia, Institute of Food Safety, Animal Health and Environment BIOR).

Trichinella spiralis (ISS 14) larvae for use in spike experiments were obtained from experimentally infected mice by the EU-RM. This work was approved by the Ethical Committee of the Dutch National Institute for Public Health and the Environment (RIVM) (DEC permit number 201200223).

For Trichinella survey in the Netherlands from October 2010 - April 2013, 369 Dutch foxes were collected by hunters from the border region with Germany in the east and Belgium in the south (Figure 1). The majority of foxes (287) was collected during the hunting season November 2010 - April 2011. Collected foxes were sent to RIVM, Bilthoven, the Netherlands. Upon arrival, fox carcasses were stored at –80 °C to inactivate the eggs of possibly present *E. multilocularis* [24] according to WHO guidelines [14]. After a minimum period of one week, carcasses were thawed at approximately 10 °C and dissected. Muscles of both lower forelegs of each fox were collected and 15 g of muscle tissue was analysed for *Trichinella*, using the validated SSM.

Validation experiments
Crucial steps of the EU-RM for the detection of Trichinella larvae are complete digestion of muscle tissue and high effectivity of the procedure to isolate *Trichinella* ML. To validate the method for detection of dead *Trichinella* larvae in frozen meat samples, the process was separated into three stages.

1. Isolation and detection of dead larvae. The efficacy of dead *Trichinella* ML isolation using EU-RM and SSM was compared by spiking dead Trichinella ML in meat digest and subsequent recovery of ML. The sequential sieving method to detect *Trichinella* larvae was further validated by adding live or dead larvae to water or *Trichinella*-free meat digest and recovery by SSM.

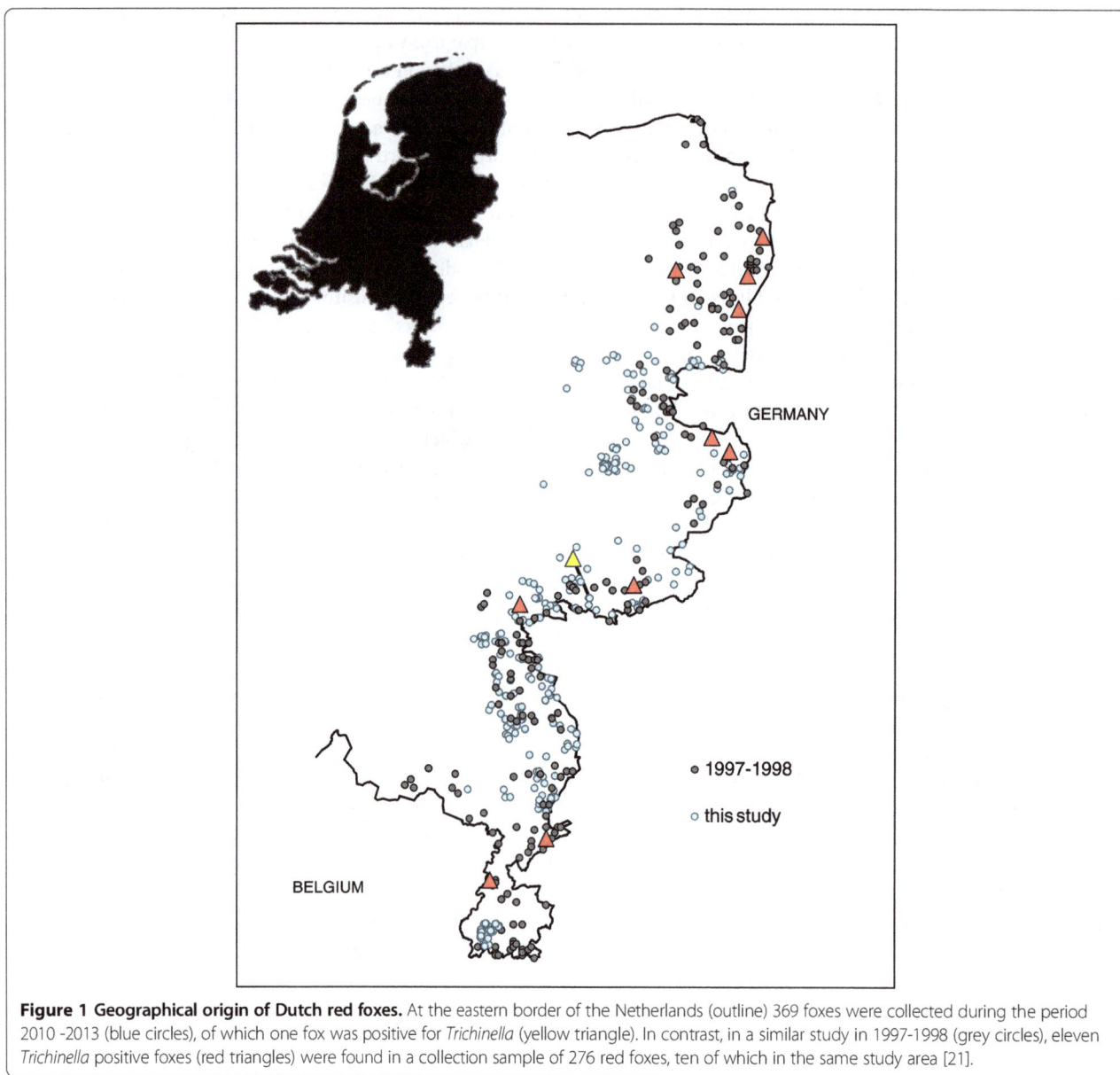

Figure 1 Geographical origin of Dutch red foxes. At the eastern border of the Netherlands (outline) 369 foxes were collected during the period 2010 -2013 (blue circles), of which one fox was positive for *Trichinella* (yellow triangle). In contrast, in a similar study in 1997-1998 (grey circles), eleven *Trichinella* positive foxes (red triangles) were found in a collection sample of 276 red foxes, ten of which in the same study area [21].

2. Feasibility of the use of *Trichinella* spiked frozen samples. Minced pork meat was spiked with live *Trichinella* larvae and subsequently, the spiked samples were frozen, to evaluate the possible effect of freezing on the recoverability of these larvae. The spiked and frozen samples were subjected to artificial digestion during 30 min according to EU 2075/2005 and subsequent detection of larvae by sequential sieving.

3. Validation of sequential sieving in relation to EU-RM. The sequential sieving method was validated by comparison of data obtained by analysis of fox forelegs using the EU-RM before freezing and data from digestion by SSM after freezing at –80 °C.

Validation of larva detection

Stainless steel sieves, approximately 18 centimetres in diameter, with mesh size 300 μm, 63 μm and 38 μm were stacked in decreasing mesh size order. A mesh size of 300 μm was used to retain undigested particles, instead of 180 μm, which is used in the EU-RM for the detection of live *Trichinella* ML. This reduced the risk of losing dead, comma shaped ML, which have typical measurements of 745-975 μm length by a width of 36 μm [25]. To validate the efficacy of the smaller mesh size sieves to retain *Trichinella* larvae, 1-39 live naked ML in tap water (BIOR, Latvia) or 1-134 dead naked ML in *Trichinella*-free fox meat digest (RIVM, Netherlands) were poured into the upper, larger mesh size sieve. Subsequently, the ML were carefully washed off the sieves with tap water using a laboratory squeeze bottle, under an angle of approximately 45 degrees. ML that concentrated in the lower rim of the sieves after washing were collected in Petri dishes in approximately 20 mL of rinse water. The number of larvae per sieve was determined microscopically. The experiments were conducted by two researchers per location (BIOR and RIVM), the first author being one of them on both locations.

This sequential sieving method to isolate dead Trichinella larvae was compared to sedimentation as used in EU-RM. For this purpose, Trichinella-free meat digest was spiked with ten dead, 6-shape to comma-shaped Trichinella larvae, which were picked randomly and transferred to approximately 2 mL tap water. Subsequently, the larvae were rinsed into 2 liter of meat digest fluid, in twenty replicate tests. The spiked fluid was either transferred to a separatory funnel and left to sediment for 30 min, after which the lower 40 mL were sedimented again for 10 min in a glass cylinder according to EU-RM, or passed through a stack of stainless steel sieves according to SSM. Residual fluids from EU-RM were passed through a 38 μm mesh size sieve, to isolate ML that did not sediment within the given time.

Feasibility of Trichinella spiked frozen samples

Six minced pork samples (100 g) were spiked with 10 live naked *T. spiralis* ML (RIVM strain, ISS14) and were frozen for two weeks at −80 °C. Three control samples spiked with 10 *Trichinella* ML were kept at +4 °C.

Validation of sequential sieving method

To evaluate possible loss of *Trichinella* ML by freezing fox carcasses, the number of *Trichinella* ML was determined in unfrozen muscle samples of individual fox upper forelegs, originating from 35 foxes collected in Latvia as described above. Briefly, 15 gram of muscle tissue per fox leg was digested according to the EU-RM, with adaptation of the digestion fluid volume to 250 mL and the use of a 1-litre separation funnel to sediment possibly present live *Trichinella* larvae.

Thirty-five *Trichinella* positive forelegs (9 - 169 ML per 15 g muscle tissue) were frozen and kept at −80 °C for one to two weeks. Following this period, deep frozen fox legs were thawed at approximately 18 °C and kept at 8 °C until analysis within 24 h and artificial digestion was performed as described above, during 40 min, to guarantee complete matrix digestion. Liberated, naked 6-shaped to comma-shaped *Trichinella* ML were isolated by sequential sieving through a stack of 300, 63 and 38 μm mesh size sieves.

Trichinella monitoring in the Netherlands

Fox carcasses were thawed at approximately 10 °C. Per individual fox, 15 g lower foreleg muscle tissue sample was isolated and pools of 4-7 foxes were digested for 40 min in 2 litre tap water of 46 °C, containing 0.5% (w/v) pepsin and 0.2% HCl (v/v) according to the EU-RM. After artificial digestion, sequential sieving through stacked stainless steel sieves with mesh size 300 μm and 63 μm was used, to isolate naked *Trichinella* ML. Foxes of pools that tested positive for *Trichinella* were retested individually using the same method.

Statistical analysis
Validation of larva detection

Trichinella ML recovery data of liquid samples that were spiked with either live or dead free ML are assumed randomly distributed. Therefore, a generalized linear model approach with Poisson link function was used to fit data with and without the factor "live/dead". Subsequently, both models were compared by likelihood ratio test to select the model with the lowest AIC-value (Akaike's Information Criterion).

The ability of EU-RM and SSM to recover dead *Trichinella* ML from spiked meat digest was compared with Fisher's Exact test.

Validation of sequential sieving method

Isolated *Trichinella* ML were counted independently by two researchers and for each fox, the average value of these two counts was used. The data were plotted and outliers were identified using Grubb's analysis of residuals for best linear fit. Identified outliers were excluded from further analysis. Average parasite numbers before and after freezing were analysed by generalized linear model approach, with negative binomial link function. This distribution allows for overdispersion, and is therefore suitable for parasite count data that typically have a contagious distribution in host tissues [26]. We checked the prerequisite of equal variances by means of the nonparametric Bartlett test of homogeneity of variances [27]. We built a model with variate "count", dependent on covariate "freezing status" with levels "frozen" or "fresh". A *p*-value below 0.05 for this covariate indicates a significant effect of freezing. Statistical analyses were performed using the software package "R", version 3.0.1 [28].

Study in a low-endemic area in the Netherlands

Lower foreleg muscles of 369 Dutch foxes were examined in pools of 4-7 animals using artificial digestion and sequential sieving through 300 and 63 μm. One single *Trichinella* sp. ML was recovered, which was stored in 5 μL sterile DNAse free water and kept at −20 °C until further use.

DNA isolation and molecular confirmation of *Trichinella* ML by Multiplex PCR

DNA was isolated using QIAGEN® QIAamp DNA Mini Kit Tissue Protocol. Of thirty foxes, a pool of five *Trichinella* ML was analysed per animal before freezing. The concentrations of extracted DNA in samples were measured with ND-1000 Spectrophotometer (NanoDrop Technologies, Inc., Wilmington, DE 19810, USA). The Multiplex PCR was directed at the ITS1, ITS2 and ESV genes as described by Zarlenga et al. [29]. PCR reactions were performed in a total volume of 30 μL, containing 15 μL 2× Master mix (PROMEGA M7505, USA), 1 μL of 10 pmol/μL oligonucleotide mixture, 4 μL of RNAse-free water and 10 μL of DNA. As positive control, *T. spiralis*, *T. britovi* and *T. nativa* DNA was used. The PCR conditions were 95 °C for 4 min followed by 35 cycles of 95 °C for 10 s, 55 °C for 30 s, 72 °C for 30 s. PCR products were analysed by QIAxcel ScreenGel 1.1.0 (Qiagen, Hilden, Germany) and identified according to banding pattern as described earlier [23,29]. This work was performed at BIOR (Riga, Latvia).

DNA isolation and molecular confirmation of *Trichinella* ML by single larvae PCR

DNA was isolated from 3-4 individual ML per Latvian red fox before and after freezing, from three individual larvae from the Latvian wild boar and from the single isolated larva from Dutch red fox according to the protocol described by Pozio et al. [30]. Briefly, 2 μL of 0.05 M TRIS-HCL pH 7.6 was added to each larva in 5 μL H2O, which was overlaid with mineral oil and heated to 90 °C for 10 min. Subsequently, 0.4 μL proteinase K and 2.6 μL H2O was added, followed by incubation at 48 °C for 3 h and finally a 10 min proteinase K inactivation step at 90 °C. A single larvae PCR directed at the 5S ribosomal rDNA intergenic region was used as described earlier [31,32], to determine the species of isolated *Trichinella* ML by DNA sequence analysis, to investigate possible occurrence of simultaneous mixed *Trichinella* infections and to evaluate the influence of freezing on DNA sequencing efficacy. 5S PCR test sensitivity was determined by PCR and agarose gel analysis of four repetitive dilution series with a range of 5 ng to 1 pg *T. britovi* control DNA. PCR amplicons were purified using standard procedures (ExoSAP-IT®, Affymetrix, Cleveland, Ohio, USA). Sequence PCR reactions were carried out on both DNA strands in 20 μL final volume containing 3 μL of amplicate, 7 μL sequence buffer, 1 μL of Big Dye Terminator and 1 μL of forward or reverse PCR primer. Sequence PCR was performed under the following conditions: 95 °C for 1 min, followed by 25 cycles of 96 °C for 10 min, 50 °C for 5 min and finally 60 °C for 4 min. Trace files of the obtained sequences were generated on an automated ABI sequencer. DNA sequences were assembled, edited manually, and analysed with BioNumerics version 7.1 (Applied Maths NV, Sint-Martens-Latem,

Belgium). Cluster analysis of the sequences was conducted using BioNumerics 7.1 with Jukes-Kantor correction setting and bootstrap analysis of 2500 replicates. Sequence homology ≥ 99% was considered proof of identity between isolates and available 5S rDNA sequences of *Trichinella* species from Genbank. This work was performed at RIVM (Bilthoven, Netherlands).

Results

Validation of larva detection

The sensitivity to detect dead *Trichinella* ML in meat digest of the EU-RM was 60% ($n = 100$), whereas the SSM performed significantly better with 92% ($n = 100$) sensitivity ($p = 6 \cdot 10^{-12}$, Fisher's Exact test) (Table 1).

Overall sensitivity of the sequential sieving to detect *Trichinella* ML was 92.9% when using dead ML ($n = 451$) and 88.9% ($n = 280$) for samples spiked with live ML. Using the recovery data of the spiked samples, a Poisson generalized linear model was fitted with and without the factor "live/dead". Comparing both models, the model without "live/dead" factor was favoured resulting from lower AIC-value (Akaike's Information Criterion) and a p-value of 0.58 after likelihood ratio testing. The best fitting model to describe the relationship between the number of spiked and counted larvae was *count* $=0.91$*spike*, the slope of which is close to, but significantly different from 1 ($p = 0.0198$) (Figure 2A).

In total 2833 dead *Trichinella* ML were isolated from 31 frozen Latvian fox forelegs by sequential sieving, of

Table 1 Recovery of dead *Trichinella* larvae spiked in meat digest

		EU 2075 2005		SSM	
	Spike	Sedimentation	Residual fluids*	63 μm	38 μm
1	10	4	6	8	0
2	10	7	3	8	1
3	10	2	8	9	0
4	10	4	5	10	0
5	10	6	3	10	0
6	10	9	1	10	0
7	10	6	3	8	0
8	10	8	2	10	0
9	10	8	2	10	0
10	10	6	4	9	0
sum:	100	60	37	92	1

Ten dead, 6-shape to comma-shaped *Trichinella* larvae were picked randomly and transferred to approximately 2 mL tap water. Subsequently, the larvae were rinsed into 2 liter of meat digest fluid. The spiked fluid was either transferred to a separatory funnel and left to sediment for 30 min according to EU 2075/2005, or passed through a stack of stainless steel sieves according to SSM. SSM performed significantly better than EU-RM for detection of dead larvae in meat digest ($p =6 \cdot 10^{-12}$, Fisher's Exact test).
* # of larvae found after sieving the residual fluids through 38 μm sieve following sedimentation.

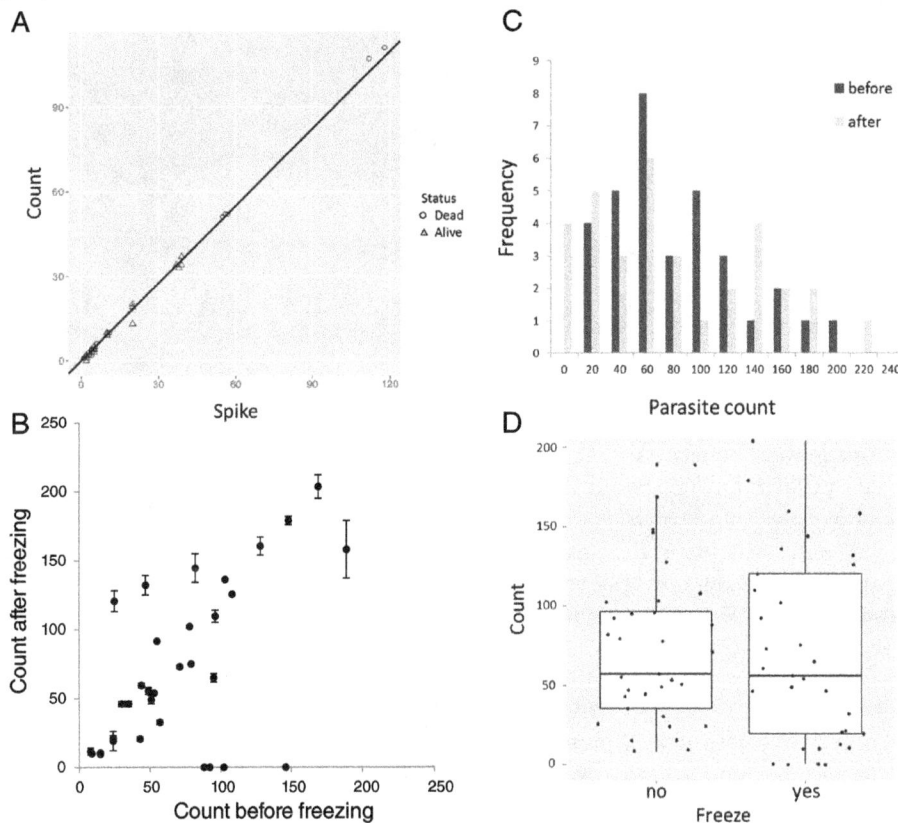

Figure 2 Recovery of dead or live *Trichinella* larvae. A. Fourty-one data points of two combined experiments using the SSM are shown: single to fourfold spikes and counts of dead larva (20 samples, RIVM) and triplicate spikes and counts of live ML (21 samples, BIOR). Identical data points from the same experiment appear as one single data point in the graph. **B.** *Trichinella* larvae were isolated using the EU-RM for live larvae (before freezing) and by the SSM for dead larvae (after freezing). Individual data points represent average values of duplicate counts by two researchers; error bars represent counts range. One identified outlier is omitted here. **C.** Parasite counts mentioned under **A** display a negative binomial distribution. **D.** Parasite counts before freezing (freeze no) and after freezing (freeze yes) overlap and median values before (57) and after (56) freezing were comparable. Top and bottom of the boxes represent 25th and 75th percentiles respectively.

which 0.4% (12 ML) passed through the 63 μm mesh size and were retrieved from the 38 μm mesh size sieve. Of live larvae, 5.8% (14 out of 243) passed through the 63 μm sieve and were collected from the underlying 38 μm sieve. From these results, it was decided to use a combination of sieves with mesh size 300 μm and 63 μm to study *Trichinella* prevalence in deep-frozen foxes from a low-endemic area (the Netherlands).

Effect of freezing on *Trichinella* larvae

Minced pork samples were spiked with free larvae (without nurse cell), to increase the precision of recovery evaluation. Detection of *T. spiralis* (RIVM strain, ISS14) ML in frozen pork samples spiked with 10 ML using artificial digestion according to EU-2075/2005 with 30 min digestion time and subsequent detection of larvae by sequential sieving, showed a sensitivity of only 48.3% (*n* =60), whereas the recovery from control samples stored at +4 °C was 80% (*n* =30) (data not shown). It was then decided to abandon this artificial line of

evaluation and to continue the validation with naturally infected fox forelegs before and after freezing, since the latter was to be used for the prevalence study in a low-endemic area.

Validation of sequential sieving method

Given the poor performance of EU-RM to detect dead Trichinella ML in meat digest, and the fact that about 6% of live ML actively pass the 63 μm sieve with SSM, it was decided to compare the most efficient method to detect live *Trichinella* ML in non-frozen meat (EU-RM) with the best method to detect dead *Trichinella* ML in frozen meat (SSM). In most cases, parasite counts in 35 Latvian fox forelegs before and after freezing were comparable (Figure 2B); in one occasion 575 *T. britovi* ML were found after freezing, against 150 prior to freezing (data not shown). This count was identified as a significant outlier in Grubb's test and therefore excluded from further analysis (G =4.5713, U =0.3476, *p* =1.3 · 10^{-7}). In four samples no ML were found after freezing against 88-146 ML before freezing, which might be related to the highly un-even distribution of *Trichinella* in host muscle tissue and the dispersed count data. Indeed, parasite counts showed a skewed frequency distribution consistent with a negative binomial distribution (Figure 2C). This was confirmed by testing these data for overdispersion (Z =6.5193, *p* =3.5 · 10^{-11}) [28]. Median parasite counts of the fox legs before and after freezing were highly similar with 57 and 56 ML respectively (Figure 2D). Variances were not significantly different (K-squared =1.6677, df =1, *p* =0.1966, non-parametric Bartlett test of homogeneity of variances) and GLM analysis of parasite counts with the variable "freeze" as factor revealed no significant difference (Z = -0.068, *p* =0.946).

Study in a low-endemic area in the Netherlands

One fox out of 369 tested positive for *Trichinella*, with one larva (Figure 3) found in a pool of six foxes. Analysis of the individual foxes that were included in the positive pool did not lead to further findings. Assuming constant prevalence over the study period, we may combine all study years, to arrive at a prevalence of 0.27% (95% CI 0.065-1.5%). Prevalence calculated only from the 287 foxes collected from November 2010 - April 2011 reached 0.35%. In contrast, analysis of 276 foxes from a previous study at the eastern border region of the Netherlands (the same region as in this present study), collected from December 1997 - March 1998 [8], revealed a significantly higher *T. britovi* prevalence of 3.9% (*p* =0.0006, Fisher's Exact Test) at a density of 0.04 - 0.71 LPG [8]. Also in the period 1969 - 1971, a significantly higher prevalence (2.8%, *n* =106) compared to this present study, was found in foxes from the same border region by digestion and subsequent sieving through sterile gauze [5], (*p* =0.036, Fisher's Exact Test).

Molecular characterization of *Trichinella* ML
Multiplex PCR
Multiplex PCR on five isolated ML each of 30 individual Latvian foxes at BIOR (Riga, Latvia) showed that 28 animals were infected with *T. britovi* and two with *T. nativa*. It is not possible however, to detect simultaneous *T. britovi* and *T. nativa* infections by multiplex PCR, since banding patterns on gel do overlap (one single band of 127 base pairs (bp) for *T. nativa* and 2 bands of 253 and 127 bp respectively for *T. britovi*).

Single larva PCR
Single larva PCR directed at 5S rDNA on three to four individual non-frozen ML per Latvian fox performed at RIVM (Bilthoven, the Netherlands), confirmed the results of multiplex PCR performed at BIOR, without any mixed *T. britovi* and *T. nativa* infection found. Of in total 96 tested non-frozen *T. britovi* ML, 90 (93.8%) were successfully sequenced, whereas only 6 out of 72 (8.3%) frozen *T.*

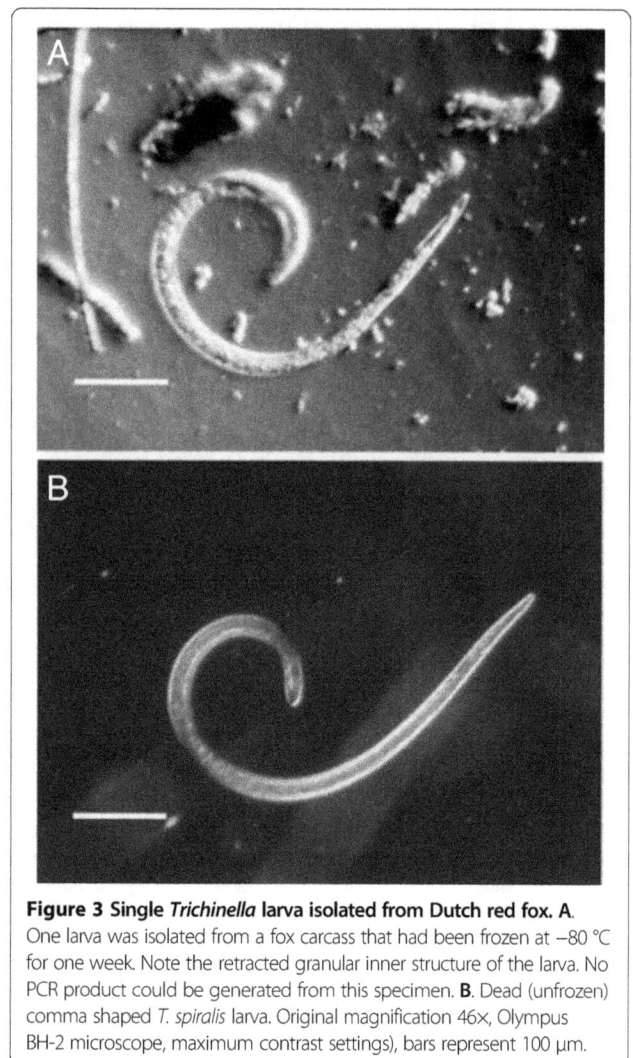

Figure 3 Single *Trichinella* larva isolated from Dutch red fox. A. One larva was isolated from a fox carcass that had been frozen at −80 °C for one week. Note the retracted granular inner structure of the larva. No PCR product could be generated from this specimen. **B**. Dead (unfrozen) comma shaped *T. spiralis* larva. Original magnification 46×, Olympus BH-2 microscope, maximum contrast settings), bars represent 100 μm.

britovi ML yielded sequences that allowed species determination (Table 2). For the more freeze-resistant *T. nativa*, six out of six non-frozen and two out of six frozen ML were successfully sequenced. The detection limit of the 5S rDNA PCR was 2.5 pg (data not shown).

The single microscopically identified *Trichinella* sp. larva that was recovered from 369 frozen lower forelegs of Dutch foxes appeared severely damaged (Figure 3) and did not result in PCR product after 5S PCR and therefore, no sequence was available for species determination of this isolate.

Discussion

A method using sequential sieving (SSM) for the detection of dead *Trichinella* ML from frozen red fox foreleg muscle was validated and was used to analyse trends in time of *Trichinella* in a Dutch red fox population. The SSM is a fast method, since two sedimentation steps of minimally 30 min primary sedimentation plus 10 min

Table 2 Species identification of Trichinella larvae

#	Animal	Multiplex PCR before freezing	Single larva 5S PCR before freezing				Single larva 5S PCR after freezing		
1	67038	*T. britovi*	*T. britovi*	*T. britovi*	*T. britovi*	*T. britovi*	NP	NP	NP
2	70414	*T. britovi*	*T. britovi*	*T. britovi*	*T. britovi*	*T. britovi*	NP	NP	NS
3	72119	*T. britovi*	*T. britovi*	*T. britovi*	*T. britovi*	*T. britovi*	NP	NP	NP
4	72407	*T. britovi*	*T. britovi*	*T. britovi*	*T. britovi*	*T. britovi*	NP	NP	NP
5	74391	*T. britovi*	*T. britovi*	*T. britovi*	NP	NP	NP	NS	NP
6	75633	*T. britovi*	*T. britovi*	*T. britovi*	*T. britovi*	*T. britovi*	NP	NP	NP
7	75068	*T. britovi*	*T. britovi*	*T. britovi*	*T. britovi*	*T. britovi*	NP	*T. britovi*	*T. britovi*
8	74497	*T. britovi*	*T. britovi*	*T. britovi*	*T. britovi*	*T. britovi*	NP	NP	NP
9	75475	*T. britovi*	*T. britovi*	*T. britovi*	*T. britovi*	*T. britovi*	*T. britovi*	NS	NS
10	75748	*T. nativa*	*T. nativa*	*T. nativa*	*T. nativa*	ND	NP	NP	NP
11	75630	*T. britovi*	*T. britovi*	*T. britovi*	*T. britovi*	ND	NP	*T. britovi*	NP
12	75638	*T. britovi*	*T. britovi*	*T. britovi*	*T. britovi*	ND	NP	NP	NP
13	75932	*T. britovi*	NP	*T. britovi*	*T. britovi*	ND	NP	NP	NP
14	75933	*T. britovi*	NP	*T. britovi*	*T. britovi*	ND	NP	NP	NP
15	75996	*T. britovi*	*T. britovi*	*T. britovi*	*T. britovi*	ND	*T. britovi*	*T. britovi*	NS
16	76148	*T. nativa*	*T. nativa*	*T. nativa*	*T. nativa*	ND	NP	*T. nativa*	*T. nativa*
17	76575	*T. britovi*	*T. britovi*	*T. britovi*	*T. britovi*	ND	NP	NP	NP
18	76580	*T. britovi*	*T. britovi*	*T. britovi*	*T. britovi*	ND	NP	NP	NP
19	76643	*T. britovi*	*T. britovi*	*T. britovi*	*T. britovi*	ND	NP	NP	NP
20	76644	*T. britovi*	*T. britovi*	NP	NP	ND	NP	NP	NP
21	76806	*T. britovi*	*T. britovi*	*T. britovi*	*T. britovi*	ND	NP	NP	NP
22	77876	*T. britovi*	*T. britovi*	*T. britovi*	*T. britovi*	ND	NP	NP	NP
23	77885	*T. britovi*	*T. britovi*	*T. britovi*	*T. britovi*	ND	NP	NP	NP
24	77958	*T. britovi*	*T. britovi*	*T. britovi*	*T. britovi*	ND	NP	NP	NP
25	78187	*T. britovi*	*T. britovi*	*T. britovi*	*T. britovi*	ND	ND	ND	ND
26	71102	*T. britovi*	*T. britovi*	*T. britovi*	*T. britovi*	ND	ND	ND	ND
27	71127	*T. britovi*	*T. britovi*	*T. britovi*	*T. britovi*	ND	ND	ND	ND
28	71128	*T. britovi*	*T. britovi*	*T. britovi*	*T. britovi*	ND	ND	ND	ND
29	74449	*T. britovi*	*T. britovi*	*T. britovi*	*T. britovi*	ND	ND	ND	ND
30	74956	*T. britovi*	*T. britovi*	*T. britovi*	*T. britovi*	ND	ND	ND	ND
31	wild boar	ND	*T. britovi*	*T. britovi*	*T. britovi*	ND	ND	ND	ND

Species identification was performed on pools of 5 larvae (multiplex PCR) and individual *Trichinella* larvae (single larva PCR). PCR on individual non-frozen larvae resulted in product for 93 out of 99 larvae (93.9%). PCR on 72 individual frozen larvae yielded PCR product for only 12 larvae, of which 8 resulted in sequence product. NP: no PCR product was formed. NS: PCR product yielded no sequence results due to poor quality of DNA. ND: not done.

secondary sedimentation (when using the EU-RM) were eliminated and were replaced by a 3-5 min sieving step in the SSM.

Dead Trichinella ML exhibit a lower sedimentation speed than live ML [4,19,20] leading to only 60% recovery of dead Trichinella ML from muscle digest using EU-RM, compared to 92% when using SSM, as is shown in this present paper. In comparison, larval counts of frozen fox foreleg muscle obtained with SSM did not differ significantly from larval counts of non-frozen fox foreleg muscle obtained with EU-RM, showing that the SSM was effective to detect dead *Trichinella* larvae. Finding or preparing

suitable samples for this type of comparison is a challenge. Henriksen [21] used minced and thoroughly mixed experimentally infected rabbit meat to evaluate the effect of freezing on recoverability of *T. spiralis* ML using disposable sieves with mesh size 350 and 20 μm to retain dead larvae. Parasite counts ranged from 82 to 124 ML in that study, irrespective of temperature treatment, despite thorough mixing. In our validation experiment, we found four negative counts after freezing of samples that contained 82-146 larvae when tested before freezing. A plausible biological explanation could be that due to uneven distribution of *Trichinella* larvae in the muscle tissue, these could be missed by chance at second sampling of the same fore-leg, near to the primary sampling site. This could also explain the same effect in the other direction, where the post-freezing count value of one sample was 383% of the pre-freezing count. The statistical analysis on the parasite counts in this present study confirmed that parasites follow a contagious distribution in tissues, necessitating GLM methods to accommodate such highly variable counts.

Detection of live and dead *Trichinella* larvae using sequential sieving showed an average sensitivity of 91% (n =451). Spiked samples with live naked or encapsulated *T. spiralis* ML provide standardized, uniform and quantifiable samples to evaluate test sensitivity of the EU-RM in routine laboratories. This type of samples are generally used by all National Reference Laboratories for *Trichinella* in Europe and elsewhere, with a quantitative sensitivity of 84% (n =2130, naked larvae) [33] and 81% - 88% (n =174 - 265, encapsulated larvae) [34] under controlled circumstances. This method however, seems less suitable to validate the SSM presented in this paper, since the test sensitivity dropped from almost 93% (validation of mesh size) to 48% (SSM, n =60) after freezing of pork samples, that had been spiked with live *T. spiralis* ML, for two weeks (at –80 °C). Test sensitivity of unfrozen spiked control samples that were stored at +4 °C was 80% (n =30). This low recovery after freezing was confirmed by a study of Nga [35], who analysed pork samples that were spiked with live *T. spiralis* ML (the same strain as was used in this present study) and were subsequently frozen at –20 °C for at least three weeks. Using the EU-RM, the test sensitivity of *Trichinella* detection was 56% (n =225) after freezing in that study, whereas the test sensitivity was 91% (n =225) for control samples that had been stored at +4 °C [35]. Dead ML were found only occasionally, indicating destruction of *T. spiralis* ML during freezing. In an earlier study, Jackson [36], demonstrated even 78% loss of *T. spiralis* larvae (compared to non-frozen samples) after freezing at –18 °C. Also in that study, dead larvae were found occasionally.

The use of free larvae without a nurse cell both in the present study and in that of Nga [35] alone, could not explain the large drop in larval recovery after freezing, since Randazzo et al. [17] found no protective effect of the nurse cell capsule against low temperature treatment. An explanation for the lower results with *T. spiralis* spiked frozen samples, could be difference in freeze tolerance between *T. spiralis* and *T. britovi* muscle larvae. Lacour et al. [18] indeed found a *T. spiralis* ML inactivation half time of 25 h at –21 °C, whereas 35 h at –21 °C were needed to inactivate half of *T. britovi* ML. However, after one week at –18 to –30 °C, both *T. spiralis* and *T. britovi* that were recovered from either experimentally infected wild boar, rat or mouse muscle tissue, were unable to infect mice [15,16,18,37]. In naturally infected carnivore muscles, the

survival time of *T. britovi* at –15 to –20 °C is considerably longer, with 3-6 months, but this trait is lost with the transfer of the parasite to experimental mice [15]. This effect might also have induced the dramatic decline in *T. spiralis* recovery after freezing in our spike experiment and that of Nga [35]. The *T. spiralis* strain that Jackson used for his freezing experiment mentioned above, was maintained for almost 40 years [36]. More importantly, these observations underscore our preference for naturally infected fox legs to validate the SSM.

In summary, we validated a fast and effective method to detect dead larvae in meat samples of wildlife. Using this method, we analysed 369 Dutch foxes, of which only one pool of six foxes was positive for *Trichinella*. In this pool, one single larva was isolated and re-tested samples of individual foxes belonging to this pool were all negative, showing a very low infection level.

The *Trichinella* prevalence found in this present study was ten times lower than that described in 1972 by Sluiters et al. [5] and in 1998 by Van der Giessen et al. [8]. Detailed literature concerning historical data regarding *Trichinella* prevalence in red fox from adjacent areas is scarce. However, in the bordering north-western part of Germany (state Hessen), the prevalence of Trichinella in red foxes in the period 1980 - 1983 was 3% (trichinoscopy, six positive, n =198), whereas in the preceding (1979 - 1980) and following period (1985 - 1987) no positive foxes were found there using artificial digestion (n =410 and 333 respectively) [38]. In Nordrhein-Westfalen, situated in-between Hessen and the Netherlands, *Trichinella* was reported in badger (*Meles meles*, 1985) and in wild boar (1988), however no prevalences were given [38]. During the hunting season of 2012, in the eastern part of Belgium (Flanders), one *Trichinella* sp. larva was found in a pool of 20 foxes and also in this occasion, it was not possible to identify an individual positive fox [13], whereas Geerts et al. [39] were not able to demonstrate *Trichinella* in 116 Belgian red foxes in 1993. The decline in *Trichinella* (*britovi*) prevalence in the Netherlands over the past 15 years fits the prevalence patterns of surrounding countries and might be driven by changing feeding habits of the opportunistic red fox in an increasingly densely populated area as the Netherlands. However, not much is known about the natural prevalence fluctuation or infection dynamics of *T. britovi* in red fox. In Slovakia, in contrast to the situation in the Netherlands, the prevalence of *Trichinella* spp. in red fox increased fourfold during the period 2000 - 2007 [12].

Efforts to identify the species of the single larva found in Dutch foxes by PCR failed, probably due to severe freezing damage, which was clearly visible microscopically. Using validation samples from naturally infected Latvian foxes, we were able to determine a success rate of only 8.3% (n =72) for molecular speciation of frozen

T. britovi ML by 5S PCR, against 94% (*n* =96) for live larvae prior to freezing. The purpose of testing frozen larvae in our setting was to determine the probability of obtaining positive identification using the 5S PCR on individual larvae that had been submitted to freezing at –80 °C for at least one week, since this information was not available in literature up to date.

Several studies report species identification of field samples that were frozen at –20 °C, using single larva multiplex PCR [10,40-43]. None of these studies however, stated the number of single larvae tested per host animal, or the success rate. One study by Pozio et al. [30] on wildlife samples frozen at –20 and –80 °C, used 5 to 10-fold single larva multiplex PCRs to identify the Trichinella species, but did not mention how many of these larvae actually were identified. The use of multiple attempts in that study implicated that it was at least anticipated to have a low success rate. Moreover, in a study in coyotes with very low *Trichinella* intensity (0.05-0.6 LPG) [44], Trichinella species identification was possible using multiplex PCR in 7 out of 9 animals after freezing of the samples at –20 °C.

The 5S PCR method displayed a test sensitivity of 2.5 pg larval DNA in our laboratory. This level is in range with a sensitivity of 1 pg DNA in a conventional PCR targeted at mitochondrial large subunit RNA of *T. spiralis* as demonstrated by Lin et al. [45]. Other methods like Q-PCR and multiplex PCR may be more sensitive than the 5S PCR, to identify sheared and otherwise damaged larval DNA after freezing, since these PCR methods usually target much smaller DNA fragments. To increase species identification sensitivity, a combination of methods may be considered.

Molecular identification of individual *Trichinella* larvae revealed two species in red fox from Latvia: *T. britovi* and *T. nativa*, without any mixed infection in 30 foxes. Malakauskas et al. [10] demonstrated *Trichinella* spp. prevalence of 29% in foxes in Latvia. In that publication, individual larvae were identified with PCR according to Pozio et al. [30], which showed a distribution of 78% *T. britovi*, 8.5% *T. nativa* and 9.3% mixed infection of the two species in 129 Latvian foxes. Although our sample size of Latvian foxes is much lower and primarily aimed at the validation of our method, we found a comparable distribution of *T. britovi* and *T. nativa*. The number of isolated *Trichinella* ML from Latvian foxes in this present study might be too low to demonstrate mixed infections.

In conclusion, this study presents a fast and effective sequential sieving method for the detection of dead *Trichinella* larvae in frozen meat. Using this method, we showed that in contrast with a study in the same area fifteen years ago using a comparable method, *Trichinella* prevalence in a Dutch red fox population was significantly lower. Moreover, this study demonstrated that the efficacy of 5S PCR

for identification of *Trichinella britovi* single larvae from meat that had been deep-frozen is not more than 8.3%. This is the first time that the effect of deep freezing on *Trichinella* species identification was quantified. To increase species identification sensitivity and at the same time generate DNA sequence information for molecular epidemiology, a combination of methods may be considered.

Competing interests
The authors declare that they have no competing interests.

Authors' contributions
FF wrote the study design, generated and analyzed parasitological data and wrote the manuscript, GD coordinated the collection of Latvia foxes, generated parasitological data and contributed to the manuscript, ZE generated parasitological data, AH advised with statistical analysis of the results AS, helped with the statistical analysis of the results JvdG wrote the project proposal, coordinated the study and contributed to the manuscript. All authors read and approved the final manuscript.

Acknowledgements
This study was financed by the Dutch Food and Product Safety Authority (NVWA). Peter Kikkert is acknowledged for practical assistance with the validation experiments and Merel Langelaar, Marieke Opsteegh, Manoj Fonville and Miriam Maas are acknowledged for their valuable contribution and help dissecting the foxes. The authors thank Sandra Witteveen of the Institute's sequencing facility for her technical assistance. We are also thankful to Margriet Montizaan of the Royal Dutch Shooting Association (KNJV) and hunters for providing red foxes. Frans van Knapen is thanked for critically reading the manuscript.

Author details
[1]National Institute for Public Health and the Environment, Centre for Zoonoses and Environmental Microbiology, Bilthoven, The Netherlands. [2]Institute of Food Safety, Animal Health and Environment "BIOR", Riga, Latvia. [3]Division Veterinary Public Health, Institute for Risk Assessment Sciences, Utrecht University, Utrecht, The Netherlands.

References
1. Pozio E: **The broad spectrum of Trichinella hosts: from cold- to warm-blooded animals.** *Vet Parasitol* 2005, **132**:3–11.
2. Pozio E, Rinaldi L, Marucci G, Musella V, Galati F, Cringoli G, Boireau P, La Rosa G: **Hosts and habitats of Trichinella spiralis and Trichinella britovi in Europe.** *Int J Parasitol* 2009, **39**:71–79.
3. European-Commission: **Regulation EC No 2075/2005 of the European parliament and of the council of 5 December 2005 laying down specific rules on official controls for Trichinella in meat.** *Off J EC L* 2005, **338**:60–82.
4. Rossi P, Pozio E: **Guidelines for the detection of Trichinella larvae at the slaughterhouse in a quality assurance system.** *Ann Ist Super Sanita* 2008, **44**:195–199.
5. Sluiters J, Ruitenberg J, Vermeulen C: **Studies on the occurrence of Trichinella spiralis in the Netherlands.** *Tijdschr Diergeneeskd* 1972, **97**:1386–1393 (In Dutch).
6. Clausen B, Henriksen SA: **The prevalence of Trichinella spiralis in foxes (Vulpes vulpes) and other game species in Denmark.** *Nord Vet Med* 1976, **28**:265–270.
7. Knapen F, Frachimont JH, Kremers AFT: *Survey of Trichinella spiralis in wild rodents (Rodentia: Muridae) and mustelids (Carnivora: Mustelidae) in the Netherlands*, Rapport nr 188802003. the Netherlands (in Dutch): National Institute for Public Health and the Environment (RIVM); 1993.
8. van der Giessen JW, Rombout Y, Franchimont HJ, La Rosa G, Pozio E: **Trichinella britovi in foxes in The Netherlands.** *J Parasitol* 1998, **84**:1065–1068.
9. Enemark HL, Bjorn H, Henriksen SA, Nielsen B: **Screening for infection of Trichinella in red fox (Vulpes vulpes) in Denmark.** *Vet Parasitol* 2000, **88**:229–237.

10. Malakauskas A, Paulauskas V, Jarvis T, Keidans P, Eddi C, Kapel CM: **Molecular epidemiology of** *Trichinella* **spp. in three Baltic countries: Lithuania, Latvia, and Estonia.** *Parasitol Res* 2007, **100:**687–693.

11. Zimmer IA, Fee SA, Spratt-Davison S, Hunter SJ, Boughtflower VD, Morgan CP, Hunt KR, Smith GC, Abernethy D, Howell M, Taylor MA: **Report of** *Trichinella spiralis* **in a red fox (***Vulpes vulpes***) in Northern Ireland.** *Vet Parasitol* 2009, **159:**300–303.

12. Hurnikova Z, Dubinsky P: **Long-term survey on** *Trichinella* **prevalence in wildlife of Slovakia.** *Vet Parasitol* 2009, **159:**276–280.

13. Claes L: **Surveillance of** *Trichinella* **in Red Fox During Oktober-December 2012.** *De Vlaams Jager* 2013, :8–9. (in Dutch).

14. WHO: **Guidelines for surveillance, prevention and control of Echinococcosis/hydatidosis.** 2nd edition. Edited by Eckert J, Gemmell MA, Matyas Z, Soulsby EJL. Geneva: WHO; 1984.

15. Pozio E, La Rosa G, Amati M: **Factors influencing the resistance of** *Trichinella* **muscle larvae to freezing.** In *Trichinellosis, Proceedings of the Eighth International Conference on Trichinellosis.* Edited by Campbell WC, Pozio E, Bruschi F. Rome, Italy: Instituto Superiore di Sanità Press; 1994:173–178.

16. Malakauskas A, Kapel CM: **Tolerance to low temperatures of domestic and sylvatic** *Trichinella* **spp. in rat muscle tissue.** *J Parasitol* 2003, **89:**744–748.

17. Randazzo VR, La Sala LF, Costamagna SR: **Effect of temperature on the viability of** *Trichinella spiralis* **larvae.** *Rev Argent Microbiol* 2011, **43:**256–262 (in Spanish).

18. Lacour SA, Heckmann A, Mace P, Grasset-Chevillot A, Zanella G, Vallee I, Kapel CM, Boireau P: **Freeze-tolerance of** *Trichinella* **muscle larvae in experimentally infected wild boars.** *Vet Parasitol* 2013, **194:**175–178.

19. Gamble HR: **Factors affecting the efficiency of pooled sample digestion for the recovery of** *Trichinella spiralis* **from muscle tissue.** *Int J Food Microbiol* 1999, **48:**73–78.

20. Dyer DC, Evje V: **A digestion-solvent technique for detecting dead trichinae.** *J Parasitol* 1971, **57:**1148–1149.

21. Henriksen SA: **Recovery of** *Trichinella spiralis* **larvae from frozen muscle samples.** *Acta Vet Scand* 1978, **19:**607–608.

22. Rombout YB, Bosch S, Van Der Giessen JW: **Detection and identification of eight** *Trichinella* **genotypes by reverse line blot hybridization.** *J Clin Microbiol* 2001, **39:**642–646.

23. Zarlenga DS, Chute MB, Martin A, Kapel CM: **A single, multiplex PCR for differentiating all species of** *Trichinella.* *Parasite* 2001, **8:**S24–S26.

24. Veit P, Bilger B, Schad V, Schafer J, Frank W, Lucius R: **Influence of environmental factors on the infectivity of** *Echinococcus multilocularis* **eggs.** *Parasitology* 1995, **110:**79–86.

25. Anderson RC: *Nematode Parasites of Vertebrates, their Development and Transmission.* Wallingford, UK: CAB International; 1992:549.

26. Alexander N: **Review: analysis of parasite and other skewed counts.** *Trop Med Int Health* 2012, **17:**684–693.

27. Bartlett M: **Properties of sufficiency and statistical tests.** *Proc R Soc A* 1937, **160:**268–282.

28. R Team: *A Language and Environment for Statistical Computing.* Vienna, Austria: R Foundation for Statistical Computing; 2008. (ISBN 3-900051-07-0): [http://www.R-project.org]

29. Zarlenga DS, Chute MB, Martin A, Kapel CM: **A multiplex PCR for unequivocal differentiation of all encapsulated and non-encapsulated genotypes of** *Trichinella.* *Int J Parasitol* 1999, **29:**1859–1867.

30. Pozio E, Casulli A, Bologov VV, Marucci G, La Rosa G: **Hunting practices increase the prevalence of** *Trichinella* **infection in wolves from European Russia.** *J Parasitol* 2001, **87:**1498–1501.

31. Bandi C, La Rosa G, Comincini S, Damiani G, Pozio E: **Random amplified polymorphic DNA technique for the identification of** *Trichinella* **species.** *Parasitology* 1993, **107:**419–424.

32. Liu LX, Blaxter ML, Shi A: **The 5S ribosomal RNA intergenic region of parasitic nematodes: variation in size and presence of SL1 RNA.** *Mol Biochem Parasitol* 1996, **83:**235–239.

33. Riehn K, Hasenclever D, Petroff D, Nockler K, Mayer-Scholl A, Makrutzki G, Lucker E: *Trichinella* **detection: identification and statistical evaluation of sources of error in the magnetic stirrer method for pooled sample digestion.** *Vet Parasitol* 2013, **194:**106–109.

34. Vallee I, Mace P, Forbes L, Scandrett B, Durand B, Gajadhar A, Boireau P: **Use of proficiency samples to assess diagnostic laboratories in France performing a** *Trichinella* **digestion assay.** *J Food Prot* 2007, **70:**1685–1690.

35. Nga VT: *Comparison of known Infected Fresh and Frozen Meat samples for the recovery of Trichinella Larvae using the Magnetic Stirrer Digestion Method,* ITM-MSTAH thesis nr 100. Antwerpen (Antwerp), Belgium: Prince Leopold Institute of Tropical Medicine; 2008.

36. Jackson G: **Recovery of** *Trichinella spiralis* **larvae.** *Br Vet J* 1977, **133:**318–319.

37. Blaga R, Cretu CM, Gherman C, Draghici A, Pozio E, Noeckler K, Kapel CM, Dida I, Cozma V, Boireau P: *Trichinella* **spp. infection in horses of Romania: serological and parasitological survey.** *Vet Parasitol* 2009, **159:**285–289.

38. Wagner JA, Schnell M, Frank W: **The occurrence of** *Trichinella* **in indigenous wildlife.** *Berl Munch Tierarztl Wochenschr* 1988, **101:**413–416 (in German).

39. Geerts S, de Borchgrave J, Vervoort T, Kumar V, de Deken R, Brandt J, Gouffaux M, Griez M, van Knapen F: **Survey on trichinellosis in slaughter pigs, wild boars and foxes in Belgium.** *Vlaams Diergeneesk Tijdsch* 1995, **64:**138–140.

40. Reichard MV, Torretti L, Snider TA, Garvon JM, Marucci G, Pozio E: *Trichinella* **T6 and** *Trichinella nativa* **in Wolverines (***Gulo gulo***) from Nunavut, Canada.** *Parasitol Res* 2008, **103:**657–661.

41. Beck R, Beck A, Kusak J, Mihaljevic Z, Lucinger S, Zivicnjak T, Huber D, Gudan A, Marinculic A: **Trichinellosis in wolves from Croatia.** *Vet Parasitol* 2009, **159:**308–311.

42. Gajadhar AA, Forbes LB: **A 10-year wildlife survey of 15 species of Canadian carnivores identifies new hosts or geographic locations for** *Trichinella* **genotypes T2, T4, T5, and T6.** *Vet Parasitol* 2010, **168:**78–83.

43. Reichard MV, Tiernan KE, Paras KL, Interisano M, Reiskind MH, Panciera RJ, Pozio E: **Detection of** *Trichinella murrelli* **in coyotes (***Canis latrans***) from Oklahoma and North Texas.** *Vet Parasitol* 2011, **182:**368–371.

44. Pozio E, Pence DB, La Rosa G, Casulli A, Henke SE: *Trichinella* **infection in wildlife of the southwestern United States.** *J Parasitol* 2001, **87:**1208–1210.

45. Lin Z, Cao J, Zhang H, Zhou Y, Deng M, Li G, Zhou J: **Comparison of three molecular detection methods for detection of** *Trichinella* **in infected pigs.** *Parasitol Res* 2013, **112:**2087–2093.

Permissions

All chapters in this book were first published in VR, by BioMed Central; hereby published with permission under the Creative Commons Attribution License or equivalent. Every chapter published in this book has been scrutinized by our experts. Their significance has been extensively debated. The topics covered herein carry significant findings which will fuel the growth of the discipline. They may even be implemented as practical applications or may be referred to as a beginning point for another development.

The contributors of this book come from diverse backgrounds, making this book a truly international effort. This book will bring forth new frontiers with its revolutionizing research information and detailed analysis of the nascent developments around the world.

We would like to thank all the contributing authors for lending their expertise to make the book truly unique. They have played a crucial role in the development of this book. Without their invaluable contributions this book wouldn't have been possible. They have made vital efforts to compile up to date information on the varied aspects of this subject to make this book a valuable addition to the collection of many professionals and students.

This book was conceptualized with the vision of imparting up-to-date information and advanced data in this field. To ensure the same, a matchless editorial board was set up. Every individual on the board went through rigorous rounds of assessment to prove their worth. After which they invested a large part of their time researching and compiling the most relevant data for our readers.

The editorial board has been involved in producing this book since its inception. They have spent rigorous hours researching and exploring the diverse topics which have resulted in the successful publishing of this book. They have passed on their knowledge of decades through this book. To expedite this challenging task, the publisher supported the team at every step. A small team of assistant editors was also appointed to further simplify the editing procedure and attain best results for the readers.

Apart from the editorial board, the designing team has also invested a significant amount of their time in understanding the subject and creating the most relevant covers. They scrutinized every image to scout for the most suitable representation of the subject and create an appropriate cover for the book.

The publishing team has been an ardent support to the editorial, designing and production team. Their endless efforts to recruit the best for this project, has resulted in the accomplishment of this book. They are a veteran in the field of academics and their pool of knowledge is as vast as their experience in printing. Their expertise and guidance has proved useful at every step. Their uncompromising quality standards have made this book an exceptional effort. Their encouragement from time to time has been an inspiration for everyone.

The publisher and the editorial board hope that this book will prove to be a valuable piece of knowledge for researchers, students, practitioners and scholars across the globe.

List of Contributors

Andrea Ladinig
Department of Large Animal Clinical Sciences, Western College of Veterinary Medicine, University of Saskatchewan, Saskatoon, SK, Canada

Joan K Lunney
U.S. Department of Agriculture, Animal Parasitic Diseases Laboratory, Beltsville Agricultural Research Center, Agricultural Research Service, Beltsville, MD, USA

Carlos JH Souza
U.S. Department of Agriculture, Animal Parasitic Diseases Laboratory, Beltsville Agricultural Research Center, Agricultural Research Service, Beltsville, MD, USA
EMBRAPA Pesca e Aquicultura, Palmas, TO, Brazil

Carolyn Ashley
Department of Large Animal Clinical Sciences, Western College of Veterinary Medicine, University of Saskatchewan, Saskatoon, SK, Canada

Graham Plastow
Department of Agricultural, Food, and Nutritional Science, Faculty of Agricultural, Life and Environmental Sciences, University of Alberta, Edmonton, AB, Canada

John CS Harding
Department of Large Animal Clinical Sciences, Western College of Veterinary Medicine, University of Saskatchewan, Saskatoon, SK, Canada

Suresh V Kuchipudi
School of Veterinary Medicine and Science, University of Nottingham, Sutton Bonington Campus, College Road, Loughborough, Nottingham, Leicestershire LE12 5RD, UK

Meenu Tellabat
School of Veterinary Medicine and Science, University of Nottingham, Sutton Bonington Campus, College Road, Loughborough, Nottingham, Leicestershire LE12 5RD, UK

Sujith Sebastian
School of Veterinary Medicine and Science, University of Nottingham, Sutton Bonington Campus, College Road, Loughborough, Nottingham, Leicestershire LE12 5RD, UK

Brandon Z Londt
Virology Department, Animal and Plant Health Agency, Weybridge, Addlestone, Surrey KT15 3NB, UK

Christine Jansen
Department of Infectious Diseases and Immunology, Faculty of Veterinary Medicine, University of Utrecht, Utrecht, The Netherlands

Lonneke Vervelde
Department of Infectious Diseases and Immunology, Faculty of Veterinary Medicine, University of Utrecht, Utrecht, The Netherlands
The Roslin Institute and R(D)SVS, University of Edinburgh, Easter Bush, Midlothian, Edinburgh EH25 9RG, UK

Sharon M Brookes
Virology Department, Animal and Plant Health Agency, Weybridge, Addlestone, Surrey KT15 3NB, UK

Ian H Brown
Virology Department, Animal and Plant Health Agency, Weybridge, Addlestone, Surrey KT15 3NB, UK

Stephen P Dunham
School of Veterinary Medicine and Science, University of Nottingham, Sutton Bonington Campus, College Road, Loughborough, Nottingham, Leicestershire LE12 5RD, UK

Kin-Chow Chang
School of Veterinary Medicine and Science, University of Nottingham, Sutton Bonington Campus, College Road, Loughborough, Nottingham, Leicestershire LE12 5RD, UK

Jose A Barasona
SaBio (Health and Biotechnology), IREC, National Wildlife Research Institute (CSIC-UCLM-JCCM), Ciudad Real, Spain

M Cecilia Latham
Landcare Research, PO Box 69040, Lincoln, Canterbury 7640, New Zealand
Estación Biológica de Doñana, Consejo Superior de Investigaciones Científicas (CSIC), Sevilla, Spain

Pelayo Acevedo
SaBio (Health and Biotechnology), IREC, National Wildlife Research Institute (CSIC-UCLM-JCCM), Ciudad Real, Spain

Jose A Armenteros
SaBio (Health and Biotechnology), IREC, National Wildlife Research Institute (CSIC-UCLM-JCCM), Ciudad Real, Spain

A David M Latham
Landcare Research, PO Box 69040, Lincoln, Canterbury 7640, New Zealand

Christian Gortazar
SaBio (Health and Biotechnology), IREC, National Wildlife Research Institute (CSIC-UCLM-JCCM), Ciudad Real, Spain

Francisco Carro
Estación Biológica de Doñana, Consejo Superior de Investigaciones Científicas (CSIC), Sevilla, Spain

Ramon C Soriguer
Estación Biológica de Doñana, Consejo Superior de Investigaciones Científicas (CSIC), Sevilla, Spain

Joaquin Vicente
SaBio (Health and Biotechnology), IREC, National Wildlife Research Institute (CSIC-UCLM-JCCM), Ciudad Real, Spain

Iacome SC Jácome
Department of Veterinary Sciences, Federal University of Paraiba, Areia, PB 58397-000, Brazil

Francisca GC Sousa
Department of Animal Science, Federal University of Paraiba, Areia, PB 58397-000, Brazil

Candice MG De Leon
Department of Animal Science, Federal University of Paraiba, Areia, PB 58397-000, Brazil

Denis A Spricigo
Department of Veterinary Sciences, Federal University of Paraiba, Areia, PB 58397-000, Brazil

Mauro MS Saraiva
Department of Veterinary Sciences, Federal University of Paraiba, Areia, PB 58397-000, Brazil

Patricia EN Givisiez
Department of Animal Science, Federal University of Paraiba, Areia, PB 58397-000, Brazil

Wondwossen A Gebreyes
Department of Veterinary Preventive Medicine, College of Veterinary Medicine, The Ohio State University, Columbus, OH 43210, USA
Veterinary Public Health and Biotechnology Global Consortium (VPH-Biotec), The Ohio State University, Columbus, OH 43210, USA

Rafael FC Vieira
Department of Veterinary Sciences, Federal University of Paraiba, Areia, PB 58397-000, Brazil

Celso JB Oliveira
Department of Animal Science, Federal University of Paraiba, Areia, PB 58397-000, Brazil
Veterinary Public Health and Biotechnology Global Consortium (VPH-Biotec), The Ohio State University, Columbus, OH 43210, USA

Helle Bielefeldt-Ohmann
School of Veterinary Science, University of Queensland, Gatton Campus, Gatton, Qld 4343, Australia
Australian Infectious Diseases Research Centre, University of Queensland, St. Lucia, Qld 4078, Australia

Natalie A Prow
Australian Infectious Diseases Research Centre, University of Queensland, St. Lucia, Qld 4078, Australia
School of Chemistry & Molecular Biosciences, University of Queensland, St. Lucia, Australia

Wenqi Wang
School of Veterinary Science, University of Queensland, Gatton Campus, Gatton, Qld 4343, Australia

Cindy SE Tan
Australian Infectious Diseases Research Centre, University of Queensland, St. Lucia, Qld 4078, Australia
School of Chemistry & Molecular Biosciences, University of Queensland, St. Lucia, Australia

Mitchell Coyle
Gatton Campus Equine Unit, University of Queensland, Gatton Campus, Gatton, Qld 4343, Australia

Alysha Douma
Gatton Campus Equine Unit, University of Queensland, Gatton Campus, Gatton, Qld 4343, Australia

Jody Hobson-Peters
Australian Infectious Diseases Research Centre, University of Queensland, St. Lucia, Qld 4078, Australia
School of Chemistry & Molecular Biosciences, University of Queensland, St. Lucia, Australia

Lisa Kidd
School of Veterinary Science, University of Queensland, Gatton Campus, Gatton, Qld 4343, Australia

Roy A Hall
Australian Infectious Diseases Research Centre, University of Queensland, St. Lucia, Qld 4078, Australia
School of Chemistry & Molecular Biosciences, University of Queensland, St. Lucia, Australia

Nikolai Petrovsky
Vaxine Pty., Ltd., Flinders Medical Centre, Adelaide, South Australia
Flinders Medical Centre and Flinders University, Bedford Park, South Australia

Andrea Ladinig
Department of Large Animal Clinical Sciences, Western College of Veterinary Medicine, University of Saskatchewan, Saskatoon, SK, Canada
University Clinic for Swine, Department for Farm Animals and Veterinary Public Health, University of Veterinary Medicine Vienna, Veterinaerplatz 1, 1210 Vienna, Austria

Wilhelm Gerner
Institute of Immunology, Department of Pathobiology, University of Veterinary Medicine Vienna, Vienna, Austria

Armin Saalmüller
Institute of Immunology, Department of Pathobiology, University of Veterinary Medicine Vienna, Vienna, Austria

Joan K Lunney
Animal Parasitic Diseases Laboratory, Beltsville Agricultural Research Center, Agricultural Research Service, U.S. Department of Agriculture, Beltsville, MD, USA

Carolyn Ashley
Department of Large Animal Clinical Sciences, Western College of Veterinary Medicine, University of Saskatchewan, Saskatoon, SK, Canada

John CS Harding
Department of Large Animal Clinical Sciences, Western College of Veterinary Medicine, University of Saskatchewan, Saskatoon, SK, Canada

Qunhui Li
Animal Infectious Disease Laboratory, College of Veterinary Medicine, Yangzhou University, Yangzhou, Jiangsu 225009, China

Xuan Wang
Animal Infectious Disease Laboratory, College of Veterinary Medicine, Yangzhou University, Yangzhou, Jiangsu 225009, China

Min Gu
Animal Infectious Disease Laboratory, College of Veterinary Medicine, Yangzhou University, Yangzhou, Jiangsu 225009, China
Jiangsu Co-innovation Center for Prevention and Control of Important Animal Infectious Diseases and Zoonoses, Yangzhou, Jiangsu 225009, China

Jie Zhu
Animal Infectious Disease Laboratory, College of Veterinary Medicine, Yangzhou University, Yangzhou, Jiangsu 225009, China

Xiaoli Hao
Animal Infectious Disease Laboratory, College of Veterinary Medicine, Yangzhou University, Yangzhou, Jiangsu 225009, China

Zhao Gao
Animal Infectious Disease Laboratory, College of Veterinary Medicine, Yangzhou University, Yangzhou, Jiangsu 225009, China

Zhongtao Sun
Animal Infectious Disease Laboratory, College of Veterinary Medicine, Yangzhou University, Yangzhou, Jiangsu 225009, China

Jiao Hu
Animal Infectious Disease Laboratory, College of Veterinary Medicine, Yangzhou University, Yangzhou, Jiangsu 225009, China
Jiangsu Co-innovation Center for Prevention and Control of Important Animal Infectious Diseases and Zoonoses, Yangzhou, Jiangsu 225009, China

Shunlin Hu
Animal Infectious Disease Laboratory, College of Veterinary Medicine, Yangzhou University, Yangzhou, Jiangsu 225009, China
Jiangsu Co-innovation Center for Prevention and Control of Important Animal Infectious Diseases and Zoonoses, Yangzhou, Jiangsu 225009, China

Xiaoquan Wang
Animal Infectious Disease Laboratory, College of Veterinary Medicine, Yangzhou University, Yangzhou, Jiangsu 225009, China
Jiangsu Co-innovation Center for Prevention and Control of Important Animal Infectious Diseases and Zoonoses, Yangzhou, Jiangsu 225009, China

Xiaowen Liu
Animal Infectious Disease Laboratory, College of Veterinary Medicine, Yangzhou University, Yangzhou, Jiangsu 225009, China
Jiangsu Co-innovation Center for Prevention and Control of Important Animal Infectious Diseases and Zoonoses, Yangzhou, Jiangsu 225009, China

Xiufan Liu
Animal Infectious Disease Laboratory, College of Veterinary Medicine, Yangzhou University, Yangzhou, Jiangsu 225009, China
Jiangsu Co-innovation Center for Prevention and Control of Important Animal Infectious Diseases and Zoonoses, Yangzhou, Jiangsu 225009, China

Ying-Ting Wang
Graduate institute of Veterinary Medicine, School of Veterinary Medicine, National Taiwan University, Taipei 10617, Taiwan

Li-En Hsieh
Graduate institute of Veterinary Medicine, School of Veterinary Medicine, National Taiwan University, Taipei 10617, Taiwan

Yu-Rou Dai
Department of Veterinary Medicine, School of Veterinary Medicine, National Taiwan University, Taipei 10617, Taiwan

Ling-Ling Chueh
Graduate institute of Veterinary Medicine, School of Veterinary Medicine, National Taiwan University, Taipei 10617, Taiwan
Department of Veterinary Medicine, School of Veterinary Medicine, National Taiwan University, Taipei 10617, Taiwan

Alix Damman
INRA, UMR1300 BioEpAR, CS 40706, F-44307 Nantes, France
Oniris, LUNAM Université, UMR BioEpAR, F-44307 Nantes, France

Anne-France Viet
INRA, UMR1300 BioEpAR, CS 40706, F-44307 Nantes, France
Oniris, LUNAM Université, UMR BioEpAR, F-44307 Nantes, France

Sandie Arnoux
INRA, UMR1300 BioEpAR, CS 40706, F-44307 Nantes, France
Oniris, LUNAM Université, UMR BioEpAR, F-44307 Nantes, France

Marie-Claude Guerrier-Chatellet
FRGDS Bourgogne, F-21000 Dijon France

Etienne Petit
FRGDS Bourgogne, F-21000 Dijon, France

Pauline Ezanno
INRA, UMR1300 BioEpAR, CS 40706, F-44307 Nantes, France
Oniris, LUNAM Université, UMR BioEpAR, F-44307 Nantes, France

Lindert Benedictus
Department of Infectious Diseases and Immunology, Faculty of Veterinary Medicine, Utrecht University, Utrecht, The Netherlands

Henny G Otten
Laboratory of Translational Immunology, University Medical Center Utrecht, Utrecht, The Netherlands

Gerdien van Schaik
GD Animal Health Service, Deventer, The Netherlands

Walter GJ van Ginkel
Laboratory of Translational Immunology, University Medical Center Utrecht, Utrecht, The Netherlands

Henri CM Heuven
Department of Clinical Sciences of Companion Animals, Faculty of Veterinary Medicine, Utrecht University, Utrecht, the Netherlands
Animal Breeding and Genomics Centre, Wageningen University, Wageningen, the Netherlands

Mirjam Nielen
Department of Farm Animal Health, Faculty of Veterinary Medicine, Utrecht University, Utrecht, The Netherlands

Victor PMG Rutten
Department of Infectious Diseases and Immunology, Faculty of Veterinary Medicine, Utrecht University, Utrecht, The Netherlands
Department of Veterinary Tropical Diseases, Faculty of Veterinary Science, University of Pretoria, Onderstepoort, South Africa

Ad P Koets
Department of Infectious Diseases and Immunology, Faculty of Veterinary Medicine, Utrecht University, Utrecht, The Netherlands
Department of Farm Animal Health, Faculty of Veterinary Medicine, Utrecht University, Utrecht, The Netherlands

Josephine Schlosser
Institute for Novel and Emerging Infectious Diseases, Friedrich-Loeffler-Institut, Südufer 10, 17493 Greifswald-Insel Riems, Germany

Martin Eiden
Institute for Novel and Emerging Infectious Diseases, Friedrich-Loeffler-Institut, Südufer 10, 17493 Greifswald-Insel Riems, Germany

Ariel Vina-Rodriguez
Institute for Novel and Emerging Infectious Diseases, Friedrich-Loeffler-Institut, Südufer 10, 17493 Greifswald-Insel Riems, Germany

Christine Fast
Institute for Novel and Emerging Infectious Diseases, Friedrich-Loeffler-Institut, Südufer 10, 17493 Greifswald-Insel Riems, Germany

Paul Dremsek
Institute for Novel and Emerging Infectious Diseases, Friedrich-Loeffler-Institut, Südufer 10, 17493 Greifswald-Insel Riems, Germany

Elke Lange
Department of Experimental Animal Facilities and Biorisk Management, Friedrich-Loeffler-Institut, Südufer 10, 17493 Greifswald-Insel Riems, Germany

Rainer G Ulrich
Institute for Novel and Emerging Infectious Diseases, Friedrich-Loeffler-Institut, Südufer 10, 17493 Greifswald-Insel Riems, Germany

Martin H Groschup
Institute for Novel and Emerging Infectious Diseases, Friedrich-Loeffler-Institut, Südufer 10, 17493 Greifswald-Insel Riems, Germany

Zhong Zou
State Key Laboratory of Agricultural Microbiology, Huazhong Agricultural University, Wuhan 430070, China
College of Veterinary Medicine, Huazhong Agricultural University, Wuhan 430070, China

Yong Hu
State Key Laboratory of Agricultural Microbiology, Huazhong Agricultural University, Wuhan 430070, China
Hubei Collaborative Innovation Center for Industrial Fermentation, Hubei University of Technology, Wuhan 430068, China

Zhigang Liu
State Key Laboratory of Agricultural Microbiology, Huazhong Agricultural University, Wuhan 430070, China
College of Veterinary Medicine, Huazhong Agricultural University, Wuhan 430070, China
College of Life Sciences, AnQing Normal University, AnQing 246011, China

Wei Zhong
State Key Laboratory of Agricultural Microbiology, Huazhong Agricultural University, Wuhan 430070, China
College of Veterinary Medicine, Huazhong Agricultural University, Wuhan 430070, China

Hangzhou Cao
State Key Laboratory of Agricultural Microbiology, Huazhong Agricultural University, Wuhan 430070, China
College of Veterinary Medicine, Huazhong Agricultural University, Wuhan 430070, China

Huanchun Chen
State Key Laboratory of Agricultural Microbiology, Huazhong Agricultural University, Wuhan 430070, China
College of Veterinary Medicine, Huazhong Agricultural University, Wuhan 430070, China

Meilin Jin
State Key Laboratory of Agricultural Microbiology, Huazhong Agricultural University, Wuhan 430070, China
College of Veterinary Medicine, Huazhong Agricultural University, Wuhan 430070, China

Guangzhi Zhang
Department of Pathology, Bacteriology and Avian Diseases, Faculty of Veterinary Medicine, Ghent University, 9820 Merelbeke, Belgium

Richard Ducatelle
Department of Pathology, Bacteriology and Avian Diseases, Faculty of Veterinary Medicine, Ghent University, 9820 Merelbeke, Belgium

Ellen De Bruyne
Department of Pathology, Bacteriology and Avian Diseases, Faculty of Veterinary Medicine, Ghent University, 9820 Merelbeke, Belgium

Myrthe Joosten
Department of Pathology, Bacteriology and Avian Diseases, Faculty of Veterinary Medicine, Ghent University, 9820 Merelbeke, Belgium

Iris Bosschem
Department of Pathology, Bacteriology and Avian Diseases, Faculty of Veterinary Medicine, Ghent University, 9820 Merelbeke, Belgium

Annemieke Smet
Department of Pathology, Bacteriology and Avian Diseases, Faculty of Veterinary Medicine, Ghent University, 9820 Merelbeke, Belgium

Freddy Haesebrouck
Department of Pathology, Bacteriology and Avian Diseases, Faculty of Veterinary Medicine, Ghent University, 9820 Merelbeke, Belgium

Bram Flahou
Department of Pathology, Bacteriology and Avian Diseases, Faculty of Veterinary Medicine, Ghent University, 9820 Merelbeke, Belgium

Xing Xie
College of Veterinary Medicine, Nanjing Agricultural University, Nanjing, China

Yan Lin
College of Veterinary Medicine, Nanjing Agricultural University, Nanjing, China

Maoda Pang
College of Veterinary Medicine, Nanjing Agricultural University, Nanjing, China

Yanbing Zhao
College of Veterinary Medicine, Nanjing Agricultural University, Nanjing, China

Dildar Hussain Kalhoro
College of Veterinary Medicine, Nanjing Agricultural University, Nanjing, China

Chengping Lu
College of Veterinary Medicine, Nanjing Agricultural University, Nanjing, China

Yongjie Liu
College of Veterinary Medicine, Nanjing Agricultural University, Nanjing, China

Annelies Maria Declercq
Department Morphology, Ghent University, Faculty of Veterinary Medicine, Salisburylaan 133, 9820 Merelbeke, Belgium

Koen Chiers
Department of Pathology, Bacteriology and Poultry diseases, Ghent University, Faculty of Veterinary Medicine, Salisburylaan 133, 9820 Merelbeke, Belgium

Wim Van den Broeck
Department Morphology, Ghent University, Faculty of Veterinary Medicine, Salisburylaan 133, 9820 Merelbeke, Belgium

Jeroen Dewulf
Department of Reproduction, Obstetrics and Herd Health, Ghent University, Faculty of Veterinary Medicine, Salisburylaan 133, 9820 Merelbeke, Belgium

Venessa Eeckhaut
Department of Pathology, Bacteriology and Poultry diseases, Ghent University, Faculty of Veterinary Medicine, Salisburylaan 133, 9820 Merelbeke, Belgium

Maria Cornelissen
Department of Basic Medical Sciences, Faculty of Medicine and Health Sciences, Ghent University, De Pintelaan 185, 9000 Ghent, Belgium

Peter Bossier
Ghent University, Laboratory of Aquaculture and Artemia Reference Center, Rozier 44, 9000 Ghent, Belgium

Freddy Haesebrouck
Department of Pathology, Bacteriology and Poultry diseases, Ghent University, Faculty of Veterinary Medicine, Salisburylaan 133, 9820 Merelbeke, Belgium

Annemie Decostere
Department Morphology, Ghent University, Faculty of Veterinary Medicine, Salisburylaan 133, 9820 Merelbeke, Belgium

Amélie Chastagner
INRA, UR346 Epidémiologie Animale, F-63122 Saint Genès Champanelle, France

Thibaud Dugat
Université Paris-Est, Ecole Nationale Vétérinaire d'Alfort, UMR BIPAR, 23 avenue du Général de Gaulle, 94706 Maisons-Alfort, France

Gwenaël Vourch
INRA, UR346 Epidémiologie Animale, F-63122 Saint Genès Champanelle, France

Hélène Verheyden
INRA, CEFS, UR035, 24 chemin de Borde Rouge - Auzeville, CS 52627, F-31326 Castanet Tolosan, France

Loïc Legrand
LABÉO - Frank Duncombe, Unite Risques Microbiens (U2RM), Normandie Universite, EA 4655 Caen, Normandy, France

Véronique Bachy
Laboratoire Vétérinaire Départemental du Rhône, Campus vétérinaire VetAgro Sup, 1 avenue Bourgelat, 69280 Marcy l'Etoile, France

Luc Chabanne
Université de Lyon, VetAgro Sup, Jeune Equipe Hémopathogènes Vectorisés, F-69280 Marcy l'Etoile, France

Guy Joncour
Groupe Vétérinaire de Callac, 26 rue du Cleumeur, 22160 Callac, France

Renaud Maillard
Ecole Nationale Vétérinaire de Toulouse, Unité pathologie des ruminants, 23 Chemin des Capelles, 31076 Toulouse, France

Henri-Jean Boulouis
Université Paris-Est, Ecole Nationale Vétérinaire d'Alfort, UMR BIPAR, 23 avenue du Général de Gaulle, 94706 Maisons-Alfort, France

Nadia Haddad
Université Paris-Est, Ecole Nationale Vétérinaire d'Alfort, UMR BIPAR, 23 avenue du Général de Gaulle, 94706 Maisons-Alfort, France

Xavier Bailly
INRA, UR346 Epidémiologie Animale, F-63122 Saint Genès Champanelle, France

Agnès Leblond
INRA, UR346 Epidémiologie Animale, F-63122 Saint Genès Champanelle, France
Département Hippique, VetAgroSup, F-69280 Marcy L'Etoile, France

Frits Franssen
National Institute for Public Health and the Environment, Centre for Zoonoses and Environmental Microbiology, Bilthoven, The Netherlands

Gunita Deksne
Institute of Food Safety, Animal Health and Environment "BIOR", Riga, Latvia

Zanda Esíte
Institute of Food Safety, Animal Health and Environment "BIOR", Riga, Latvia

Arie Havelaar
National Institute for Public Health and the Environment, Centre for Zoonoses and ernvironmental Microbiology, Bilthoven, The Netherlands
Division Veterinary Public Health, Institute for Risk Assessment Sciences, Utrecht University, Utrecht, The Netherlands

Arno Swart
National Institute for Public Health and the Environment, Centre for Zoonoses and Environmental Microbiology, Bilthoven, The Netherlands

Joke van der Giessen
National Institute for Public Health and the Environment, Centre for Zoonoses and Environmental Microbiology, Bilthoven, The Netherlands